# TEXTBOOK OF PEDIATRICS

## VOLUME 1

## FOUNDATIONS OF CHILD HEALTH AND DEVELOPMENT

**Dr. Maruf Tinsae**

ALLIED HEALTH PRESS

**Textbook of Pediatrics Volume 1**

**Foundations of Child Health and Development**

*Author:* **Dr. Maruf Tinsae**

Allied Health Press
4164 Lakeshore Road
Burlington ON L7L 1A4
Canada
www.alliedhealthpress.com
Email: orders@arclereducation.com


**ISBN:** 978-1-77956-844-1



Allied Health Press publishes wide variety of books and eBooks. For more information about Allied Health Press and its products, visit our website at www.alliedhealthpress.com

# ABOUT THE AUTHOR

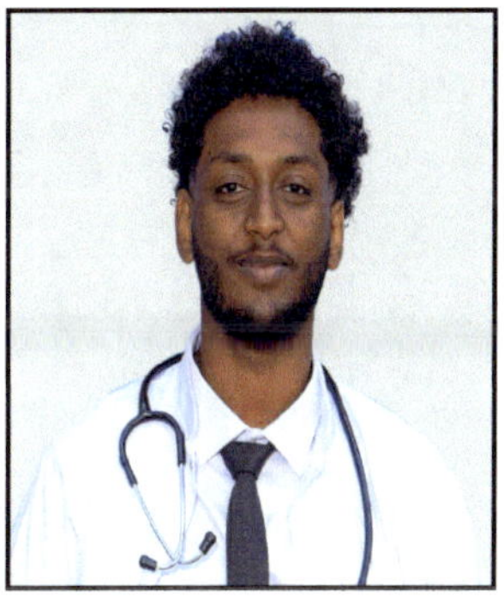

**Dr. Maruf Tinsae** is a Medical Doctor and current Internal Medicine Resident with over fi ve years of clinical experience. He obtained his Doctor of Medicine degree from Hawassa University,Ethiopia in 2020. His professional journey includes roles as a physician at Black Lion Hospital, HUSCH, and Panesiya General Hospital, where he has been actively involved in patient care, medical training, and academic contributions.

His areas of expertise include clinical assessment, diagnosis, and management of diverse medical conditions. In addition, he is deeply engaged in medical writing, journal and book reviews, authorship, and research. He is one of the writers of the MedStar Book Series, one of the largest and most recognized medical short guide collections in Ethiopia, contributing to accessible and practical medical knowledge for healthcare professionals.

# Brief Table of Contents


| | |
|---|---|
| 1. Introduction to Pediatrics | 1 |
| 2. Pediatric Growth and Development | 31 |
| 3. Pediatric Nutrition | 59 |
| 4. Immunization and Preventive Care | 93 |
| 5. Neonatology: Care of the Newborn | 125 |
| 6. Pediatric Infectious Skin Diseases | 161 |
| 7. Pediatric Respiratory Disorders | 187 |
| 8. Pediatric Gastroenterology | 219 |
| 9. Pediatric Hematology and Oncology | 253 |
| 10. Pediatric Endocrinology | 285 |
| 11. Pediatric Neurology | 317 |
| 12. Pediatric Cardiovascular Disorders | 351 |
| Index | 377 |

## Chapter Openers

A list of Chapter Outline is presented providing a brief Introduction to what will be covered in the chapter.

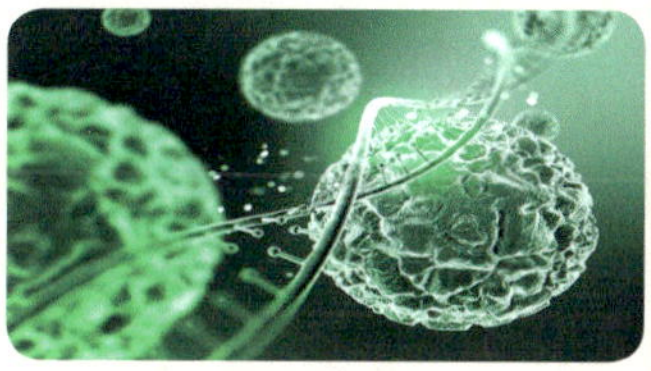

**Introduction**

Often referred to as the science of life, biology is a broad field of study aimed at comprehending the several kinds of life on Earth, from tiny creatures to sophisticated multicellular entities. Comprising several subfields, including molecular biology, ecology, and evolutionary biology, each of which advances our knowledge of living systems, this field clarifies the mechanisms controlling life events, including development, reproduction, and interaction with the surroundings, which is the central goal of biology. Moreover, biology fills in the void between the natural sciences and medicine by offering a necessary understanding of health, illness, and the interactions between organisms and their environments. Dealing with urgent global issues such as climate change, biodiversity loss, and new diseases depends on an awareness of these complex biological interactions, therefore highlighting the critical part biology plays in modern civilization. Fundamentally, biology explores and tests ideas about the living world using the scientific method. Through methodical observation and experimentation,

LEARNING OBJECTIVES

**After studying this chapter, you will be able to:**

1. Discuss the scientific method in biology;
2. Explain the cell theory;
3. Discuss the genetics and heredity;
4. Evolution and natural selection;
5. Focus on ecology and ecosystems;
6. Learn about human biology;
7. Evaluate the plant biology;
8. Explain the microbiology;
9. Focus on current trends in biology.

**1.1. The Scientific Method in Biology**

**Learning Outcome**

1. Describe the steps of the scientific method;
2. Focus on hypothesis formation;
3. Learn about experimental design.

## Learning Outcomes

The beginning of each section of every chapter contains a set of Learning Outcomes that inform students of concepts they should understand. These outcomes help students understand what they should be able to do if they have mastered the material in that section.

## Test Your Knowledge

Throughout each chapter, Test Your Knowledge cues you to note which topics have been covered and to self-test your understanding of the material presented.

**Test Your Knowledge**

1. Explain why correlation does not imply causation in scientific experiments.
2. How does the scientific method help reduce the influence of personal opinions in research?

## Chapter Summary

The Summary Section appear at the end of each chapter and summarize main concepts covered throughout the chapter. These points provide key concepts in an engaging and meaningful way.

**Summary**

The investigation of biological principles highlights the importance of a comprehensive view of life by reflecting the intricate interactions that occur within living systems. The complexity of biology goes beyond individual species or systems, as this essay highlights; it also includes the interactions that mold ecosystems and affect biodiversity. Researchers can conduct in-depth analyses of metabolomic data using sophisticated technologies like MetaboAnalyst, which offer insights into the molecular mechanisms underlying these interactions. As demonstrated by the developments in MetaboAnalyst, for example, the integration of diverse omics data promotes a thorough understanding of metabolic pathways and helps identify important biological markers necessary for research on development and disease (Chong et al., 2018). Additionally, the phenomenon of ecological invasions is a key component of biological research and a vital field of study. The introduction of non-native species into unfamiliar habitats has significant ramifications and calls for multidisciplinary management strategies. Examining the origins and effects of these biological incursions, invasion science has become a crucial field that highlights the need to comprehend ecological dynamics and community interactions. As interest in biological invasions increases, new findings are emerging that put conventional ecological theories and practices to the test. The importance of incorporating various scientific viewpoints is shown by this developing discipline, which also highlights how invasive species shape ecosystems and advances our knowledge of ecological resilience (David et al., 2013). When taken as a whole, these discoveries from invasion science and metabolomics highlight the value of multidisciplinary biology research. Fostering cross-disciplinary collaboration and utilizing technological breakthroughs to improve our comprehension of intricate biological interactions are crucial as we look to the future of biological research. In addition to deepening our understanding of the complexities of life, this method lays the groundwork for tackling urgent environmental issues. Future studies can ensure the continued relevance of biology in a world that is constantly changing by acknowledging the interconnection of biological systems and opening the door to creative solutions that support sustainability and biodiversity conservation. We might imagine a thorough comprehension of life that serves both academia and society at large through ongoing investigation and integration of scientific knowledge.

## Knowledge Assessment

The chapter includes material designed to review and reinforce each content. It includes Critical Thinking Questions to help test of your understanding of information presented in the chapter and Short answer Questions to review your understanding of the key concepts presented in the chapter.

### Critical Thinking Questions

1. **Who is known as the "Father of Modern Biology"?**
   a. Aristotle
   b. Charles Darwin
   c. Gregor Mendel
   d. Louis Pasteur
2. **What is the basic unit of life?**
   a. Atom
   b. Molecule
   c. Cell
   d. Organism
3. **Which branch of biology studies the interaction of organisms with their environment?**
   a. Genetics
   b. Ecology
   c. Physiology
   d. Botany
4. **Which macromolecule is the main source of energy for living organisms?**
   a. Proteins
   b. Lipids
   c. Carbohydrates
   d. Nucleic acids
5. **DNA is primarily responsible for which function in living organisms?**
   a. Energy production
   b. Protein synthesis
   c. Storing genetic information
   d. Regulating body temperature

### Short Answer Questions

1. What is biology, and why is it important to study biology?
2. What are the three main domains of life, and how are they different from one another?
3. Define homeostasis and give an example of how it works in living organisms.
4. What is the cell theory, and why is it fundamental to biology?
5. How do autotrophs and heterotrophs differ in the way they obtain energy?
6. What is the scientific method, and how is it applied in biological research?
7. Discuss how biology helps address global challenges such as climate change, disease, and food security.
8. Explain the levels of biological organization from the smallest unit to the largest. Provide examples at each level.
9. Describe the relationship between structure and function in biology, giving specific examples from cells or organs.
10. How has the discovery of genetics shaped our understanding of inheritance and variation among organisms?

## Supplementary Materials

**Key Terms:** A list of key terms is given for quick reference

### KEY TERMS FROM THIS CHAPTER

| | | |
|---|---|---|
| Annotation enrichment analysis | Biological structure | Cell |
| Cell theory | Cellular structure | Ecology |
| Ecosystems | Genetics | Human biology |
| Microbiology | Natural selection | Organism |
| Plant biology | | |

**Further Resources:** Recommendations for additional readings, websites, and multimedia resources.

### References


1. Argelaguet, R., Velten, B., Arnol, D., Dietrich, S., Zenz, T., Marioni, J. C., Buettner, F., et al. (2018). Multi-omics factor analysis—A framework for unsupervised integration of multi-omics data sets. *Molecular Systems Biology, 14*. https://doi.org/10.15252/msb.20178124.
2. Bacher, S., Blackburn, T. M., Essl, F., & Genovesi, P. (2017). *Socio-Economic Impact Classification of Alien Taxa (SEICAT)*. https://core.ac.uk/download/286567949.pdf (accessed on 8th March 2025).
3. Barnett, R., Brace, S., Cucchi, T., & Dobney, K. (2013). *Divergent Evolutionary Processes Associated with Colonization of Offshore Islands*. https://core.ac.uk/download/20664364.pdf (accessed on 8th March 2025).

# Detailed Table of Contents

*List of Figures* xvii
*Preface* xxv

CHAPTER 1

## Introduction to Pediatrics 1

**Introduction** 1
**1.1. Growth and Development in Pediatrics** 5
1.1.1. Stages of Child Development 5
1.1.2. Milestones in Physical Growth 6
1.1.3. Cognitive Development in Children 6
1.1.4. Emotional and Social Development 6
1.1.5. Factors Influencing Growth 7
1.1.6. Growth Disorders and Their Management 7
1.1.7. Role of Nutrition in Development 8
1.1.8. Importance of Regular Check-Ups 8
1.1.9. Developmental Screening Tools 8
**1.2. Common Pediatric Illnesses** 9
1.2.1. Overview of Acute Illnesses 10
1.2.2. Chronic Conditions in Children 10
1.2.3. Infectious Diseases Affecting Children 11
1.2.4. Allergies and Asthma in Pediatrics 11
1.2.5. Pediatric Obesity and Its Implications 11
1.2.6. Mental Health Issues in Children 12
1.2.7. Preventive Care and Vaccination 12
1.2.8. Management of Pediatric Emergencies 13
1.2.9. Role of Family in Managing Illness 13
**1.3. Pediatric Healthcare Systems** 14
1.3.1. Structure of Pediatric Healthcare Services 14
1.3.2. Pediatric Primary Care versus Specialty Care 15
1.3.3. Role of Hospitals in Pediatric Care 15
1.3.4. Pediatric Emergency Services 15
1.3.5. Community Health Initiatives for Children 16
1.3.6. Access to Pediatric Care 16
1.3.7. Insurance and Pediatric Healthcare 17
1.3.8. Telemedicine in Pediatrics 17
1.3.9. Future Directions in Pediatric Healthcare 17
**1.4. Ethical Considerations in Pediatrics** 18
1.4.1. Informed Consent in Pediatric Care 18
1.4.2. Confidentiality and Privacy Issues 19
1.4.3. Ethical Dilemmas in Pediatric Treatment 19
1.4.4. Role of Parents in Decision-Making 20
1.4.5. Pediatric Research Ethics 20
1.4.6. Cultural Competence in Pediatric Care 20
1.4.7. End-of-Life Decisions for Children 21
1.4.8. Advocacy for Child Health Rights 21
1.4.9. Balancing Risks and Benefits in Treatment 22
**Summary** 23
**References** 25

CHAPTER 2

## Pediatric Growth and Development 31

**Introduction** 31
**2.1. Physical Growth in Children** 35
2.1.1. Stages of Physical Growth 35

2.1.2. Growth Patterns in Infancy 36
2.1.3. Growth Spurts During Childhood 36
2.1.4. Role of Nutrition in Physical Growth 36
2.1.5. Impact of Genetics on Growth 37
2.1.6. Measurement of Growth (Height, Weight, BMI) 37
2.1.7. Common Growth Disorders 37
2.1.8. Importance of Regular Health Check-Ups 38
2.1.9. Growth Charts and Their Interpretation 38
**2.2. Cognitive Development 39**
2.2.1. Overview of Cognitive Development Theories 39
2.2.2. Piaget's Stages of Cognitive Development 40
2.2.3. Role of Play in Cognitive Growth 40
2.2.4. Language Acquisition Milestones 40
2.2.5. Impact of Environment on Cognitive Skills 41
2.2.6. Assessment of Cognitive Development 41
2.2.7. Common Cognitive Developmental Delays 42
2.2.8. Importance of Early Childhood Education 42
2.2.9. Technology's Influence on Cognitive Development 42
**2.3. Social and Emotional Development 43**
2.3.1. Definition of Social and Emotional Development 44
2.3.2. Attachment Theory and Its Significance 44
2.3.3. Development of Self-Regulation Skills 44
2.3.4. Role of Family in Social Development 45
2.3.5. Peer Relationships and Their Impact 45
2.3.6. Emotional Milestones in Early Childhood 46
2.3.7. Effects of Trauma on Emotional Development 46
2.3.8. Importance of Social Skills Training 46
2.3.9. Cultural Influences on Social Development 47
**2.4. Behavioral Development 48**
2.4.1. Understanding Typical Behavioral Patterns 48
2.4.2. Role of Parenting Styles in Behavior 49
2.4.3. Common Behavioral Issues in Children 49
2.4.4. Strategies for Positive Behavior Reinforcement 49
2.4.5. Impact of Screen Time on Behavior 50
2.4.6. Behavioral Assessments and Interventions 50
2.4.7. Importance of Consistency in Discipline 51
2.4.8. Role of Schools in Behavioral Development 51
2.4.9. Long-Term Effects of Childhood Behavior 51
**Summary 53**
**References 55**

CHAPTER 3

## Pediatric Nutrition 59

**Introduction 59**
**3.1. Nutritional Requirements by Age Group 63**
3.1.1. Infants (0–12 Months) 64
3.1.2. Toddlers (1–3 Years) 65
3.1.3. School-Age Children (4–12 Years) 65
**3.2. Common Nutritional Deficiencies in Children 67**
3.2.1. Iron Deficiency Anemia 67
3.2.2. Vitamin D Deficiency 68
3.2.3. Calcium Deficiency 69
**3.3. The Role of Breastfeeding 71**
3.3.1. Benefits of Breastfeeding for Infants 72
3.3.2. Recommended Duration of Breastfeeding 73
3.3.3. Challenges and Solutions for Breastfeeding Mothers 74
**3.4. Introduction of Solid Foods 75**
3.4.1. Guidelines for Introducing Solids 76
3.4.2. Common First Foods and Their Nutritional Value 76
3.4.3. Signs of Readiness for Solid Foods 77
**3.5. Impact of Nutrition on Child Development 78**
3.5.1. Physical Growth and Development 79
3.5.2. Cognitive Development and Learning 80
3.5.3. Emotional and Social Development 81
**3.6. Addressing Pediatric Obesity 82**
3.6.1. Causes and Risk Factors of Pediatric Obesity 83
3.6.2. Strategies for Prevention and Management 84
3.6.3. Role of Family and Community in Promoting Healthy Habits 85
**Summary 87**
**References 90**

CHAPTER 4

## Immunization and Preventive Care 93

**Introduction 93**
**4.1. Historical Context of Immunization 96**
4.1.1. Early Methods of Disease Prevention 97

4.1.2. Development of Vaccines 97

4.1.3. Impact of Immunization on Public Health 98

**4.2. Types of Vaccines 99**

4.2.1. Live Attenuated Vaccines 100

4.2.2. Inactivated Vaccines 101

4.2.3. mRNA Vaccines 102

**4.3. Benefits of Immunization 103**

4.3.1. Individual Health Protection 104

4.3.2. Community Immunity (Herd Immunity) 104

4.3.3. Economic Benefits of Vaccination Programs 105

**4.4. Challenges in Immunization 106**

4.4.1. Vaccine Hesitancy and Misinformation 107

4.4.2. Access to Vaccines in Underserved Populations 108

4.4.3. Global Disparities in Vaccination Rates 109

**4.5. Preventive Care Beyond Immunization 110**

4.5.1. Regular Health Screenings 111

4.5.2. Lifestyle Modifications for Disease Prevention 112

4.5.3. Role of Healthcare Providers in Preventive Care 113

**4.6. Policy and Legislation 114**

4.6.1. Government Mandates for Vaccinations 115

4.6.2. Role of Public Health Organizations 116

4.6.3. Ethical Considerations in Immunization Policies 117

**Summary 119**

**References 122**

CHAPTER 5

**Neonatology: Care of the Newborn 125**

**Introduction 125**

**5.1. Developmental Stages of Newborns 129**

5.1.1. Premature versus Full-Term Infants 130

5.1.2. Physiological Changes at Birth 131

5.1.3. Key Milestones in the First Month 132

**5.2. Common Neonatal Conditions 133**

5.2.1. Respiratory Distress Syndrome 134

5.2.2. Jaundice in Newborns 135

5.2.3. Infections and Sepsis 136

**5.3. Neonatal Assessment and Monitoring 137**

5.3.1. Apgar Score and Its Significance 138

5.3.2. Physical Examination Techniques 139

5.3.3. Monitoring Vital Signs and Growth 140

**5.4. Nutritional Needs of Newborns 141**

5.4.1. Breastfeeding Benefits and Challenges 142

5.4.2. Formula Feeding Guidelines 142

5.4.3. Nutritional Requirements for Preterm Infants 143

**5.5. Neonatal Intensive Care Unit (NICU) 145**

5.5.1. Role and Function of the NICU 145

5.5.2. Common Interventions and Technologies Used 146

5.5.3. Family Involvement in NICU Care 147

**5.6. Ethical Considerations in Neonatology 148**

5.6.1. Decision-Making in Critical Care Situations 149

5.6.2. End-of-Life Care and Palliative Options 150

5.6.3. Informed Consent and Parental Rights 151

**Summary 153**

**References 156**

CHAPTER 6

**Pediatric Infectious Skin Diseases 161**

**Introduction 161**

**6.1. Common Pediatric Infectious Skin Diseases 164**

6.1.1. Impetigo: Causes and Symptoms 165

6.1.2. Chickenpox: Transmission and Prevention 165

6.1.3. Hand, Foot, and Mouth Disease: Overview 166

6.1.4. Ringworm: Diagnosis and Treatment 166

6.1.5. Scabies: Symptoms and Management 166

6.1.6. Molluscum Contagiosum: Characteristics 167

6.1.7. Candidiasis: Risk Factors in Children 167

6.1.8. Erysipelas: Clinical Presentation 168

6.1.9. Herpes Simplex Virus Infections: Types and Effects 168

**6.2. Diagnosis and Clinical Evaluation 169**

6.2.1. Importance of Accurate Diagnosis 169

6.2.2. Common Diagnostic Methods 169

6.2.3. Role of Medical History in Diagnosis 170

6.2.4. Physical Examination Techniques 170

6.2.5. Laboratory Tests and Their Significance 171

6.2.6. Differential Diagnosis Considerations 171

6.2.7. Challenges in Diagnosing Skin Diseases in Children 171

6.2.8. Use of Imaging Studies in Complex Cases 172

6.2.9. Referral to Specialists When Necessary 173

**6.3. Treatment and Management Strategies 173**

6.3.1. Overview of Treatment Options 174

6.3.2. Topical Treatments: Types and Applications 174

6.3.3. Oral Medications: Indications and Usage 175

6.3.4. Role of Antibiotics in Treatment 175

6.3.5. Importance of Adherence to Treatment Plans 175

6.3.6. Management of Complications 176

6.3.7. Supportive Care and Symptom Relief 176

6.3.8. Education for Parents and Caregivers 177

6.3.9. Follow-Up Care and Monitoring 177

**6.4. Prevention and Public Health Implications 178**

6.4.1. Importance of Vaccination in Prevention 178

6.4.2. Hygiene Practices to Reduce Transmission 179

6.4.3. Role of Schools in Disease Prevention 179

6.4.4. Community Awareness and Education Programs 179

6.4.5. Impact of Socioeconomic Factors on Disease Prevalence 180

6.4.6. Strategies for Outbreak Management 180

6.4.7. Importance of Early Detection and Reporting 181

6.4.8. Collaboration with Public Health Agencies 181

6.4.9. Future Directions in Prevention Research 182

**Summary 183**

**References 185**

CHAPTER 7

**Pediatric Respiratory Disorders 187**

**Introduction 187**

**7.1. Anatomy and Physiology of the Pediatric Respiratory System 191**

7.1.1. Differences Between Pediatric and Adult Respiratory Systems 192

7.1.2. Developmental Changes in the Respiratory System 193

7.1.3. Impact of Anatomy on Disease Presentation and Management 194

**7.2. Common Pediatric Respiratory Disorders 195**

7.2.1. Asthma: Prevalence and Pathophysiology 196

7.2.2. Bronchiolitis: Causes and Clinical Features 197

7.2.3. Pneumonia: Types and Treatment Approaches 198

**7.3. Assessment and Diagnosis 199**

7.3.1. Clinical Signs and Symptoms of Respiratory Disorders 200

7.3.2. Diagnostic Tools and Techniques Used in Pediatrics 201

7.3.3. Importance of Family History and Environmental Factors 201

**7.4. Nursing Interventions and Management 203**

7.4.1. Role of Nursing in Acute and Chronic Management 204

7.4.2. Medication Administration and Monitoring 204

7.4.3. Education and Support for Families 205

**7.5. Complications and Challenges 206**

7.5.1. Potential Complications of Untreated Respiratory Disorders 207

7.5.2. Challenges in Pediatric Patient Compliance 208

7.5.3. Socioeconomic Factors Affecting Care and Outcomes 209

**7.6. Current Research and Advances in Treatment 210**

7.6.1. Innovations in Pharmacological Treatments 211

7.6.2. Emerging Therapies and Technologies 211

7.6.3. Importance of Ongoing Research in Pediatric Nursing 212

**Summary 214**

**References 217**

CHAPTER 8

**Pediatric Gastroenterology 219**

**Introduction 219**

**8.1. Anatomy and Physiology of the Pediatric Gastrointestinal System 223**

8.1.1. Differences Between Pediatric and Adult Gastrointestinal Anatomy 224

8.1.2. Developmental Changes in the Gastrointestinal System 225

8.1.3. Common Physiological Functions and Their Significance 226

**8.2. Common Gastrointestinal Disorders in Children** **227**
8.2.1. Gastroesophageal Reflux Disease (GERD) 228
8.2.2. Inflammatory Bowel Disease (IBD) 229
8.2.3. Celiac Disease and Gluten Sensitivity 229
**8.3. Diagnostic Approaches in Pediatric Gastroenterology** **231**
8.3.1. Clinical Evaluation and History Taking 232
8.3.2. Imaging Techniques and Their Applications 232
8.3.3. Endoscopic Procedures and Their Relevance 233
**8.4. Treatment Modalities in Pediatric Gastroenterology** **235**
8.4.1. Pharmacological Treatments and Their Indications 235
8.4.2. Nutritional Management and Dietary Interventions 236
8.4.3. Surgical Options for Severe Gastrointestinal Conditions 237
**8.5. Impact of Gastrointestinal Disorders on Child Development** **239**
8.5.1. Physical Growth and Nutritional Status 240
8.5.2. Psychological Effects and Emotional Well-Being 241
8.5.3. Social Implications and Quality of Life 241
**8.6. Advances in Pediatric Gastroenterology** **243**
8.6.1. Emerging Research and Clinical Trials 244
8.6.2. Innovations in Diagnostic Technologies 245
8.6.3. Future Directions in Treatment and Management 245
**Summary** **247**
**References** **250**

CHAPTER 9

## Pediatric Hematology and Oncology 253

**Introduction** **253**
**9.1. Overview of Hematological Disorders in Children** **256**
9.1.1. Common Hematological Disorders 257
9.1.2. Symptoms and Diagnosis 258
9.1.3. Treatment Options and Management 259
**9.2. Overview of Oncological Disorders in Children** **260**
9.2.1. Types of Pediatric Cancers 261
9.2.2. Early Signs and Diagnostic Procedures 262
9.2.3. Treatment Modalities and Their Implications 262
**9.3. The Role of Pediatric Hematologists and Oncologists** **263**
9.3.1. Education and Training Requirements 264
9.3.2. Responsibilities in Patient Care 265
9.3.3. Collaboration with Multidisciplinary Teams 266
**9.4. Advances in Research and Treatment** **267**
9.4.1. Recent Breakthroughs in Pediatric Hematology 268
9.4.2. Innovations in Cancer Treatment for Children 269
9.4.3. The Impact of Clinical Trials on Patient Outcomes 269
**9.5. Psychological and Social Impacts on Patients and Families** **271**
9.5.1. Emotional Challenges Faced by Children 271
9.5.2. Support Systems for Families 272
9.5.3. Long-Term Effects of Treatment on Quality of Life 273
**9.6. Ethical Considerations in Pediatric Hematology and Oncology** **275**
9.6.1. Informed Consent and Decision-Making 275
9.6.2. Balancing Treatment Benefits and Risks 276
9.6.3. The Role of Palliative Care 277
**Summary** **279**
**References** **282**

CHAPTER 10

## Pediatric Endocrinology 285

**Introduction** **285**
**10.1. Hormonal Development in Children** **289**
10.1.1. Stages of Hormonal Development from Infancy to Adolescence 290
10.1.2. Role of Hormones in Growth and Development 291
10.1.3. Impact of Hormonal Imbalances During Developmental Stages 292
**10.2. Common Endocrine Disorders** **293**
10.2.1. Diabetes Mellitus in Children 294

10.2.2. Growth Hormone Deficiency 294
10.2.3. Thyroid Disorders in Pediatric Patients 295
**10.3. Diagnosis of Endocrine Disorders 296**
10.3.1. Clinical Evaluation and Patient History 297
10.3.2. Laboratory Tests and Imaging Studies 298
10.3.3. Importance of Early Diagnosis for Treatment Outcomes 299
**10.4. Treatment Options in Pediatric Endocrinology 300**
10.4.1. Hormone Replacement Therapies 301
10.4.2. Lifestyle Modifications and Dietary Interventions 301
10.4.3. Surgical Options for Endocrine Disorders 302
**10.5. Psychological and Social Implications 303**
10.5.1. Impact of Endocrine Disorders on Mental Health 304
10.5.2. Social Challenges Faced by Affected Children 305
10.5.3. Importance of Family Support and Counseling 306
**10.6. Advances in Pediatric Endocrinology 307**
10.6.1. Recent Research and Clinical Trials 308
10.6.2. Technological Advancements in Treatment 309
10.6.3. Future Directions in Pediatric Endocrine Care 310
**Summary 311**
**References 314**

CHAPTER 11

## Pediatric Neurology 317

**Introduction 317**
**11.1. Developmental Milestones and Neurological Assessment 321**
11.1.1. Key Developmental Milestones in Childhood 322
11.1.2. Techniques for Neurological Assessment in Children 323
11.1.3. Importance of Early Detection and Intervention 324
**11.2. Common Pediatric Neurological Disorders 325**
11.2.1. Epilepsy and Seizure Disorders 326
11.2.2. Cerebral Palsy and Its Implications 327
11.2.3. Neurogenetic Disorders and Their Impact 328
**11.3. Diagnostic Tools and Techniques 329**
11.3.1. Imaging Techniques: MRI and CT Scans 330
11.3.2. Electroencephalography (EEG) in Diagnosis 331
11.3.3. Genetic Testing and Its Role in Pediatric Neurology 332
**11.4. Treatment Approaches in Pediatric Neurology 333**
11.4.1. Pharmacological Treatments and Their Effectiveness 334
11.4.2. Surgical Interventions for Neurological Conditions 334
11.4.3. Role of Rehabilitation Therapies in Recovery 335
**11.5. Challenges in Pediatric Neurology 336**
11.5.1. Ethical Considerations in Treatment Decisions 337
11.5.2. Access to Care and Disparities in Treatment 338
11.5.3. Psychological Impact on Patients and Families 339
**11.6. Recent Advances in Pediatric Neurology 340**
11.6.1. Innovations in Treatment Methodologies 341
11.6.2. Research Trends in Pediatric Neurological Disorders 342
11.6.3. The Role of Technology in Enhancing Patient Care 343
**Summary 345**
**References 348**

CHAPTER 12

## Pediatric Cardiovascular Disorders 351

**Introduction 351**
**12.1. Common Pediatric Cardiovascular Disorders 354**
12.1.1. Congenital Heart Defects 355
12.1.2. Myocarditis and Pericarditis 355
12.1.3. Arrhythmias in Children 356
12.1.4. Cardiogenic Shock 357
12.1.5. Pulmonary Embolism 357
12.1.6. Aortic Dissection 357
12.1.7. Hypertrophic Cardiomyopathy 358
12.1.8. Heart Failure in Pediatric Patients 358
12.1.9. Cardiac Arrest in Children 359
**12.2. Clinical Presentation and Diagnosis 359**

12.2.1. Signs and Symptoms of Cardiovascular Disorders 360
12.2.2. Importance of History-Taking in Pediatric Patients 360
12.2.3. Physical Examination Techniques 361
12.2.4. Diagnostic Imaging Modalities 361
12.2.5. Laboratory Tests and Biomarkers 361
12.2.6. Differential Diagnosis Considerations 362
12.2.7. Role of Telemedicine in Diagnosis 362
12.2.8. Challenges in Diagnosing Pediatric Patients 363
12.2.9. Importance of Early Diagnosis for Outcomes 363
**12.3. Management and Treatment Strategies 364**
12.3.1. Initial Assessment and Stabilization 364
12.3.2. Pharmacological Interventions 365
12.3.3. Role of Advanced Cardiac Life Support (ACLS) 365
12.3.4. Surgical Interventions and Procedures 365
12.3.5. Post-Emergency Care and Monitoring 366
12.3.6. Family Involvement in Treatment Decisions 366
12.3.7. Multidisciplinary Approach to Care 366
12.3.8. Long-Term Management and Follow-Up 367
12.3.9. Ethical Considerations in Treatment 367
**12.4. Prevention and Education 368**
12.4.1. Importance of Preventive Care in Pediatrics 368
12.4.2. Screening for Congenital Heart Disease 369
12.4.3. Parental Education on Warning Signs 369
12.4.4. Community Awareness Programs 370
12.4.5. Role of Schools in Health Education 370
12.4.6. Guidelines for Physical Activity in Children 370
12.4.7. Vaccination and Its Impact on Cardiovascular Health 371
12.4.8. Research on Prevention Strategies 371
12.4.9. Future Directions in Pediatric Cardiovascular Health 371
**Summary 373**
**References 375**
**INDEX 377**

# LIST OF FIGURES

Figure 1.1. pediatrics is the branch of medicine that focuses on the medical care of infants, children, and adolescents

Figure 1.2. The scope of pediatric practice encompasses a multifaceted approach to child health

Figure 1.3. The differences between pediatrics and adult medicine

Figure 1.4. Overview of pediatric subspecialties

Figure 1.5. The growth and development in pediatrics

Figure 1.6. Milestones in physical growth

Figure 1.7. Growth in pediatric populations

Figure 1.8. A pediatrician interacting with a mother and her baby during a check-up, emphasizing the importance of early childhood healthcare

Figure 1.9. Common pediatric illnesses

Figure 1.10. Chronic conditions in children

Figure 1.11. Child wearing a protective face mask and gown, symbolizing pediatric precautions against infectious diseases

Figure 1.12. The mental health of children has emerged as a critical concern in pediatrics

Figure 1.13. Medical team transporting a child on a hospital stretcher during a pediatric emergency, highlighting the urgency and care involved in critical pediatric situations

Figure 1.14. Pediatric healthcare systems

Figure 1.15. The role of hospitals in pediatric care extends beyond immediate medical intervention

Figure 1.16. Access to pediatric care is a critical component of child health

Figure 1.17. Future directions in pediatric healthcare

Figure 1.18. Informed consent in pediatric care is a nuanced process

Figure 1.19. A healthcare provider discusses medical information with a multi-generational family, emphasizing shared decision-making in a clinical setting

Figure 1.20. A pediatrician engages in a shared decision-making discussion with a family, fostering collaborative care in a clinical setting

Figure 2.1. Pediatric growth and development

Figure 2.2. A child points to a smiling face during an emotional recognition activity with a therapist, supporting social-emotional development in a clinical or educational setting

Figure 2.3. The significance of early intervention in pediatric growth and development

Figure 2.4. Physical growth in children

Figure 2.5. The growth patterns in infancy
Figure 2.6. Children enjoy a variety of fresh fruits, promoting healthy eating habits and balanced nutrition in early childhood
Figure 2.7. Common growth disorders
Figure 2.8. Young children engage in a hands-on sensory activity involving colorful beads, fostering cognitive development and collaborative learning in a classroom maker space
Figure 2.9. Piaget's stages of cognitive development
Figure 2.10. Impact of environment on cognitive skills
Figure 2.11. Importance of early childhood education
Figure 2.12. Toddlers play collaboratively with building blocks in an early childhood setting, supporting social interaction and fine motor development
Figure 2.13. Development of self-regulation skills
Figure 2.14. A young child appears frustrated during playtime, highlighting the importance of supporting social-emotional wellness and self-regulation in early childhood settings
Figure 2.15. The acquisition of social skills stands as a critical component influencing a child's overall well-being and academic success
Figure 2.16. A pediatrician gently supports a smiling infant during a wellness check, illustrating the importance of compassionate care in early childhood health
Figure 2.17. Common behavioral issues in children
Figure 2.18. The behavioral assessments and interventions play a critical role in understanding and enhancing children's overall well-being
Figure 2.19. A young girl stands between two adults pulling her in opposite directions, symbolizing the emotional impact of parental conflict or divorce on children
Figure 3.1. The pediatric nutrition
Figure 3.2. Two young children eat a nutritious meal together at a kitchen table, reinforcing healthy eating habits and independence in early childhood
Figure 3.3. The nutritional requirements of children vary significantly across different age groups
Figure 3.4. Essential nutrition for infants and toddlers
Figure 3.5. A smiling child enjoys a balanced meal with family, promoting healthy nutrition and positive mealtime experiences in childhood
Figure 3.6. Nutritional deficiencies in children
Figure 3.7. Iron-deficiency anemia
Figure 3.8. Vitamin D deficiency has emerged as a significant concern in the context of pediatric nutrition
Figure 3.9. A baby drinks milk from a glass while seated in a highchair, supporting early childhood nutrition and calcium intake for healthy growth and development
Figure 3.10. The role of breastfeeding
Figure 3.11. Benefits of breastfeeding for infants

Figure 3.12. A mother breastfeeds her infant in a calm, supportive environment, highlighting the importance of maternal bonding and optimal infant nutrition
Figure 3.13. A baby is spoon-fed soft food while seated in a highchair, representing the transition to solid foods and the development of healthy eating habits in infancy
Figure 3.14. Common first foods and their nutritional value
Figure 3.15. Impact of nutrition on child development
Figure 3.16. Cognitive development and learning
Figure 3.17. A healthcare professional measures a smiling child's waist circumference as part of a wellness assessment, emphasizing the importance of healthy lifestyle habits and positive body image
Figure 3.18. Risk factors, clinical consequences, prevention, and treatment of childhood obesity
Figure 4.1. A smiling toddler sits comfortably during a preventive checkup as a healthcare provider uses a stethoscope, illustrating a positive pediatric care experience
Figure 4.2. Preventive care serves as the cornerstone of public health
Figure 4.3. Early methods of disease prevention
Figure 4.4. A healthcare professional administers a vaccination to a smiling infant, emphasizing the role of immunization in promoting early childhood health and disease prevention
Figure 4.5. The development of vaccines has revolutionized public health
Figure 4.6. A healthcare provider prepares to administer a vaccine to a young girl, underscoring the importance of routine immunizations in childhood disease prevention
Figure 4.7. Immunization represents one of the most significant advancements in public health
Figure 4.8. Community immunity, commonly referred to as herd immunity
Figure 4.9. The landscape of immunization is fraught with multiple challenges that significantly hinder effective vaccination programs
Figure 4.10. Access to vaccines remains a critical challenge for under served populations
Figure 4.11. A healthcare provider administers a vaccine to a toddler, illustrating a supportive approach to pediatric immunization
Figure 4.12. Lifestyle modifications play a critical role in disease prevention
Figure 4.13. Policy and legislation
Figure 4.14. Role of public health organizations
Figure 5.1. Neonatology, a subspecialty of pediatrics
Figure 5.2. Definition and scope of neonatology
Figure 5.3. Neonatal care is imperative for ensuring the health and well-being of newborns
Figure 5.4. The developmental stages of newborns are critical in the context of neonatology
Figure 5.5. Premature versus full-term infants
Figure 5.6. Physiological changes at birth
Figure 5.7. Key milestones in the first month
Figure 5.8. The management of common neonatal conditions
Figure 5.9. Respiratory distress syndrome

Figure 5.10. The incidence of jaundice in newborns

Figure 5.11. Neonatal assessment and monitoring

Figure 5.12. Physical examination techniques

Figure 5.13. A smiling infant is surrounded by a colorful assortment of fruits, vegetables, and baby food, highlighting the importance of balanced nutrition in early childhood development

Figure 5.14. In the realm of neonatal care, formula feeding guidelines are critical in ensuring that infants receive adequate nutrition

Figure 5.15. The neonatal intensive care unit (NICU)

Figure 5.16. A young girl uses a digital tablet for communication with the support of a caregiver, illustrating assistive technology in speech and language development for children with special needs

Figure 5.17. A newborn in a neonatal intensive care unit (NICU) is monitored using medical sensors on the foot, highlighting the critical care and technology used to support premature or medically fragile infants

Figure 5.18. The provision of end-of-life care and palliative options within the field of neonatology

Figure 6.1. The complex landscape of pediatric infectious skin diseases presents significant challenges to healthcare providers

Figure 6.2. Infectious skin diseases are prevalent among pediatric populations

Figure 6.3. A mother helps her children wash their hands at a kitchen sink, promoting hygiene practices essential for preventing illness and supporting family health

Figure 6.4. Chickenpox: Transmission and prevention

Figure 6.5. Hand, foot, and mouth disease can cause an itchy rash, painful sores, and blisters

Figure 6.6. An infant's abdomen shows a widespread rash associated with scabies, a contagious skin condition caused by mites, highlighting the need for early diagnosis and treatment

Figure 6.7. Clinical Presentation of Erysipelas

Figure 6.8. A medical professional performs an ultrasound scan on an infant's arm, demonstrating the use of noninvasive imaging techniques in pediatric diagnostics

Figure 6.9. A systematic approach to physical examination techniques

Figure 6.10. A close-up of a baby's arm shows a red, bumpy rash, commonly indicative of a skin condition such as eczema or heat rash, emphasizing the need for dermatological care in infants

Figure 6.11. Effective treatment and management strategies for pediatric infectious skin diseases

Figure 6.12. An adult applies medicated ointment to a child's skin lesions, showing treatment for impetigo, a common and highly contagious bacterial skin infection in children

Figure 6.13. Importance of adherence to treatment plans

Figure 6.14. Education for parents and caregivers plays a crucial role in managing pediatric infectious skin diseases

Figure 6.15. Vaccination plays a crucial role in the prevention of pediatric infectious skin diseases

Figure 6.16. A large group of children and young women participates in a Social Safety Awareness Program, holding informational pamphlets aimed at promoting education on personal safety and empowerment

Figure 6.17. Effective outbreak management is crucial in controlling pediatric infectious skin diseases
Figure 6.18. A young girl smiles while receiving a vaccination from a healthcare worker, with another provider offering reassurance, highlighting the role of public health outreach in community-based pediatric care
Figure 7.1. Pediatric respiratory disorders represent a significant area of concern
Figure 7.2. A pediatric healthcare provider uses a stethoscope to examine an infant during a checkup, reflecting attentive and compassionate clinical care
Figure 7.3. The role of is paramount in the comprehensive management of pediatric respiratory disorders
Figure 7.4. Anatomy and physiology of the pediatric respiratory system
Figure 7.5. Developmental changes in the respiratory system
Figure 7.6. Common pediatric respiratory disorders
Figure 7.7. Pediatric asthma
Figure 7.8. Pediatric bronchiolitis
Figure 7.9. Pneumonia in children
Figure 7.10. Clinical signs and symptoms of respiratory disorders
Figure 7.11. Importance of family history and environmental factors
Figure 7.12. Nursing interventions and management
Figure 7.13. Medication administration and monitoring
Figure 7.14. Supporting developmental growth through play-based learning
Figure 7.15. Challenges in pediatric patient compliance
Figure 7.16. Current research and advances in treatment
Figure 7.17. Emerging therapies and technologies
Figure 8.1. Pediatric gastroenterology: medical specialty managing children's digestive and nutritional health.
Figure 8.2. The scope of pediatric gastroenterology
Figure 8.3. Overview of common gastrointestinal disorders in children
Figure 8.4. The differences in gastrointestinal anatomy between pediatrics and adults is crucial for pediatric gastroenterology
Figure 8.5. A healthcare provider performs an abdominal examination on a young child, demonstrating pediatric assessment in the context of gastrointestinal care
Figure 8.6. Common gastrointestinal disorders in children
Figure 8.7. Understanding gastroesophageal reflux disease (GERD)
Figure 8.8. Inflammatory bowel disease (IBD)
Figure 8.9. A healthcare provider evaluates a young boy experiencing abdominal discomfort, illustrating a clinical consultation in pediatric gastroenterology
Figure 8.10. Imaging techniques and their applications

Figure 8.11. Endoscopic procedures play a pivotal role in the field of pediatric gastroenterology
Figure 8.12. Pharmacological treatments and their indications
Figure 8.13. Surgical options for severe gastrointestinal conditions
Figure 8.14. A young girl covers her mouth, appearing nauseous, which may indicate symptoms of an underlying gastrointestinal issue
Figure 8.15. Physical growth and nutritional status
Figure 8.16. Social implications and quality of life
Figure 8.17. Advancement in pediatric gastroenterology
Figure 8.18. A scientist records observations in a laboratory surrounded by microscopes and glassware containing blue solutions, representing active research and experimentation in a clinical or biomedical setting
Figure 8.19. The future of treatment and management in pediatric gastroenterology
Figure 9.1. The field of pediatric hematology and oncology encompasses a wide range of conditions affecting children
Figure 9.2. The specialized field of pediatric hematology and oncology focuses on the diagnosis
Figure 9.3. Overview of hematological disorders in children
Figure 9.4. Common hematological disorders
Figure 9.5. A healthcare provider discusses medical information with a patient, emphasizing shared decision-making and informed consent in a clinical consultation
Figure 9.6. Types of pediatric cancers
Figure 9.7. Treatment modalities and their implications
Figure 9.8. Education and training requirements for pediatric hematology and oncology
Figure 9.9. Collaboration with multidisciplinary teams
Figure 9.10. Recent breakthroughs in pediatric hematology
Figure 9.11. The impact of clinical trials on patient outcomes
Figure 9.12. Emotional challenges faced by children diagnosed with hematological or oncological conditions
Figure 9.13. The long-term effects of treatment for pediatric cancers significantly impact the quality of life as survivors grow into adulthood
Figure 9.14. Informed consent and decision-making
Figure 9.15. Balancing treatment benefits and risks
Figure 10.1. Pediatric endocrinology encompasses the study and management of hormonal disorders in children
Figure 10.2. The significance of endocrine health in children
Figure 10.3. A smiling infant undergoes a routine checkup as a healthcare provider listens to the chest with a stethoscope, highlighting the importance of regular pediatric assessments
Figure 10.4. Stages of hormonal development from infancy to adolescence
Figure 10.5. Hormones play a pivotal role in the growth and development of children
Figure 10.6. The study of common endocrine disorders

Figure 10.7. Growth hormone deficiency (GHD) in pediatric patients poses significant challenges for healthcare professionals in the field of pediatric endocrinology

Figure 10.8. Fostering a positive and engaging experience in pediatric care

Figure 10.9. Laboratory tests and imaging studies

Figure 10.10. The treatment options in pediatric endocrinology

Figure 10.11. Lifestyle modifications and dietary interventions

Figure 10.12. Psychological and social implications

Figure 10.13. Social challenges faced by affected children

Figure 10.14. Demonstration of compassionate care in a clinical setting

Figure 10.15. Technological advancements in treatment

Figure 11.1. Pediatric neurology serves as a critical sub-field within the broader discipline of neurology

Figure 11.2. Importance of studying neurological disorders in children

Figure 11.3. The focus on pediatric neurological development and assessment

Figure 11.4. Key developmental milestones in childhood

Figure 11.5. Techniques for neurological assessment in children

Figure 11.6. The significance of early detection and intervention in pediatric neurology cannot be overstated

Figure 11.7. Demonstrating the assessment of pediatric neurological or developmental conditions

Figure 11.8. Epilepsy and seizure disorders represent a significant aspect of pediatric neurology

Figure 11.9. Cerebral palsy and its implications

Figure 11.10. Diagnostic tools and techniques

Figure 11.11. Electroencephalography (EEG) in diagnosis

Figure 11.12. Treatment approaches in pediatric neurology

Figure 11.13. Surgical interventions for neurological conditions in the pediatric population

Figure 11.14. The field of pediatric neurology faces numerous challenges that significantly impact diagnosis

Figure 11.15. Pediatric emergency care and injury management

Figure 11.16. Recent advances in pediatric neurology have significantly improved the understanding and management of various neurological disorders affecting children

Figure 11.17. Innovations in treatment methodologies

Figure 11.18. Pediatric neurological development and the complexity of brain function in early childhood

Figure 12.1. Pediatric cardiovascular disorders

Figure 12.2. The common pediatric cardiovascular conditions

Figure 12.3. Significance of research and advancements in treatment

Figure 12.4. Congenital heart defects in children

Figure 12.5. Pediatric pericarditis

Figure 12.6. Arrhythmia in children
Figure 12.7. Pulmonary embolism
Figure 12.8. Hypertrophic cardiomyopathy
Figure 12.9. Heart failure in pediatric patients
Figure 12.10. Signs and symptoms of cardiovascular disorders
Figure 12.11. The use of pediatric-friendly imaging technology for a comfortable diagnostic experience
Figure 12.12. The role of telemedicine in the diagnosis of pediatric cardiovascular disorders has been transformative
Figure 12.13. Management and treatment strategies
Figure 12.14. The role of advanced cardiac life support (ACLS) in pediatric cardiovascular disorders
Figure 12.15. Family involvement in treatment decisions
Figure 12.16. An illustration portrays a physician examining a child while a clergyman and a lawyer observe, symbolizing the ethical, spiritual, and legal dimensions involved in pediatric medical decision-making
Figure 12.17. Screening for congenital heart disease
Figure 12.18. Role of schools in health education
Figure 12.19. Emergency care for pediatric heat-related illness

# PREFACE

Pediatrics encompasses the entire range of diseases and health in children, infants , and adolescents , recognizing that growth and development progress along distinct patterns that differ from those of adults. During the early life period, body systems mature at an accelerated pace, and how youthful bodies react to disease, heal, and adjust are influenced by a range of factors, including genetics, diet, and environmental exposures. Healthcare professionals need to appreciate how childhood illnesses are presented differently, how developmental milestones inform clinical assessment, and how preventive interventions can alter the life course. In managing young patients, there is a need to balance demands for the urgency of treatment with long-term consequences of treatment, with an eye to both short-term outcomes as well as the root system architecture of early child experience in shaping lifelong health.

More than the absence of illness is child health. It encompasses creating growth and development of the body, enabling optimal cognitive and emotional development, and engaging with families as the hub of a child's care. Collaborative practice among doctors, nurses, dietitians, therapists, and social workers is essential in giving each child holistic care. A focus on preventive care, such as frequent immunizations, growth monitoring, and anticipatory guidance, prevents complications and sets the stage for a healthy adolescence and adulthood. Recognizing that social determinants, such as family, access to healthcare, and community resources, strongly influence outcomes, pediatric practice combines medical expertise with advocacy to give all children the opportunity to fulfill their potential.

This volume, *Textbook of Pediatrics: Volume 1*, offers systematic and thorough coverage of major pediatric medicine subjects from basic principles to special topics. This work is aimed at medical students, residents, and practitioners alike and offers cutting-edge, evidence-based practice, principles of diagnosis, and practice of management. Every chapter has been carefully constructed to ensure both conceptual correctness and practical application, making this work a reliable guide for both scholarly learning and clinical practice.

Chapter 1 introduces pediatric principles with a history of the profession, key concepts in child growth and development, and the framework for clinical assessment in children. Chapter 2 focuses on growth and developmental stages, including physical milestone monitoring, neuro developmental screening, and the role of nutrition in development. Chapter 3 highlights the fundamentals of pediatric nutrition, covering breastfeeding, formula feeding, weaning regimens, and the management of nutritional deficiencies. Chapter 4 presents immunization schedules and preventive care measures, emphasizing vaccine mechanisms, the risk–benefit ratio, and strategies for addressing vaccine hesitancy. Chapter 5 explores neonatology and newborn care, including initial stabilization, thermoregulation, and the management of common neonatal conditions such as jaundice and hypoglycemia. Chapter 6 reviews infectious dermatoses in children, from diaper dermatitis to impetigo, with guidelines for diagnosis, treatment, and prevention of transmission. Chapter 7 addresses respiratory illnesses, including acute bronchiolitis, asthma management, and respiratory support modalities. Chapter 8 examines pediatric gastroenterology through the evaluation of abdominal pain, diarrhea, malabsorption syndromes, and liver function abnormalities. Chapter 9 discusses hematology and oncology, including the evaluation of anemia, bleeding disorders, and the basics of pediatric cancer diagnosis and treatment. Chapter 10 covers endocrine disorders such as growth hormone deficiency, thyroid disease, and diabetes mellitus. Chapter 11 focuses on pediatric neurology, including seizure management, neurodevelopmental disorders, and approaches to pediatric headaches. Finally, Chapter 12 explores cardiovascular disease, including congenital heart abnormalities, acquired heart conditions, and principles of pediatric cardiac imaging and intervention.

The book is primarily written for medical students, providing clear explanations of essential topics. Residents and fellows will find detailed management protocols useful during clinical rotations, while pediatricians and family practitioners will appreciate concise, up-to-date summaries of treatment and prevention. Allied health professionals—including physician assistants, nurses, and nutritionists—will recognize the importance of multidisciplinary collaboration in pediatric care. Ultimately, this book aims to support all healthcare providers working with children by offering evidence-based knowledge and practical approaches for effective and empathetic care.

# INTRODUCTION TO PEDIATRICS

# 1

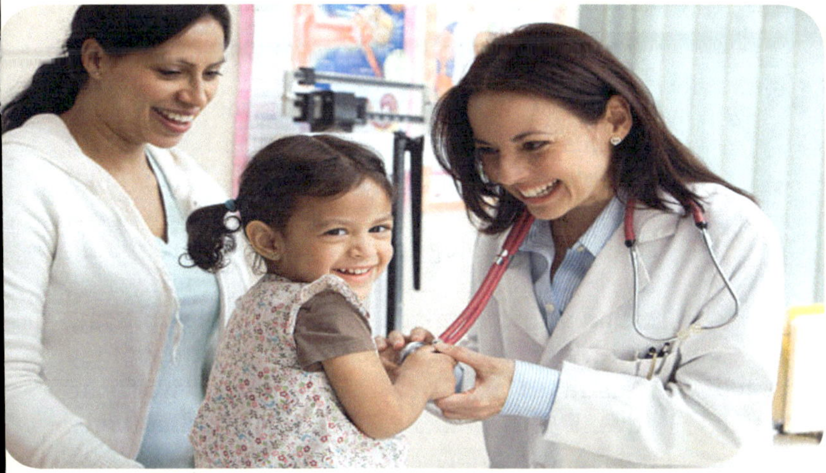

## LEARNING OBJECTIVES

**After studying this chapter, you will be able to:**

1. Discuss the growth and development in pediatrics;
2. Explain the common pediatric illnesses;
3. Know pediatric healthcare systems;
4. Understand ethical considerations in pediatrics.

## Introduction

In understanding the significance of pediatrics, recognizing the evolving nature of children's health and the pivotal role pediatricians play in addressing the many challenges faced by young patients is key. The current pediatric mental health crisis affirms the necessity for comprehensive training of the health care professionals so that they can screen, diagnose, and treat mental and behavioral health illness appropriately, and from statistics, approximately one in five children has a discernible problem. While the COVID-19 pandemic widened existing inequalities, pediatricians have been placed at the center of managing multi-faceted requirements in their areas, and it is thus important that they are adequately equipped with the necessary knowledge and expertise in mental care (Meyers et al., 2022). Innovative learning methods, such as virtual and augmented reality, are being piloted to enhance medical education, particularly in low-resource settings, by providing effective and ethical interactive learning (Barteit et al., 2021).

## Definition of Pediatrics

Pediatrics is a specialized field of medicine that is concerned with the overall health care of infants, children, and adolescents, usually considered to be people from birth until 18 years of age. Pediatrics involves a wide range of health problems, from preventive health care to diagnosis, treatment, and management of acute and chronic diseases common to younger people.

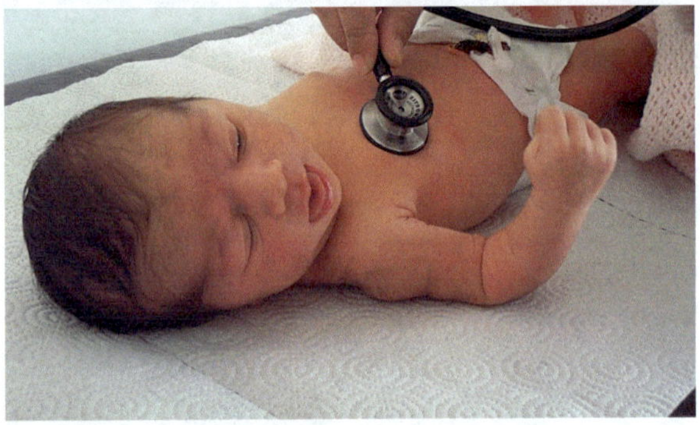

**Figure 1.1.** Pediatrics is a specialized branch of medicine dedicated to the comprehensive health care of infants.

*Source:* https://upload.wikimedia.org/wikipedia/commons/0/08/Newborn_Examination_1967.jpg.

Pediatricians play an important role in not just addressing the medical concerns of their patients but also addressing the psychosocial determinants that impact child health, such as family dynamics and developmental milestones. Emphasized in educational interventions in addressing issues among health care providers, such as underrepresented minorities in medicine, is the importance of addressing these determinants as a response to systemic issues pertinent in such a practice area (Austin et al., 2016). Furthermore, shifting patterns of treatment, including advances in genetic screening and treatment patterns, represent the dynamic nature of practice among children (Srivastava et al., 2020). These aspects emphasized the importance of pediatrics as an essential component of the health system (Figure 1.1).

## Importance of Pediatric Medicine

The significance of pediatrics lies in its regard for the unique physiological and developmental needs of children, which are significantly different from adults. Pediatrics not only encourages medical intervention based on age but also preventive medicine, focusing on resolving health issues at an early stage before they worsen. Therapeutic drug monitoring included in the treatment of children is especially significant, as it will be able to enhance the efficacy of individual therapy and decrease side effects. For instance, sensor technology advancements are going to revolutionize therapeutic drug monitoring by measuring on-site regularly following the children's special needs for pharmacology (Austin et al., 2016). Additionally, with the advent of IoT and smart health technologies in pediatrics, there is a platform where data can enhance patient outcomes in real-time to ensure safety and effective care (Austin et al., 2016). Pediatric medicine is thus important not just for the delivery of immediate health but also for the development of long-term well-being in the pediatric population.

## Historical Development of Pediatrics

Pediatrics' own historical development has been fairly dramatic throughout, showing a progression of changing society and advancing medical science. Initially, pediatric care had a lot of involvement with the delivery of general medicine and even had very little specialized knowledge regarding infant and child illness and growth. Over time, an awareness of children's distinctive health requirements led to pediatrics becoming established as a distinct medical specialty during the late 19$^{th}$ and early 20$^{th}$ centuries. Profession leaders supported differentiated approaches to child health, focusing on prevention and surveillance of development, further guided by resilience science, with its identification of how childhood adversities influence a lifetime of development and the imperative for proactive pediatric practice (Austin et al., 2016). Moreover, with the demystification of the walls of traditional data storytelling, current pediatricians now strive to make sense of child health in the arena of broader social determinants, calling for equity in the availability of care (Catherine et al., 2020).

## Scope of Pediatric Practice

The extent of pediatric practice involves a broad model for the approach to child health, one that not only focuses on medical care but also developmental and preventive care across a child's lifespan. Pediatric care providers must be skilled in delivering and managing comprehensive care.

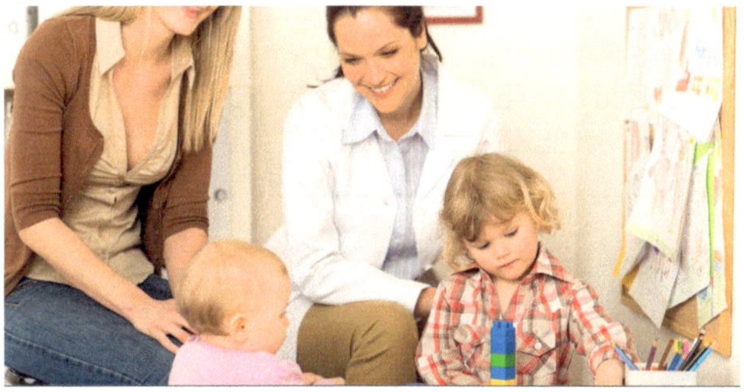

**Figure 1.2.** The scope of pediatric practice encompasses a multifaceted approach to child health.

*Source:* https://ilchiro.org/wp-content/uploads/2019/06/cbi-0216-040_017_310312-1280x640.jpg.

That is tailored to meet the unique needs of children, especially those who have significant risk factors, such as in programs like the SCVHHS BRIDGE program, which deals with the crucial care transition from the Neonatal Intensive Care Unit (NICU) to home for high-risk infants (Patel et al., 2015). In addition, successful care coordination among health care, educational services, and family support is essential to enhance pediatric outcomes, suggesting a structured type of care coordination that can optimize general child growth (Jeanne et al., 2009). Therefore, the domain of pediatric practice includes more than direct health interventions, necessitating the engagement of various stakeholders to ensure the wholesome growth and well-being of children (Figure 1.2).

## Pediatricians' Role in Healthcare

Pediatricians are a critical component of the health care network as the principal caregivers for infants, teenagers and children, who represent a distinct group with inherent physiological and psychological needs. They are responsible for monitoring development and growth, diagnosing disease and managing it, and providing preventive services, such as immunizations and health education. The COVID-19 pandemic has revealed the true spirit of pediatricians, as they adapted their practice to maintain continuity of care and meet emerging challenges.

For instance, the majority of pediatricians used telehealth platforms to maintain their interface with patients amid social distancing, clearly indicating their resilience and commitment to health care delivery (Somekh et al., 2020). In addition, pediatricians are pivotal in developing resilience in children according to resilience science principles that emphasize supportive systems and environments essential for healthy development (Austin et al., 2016). Thus, the multifaceted role of pediatricians not only meets short-term health demands but also constructs long-term wellness among the pediatric population.

## Differences Between Pediatrics and Adult Medicine

There is a need to recognize the differences between internal medicine and pediatrics to provide complete healthcare. One of the most important differences is the developmental stage of pediatric patients, which significantly influences the management of their medical cases.

Unlike adults, children's physiological and psychological parameters continually change due to development and growth, necessitating varied therapy and diagnostic strategies. Furthermore, child treatment frequently involves a family-based model, where parents or guardians are directly involved in decision-making. Pediatric health presents unique challenges, as children are particularly vulnerable to conditions that can affect both growth and development. Eating disorders are one such example, with long-term consequences that extend into physical and psychosocial domains (Austin et al., 2016). Moreover, the pediatric population is at increased risk for various diseases and mental health conditions, underscoring the need for advocacy and strong support systems within healthcare (Austin et al., 2016). These distinctions highlight the imperative for specialized training and pediatric-specific approaches to medical care (Figure 1.3).

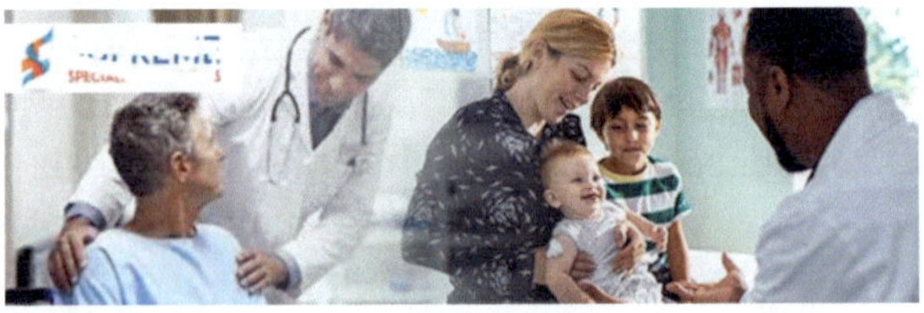

**Figure 1.3.** The differences between pediatrics and adult medicine.

*Source:* https://www.supremehospitals.in/wp-content/uploads/2024/12/Understanding-the-Key-Differences-Between-Paediatrics-and-Adult-Medicine-blog.jpg.

## Overview of Pediatric Subspecialties

Pediatric subspecialties form a vital component of pediatric care, addressing the various complex health issues that children acquire at various stages of development. At their growth phases, these subspecialties are supposed to provide specialized training in departments like pediatric cardiology, oncology, and neurology to make certain that children receive adequate and effective treatment for their respective medical conditions. For instance, pediatric oncology encourages the importance of family-centered education in managing diagnoses, observing that families require time to process blow-by-blow information while they devise ways to take care of their child (Landier et al., 2016). Moreover, the growth of pediatric subspecialties reflects a growing requirement for knowledge and expertise, evidenced by trends in other branches of medicine. An example of this includes the increased interest among neurology trainees in specialties like movement disorders and epilepsy, indicative of the demand for alignment between future interest and population need (Zis et al., 2018). This ongoing change underscores the importance of pediatric subspecialties in enhancing child health outcomes (Figure 1.4).

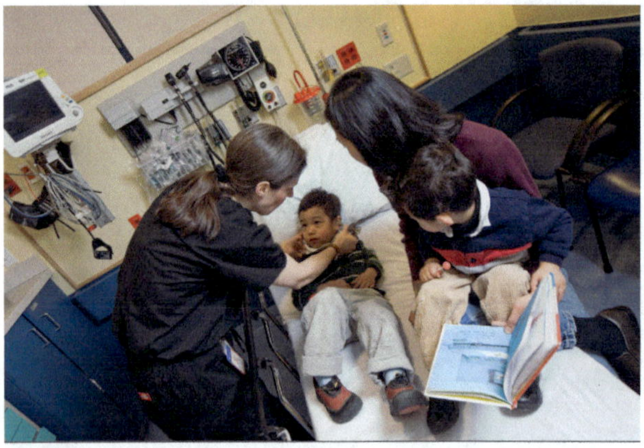

**Figure 1.4.** Overview of pediatric subspecialties.

*Source:* https://res.cloudinary.com/ysm/image/upload/yms/prod/c3b1195f-dd0f-44c9-af32-da2e853b25b6.

### Current Trends in Pediatric Care

With advancements in pediatric healthcare, emerging trends give growing importance to health equity and access to new treatments for chronic diseases that are prevalent among children. The growing realization of inequalities in health outcomes has led to measures eliminating these inequities, primarily among poorer communities. For instance, a rise in health equity publications, as recorded in reviews such as Troyer et al. (2024), signifies a need for more extensive, in-depth studies on disparities of pediatric patients. Furthermore, studies on diseases like sickle cell disease show significant differences in the outpatient treatment, with hematologists being the primary providers in children and adults relying largely on emergency services (Ogunsile et al., 2017). This imbalance emphasizes the need for increased access to specialist care during childhood and underscores that high-intensity interventions would significantly contribute to enhancing children's health outcomes as well as pushing equity in children's healthcare coverage.

## 1.1. Growth and Development in Pediatrics

**Learning Outcome**

1. Stages of child development;
2. Milestones in physical growth;
3. Cognitive development in children;
4. Emotional and social development;
5. Factors influencing growth;
6. Growth disorders and their management;
7. Role of nutrition in development;
8. Importance of regular check-ups;
9. Developmental screening tools.

Growth and development in pediatrics should be understood as the process of recognizing the wide spectrum of normal childhood wellness and identifying specific problems that may arise. Early growth patterns are strongly influenced by genetic, nutritional, and environmental factors. Deviations can be observed in several conditions, such as Turner syndrome, which is associated with endocrine complications requiring careful management, and Down syndrome, which involves distinctive developmental challenges. Both highlight the need for specialized approaches to ensure optimal outcomes from infancy through adolescence (Sabbadin et al., 2024). Furthermore, intrauterine growth restriction (IUGR) is one of the most important concerns since it affects neonatal morbidity and development in the long term. IUGR leads to conditions such as hypoglycemia, and this highlights the need for pediatricians to monitor and act upon such conditions closely (Laljibhai et al., 2024). Last but not least, a holistic approach to monitoring growth and development is most critical in pediatrics to allow every child to have their specific needs addressed optimally and with compassion (Figure 1.5).

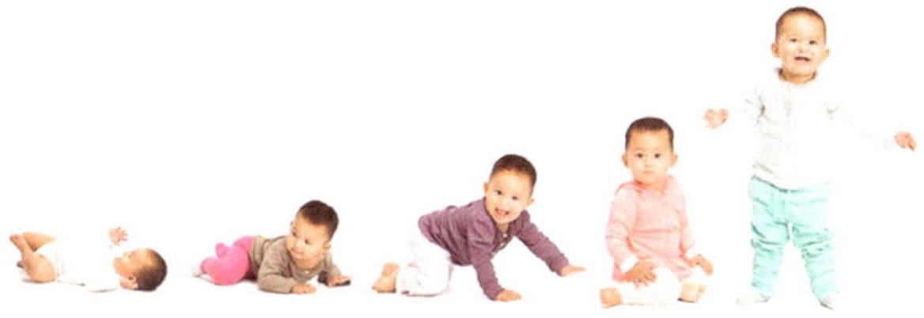

**Figure 1.5.** The growth and development in pediatrics.

*Source:* https://drsupriyawakchaure.com/images/child-growth-development-assessment-evaluation.jpg.

### 1.1.1. Stages of Child Development

Understanding the phases of child development is crucial for pediatricians as it is used for diagnosis and intervention. Development occurs in several areas, including physical, cognitive, and social-emotional development, each progressing through identifiable phases. From infancy with the creation of attachment and basic trust, continuing through early childhood with the combative attainment of cognitive abilities and social skills, each phase builds upon the preceding one to establish ensuing skills and behaviors. For instance, as children engage with the world around them, what they go through can influence mental health trajectories; research has established that overuse of social media is linked with increased depression and anxiety among adolescents, emphasizing that these activities need to be monitored (Ari, 2021). In addition, tracking development milestones may be used to assess disorders like autism spectrum disorder (ASD), which is required for early intervention (Baio et al., 2018). Therefore, understanding these phases enables healthcare professionals to promote healthier development results.

### 1.1.2. Milestones in Physical Growth

Understanding physical development milestones is crucial in pediatric medicine, as they serve as key indicators of a child's overall development and future health. The first 1,000 days of life are particularly critical, with optimal nutrition forming the foundation for growth parameters and cognitive development. Children who receive adequate early nutritional care demonstrate not only improved height and weight outcomes but also enhanced cognitive functioning and reduced morbidity, underscoring the strong link between nutrition and development (Ari, 2021). In contrast, pediatric oncology illustrates how growth milestones can be disrupted, as cancer treatments often lead to delays in sensory and motor skills due to their side effects (Schmidli et al., 2025). Continuous monitoring and targeted interventions are therefore essential to safeguard both physical and psychological wellness throughout early childhood (Figure 1.6).

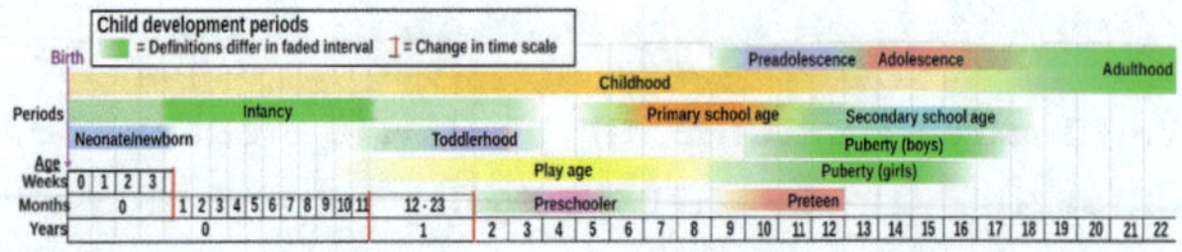


**Figure 1.6.** Milestones in physical growth.

Source: By Mikael Häggström - Own work, Public Domain, https://commons.wikimedia.org/w/index.php?curid=7209351

### 1.1.3. Cognitive Development in Children

Cognitive development in children is a multi-factorial phenomenon with various biological, environmental, and social determinants and, hence, a critical field of study for pediatrics. Its multi-factorial nature is most dramatically emphasized in the example of preterm children, who will have high chances of developing severe neuro-developmental disability. As highlighted in the literature, many preterm birth survivors not only face serious neurological disabilities but also subtle cognitive impairments that persist into childhood and adult life (Mento et al., 2015). Traditional measures of assessment are often incapable of identifying subtle impairments, thus highlighting the importance of effective developmental screenings. Recent studies have identified the moderating role of environmental determinants, such as academic success, in reducing these cognitive challenges in late preterm infants, further showing that particular interventions can decrease the risks (Drotar et al., 2008). Pediatric practitioners must understand these dynamics in supporting cognitive development and addressing the individualized needs of each child.

### 1.1.4. Emotional and Social Development

It is crucial to understand pediatric social and emotional development because it profoundly affects a child's overall health and future opportunities. Adverse childhood experiences and the social determinants of health (SDOH) are especially critical in determining developmental pathways. Research has indicated that children who experience traumatic events have a high risk for every type of health disparity, potentially impairing their social and emotional development (Corvini et al., 2018). Particularly, the foster care population most perfectly reflects the need for specialized approaches to address the challenges because the majority of the children have cumulative health issues and developmental delays due to experiencing traumas (Blake et al., 2019). Pediatric practitioners should therefore employ trauma-informed models of care that are attuned to the impact of the experiences so that interventions not only address but also foster the child's emotional and social welfare. This integrated knowledge promotes healthier growth and fosters resilience among at-risk groups.

### 1.1.5. Factors Influencing Growth

Child population growth is influenced by many factors, such as genetic, nutritional, and environmental factors. Genetic background is of gigantic significance, as growth patterns and final height potential can be determined by inherited factors. Nutritional supply is also a significant determinant; proper access to adequately balanced diets containing sufficient amounts of all essential nutrients, such as proteins, vitamins, and minerals, will ensure optimal growth, and shortages will retard growth and develop health issues. Environmental determinants like socioeconomic status and housing also affect the patterns of growth through their impact on health care and nutritional access. Chronic diseases, particularly those related to gastrointestinal absorption, can also affect growth by impairing nutritional uptake and metabolic processes. As is the case in diseases like food protein-induced enterocolitis, such illnesses need to be monitored and controlled to ensure healthy growth patterns in the affected children (Ari, 2021). Lastly, understanding such intricate influences is needed by pediatric healthcare professionals in order to ensure healthy development (Figure 1.7).

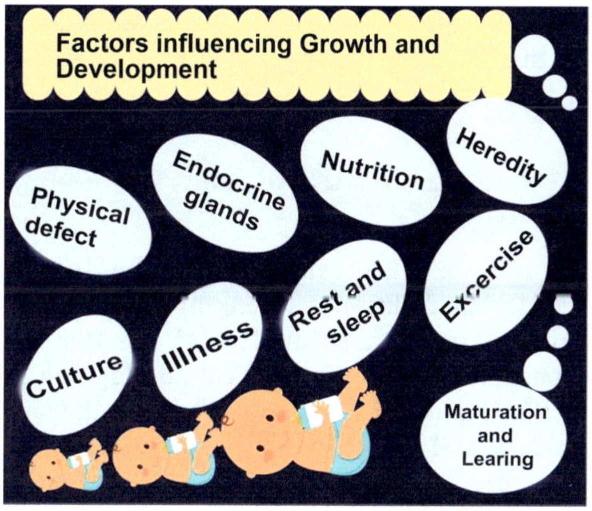


**Figure 1.7.** Growth in pediatric populations.

*Source:* https://i0.wp.com/educom360.com/wp-content/uploads/2022/09/Factors-2Binfluencing-2BGrowth-2Band-2BDevelopment.png.

### 1.1.6. Growth Disorders and Their Management

Growth disorders are a significant pediatric concern that impact the overall well-being, development, and quality of life of a child. Achondroplasia and Turner syndrome illustrate the complexity of managing growth-related problems. Turner syndrome, a chromosomal disorder affecting females, is characterized by short stature, gonadal dysgenesis, and associated cardiovascular and endocrine complications, emphasizing the need for early diagnosis and lifelong management (Shams, 2025). In contrast, achondroplasia—the most common cause of dwarfism—results from genetic mutations leading to disproportionate short stature and additional medical complications. Current treatment strategies include growth hormone therapy and surgical approaches such as limb lengthening, though these methods have limitations and potential risks (Zis et al., 2018). A multidisciplinary approach that integrates medical, psychological, and social support is therefore fundamental in addressing the multifaceted challenges of growth disorders in children.

### 1.1.7. Role of Nutrition in Development

Nutrition is a key component in the growth and development of children, influencing both physical status and intellectual functioning. Proper nutrition during critical developmental phases, infancy, and early childhood, enhances fundamental body function and substantially enhances learning potential and emotional status. Maintenance of sufficient macro-nutrient and miicronutrientconsumption ensures maximum brain development, with deficiency linked to cognitive dysfunction and behavioral disorders. Besides, a balanced diet will prevent obesity and obesity-related diseases that are increasingly common in children. The importance of nutrition also extends to prevention against conditions such as obstructive sleep apnea syndrome (OSAS), which is a condition that could be triggered by obesity (Ari, 2021). Meeting nutritional needs is thus not a matter of nutritional sufficiency, but an integrated process with impact on long-term health and developmental outcomes in children (Ève et al., 2013).

### 1.1.8. Importance of Regular Check-Ups

Regular check-ups are of utmost importance in pediatrics since they provide an opportunity for early detection and treatment of health issues, which ultimately contribute to better long-term results. The visits provide a structured channel by which the medical practitioner can monitor a child's development, assess growth patterns, and identify any pre-existing issues of obesity, which is a critical public health issue among most children today. Joint recommendations, as given in a consensus statement by the Polish Society of Pediatrics, emphasize the highest priority of primary care in preventing obesity as well as in treating obesity through lifestyle interventions like diet and physical activity (Mazur et al., 2022). Moreover, regular check-ups play an essential role in the management of chronic diseases, including asthma, where the proper choice of device and training has a real impact on the effectiveness of treatment (Ari, 2021). Consequently, these regular checks not only educate parents but also create a proactive approach to children's health, addressing problems prior to their becoming complications (Figure 1.8).

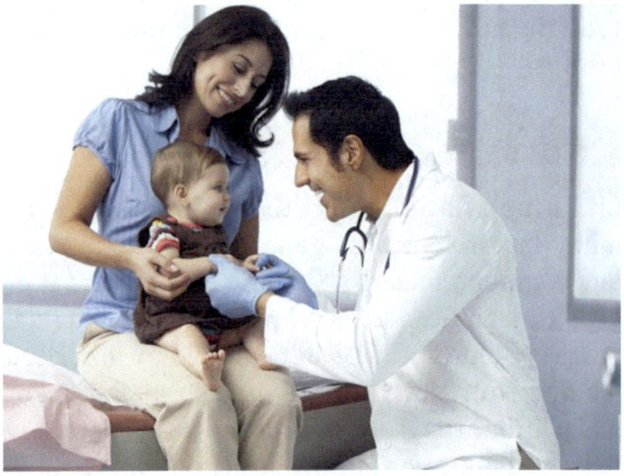

**Figure 1.8.** A pediatrician interacting with a mother and her baby during a check-up, emphasizing the importance of early childhood healthcare.

*Source:* https://prempediatrics.com/wp-content/uploads/pediatrician-1904.jpg.

### 1.1.9. Developmental Screening Tools

For pediatrics, developmental screening tools are critical to the detection of children who are at risk for developmental delay and disability, such as autism spectrum disorder

(ASD). Tools such as the Modified Checklist for Autism in Toddlers (M-CHAT) allow for early detection by way of standardized measurement during well-child visits, typically at 18 and 24 months of age. This proactive approach is in line with the American Academy of Pediatrics' suggestion of emphasizing early intervention as being key for improving long-term outcomes in affected children. Implementation of native tools of assessment, as suggested in government guidelines, also provides more cultural compatibility and access in diverse populations (Subramanyam et al., 2019). Furthermore, newer advances in resilience science underscore the importance of developing protective factors in children and the environment around them, illustrating the potential for early detection and targeted interventions to enhance resilience and construct improved developmental paths (Ari, 2021).

## Test Your Knowledge

1. What is the difference between constitutional growth delay and pathological short stature?
2. Why is regular plotting of height and weight on a growth chart important in pediatrics?

## 1.2. Common Pediatric Illnesses

**Learning Outcome**

1. Overview of acute illnesses;
2. Chronic conditions in children;
3. Infectious diseases affecting children;
4. Allergies and asthma in pediatrics;
5. Pediatric obesity and its implications;
6. Mental health issues in children;
7. Preventive care and vaccination;
8. Management of pediatric emergencies;
9. Role of family in managing illness.

Familiarity with such typical pediatric diseases is of paramount importance in pediatric practice since they pose unique diagnostic and therapeutic challenges. Some of the most frequent childhood diseases are respiratory disease, gastroenteritis, and conditions like asthma and obesity, and they have far-reaching implications for healthy child development. For instance, respiratory syncytial virus (RSV) and influenza are usually seasonal in nature, leading to high hospitalization rates for bronchiolitis and pneumonia. The changing COVID-19 pandemic has even created this scenario more intricate, with a noteworthy reduction in the presentation of respiratory illness observed from nonpharmaceutical interventions (Taylor et al., 2021). In addition, chronic illnesses like asthma continue to affect millions of children, necessitating a holistic management strategy taking both short-term and long-term care into account. The addition of updated clinical guidelines, including those by the American Diabetes Association, reinforces the importance of preventive care in the management of such common childhood conditions (Nuha et al., 2022) (Figure 1.9).

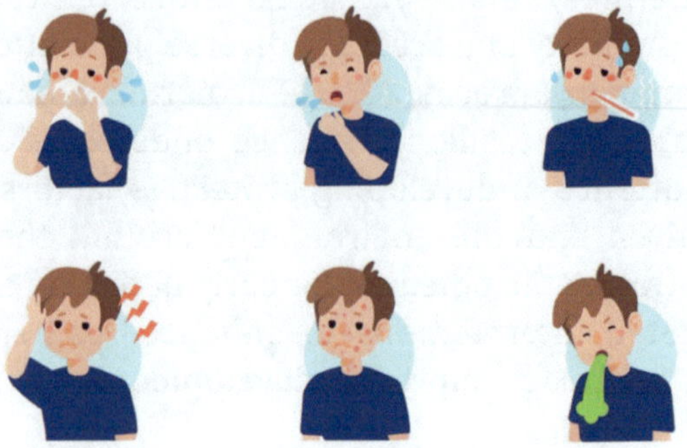

**Figure 1.9.** The common pediatric illnesses.

*Source:* https://www.lotusmedicalcentre.com.au/wp-content/uploads/2022/02/7-Common-Childhood-Illnesses-and-Their-Treatments-1024x683.jpg.

## 1.2.1. Overview of Acute Illnesses

Pediatric populations of acute illness are characterized by distinctive challenges that require immediate identification and specific interventions. Acute watery diarrhea and Kawasaki disease are examples of the range of acute diseases that target children. Acute watery diarrhea remains a primary concern of health in children between six months to five years, with studies indicating that zinc supplementation can cure such cases significantly within shorter durations, thereby improving outcomes of acute diarrheal disease (Jahan et al., 2025). Conversely, Kawasaki disease, an acute febrile illness with vasculitis features, requires rapid diagnosis before severe conditions like coronary artery damage (Mateiko et al., 2025) can occur. The differential clinical picture of these illnesses highlights the importance of careful pediatric care, whereby doctors must work through the complexities of symptomology and treatment outcomes in a bid to give the best recovery to the pediatric population. An understanding of these acute conditions thus forms a vital part of pediatrics.

## 1.2.2. Chronic Conditions in Children

Chronic conditions in children, including allergies and functional gastrointestinal disorders, are among the most significant problems in pediatrics. Allergic disorders, and particularly cow's milk protein allergy (CMPA), have been rising in prevalence and have been linked to a number of early-life factors such as prematurity and antibiotic exposure, which may disrupt gut microbiota development (Burgos et al., 2022). Furthermore, chronic functional constipation appears as an extensive condition that leads to numerous referrals to pediatric gastroenterologists and subsequently causes a lot of strain on the afflicted children (Faramarzian et al., 2021).

The chronic diseases can be managed by concerted efforts by all the healthcare providers, such as pediatricians, allergists, and nutritionists, who join forces to come up with proper treatment plans. Early intervention, particularly that for modulating gut microbiota and education intervention programs, can significantly improve the health status and quality of life for children with such chronic conditions, and evidence is emerging to acknowledge the significance of a combined pediatric care strategy (Figure 1.10).

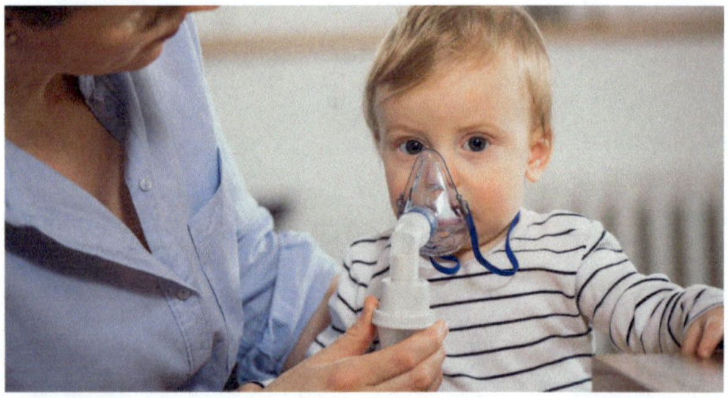

**Figure 1.10.** Chronic conditions in children.

*Source:* https://www.kernodle.com/wp-content/uploads/2020/02/Kernodle-Pediatrics_Chronic-and-Acute-Illness.jpeg.

### 1.2.3. Infectious Diseases Affecting Children

Infectious diseases are a strong threat to children's populations, which are often accompanied by severe health outcomes and complications. Viral infections to bacterial pathogens as well and parasitic diseases are likely to result from poor sanitation and restricted healthcare access. Research highlighted the connection between parental consciousness and the dental health of kids, indicating that myths about the treatment of milk teeth significantly correlate with greater caries in children, which is a common dental infection. In addition to this, recent viruses, such as SARS-CoV-2, have exhibited the weaknesses of children in today's health system.

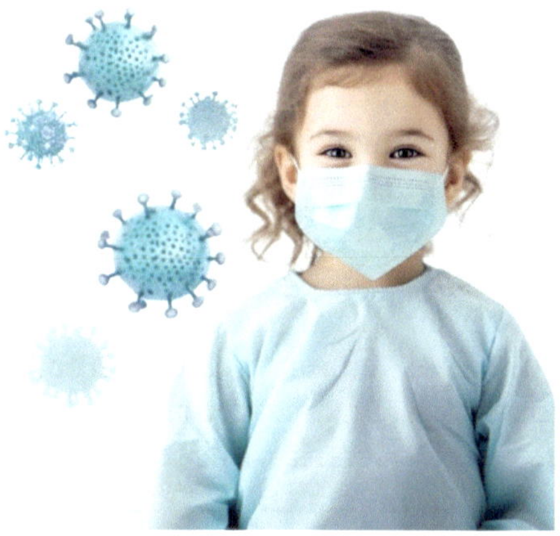

**Figure 1.11.** Child wearing a protective face mask and gown, symbolizing pediatric precautions against infectious diseases.

*Source:* https://suryahospitals.com/blog/66de89644a876large-types-of-pediatric-infectious-diseases.webp.

Though the attack rates of severe illness are lower among younger individuals, risk factors for transmission and the occurrence of related conditions like multisystem inflammatory syndrome justify the application of special public health interventions, such as pediatric vaccination drives (Stanley et al., 2021). These findings emphasize the importance of comprehensive pediatric care directed at both infectious disease prevention and control (Figure 1.11).

### 1.2.4. Allergies and Asthma in Pediatrics

Asthma and allergies among children remain a major public health concern, particularly in urban populations. Studies indicate that rural living provides protective factors, as children exposed to diverse diets and farming environments have lower rates of allergic disorders (Wang et al., 2025). However, with rapid urbanization—especially in emerging economies such as China—there has been a staggering rise in allergic diseases, often compounded by inadequate management and limited access to healthcare (Wang et al., 2025). Furthermore, research on asthma control in children revealed that more than half of the participants experienced uncontrolled symptoms, with socioeconomic status and limited awareness of triggers identified as key contributing factors. These findings highlight the urgent need for strengthened education programs and improved access to healthcare to effectively control and prevent the burden of asthma and allergies in pediatric populations.

### 1.2.5. Pediatric Obesity and Its Implications

The rising epidemic of childhood obesity is a significant public health issue with wide-ranging implications for the health and well-being of children and adolescents. A state of physical discordance between requirements and caloric needs, obesity not only puts young people at risk of a multitude of physical health issues but also negatively affects their psychological and social development. According to Alvina et al. (2021), other obesity-related disorders such as Type 2 Diabetes Mellitus, high blood pressure, and psychiatric disorders, including eating disorders, have also spread among youth. The consequences extend beyond direct health hazards; they also affect academic performance and overall well-being. Despite the complexities of treatment, with treatments often laid down based on lifestyle modification, holistic interventions are necessary to address both the physiological and psychosocial aspects of this disorder. As clinicians struggle through the intricacies, utilization of evidence-based guidelines, such as those established by the American Diabetes Association, becomes a requisite for successful management (Nuha et al., 2022).

### 1.2.6. Mental Health Issues in Children

The child's psychological well-being is an increasingly important concern in pediatrics, especially following the recent worldwide problems, such as the COVID-19 crisis. Empirical reports indicate the high prevalence of children's behavioral and emotional disorders at that time, mentioning the psychological impact of social isolation and disruption of routines (Somekh et al., 2020). The pandemic has prompted elevated anxiety, depression, and symptoms of stress, disproportionately impacting vulnerable groups such as those with underlying health issues. Moreover, perinatal period issues, such as the mental health of mothers during infectious diseases, point towards the likelihood of adverse outcomes in newborns, as seen in diseases where mothers are infected by agents such as COVID-19 (Zhu et al., 2020). These are issues that highlight the imperative importance of pediatricians prioritizing mental health screenings and interventions, incorporating holistic care that addresses physical and psychological health in kids. Such a balanced strategy is crucial to foster resilience and optimal development in children (Figure 1.12).

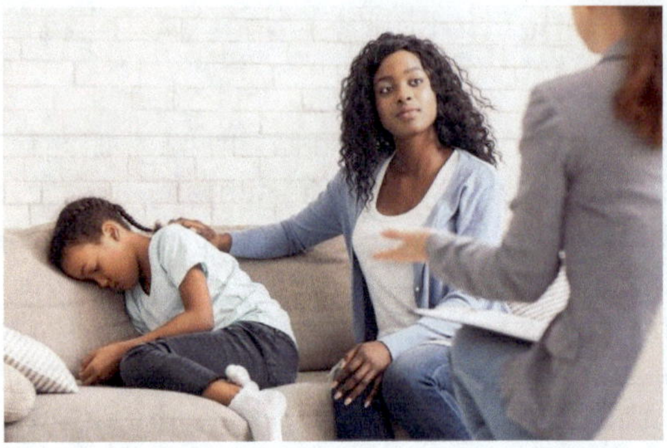

**Figure 1.12.** The mental health of children has emerged as a critical concern in pediatrics.

*Source:* https://www.vachhanihospital.com/blog/wp-content/uploads/2024/01/Mental-Health-in-Pediatrics.jpg.

### 1.2.7. Preventive Care and Vaccination

Preventive care and immunization are the foundation of pediatric wellness, significantly reducing the incidence of infectious diseases among children. Immunization not only protects children from disease but also assists in the development of herd immunity, which shields communities from outbreaks of measles, mumps, and rubella. The importance of vaccination is further generated by evidence stating that bacterial infections, despite the evolution of immunization, remain prevalent among children, thereby there is an ongoing necessity to prioritize vaccination campaigns to negate risk factors of severe diseases such as meningitis and pneumonia (Ahmad et al., 2025; Moon et al., 2025). Moreover, adding preventive practices, such as routine health examinations and education on good lifestyle routines, enhances the effectiveness of vaccinations. This coordinated approach of preventive care ensures children are better protected from infectious as well as non-infectious diseases, eventually resulting in a healthier generation and alleviating the workload of healthcare systems.

### 1.2.8. Management of Pediatric Emergencies

Effective management of pediatric emergencies is crucial in minimizing morbidity and mortality among children because of their unique physiologic response and developmental considerations. Pediatric practitioners must be adept at the recognition of the vast range of potential emergencies, ranging from respiratory distress with asthma wheezing to concerns for underlying conditions such as immune thrombocytopenia.

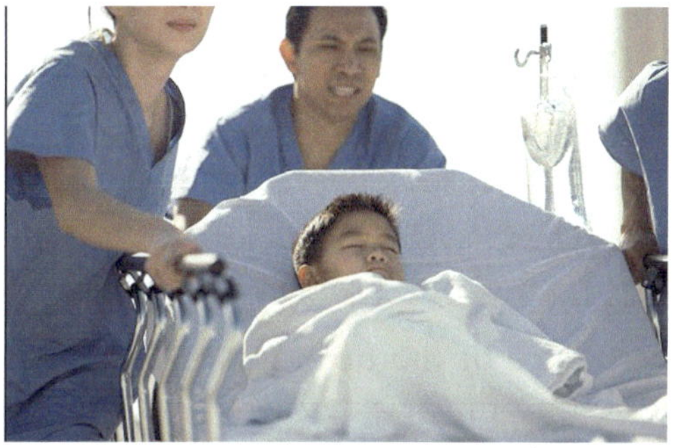

**Figure 1.13.** Medical team transporting a child on a hospital stretcher during a pediatric emergency, highlighting the urgency and care involved in critical pediatric situations.

*Source:* https://media.fmp-data.bliss.build/images/What_is_Pediatric_Emergency.format-jpeg.jpegquality-75.jpg.

Childhood asthma is one example of this, which requires a subtle strategy from acute care in the emergency room to chronic outpatient treatment (James et al., 2020). Skill in timely diagnosis and use of treatment modalities, including medication management and education of parents on how to recognize symptoms, is essential here. Second, evidence-based guidelines for conditions like immune thrombocytopenia encourage personalized care plans with a focus on family-shared decision-making (Neunert et al., 2019). Accordingly, pediatric emergency training that is holistic in scope prepares providers to address both immediate clinical issues and long-term care implications effectively (Figure 1.13).

### 1.2.9. Role of Family in Managing Illness

In children's care, the family plays a pivotal role in sickness management because they are not only primary carers but also key decision-makers along the treatment pathway. Families must navigate often complex health systems, particularly when children transfer from child to adult services, where their experience can have a significant effect on continuity of care for patients with chronic illness. There is evidence to indicate a literature gap that is expansive on effective transition programs, and there is a necessity for evidence-based guidelines responsive to the unique dynamics of family involvement in palliative care scenarios (Adi et al., 2009). Families may also advocate for their children's needs, providing a conducive environment that facilitates adherence to treatment plans. This family engagement is important because it lays the foundation for the psychological and emotional health of pediatric patients, consequently affecting health outcomes. Therefore, a knowledge of family dynamics is important for enhancing pediatric healthcare provision (Feinstein et al., 1963).

## Test Your Knowledge

1. What is the role of family in managing behavioral problems in children?
2. What is the first step in managing a child with respiratory distress in an emergency setting?

# 1.3. Pediatric Healthcare Systems

**Learning Outcome**

1. Structure of pediatric healthcare services;
2. Pediatric primary care vs. Specialty care;
3. Role of hospitals in pediatric care;
4. Pediatric emergency services;
5. Community health initiatives for children;
6. Access to pediatric care;
7. Insurance and pediatric healthcare;
8. Telemedicine in pediatrics;
9. Future directions in pediatric healthcare.

While learning Pediatric Healthcare Systems, one must keep in mind family-oriented care as the core of treatment models. The literature highlights the importance of interweaving family involvement into clinical decisions, especially in the intensive care unit, where the family's emotional and psychological support is directly involved in shaping child health outcomes. Guidelines determined by a multidisciplinary advisory group emphasize the significance of encouraging optimal communication and working practices that maximize family presence and assistance within the pediatric ICU environment (Judy et al., 2016).

Moreover, aside from that, with the advancement of pediatric medicine, the use of rigorous reporting guidelines, such as those outlined in the TRIPOD Statement, arises as necessary in developing predictive models that will be capable of quantifying the effect of interventions on children's health outcomes (Moons et al., 2015). By narrowing the gap between evidence-based advice and practice, health systems have the ability to improve considerably both the quality of care provided and the overall healthcare experience for children and families (Figure 1.14).

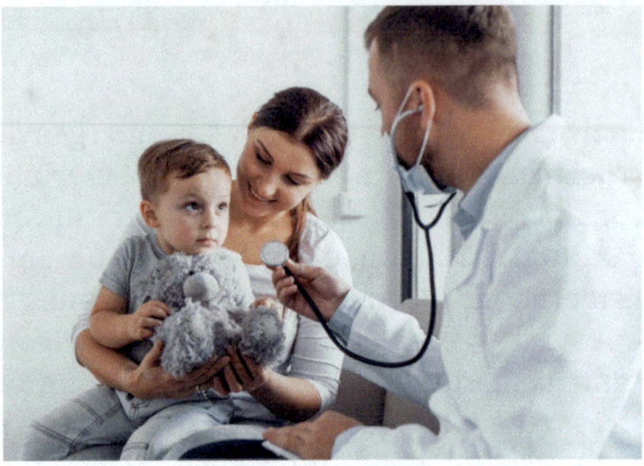

**Figure 1.14.** Pediatric healthcare systems.

*Source:* https://brhealthcare.in/uploads/blogs/1715716190_health-care-scaled-1-2048x1365.jpg.

## 1.3.1. Structure of Pediatric Healthcare Services

The structure of the health care of children is complex, due to the need to deliver especially adapted care to match the child's medical, emotional, and developmental needs. This is generally made up of a variety of institutions and practices that focus on pediatric care, e.g., specialized children's hospitals, outpatient centers, and general practices with pediatric orientations. At the core of effective pediatric practice is the application of shared decision-making (SDM), already widely embraced for its significance yet not yet fully exploited across practices. The identified hindrances in the healthcare system, from resistance by providers to the lack of extensive systems that support, hinder complete SDM adoption in pediatrics (Boland et al., 2019). Besides, training programs, such as those associated with the I-PASS Handoff Curriculum, emphasize the need for standard communication and continuity of care in various healthcare settings, and how education with scope and systemic change can enhance the landscape of pediatric healthcare (Jennifer et al., 2019).

### 1.3.2. Pediatric Primary Care versus Specialty Care

In attempting to understand the landscape of pediatric care, the dichotomy between specialty care and primary care becomes something to take into account. Pediatric primary care is the initial encounter for families, one that emphasizes the health and development of children on an overall basis through prevention, preventive check-ups, and the handling of common illnesses. On the other hand, specialty care addresses specific health concerns or complex cases requiring professional competencies, e.g., pediatric cardiology or endocrinology. Such a demarcation points to a need for a well-coordinated healthcare system that, in addition to prioritizing access to quality care, prioritizes social determinants affecting child health outcomes. For instance, successful interventions can include establishing communities of opportunity to eliminate systemic inequalities, so that every child possesses the resources required to develop and thrive (David et al., 2019). This dialogue between these two sides of pediatric care is crucial to construct a health system that effectively caters to various needs (Adam et al., 2018).

### 1.3.3. Role of Hospitals in Pediatric Care

The role of hospitals in the treatment of children is more than just the provision of emergency medical attention and encompasses wide-ranging management of the welfare and health of children. The facilities are central sites for the implementation of evidence-based treatment guidelines, as illustrated through studies on their efficacy in the treatment of conditions such as asthma among children treated in hospitals (Cabana et al., 2021). By assuming formal pathways, hospitals enhance the caliber of care, facilitate interdisciplinary collaboration, and make it easier for families to gain access to education materials that they need. Hospitals also play a major role in facilitating transfer from child to adult services for young people with chronic or limiting conditions. However, research indicates inconsistencies in the continuity and quality of care during this transition process, indicating that many pediatric programs have failed to develop standardized transition policies, which can impact the ongoing care provided to these patients (Adi et al., 2009). Hospitals must thus fill these gaps to fulfill their important role in pediatric care (Figure 1.15).

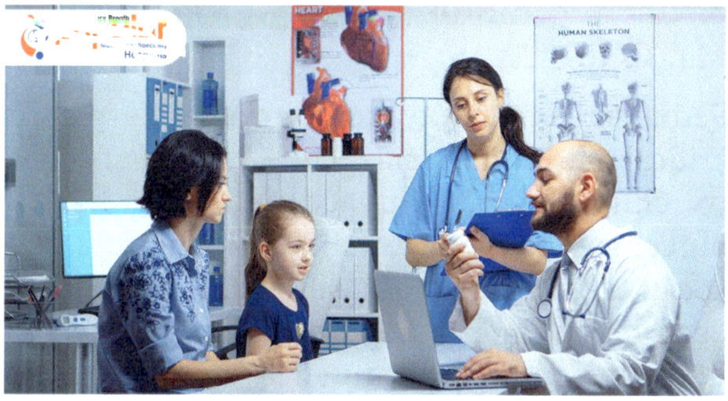

**Figure 1.15.** The role of hospitals in pediatric care extends beyond immediate medical intervention.

*Source:* https://www.popularhospital.in/blog/wp-content/uploads/2023/06/Pediatric-Department-in-Hospital-for-Best-Children-Care.jpeg.

### 1.3.4. Pediatric Emergency Services

Children's emergency care plays an essential role in meeting children's immediate health care needs, providing specialized care that differs tremendously from that of adults in emergency practice. The services must operate effectively within a health system focused on the safety and satisfaction of families and child patients. Evidence shows that a high proportion, approximately 40%, of children who present in pediatric acute assessment units can be appropriately treated without being an inpatient, thereby reducing hospital congestion and unnecessary admissions' expense (Ogilvie et al., 2005). Second, the successful implementation of community-based models, such as those demonstrated by Texas Children's Pediatrics' Community Cares program, illustrates the importance of accessibility and accessible delivery of care within populations that are otherwise underserved (Austin et al., 2016). Rendering these emergency services efficient and accessible remains a critical challenge and opportunity for pediatric care, extending into long-term children's health outcomes.

### 1.3.5. Community Health Initiatives for Children

Pediatric community health programs play a critical role in addressing the multiple challenges to children that impact pediatric health outcomes. The programs usually address the social determinants of health (SDH), including economic, environmental, and psychosocial determinants that influence the health of children. Advocacy plays a critical role in such initiatives as pediatricians and health care professionals attempt to engage communities in improving levels of health. Curriculum that teach advocacy as part of pediatrics demonstrate considerable benefit, students achieve higher levels of knowledge about SDH and advocacy skills after directed training (Melanie et al., 2019). Moreover, universal surveillance systems like the Autism and Developmental Disabilities Monitoring (ADDM) Network provide valuable data regarding the prevalence and characteristics of developmental disorders in children that help intervention (Baio et al., 2018). By centering on such community-oriented work, health workers can play an important role in molding healthier surroundings for children, ultimately leading to a fairer health landscape.

### 1.3.6. Access to Pediatric Care

Pediatric access is an important component of child health, whose goal is to provide children with immediate and appropriate medical treatment specifically responsive to their developmental needs. However, there are still critical barriers, particularly among under-served populations where the healthcare infrastructure is limited. In Sub-Saharan Africa, for instance, the majority of public health centers struggle to respond to the evolving health needs of children because there is inadequate data-informed practice in pediatrics. As evident through the failure to utilize critical health information, the failure to establish evidence-based systems of pediatric care results in decreased access and quality of care (Batani et al., 2022). Conversely, effective training in communication skills, especially pediatric palliative care, is regarded as essential in confidence-building among medical students and residents. It has been shown through research that such training enhances the ability to conduct sensitive conversations with families, ultimately bringing improved overall access to and outcomes of care for children with severe health conditions (Cowfer et al., 2020) (Figure 1.16).

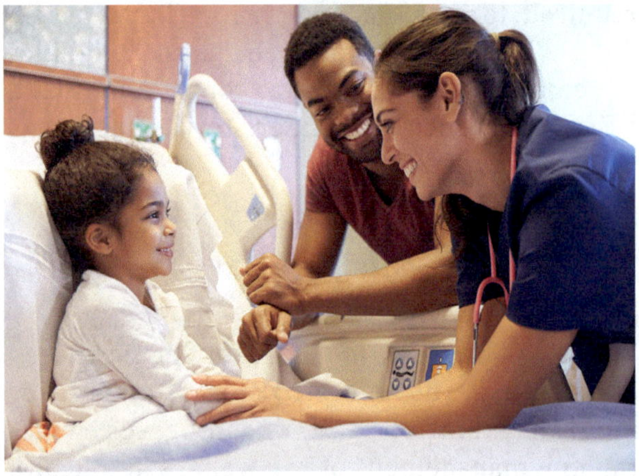

**Figure 1.16.** Access to pediatric care is a critical component of child health.

*Source:* https://cdn.prod.website-files.com/66d8b133b75a59cb016e9476/6744a55cbe2300ef7a0b266e_6706eb58168dd9d4c99388d9_66f078c916118a1c2f922eb9_pediatric-sepsis.jpeg.

### 1.3.7. Insurance and Pediatric Healthcare

The interplay of pediatric healthcare and insurance is critical to the provision of access to proper medical care for children. It is shown in research that insurance payor status strongly affects the timeliness and quality of care provided to pediatric patients. Publicly insured or uninsured children, for instance, face delays in accessing healthcare services, with delays in receiving treatment extending several times longer than for privately insured children.

These delays increase the severity of child sports-related injuries to lead to poorer health outcomes and complications (Katherine et al., 2025). Even vaccine utilization, such as the 13-valent pneumococcal vaccine, has cited a shift in healthcare use and expense, demonstrating improved preventive outcomes with good insurance coverage (Yen et al., 2025). Finally, eliminating disparities in insurance coverage is critical to ensuring fair pediatric treatment and overall health outcomes for vulnerable populations.

### 1.3.8. Telemedicine in Pediatrics

The development of telemedicine in pediatrics is an important shift in delivering healthcare to children, particularly highlighted by difficulties seen during the COVID-19 pandemic. Telemedicine not only expands access to pediatric care for families in remote or underserved populations but also assures that logistical barriers such as travel and lost work or school time are broken.

However, some factors hinder the full implementation of telemedicine strategies. Strong evidence highlights the fact that technical and infrastructure restrictions, as well as psychological and personal problems of healthcare professionals, constitute the principal obstacles to adoption in clinical practice (Israel et al., 2023). Conversely, the potential for combining emerging technologies, including metaverse application use, creates new possibilities for the delivery of comprehensive care in pediatrics (Bansal et al., 2022). This combined approach is necessary for building strong, adaptable healthcare systems that are sensitive to evolving needs among pediatric populations.

### 1.3.9. Future Directions in Pediatric Healthcare

With pediatric medicine advancing, future growth must be geared toward total management plans that encompass preventive interventions and future health issues in children.

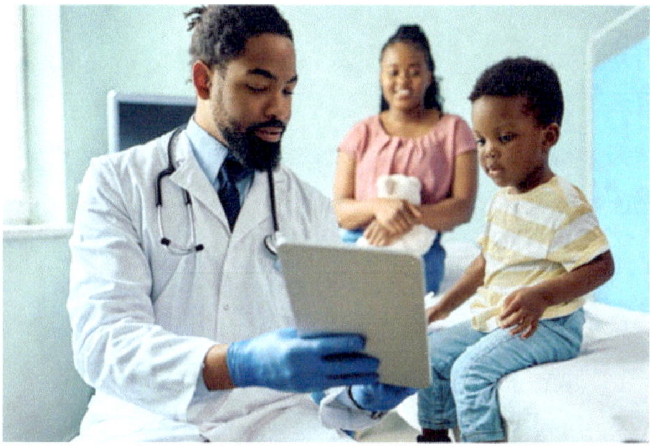

**Figure 1.17.** Future directions in pediatric healthcare.

*Source:* https://www.childrenshospitals.org/-/media/images/global/large-card/ai_future_of_pediatric_health.jpg.

The American Academy of Pediatrics' Bright Futures program is a good example of an excellent framework for providing quality pediatric care through systematic provision via well-child visits and universal screening, thereby enhancing immunization rates and the detection of developmental delay (Davis et al., 2016). Furthermore, fighting vaccine refusal remains vital, particularly in areas with considerably low vaccine levels where influential factors of parental decision-making on vaccinations have been established. Such barriers can provide information to healthcare providers to create education programs that effectively fight against misinformation and encourage preventive interventions, such as the influenza vaccine, important in reducing morbidity and mortality of childhood diseases (Leder et al., 2015). Thus, pediatric care in the future needs to concentrate on following defined guidelines and also solve issues in society regarding vaccine uptake (Figure 1.17).

## Test Your Knowledge

1. Why is a multidisciplinary team important in pediatric hospital care?
2. How do Anganwadi centers contribute to pediatric healthcare at the community level?

## 1.4. Ethical Considerations in Pediatrics

**Learning Outcome**

1. Informed consent in pediatric care;
2. Confidentiality and privacy issues;
3. Ethical dilemmas in pediatric treatment;
4. Role of parents in decision-making;
5. Pediatric research ethics;
6. Cultural competence in pediatric care;
7. End-of-life decisions for children;
8. Advocacy for child health rights;
9. Balancing risks and benefits in treatment.

The landscape of children's practice is awash with unique ethical dilemmas that require careful consideration of the rights and interests of children. Foremost among them is striking a balance between the child's best interests, parental rights, and societal expectations, an impossibly fine balancing act requiring sensitivity and ethical expertise. Pediatric practitioners often use guidelines such as the American Academy of Pediatrics (AAP) Bright Futures (BF) to standardize care and optimize health outcomes in children as they move through these waters of morality (Davis et al., 2016). Secondly, children and their families' involvement in decision-making is also important as it acknowledges the child's agency and facilitates a collaborative health care approach that caters to ethical considerations as elaborated in pediatric nursing books (Bagnasco et al., 2016). Developing frameworks to enhance compliance with ethical principles while delivering quality care is a priority area in pediatric practice, ensuring the most vulnerable cohorts receive the respect and dignity they deserve.

### 1.4.1. Informed Consent in Pediatric Care

Pediatric informed consent is a delicate procedure of balancing the rights and autonomy of children against their protection and well-being. As children are legally unable to provide consent for medical interventions, health care professionals must engage not only the parents or guardians but also the pediatric patients in order to hear their opinions as well. This participatory approach not only promotes ethical practice but equips young patients with the information required to assist in informing healthcare decisions as they age. As a testament to growing pediatric-specialized training programs that enhance provider knowledge, compassion, and confidence when addressing such complexities, there is a specific demand for applicable educational resources that are capable of addressing the unique aspects of informed consent in the pediatric patient population (Garg et al., 2021). Furthermore, within the field of an emerging health hazard, such as that posed by COVID-19, strict adherence to informed consent processes becomes a top priority, highlighting the dynamic practice of pediatric medicine (Zachariah et al., 2020) (Figure 1.18).

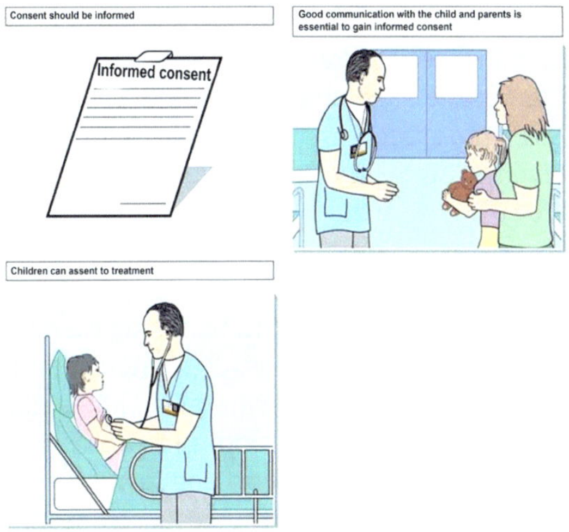


**Figure 1.18.** Informed consent in pediatric care is a nuanced process.

*Source:* https://i0.wp.com/nursekey.com/wp-content/uploads/2018/10/c06f001.jpg?w=960.

## 1.4.2. Confidentiality and Privacy Issues

Confidentiality and privacy are of utmost concern in pediatrics, particularly when working with sensitive issues such as sexually transmitted infections (STIs) and adherence to medical regimens. The unique vulnerabilities of adolescent patients necessitate the careful consideration of how information about their health is managed, as mismanagement will deter them from presenting for care when they need it. Research indicates that pediatric primary care settings can enhance STI risk screening by creating an even more private and confidential setting, which is valuable in establishing open communication between providers and patients (Fahd et al., 2023). Also, electronic monitoring (EM) of adherence is problematic from an ethical standpoint with regard to privacy and autonomy. Health care professionals should proactively manage the complexities of informed consent and confidentiality in a manner that supports patient trust and treatment adherence and ensures that their use does not erode these (Rich et al., 2022). Therefore, confidentiality is crucial to ensuring healthcare participation by children to the fullest.

## 1.4.3. Ethical Dilemmas in Pediatric Treatment

Handling the ethical dilemmas in pediatric care involves a tactful understanding of both the patient's medical needs and the family context. Clinical professionals constantly grapple with reconciling granting parents' desires with advocating the best interests of the child. Such conflict is more pronounced in extreme circumstances where relatives' involvement can make or break the child's handling. For instance, while the involvement of parents in treatment may provide psychological comfort, it can also introduce tensions around decision-making, particularly in the case of severe illness when treatment options are ethically questionable.

Evidence indicates that interaction with families in care is driving enhanced outcomes, but still remains confronted by challenges for healthcare practitioners with varying practice backgrounds and levels of education, producing conflicting perceptions of the parent's role within pediatric settings (Angelopoulou et al., 2023). Furthermore, given that pediatric conditions overlap with intricate ethical issues, discussion and education on clinical ethics in pediatrics remain essential to good practice (Frankel et al., 2005).

### 1.4.4. Role of Parents in Decision-Making

The parent's role in pediatric decision-making is central and governs not just the child's health outcomes but also the health care experience as a whole. Parents are the backbone advocates, translating their children's needs and wants within the clinical setting.

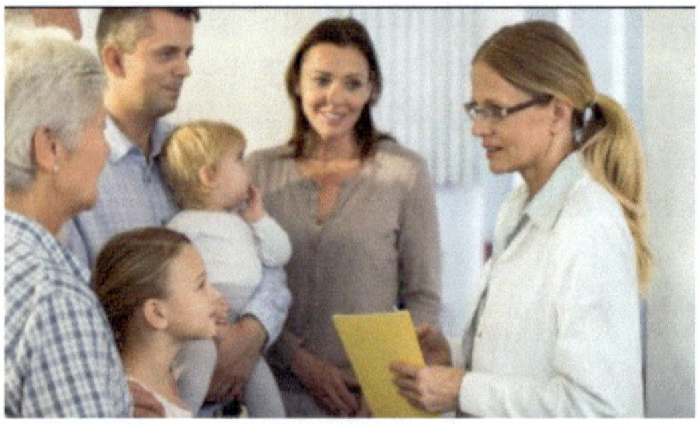

**Figure 1.19.** A healthcare provider discusses medical information with a multigenerational family, emphasizing shared decision-making in a clinical setting.

*Source:* https://www.healthychildren.org/SiteCollectionImagesArticleImages/SDM_family_Doc.jpg.

Despite the pervasive impact of shared decision-making (SDM) in adult health, its usage in pediatrics is non-uniform as revealed in studies, which identify many facilitators and barriers across various perspectives, e.g., observers and clinicians (Boland et al., 2019). Besides, advances in resilience science reveal active parental involvement since building resilience in children often relies on healthy family relationships and decision-making processes. Parents involved in collaborative strategies will be more likely to support their children's adaptation to illness, underlining the crucial role they have to promote healthy development across the lifespan (Ann et al., 2018). Thus, learning the nuances of parent involvement is essential for maximizing pediatric care (Figure 1.19).

### 1.4.5. Pediatric Research Ethics

In pediatric research, ethical considerations are of paramount importance, especially when recruiting vulnerable groups such as children with chronic illnesses. Enrolling pediatric patients in clinical trials remains a persistent challenge, with clinicians often facing barriers such as limited awareness of available trials, uncertainty about potential risks, and logistical difficulties for families (Benjamin et al., 2018). Furthermore, studies like Charting the Territory highlight the complex biopsychosocial processes that families experience in the context of chronic illness, underscoring the ethical sensitivities involved in engaging them in research (Siden et al., 2010). A thorough understanding of these challenges is essential to safeguarding the rights and well-being of pediatric participants, ensuring truly informed consent, and fostering respectful collaboration with families. Ultimately, the field must prioritize ethical principles that balance respect for children's developing autonomy with consideration of caregiver concerns and the broader complexities of the research setting.

### 1.4.6. Cultural Competence in Pediatric Care

Pediatric cultural competence is essential in order to effectively address the needs of children of different cultures. As increasing numbers of patients are treated by healthcare workers of multicultural heritage, awareness of and sensitivity toward differences allows for an excellent quality of service offered. Evidence shows that minority or low-income children experience disparities in the utilization of adequate health care, which compromises their health status. This is best evident in oral health, as untreated dental caries prevalence is higher among such groups, which reflects broader socio-economic disparities (Leder, 2015). Moreover, the inclusion of technology such as telehealth has emerged as an essential pediatric approach, especially during times of public health crises, such as the COVID-19 pandemic. Although telehealth shows promise in wider accessibility, determining the most suitable applications for diverse pediatric populations remains a challenge (Camden et al., 2020). Maximizing cultural competence is therefore essential in ensuring equitable health outcomes in pediatric practice.

### 1.4.7. End-of-Life Decisions for Children

In pediatrics, end-of-life decisions in children are an extremely emotional and ethically delicate topic that deserves scrupulous consideration from healthcare professionals. The enactment of such bills as the Korean LST Decision Act has dramatically influenced the end-of-life decision-making (EOLDM) in pediatric situations, moving toward more prompt and structured discussions of life-sustaining treatment. As shown in a study conducted at Kyungpook National University Children's Hospital, its enactment led to a significant decrease in hospital lengths of stay and a unique increase in proactive withdrawal of life-sustaining treatment decisions, representing improved compassionate and responsive care (Roh et al., 2024). Also, feedback from Croatian medical practitioners illustrates the challenge faced within pediatric intensive care units, where morally questionable attitudes toward restriction of life-sustaining treatment portray the need for more defined guidelines and supportive systems in the care of such sensitive issues (Ćurković et al., 2024). These findings carry significance for the imperative of integrating ethical considerations and professional support within pediatric end-of-life care (Figure 1.20).

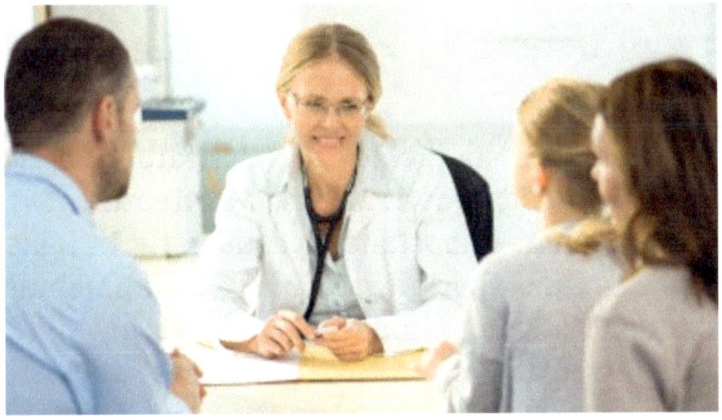

**Figure 1.20.** A pediatrician engages in a shared decision-making discussion with a family, fostering collaborative care in a clinical setting.

*Source:* https://www.healthychildren.org/SiteCollectionImages/SDM_family_HC.jpg.

### 1.4.8. Advocacy for Child Health Rights

In pediatrics, a mandate to uphold child health rights is a vocation imperative to the profession, so that every child gets access to essential health care and services. Since about half of the 70.8 million displaced individuals in the world comprise children, the healthcare profession is likewise under greater obligation to attend to the specific problems of such vulnerable groups, including trauma and unavailability of appropriate healthcare (Umbereen et al., 2020). Child health rights promotion not only involves ensuring physical needs but also social and emotional well-being as a reflection of equity and accessibility principles enunciated by various human rights platforms (Leder, 2015). It is a collaborative process involving healthcare professionals, policymakers, and populations in efforts to advocate for children's rights, enhance healthcare resources, and adopt holistic care strategies. By advocating these rights, pediatricians can substantially enhance health and quality-of-life outcomes for children all over the globe and thus carry out their ethical responsibility to this most valuable of populations.

### 1.4.9. Balancing Risks and Benefits in Treatment

For pediatric medicine, the delicate tipping point between benefit and risk of treatment is of paramount importance, particularly in light of the unique physiological and developmental characteristics of children. As a case in point, when treating conditions such as obesity, treatments are compelled to weigh possible health benefits against risks from adverse effects of treatments or changes in diet (Dennis et al., 2017). Second, when managing illnesses like thyrotoxicosis, clinicians face the challenge of making decisions regarding safe and effective treatments, particularly for vulnerable groups like pregnant women and children (Douglas et al., 2016). This not only involves critical evaluation of best evidence practices and clinical guidelines, but also active collaboration with patients and families to honor their values and fears. Thus, the successful management of childhood conditions hinges on the capability of clinicians to thread through these issues, finally working towards optimizing health outcomes while minimizing the potential for harm.

## Test Your Knowledge

1. Who provides informed consent for medical procedures in children, and why is assent from the child also important?
2. How can healthcare providers demonstrate cultural competence and advocate for a child's health rights in a diverse community setting?

## SUMMARY

It is necessary to note the inter-disciplinary collaboration in achieving maximum health outcomes for children. As pediatric care evolves, the co-mingling of specialties like emergency medicine and mental health services is more vital. The quick observations included in publications by Smulski et al. (2019) highlight the importance of detecting and avoiding errors in pediatric imaging that can greatly affect diagnosis and therapeutic outcomes. In addition, mental health interventions, as Marsh et al. (2019) strongly demonstrate the necessity of making use of technology-based solutions in order to bridge common barriers and, in turn, increase pediatric populations' access to care. The future of pediatric healthcare thus depends not only on advances in clinical knowledge but also on building cooperative systems that leverage diverse expertise. This commitment to collaboration will ensure a more consolidated effort, appropriately responding to the multiaspected needs of children in various healthcare settings.

In pediatric practice, effective communication between caregivers and healthcare professionals is paramount, particularly in complex clinical cases in multidisciplinary settings. A significant development in this arena is the production of after-visit summaries (AVS), which summarize necessary patient instructions, reducing caregiver information overload. There is evidence that AVS compliance may be significantly increased and significantly enhance communication outcomes, as experienced with an increase in completion rates from 39.4% to 85.0% following targeted education of providers to simplify medical terminology (Ari, 2021). Differences in the treatment of common pediatric conditions, such as wrist fractures, identify the importance of a worldwide agreed-upon best practice. This gap highlights the need for greater research, and in particular, randomized controlled clinical trials, to create evidence-based treatment protocols that can ensure high-quality care regardless of variable healthcare systems (Labianca et al., 2024). Interoperability between structured communication tools and evidence-based practices is thus the cornerstone of pediatric care improvement.

## KEY TERMS FROM THIS CHAPTER

- Adverse childhood experiences (ACEs)
- Childhood diseases
- Diagnose
- Health equity
- Health measures
- Healthcare
- Mental health
- Neurology
- Childhood
- Cognitive development
- Health education
- Health interventions
- Health professionals
- Medicine
- Milestones
- Oncology

## CRITICAL THINKING QUESTIONS

1. **Pediatrics is the branch of medicine that deals with:**
   a. Only newborn care
   b. Treatment of adults
   c. Medical care of children and adolescents
   d. Elderly care
2. **The neonatal period is defined as:**
   a. First 3 months of life
   b. Birth to 28 days
   c. 1 month to 1 year
   d. Birth to 1 year
3. **Which of the following is a primary goal of pediatrics?**
   a. Geriatric care
   b. Disease management only
   c. Promoting optimal growth and development
   d. Cosmetic treatment
4. **A child is considered a toddler between the ages of:**
   a. 0–1 year
   b. 1–3 years
   c. 3–5 years
   d. 6–12 years
5. **Who is regarded as the "Father of Modern Pediatrics"?**
   a. Hippocrates
   b. William Osler
   c. Abraham Jacobi
   d. Thomas Syndenham

### Short Answer Questions

1. What is the age classification in pediatrics?
2. Differentiate between neonate, infant, toddler, and adolescent.
3. What is the importance of growth and development monitoring in children?
4. What are the components of a well-baby visit?
5. What are growth charts, and how are they used in pediatrics?
6. Explain the concept of family-centered care in pediatrics.

### *Answers to Critical Thinking Questions*

1. (c) 2. (b) 3. (c) 4. (b) 5. (c)

## REFERENCES


1. Landier, W., Ahern, J., Barakat, L. P., Bhatia, S., Bingen, K. M., Bondurant, P. G., Cohn, S. L., Dobrozsi, S. K., Haugen, M., Herring, R. A., Hooke, M. C., Martin, M., Murphy, K., Newman, A. R., Rodgers, C. C., Ruccione, K. S., Sullivan, J., Weiss, M., Withycombe, J., Yasui, L., ... Hockenberry, M. (2016). Patient/Family Education for Newly Diagnosed Pediatric Oncology Patients. *Journal of pediatric oncology nursing : official journal of the Association of Pediatric Oncology Nurses, 33*(6), 422–431. https://doi.org/10.1177/1043454216655983 (accessed on 16th June 2025).
2. Ahmad, F. A., Chan, P., McGovern, C., Dickey, V., Foraker, R., & McKay, V. (2023). Adapting an electronic STI risk assessment program for use in pediatric primary care. *Journal of Primary Care & Community Health, 14*. https://www.semanticscholar.org/paper/f475e24c664cd5c3ebb1d92993346dcb4a3ebef4 (accessed on 16th June 2025).
3. Alvina, R., Kansra, A. R., Lakkunarajah, S., & Jay, M. S. (2021). Childhood and adolescent obesity: A review. *Frontiers in Pediatrics, 8*. https://doi.org/10.3389/fped.2020.581461 (accessed on 16th June 2025).
4. Siden, H., Steele, R., Brant, R., Cadell, S., Davies, B., Straatman, L., Widger, K., & Andrews, G. S. (2010). Designing and implementing a longitudinal study of children with neurological, genetic or metabolic conditions: charting the territory. *BMC pediatrics, 10*, 67. https://doi.org/10.1186/1471-2431-10-67(accessed on 16th June 2025).
5. Ari, A. (2021). A path to successful patient outcomes through aerosol drug delivery to children: A narrative review. *Annals of Translational Medicine, 9*, 593–593. https://doi.org/10.21037/atm-20-1682 (accessed on 16th June 2025).
6. Ates, H. C., Roberts, J., Lipman, J., Cass, A. E. G., Urban, G., & Dincer, C. (2020). On-site therapeutic drug monitoring. *Trends in Biotechnology, 38*, 1262–1277. https://doi.org/10.1016/j.tibtech.2020.03.001 (accessed on 16th June 2025).
7. Bagnasco, A., Barisone, M., Bressan, V., Cadorin, L., et al. (2016). Ethical dimensions of pediatric nursing: A rapid evidence assessment. https://core.ac.uk/download/151162979.pdf (accessed on 16th June 2025).
8. Baio, J., Wiggins, L. D., Christensen, D., Maenner, M. J., Daniels, J. L., Warren, Z., Kurzius-Spencer, M., et al. (2018). Prevalence of autism spectrum disorder among children aged 8 years–Autism and Developmental Disabilities Monitoring Network, 11 sites, United States, 2014. *MMWR Surveillance Summaries, 67*, 1–23. https://doi.org/10.15585/mmwr.ss6706a1 (accessed on 16th June 2025).
9. Barteit, S., Lanfermann, L., Bärnighausen, T., Neuhann, F., & Beiersmann, C. (2021). Augmented, mixed, and virtual reality-based head-mounted devices for medical education: Systematic review. *JMIR Serious Games, 9*, e29080–e29080. https://doi.org/10.2196/29080 (accessed on 16th June 2025).
10. Batani, J., & Maharaj, M. (2022). Towards data-driven pediatrics in Zimbabwe. https://doi.org/10.1109/icabcd54961.2022.9855907 (accessed on 16th June 2025).
11. Blake, C. P., Graham, C., & Graham, C. P. (2019). Screening for trauma in the foster care community. https://core.ac.uk/download/286729709.pdf (accessed on 16th June 2025).

12. Cabana, M. D., Cattamanchi, A., Gupta, N., Jennings, T., et al. (2021). Implementing pediatric inpatient asthma pathways. https://core.ac.uk/download/323082497.pdf (accessed on 16th June 2025).

13. Zis, P., Macerollo, A., Sauerbier, A., Papp, V., Klingelhoefer, L., & Cock, H. R. (2018). Subspecialty preferences among neurologists of the future. *European journal of neurology*, *25*(3), 597–601. https://doi.org/10.1111/ene.13526 (accessed on 16th June 2025).

14. D'Ignazio, C., & Klein, L. (2020). *Data Feminism*. The MIT Press eBooks. https://doi.org/10.7551/mitpress/11805.001.0001 (accessed on 16th June 2025).

15. Davidson, J. E., Aslakson, R. A., Long, A. C., Puntillo, K., Kross, E. K., Hart, J. L., Cox, C. E., et al. (2016). Guidelines for family-centered care in the neonatal, pediatric, and adult ICU. *Critical Care Medicine, 45*, 103–128. https://doi.org/10.1097/ccm.0000000000002169 (accessed on 16th June 2025).

16. Drotar, D., Dworkin, P., & Stancin, T. (2008). Pediatric developmental screening: Understanding and selecting screening instruments. https://core.ac.uk/download/71353748.pdf (accessed on 16th June 2025).

17. Faramarzian, Z., Kargar, M., Dehghani, S., & Zare, N. (2021). Management of functional constipation in pediatrics based on nurse educational intervention. *Journal of Health Sciences and Surveillance System, 9*, 111–117. https://www.semanticscholar.org/paper/c2961ba1cde9887f9c425d3656ac9e6a51414f9c (accessed on 16th June 2025).

18. Feinstein, B., Frum, C., Miller, P. C., Rice, R., et al. (1963). Mothers of children with congenital heart defects: The effects of ethnicity and education on perceptions, attitudes and feelings; (Implications for social work practice). https://open.bu.edu/bitstream/2144/4161/2/Feinstein_1963_web.pdf (accessed on 16th June 2025).

19. Frankel, L., Goldworth, A., Rorty, M., & Silverman, W. (2005). Ethical dilemmas in pediatrics: References. https://www.semanticscholar.org/paper/a0513d66eb4d4e37bcd4615cbf8b303d753b7370 (accessed on 16th June 2025).

20. Hornberger, L. L., Lane, M., Breuner, C. C., Alderman, E. M., Grubb, L. K., et al. (2020). Identification and management of eating disorders in children and adolescents. *Pediatrics, 147*. https://doi.org/10.1542/peds.2020-040279 (accessed on 16th June 2025).

21. Jahan, A., Mir, H., Mohammad, J., & Jahan, F. (2025). The effect of zinc supplementation on the duration of acute watery diarrhea in children age 6 months to 5 years old. *Indus Journal of Bioscience Research*. https://www.semanticscholar.org/paper/8e03bde9f7b7db46f4fef9f453f5a86936142eff (accessed on 16th June 2025).

22. Keles, B., McCrae, N., & Grealish, A. (2019). A systematic review: The influence of social media on depression, anxiety and psychological distress in adolescents. *International Journal of Adolescence and Youth, 25*, 79–93. https://doi.org/10.1080/02673843.2019.1590851 (accessed on 16th June 2025).

23. Leder, L. (2015). Vaccination hesitation: Investigation why parents decline pediatric influenza vaccines in Juneau, Alaska. https://core.ac.uk/download/162577318.pdf (accessed on 16th June 2025).

24. Marcus, C. L., Brooks, L. J., Draper, K. A., Gozal, D., Halbower, A. C., Jones, J. K. N., Schechter, M. S., et al. (2012). Diagnosis and management of childhood obstructive sleep apnea syndrome.

*Pediatrics, 130*, 576–584. https://doi.org/10.1542/peds.2012-1671 (accessed on 16th June 2025).

25. Marsh, M. C., Supples, S., McLaurin-Jiang, S., Brown, C. L., & Linton, J. M. (2019). Introducing the concepts of advocacy and social determinants of health within the pediatric clerkship. *MedEdPORTAL*. https://doi.org/10.15766/mep_2374-8265.10798 (accessed on 16th June 2025).
26. McAllister, J. W., Popp, J., & Antonelli, R. (2009). Making care coordination a critical component of the pediatric health system: A multidisciplinary framework. https://core.ac.uk/download/71352885.pdf (accessed on 16th June 2025).
27. Mento, G., & Nosarti, C. (2015). The case of late preterm birth: Sliding forwards the critical window for cognitive outcome risk. https://core.ac.uk/download/84923605.pdf (accessed on 16th June 2025).
28. Metz, J. B., & Burns, R. (2020). Pediatric boot camp series: Longitudinal care for a child with asthma—From the emergency department to outpatient clinic. *MedEdPORTAL*. https://doi.org/10.15766/mep_2374-8265.10906 (accessed on 16th June 2025).
29. Meyers, N., Maletz, B., Berger-Jenkins, E., Lane, M., Shindle, E., Costich, M., Caddle, S., et al. (2022). Mental health in the medical home: A longitudinal curriculum for pediatric residents on behavioral and mental health care. *MedEdPORTAL*. https://doi.org/10.15766/mep_2374-8265.11270 (accessed on 16th June 2025).
30. Moon, J. Y., El Labban, M., Gajic, O., & Odeyemi, Y. (2025). Strategies for preventing and reducing the impact of acute respiratory failure from pneumonia. *Expert Review of Respiratory Medicine, 19*, 205–221. https://www.semanticscholar.org/paper/4837bac6cd99d07df7a1a1161350cb1601f08d0d (accessed on 16th June 2025).
31. Nehal, U. S., Kanahara, S., Tanabe, M., Hayner, G., & Nelson, B. D. (2020). Pediatric refugee health care delivery in the community setting: An educational workshop for multidisciplinary family-centered care during resettlement. *MedEdPORTAL*. https://doi.org/10.15766/mep_2374-8265.10988 (accessed on 16th June 2025).
32. Neunert, C., Terrell, D. R., Arnold, D. M., Buchanan, G. R., Cines, D. B., Cooper, N., Cuker, A., et al. (2019). American Society of Hematology 2019 guidelines for immune thrombocytopenia. *Blood Advances, 3*, 3829–3866. https://doi.org/10.1182/bloodadvances.2019000966 (accessed on 16th June 2025).
33. Northridge, M. E., Kumar, A., & Kaur, R. (2020). Disparities in access to oral health care. *Annual Review of Public Health, 41*, 513–535. https://doi.org/10.1146/annurev-publhealth-040119-094318 (accessed on 16th June 2025).
34. O'Toole, J. K., Starmer, A. J., Calaman, S., Campos, M. L., Hepps, J., Lopreiato, J., Patel, S. J., et al. (2019). I-PASS mentored implementation handoff curriculum: Champion training materials. *MedEdPORTAL*. https://doi.org/10.15766/mep_2374-8265.10794 (accessed on 16th June 2025).
35. Ogilvie, D. (2005). Hospital-based alternatives to acute pediatric admission: A systematic review. https://core.ac.uk/download/1393372.pdf (accessed on 16th June 2025).
36. Patel, R. (2015). Pediatric nurse practitioner home visitation is associated with a decrease in home care and healthcare utilization errors in high-risk infants. https://core.ac.uk/download/129532636.pdf (accessed on 16th June 2025).

37. Plotkin, S. A., & Levy, O. (2021). Considering mandatory vaccination of children for COVID-19. *Pediatrics, 147*. https://doi.org/10.1542/peds.2021-050531 (accessed on 16th June 2025).

38. Rich, K., Pai, A. L. H., Varnell, C. D., Hooper, D., Eckhardt, C., & Modi, A. (2022). Electronic monitoring of adherence in clinical care: Ethical and practical considerations. *Clinical Practice in Pediatric Psychology, 10*, 452–461. https://www.semanticscholar.org/paper/7d8dbf1a4c00c775739499d8aadab45f0325ac29 (accessed on 16th June 2025).

39. Roh, D., Kwon, J., Lim, Y., & Kim, Y. (2024). Changes in pediatric end-of-life process after the enforcement of the act on life-sustaining treatment decisions—The experience of a single children's hospital. *Healthcare, 12*. https://www.semanticscholar.org/paper/23c8828eccd3cf63541eb1ae9e50d069d6f9f3c3 (accessed on 16th June 2025).

40. Ross, D. S., Burch, H. B., Cooper, D. S., Greenlee, M. C., Laurberg, P., Maia, A. L., Rivkees, S. A., et al. (2016). 2016 American Thyroid Association guidelines for diagnosis and management of hyperthyroidism and other causes of thyrotoxicosis. *Thyroid, 26*, 1343–1421. https://doi.org/10.1089/thy.2016.0229 (accessed on 16th June 2025).

41. Sabbadin, C., Marin, L., Manso, J., Mozzato, C., Camozzi, V., Andrisani, A., Sacchetti, C., et al. (2024). Transition from pediatrics to adult health care in girls with Turner syndrome. *Expert Review of Endocrinology & Metabolism, 19*, 229–240. https://www.semanticscholar.org/paper/b66b778a892e20b4294ed3406bbc0d70dc101a85 (accessed on 16th June 2025).

42. Schmidli, B., Hammadou, C., Schindera, C., von der Weid, N. X., Tacke, U., Faude, O., Koch, S., et al. (2025). The importance of specific exercise therapy in pediatric oncology. *Current Issues in Sport Science (CISS)*. https://www.semanticscholar.org/paper/a85e8fce7912ce96a8d9584413237846ae5fa481 (accessed on 16th June 2025).

43. Simone, A. M., Simone, M., Block, L., & LaVine, N. (2020). Contract negotiation skills: A workshop for women in medicine. *MedEdPORTAL*. https://doi.org/10.15766/mep_2374-8265.10910 (accessed on 16th June 2025).

44. Smulski, S., & Faraoni, D. (2019). A review of errors in emergency and trauma radiology. *Anesthesia & Analgesia*. https://www.semanticscholar.org/paper/21a750f7affbdccd2275c4875e6f8c6121f778bd (accessed on 16th June 2025).

45. Squires, J. E., & Balistreri, W. F. (2017). Hepatitis C virus infection in children and adolescents. *Hepatology Communications, 1*, 87–98. https://doi.org/10.1002/hep4.1028 (accessed on 16th June 2025).

46. Styne, D. M., Arslanian, S., Connor, E. L., Farooqi, I. S., Murad, M. H., Silverstein, J., & Yanovski, J. A. (2017). Pediatric obesity—Assessment, treatment, and prevention: An Endocrine Society clinical practice guideline. *The Journal of Clinical Endocrinology & Metabolism, 102*, 709–757. https://doi.org/10.1210/jc.2016-2573 (accessed on 16th June 2025).

47. Villagra Rivera, N., Feldman, E. A., Augustin, D. A., Cáceres, W., Gans, H. A., & Blankenburg, R. (2021). Do I belong here? Confronting imposter syndrome at an individual, peer, and institutional level in health professionals. *MedEdPORTAL*. https://doi.org/10.15766/mep_2374-8265.11166 (accessed on 16th June 2025).

48. Wang, Y., Yang, J., Lai, X., Leung, A., Xing, Y., & Wong, G. (2025). Early origins of asthma and allergies: Clues from studies in China. *Clinical and Experimental Allergy: Journal of the British Society for Allergy and Clinical Immunology*. https://www.semanticscholar.org/paper/f6e9375646d9c9f457dd802628342bdb51d1bfbd (accessed on 16th June 2025).

49. Williams, D. R., & Cooper, L. A. (2019). Reducing racial inequities in health: Using what we already know to take action. *International Journal of Environmental Research and Public Health, 16*, 606–606. https://doi.org/10.3390/ijerph16040606 (accessed on 16th June 2025).

50. Zhu, H., Wang, L., Fang, C., Peng, S., Zhang, L., Gui-ping, C., Xia, S., et al. (2020). Clinical analysis of 10 neonates born to mothers with 2019-nCoV pneumonia. *Translational Pediatrics, 9*, 51–60. https://doi.org/10.21037/tp.2020.02.06 (accessed on 16th June 2025).

# PEDIATRIC GROWTH AND DEVELOPMENT

# 2

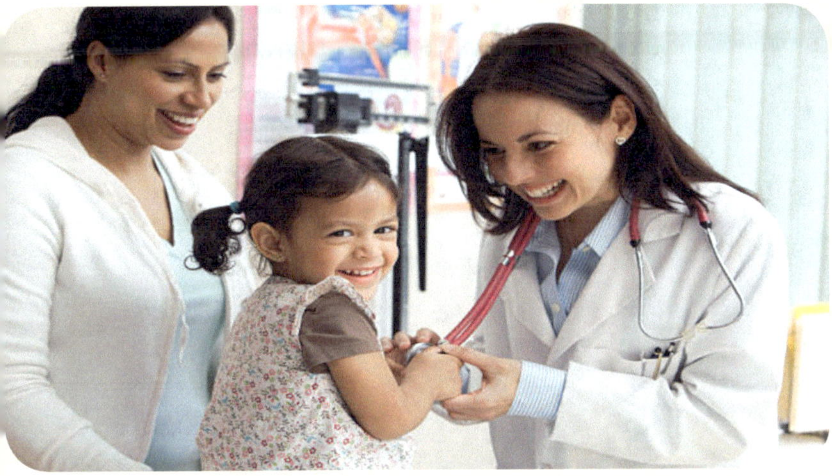

## LEARNING OBJECTIVES

**After studying this chapter, you will be able to:**

1. Discuss the physical growth in children;
2. Focus on cognitive development;
3. Explain the social and emotional development;
4. Know behavioral development.

## Introduction

The multidimensional process of child growth and development is a unified component of human existence that has a direct influence on physical and psychological patterns of health. Children have grown rapidly since birth, with their general well-being and social adaptation relying on their progress. The process is marked by principal milestones, including the development of motor functions, growth of cognition, and the formation of emotions. Understanding the various stages of this development provides perspective on the scope of factors that determine a child's trajectory, from genetics to environment. This chapter aims to look into the intricate aspects of pediatric development, such as the dynamic interplay between biological development and socialization, and their implications on overall health across life. By examining normative trends and potential disruption in development, we can better appreciate the relevance of fostering interventions in early childhood (Figure 2.1).

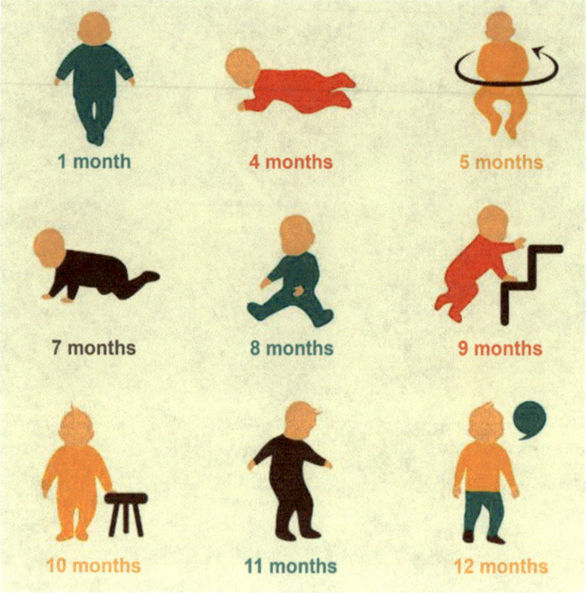


**Figure 2.1.** Pediatric growth and development.

Source: https://cdn.vectorstock.com/i/1000v/84/35/baby-development-child-growth-milestones-vector-46538435.jpg.

## Definition of Pediatric Growth and Development

The development and growth of children involve physical, emotional, social, and mental changes during infancy to adolescence. This broad idea keeps in mind that development brings not only measurable changes in weight and height but also food for thought regarding the interdependent nature of developmental phases and health outcomes. For instance, there is critical development of the brain during early childhood, which lays the foundation for learning and behavior. As children mature, their rate of growth can be influenced by various factors, including genetics, diet, and the environment. The prevalence of hypertension in children, as indicated by Lurbe et al. (2016), highlights the importance of monitoring growth parameters to prevent complications of long-term growth. Similarly, studies by Selma et al. (2015) indicate how early growth indicators can predict impending health issues, demonstrating that childhood growth is comprehensible and indispensable not only for present-day health assessments but also for health management for a lifetime.

## Importance of Studying Pediatric Growth

Understanding pediatric development is essential to optimizing health outcomes, particularly for high-risk newborns at discharge from the neonatal intensive care unit. Programs like the SCVHHS BRIDGE program demonstrate how targeted interventions can address the risk vulnerabilities of such infants.

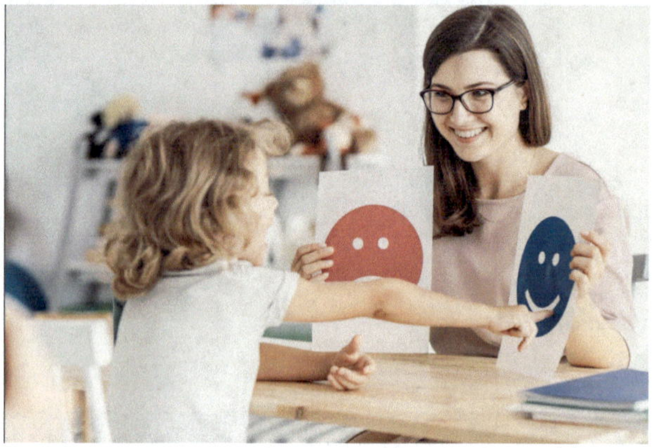

**Figure 2.2.** A child points to a smiling face during an emotional recognition activity with a therapist, supporting social-emotional development in a clinical or educational setting.

*Source:* https://keystoneacademic-res.cloudinary.com/image/upload/element/14/149099_UNylpchilddev.jpg.

By minimizing home care errors and optimizing caregiver instruction, the program promotes both infant development and access to health care following discharge (Patel et al., 2015). As pediatric growth is not only a body process but also encompasses emotional and psychological well-being, there should be a holistic approach. For instance, adolescents with chronic diseases like sickle cell disease will employ religiosity and spirituality as coping mechanisms, which can significantly impact their overall health experience (Belknap et al., 2016). These dimensions highlight the significance of addressing pediatric growth in an integrated manner, since they are important in revealing clinical practices and guiding policies that promote resilience and long-term well-being in children. It is essential to understand these for gaining beneficial developmental pathways throughout childhood and into adolescence (Figure 2.2).

## Overview of Developmental Milestones

Children grow through a sequence of developmental milestones that outline fundamental cognitive, physical, and emotional skills. These milestones serve as essential benchmarks, enabling healthcare professionals and caregivers to assess whether a child is growing normally. For instance, infants begin demonstrating feeding skills, which can be particularly challenging for children with neurodevelopmental disabilities. A study conducted on infants with Down syndrome highlights that over half of the participants under investigation had significant feeding and swallowing disorders, which needed to be assessed and managed (Bull et al., 2019). Physical development is not the only aspect included in milestones; there is also social and psychological development, as witnessed in the emotional responses parents have towards conditions such as hearing loss. It has been established that parents with hearing-impaired children have varied quality of life experiences, further emphasizing the need for personalized assistance in managing such challenges (Grima et al., 2015). Ultimately, achieving such milestones is of core significance in supporting healthy child growth and addressing potential issues at an early stage.

## Factors Influencing Growth and Development

In comprehending drivers of growth and development in children, it is essential to ensure optimal health outcomes. An interdisciplinary examination reveals that biological as well as environmental considerations play significant roles in shaping paths of development. For instance, socio- demographic influences such as socioeconomic status can have a profound impact on cognitive and physical development, as evidenced by a study following patterns of development across various groups. Through this research, low birth weight and preterm children grew catch-up but were still impacted in terms of cognitive function, with males consistently scoring lower than females. Moreover, the interactional complexity between brain maturation and the environment highlights the significance of critical periods of intervention, particularly during infancy and early childhood. Through identifying these influential factors, for instance, adverse birth outcomes, pediatric health workers can use certain mechanisms to support good growth and development, optimizing children's long-term results (Aguate et al., 2023; Alex et al., 2024).

## Significance of Early Intervention

The value of early intervention in childhood development and growth is better appreciated as a means to correct many of the health problems that arise in adolescence. Early intervention has the potential to significantly lower the risk for chronic conditions later on, such as obesity and its accompanying metabolic dysfunction, which have profound long-term health consequences. For instance, children who engage in binge eating exhibit high levels of metabolic syndrome, and this warrants interventions that ought to be started early enough to reverse adverse lifestyle choices (Miller, 2012). In addition, knowledge concerning respiratory function during infancy is important; failure here could result in a lifetime of respiratory problems because of damage that is done early in life (Stocks, 2004). These results underscore the need for universal screening and prevention interventions, which can maximize physical and psychological well-being in children. Ultimately, investment in early intervention not only enhances health outcomes now but also lays the foundation for healthier populations as adults (Figure 2.3).

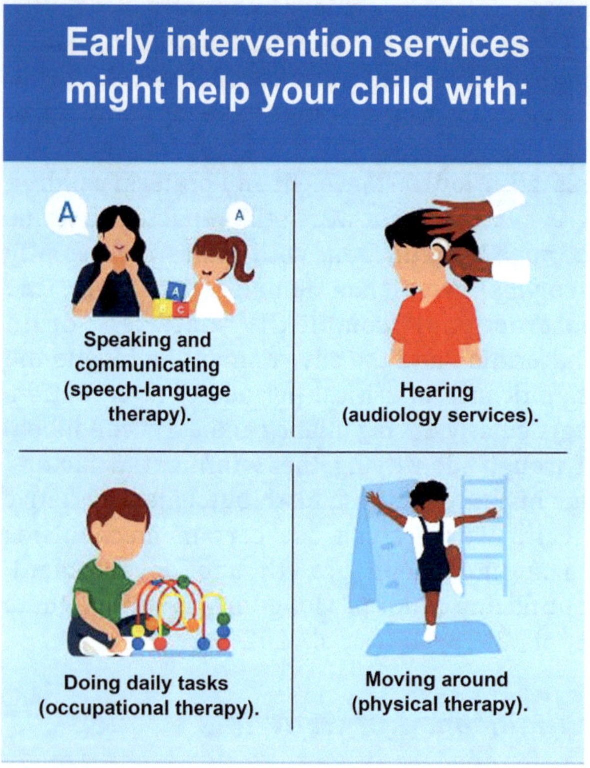


**Figure 2.3.** The significance of early intervention in pediatric growth and development.

*Source:* https://my.clevelandclinic.org/-/scassets/images/org/health/articles/early-intervention?io=transform:fit,width:780.

## Role of Healthcare Professionals

In pediatric development and growth, healthcare professionals play a replaceable role, and this cannot be offered by others. They collaborate with families, schools, and community agencies to ensure a comprehensive strategy in children's health. Coordination among the stakeholders, such as healthcare professionals, educators, and support systems, is needed to facilitate maximum development. As has been discussed in the literature, a top-down model of pediatric care coordination consolidates these elements, deeply enhancing the support offered for children and families (Jeanne et al., 2009). Moreover, the childhood obesity programs emphasize the contributions of these professionals to resolving complex health issues, taking steps to guarantee policies that encompass not just clinical care but also community participation and education (Cooper et al., 2008). In the end, the active involvement of healthcare workers is essential for unraveling the intricacies of child development and ensuring children achieve their highest potential.

## Societal Implications of Pediatric Growth

Understanding the social effects of child development is crucial when creating comprehensive child development models. The growth of children influences not only a person's health status but also overall society dynamics, like schooling performance and national income productivity. Lower growth due to malnutrition or persistent disease can lead to increased healthcare costs and reduced workforce efficiency, jeopardizing national economic stability. Studies indicate that prolonged breastfeeding, as desirable for infant development, can also be associated with the development of early childhood caries (ECC) when it exceeds 12 months, and emphasis is given to education on balanced nutrition (Dean et al., 2018). Furthermore, creating early childhood policy on the basis of strengthening relationships, safe settings, and healthy eating is key to developing lifetime health and protecting against sickness (Cooper et al., 2008). Thus, the mutual interdependence of child development and societal development highlights the imperative for targeted interventions and aggressive public health interventions.

# 2.1. Physical Growth in Children

**Learning Outcome**

1. Stages of physical growth;
2. Growth patterns in infancy;
3. Growth spurts during childhood;
4. Role of nutrition in physical growth;
5. Impact of genetics on growth;
6. Measurement of growth (height, weight, BMI);
7. Common growth disorders;
8. Importance of regular health check-ups;
9. Growth charts and their interpretation.

The development of the body in children is a complex process influenced by a variety of factors like genes, diet, and the environment. Children develop and grow at very high rates during their initial years of life, establishing the foundation for their overall health and well-being. The need to intervene early in life when dealing with growth issues is emphasized by the way in which the development of the body in children has an impact on their psychological and emotional well-being.

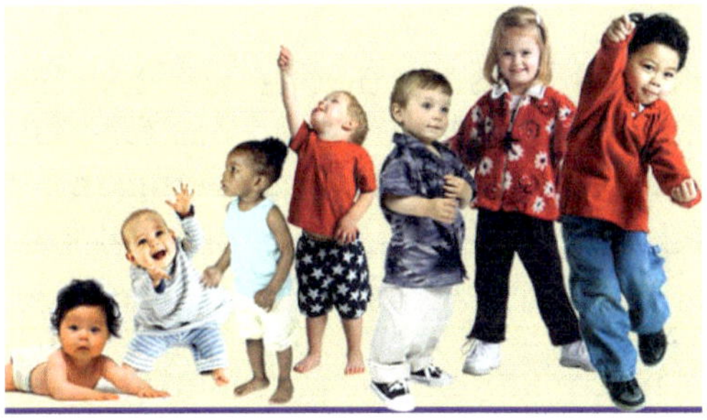

**Figure 2.4.** Physical growth in children.

*Source:* https://external-content.duckduckgo.com/iu/?u=https%3A%2F%2Fpppfchildren.files.wordpress.com%2F2011%2F06%2Finteractive2.jpg&f=1&nofb=1&ipt=b044dd862465b1e7d5c8d2a53854b81dd5202230fc42c9eb99867702e7067347&ipo=images.

For instance, alopecia can happen at this crucial phase, affecting the self-esteem and social interactions of children, which can affect normal mental and physical growth (Al-Refu et al., 2017). Conversely, some complications like pediatric multiple sclerosis may raise specific issues that affect growth, not only physically but also mentally, leading to learning and daily functioning problems (Tarantino et al., 2024). Thus, an understanding of the physical growth process as a complex phenomenon is essential for healthy child development promotion (Figure 2.4).

## 2.1.1. Stages of Physical Growth

Understanding the physical growth phases is important to the overall evaluation of pediatric health and development. Every stage, beginning at infancy and progressing to adolescence, is characterized by particular physical, emotional, and intellectual changes required for achieving overall wellness.

For instance, in early childhood, growth is fast-paced and needs adequate nutrition to support bone building; research has shown a direct correlation between egg consumption and the strength of cortical bone in children, pinpointing the nutritional needs at this stage of early development (Coheley et al., 2018). In adolescence, children experience hormonal balance changes that cause growth spurts, which can even be influenced by factors in the environment. The interaction between school, family, and community environments significantly determines a child's physical development trajectory as suggested by studies linking playing in schools to symptoms of ADHD, hence placing emphasis on the complex ecological determinants of development (Nguyen et al., 2018). Thus, identification of these diverse phases serves to create improved developmental outcomes.

### 2.1.2. Growth Patterns in Infancy

A clear understanding of infant growth patterns is central to promoting optimal pediatric health. Infants experience rapid growth during the first year of life, with nutrition playing a crucial role in shaping these patterns. Variability in weight-for-length growth curves across this period provides important insights into infant development. For example, a study identified three distinct growth trajectories—low and stable, rapid, and moderate—while noting that maternal and feeding behaviors did not differ significantly among them (Lopez-Cepero et al., 2017). The nutritional foundation established during infancy not only influences immediate well-being but also affects long-term risks of obesity and chronic disease. Meeting nutritional requirements is therefore critical, not only in terms of energy but also micronutrients such as iron and vitamin D, which are particularly vulnerable to deficiency during infancy (Binns et al., 2017). Recognizing these growth patterns is essential to designing interventions that support healthy developmental trajectories (Figure 2.5)..

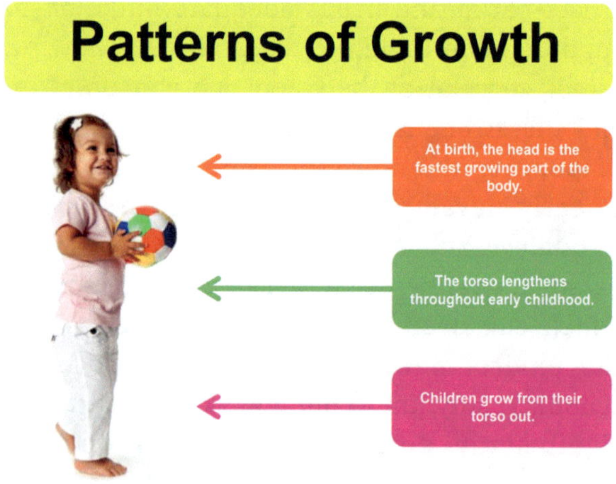


**Figure 2.5.** The growth patterns in infancy.

*Source:* https://activeearlyhealthybites.wordpress.com/wp-content/uploads/2014/01/slide8.png.

### 2.1.3. Growth Spurts During Childhood

Growth spurts are sensitive phases in the growth of children, reflecting the passage through the various phases of childhood to adolescence. Spurts are characterized by an abrupt increase in body height and weight, typically occurring during infancy, early childhood, and adolescence. Studies point out that the severity and duration of such spurts can differ immensely based on various factors, including health condition and background diet. For example, perinatally acquired HIV adolescents who began antiretroviral therapy (ART) at older ages or with prior stunting had more delayed and attenuated growth spurts than their healthier peers (Aké-Assi et al., 2023). In addition, studies have confirmed that children beginning ART with lower height-for-age z-scores experience later and less prominent growth spurts (Abou-Rayyah et al., 2019). These results highlight the intricate interaction between health states and growth trajectories, and the requirement for intervention that is aimed at optimal growth during important developmental windows.

### 2.1.4. Role of Nutrition in Physical Growth

Nutritional consumption is key to physical development in children and has far-reaching implications for overall development. It is during early childhood that growth patterns are established, and these can have long-term health implications later on in life. Proper nutrition, with a macronutrient and micronutrient balance, is associated with optimal growth patterns, but improper nutrition leads to stunted growth and developmental lags. Studies have established that diets consisting of critical vitamins and minerals, particularly during periods of increasing growth, are essential in preventing conditions such as precocious puberty, a condition linked to nutritional status (Calcaterra et al., 2021). Further, the shielding effects were emphasized for breastfeeding in preventing early onset puberty, as well as preventing childhood obesity (Negeri et al., 2024). Hence, promoting healthy eating among children is imperative to ensure assured growth and development during the developing years (Figure 2.6).

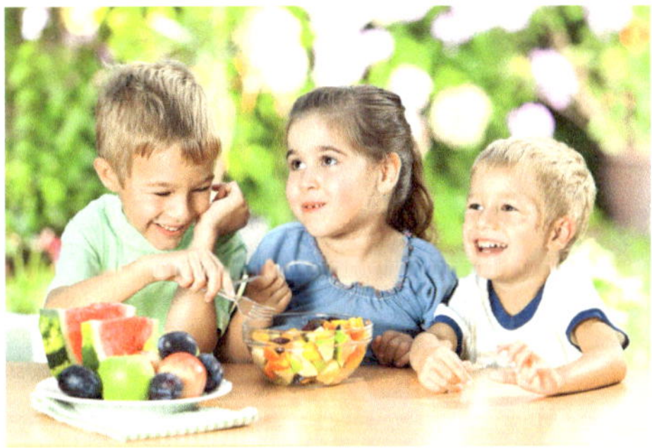

**Figure 2.6.** Children enjoy a variety of fresh fruits, promoting healthy eating habits and balanced nutrition in early childhood.

*Source:* http://www.childteaching.com/wp-content/uploads/2015/09/child-nutrition2.jpg.

### 2.1.5. Impact of Genetics on Growth

In children's development and growth, genetics plays a significant role in determining a person's growth pattern, height, and overall physical development. Research has revealed that genetics accounts for a great percentage of the variance in children's growth rate and influences not just their height but also the timing of the onset of developmental milestones. For instance, there are some gene variations that have been linked with height, weight, and body composition, highlighting the necessity of family histories in assessing children's growth patterns. In addition, the interaction between genetics and the environment, such as nutrition and exercise, further complicates this connection. A longitudinal study of genetic factors reveals that the clinical trajectory of growth-related disorders can be substantially different in children with genetic predispositions (Gupta et al., 2018). Thus, the detection of such genetic factors allows health professionals to tailor interventions to suit individual children, maximizing growth as per the child's specific genetic makeup (Kinney et al., 2007).

### 2.1.6. Measurement of Growth (Height, Weight, BMI)

The measurement of growth indicators such as height, weight, and body mass index (BMI) is critical in identifying pediatric development and screening for linked health issues at an early age. The anthropometric findings provide an indication of a child's nutritional status and overall health trend. For instance, a study of pediatric Crohn's disease found significant differences in z-scores in anthropometrics, with medicines having profound impacts on growth patterns, particularly in weight and BMI (Gupta et al., 2018). Second, the frequency with which children have high blood pressure lends credence to the inclusion of growth measures in predicting long-term health outcomes, such as the development of hypertension later on (Falkner et al., 2018). By monitoring regularly, the alterations in such indicators, healthcare workers are able to implement timely interventions such that the children achieve maximum growth and development while addressing any underlying medical complications they develop during these initial years.

### 2.1.7. Common Growth Disorders

Pediatric growth disorders are a significant issue in the area of pediatric growth and development. Growth disorders may lead to short stature, obesity, or delay in puberty and are caused by a multifactorial interplay of environmental, hormonal, and genetic factors. A classic illustration of such a multisystem condition is resistance to thyroid hormone, an infrequent disorder due to mutations in the thyroid hormone receptor. One of the cases involving a boy who was two years old revealed elevated thyroid hormone levels but regular growth patterns, and therefore, the significance of extensive assessment in atypical presentations (Rawan et al., 2024). Additionally, professionals most often face challenges when applying evidence-based interventions when working with children with autism spectrum disorder, thus making growth assessment and intervention challenging (Bryden et al., 2018). As early detection and control are crucial, it is essential to know these common growth disorders to encourage healthy growth among children (Figure 2.7).

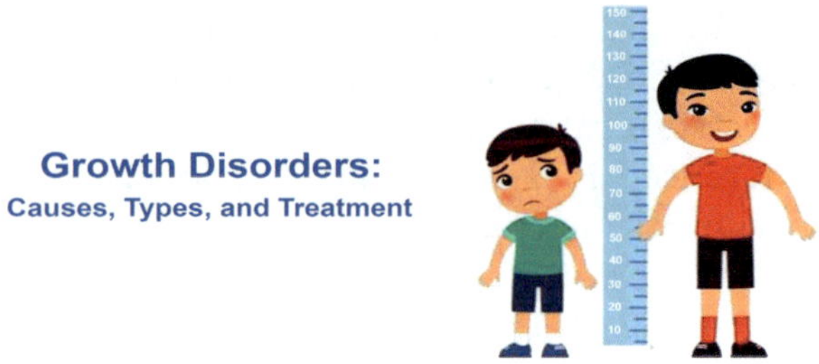


**Figure 2.7.** Common growth disorders.

*Source:* https://www.sprintdiagnostics.in/blog/images/growth-disorder-causes-types-treatment.webp.

## 2.1.8. Importance of Regular Health Check-Ups

Regular check-ups are imperative in the area of pediatric growth and development because they enable the discovery at an early stage of any expected health issues and monitoring of development milestones. Through regular screenings, medical professionals can measure a child's physical, emotional, as well as intellectual development to ensure abnormalities are screened on time. This proactive step not only encourages a healthy path of development but also lays the foundation for sustained practice of health. Interventions that integrate early learning, healthcare, and family support have documented positive outcomes, as per research which emphasizes the interlinkage between child health and school readiness (Bruner et al., 2007). Moreover, regular health check-ups can promote closer contact between healthcare workers and families, enhancing prevention as well as healthy living habits. Basically, routine check-ups are a critical component of a comprehensive strategy to optimize pediatric well-being and ensure healthy development of children in early phases.

## 2.1.9. Growth Charts and Their Interpretation

Growth charts are much valuable monitoring instrument for tracking the physical development of children in order to ascertain whether a child's development pattern agrees with pre-established norms. Charts are utilized to assess parameters like height, weight, and body mass index (BMI), hence providing a graphical representation of a child's development compared to other children. These graphs need to be read in terms of a nuanced understanding of a number of factors, such as age, sex, and family history, since any deviation from the norm would signify potential illness. For example, an extreme deviation would warrant inspection or intervention, consistent with broader pediatric health assessment evident in the Human Phenotype Ontology and standardization across medical specialties (Sebastian et al., 2020). Furthermore, new diagnostic approaches like those utilized in neurological infection cases underscore the significance of accurate growth tracking for complete-scale pediatric practice (Miller et al., 2019).

### Test Your Knowledge

1. At what age does the most rapid growth occur in children, and when are typical growth spurts observed?
2. Which parameters are commonly used to assess physical growth in children, and how is BMI calculated?

## 2.2. Cognitive Development

**Learning Outcome**

1. Overview of cognitive development theories;
2. Piaget's stages of cognitive development;
3. Role of play in cognitive growth;
4. Language acquisition milestones;
5. Impact of environment on cognitive skills;
6. Assessment of cognitive development;
7. Common cognitive developmental delays;
8. Importance of early childhood education;
9. Technology's influence on cognitive development.

Cognitive development in children is an important domain of total development that affects school achievement and life quality. Cognitive development may be affected by numerous diseases, such as congenital heart disease (CHD) and multiple sclerosis (MS), which surprisingly affect neuropsychological development in children.

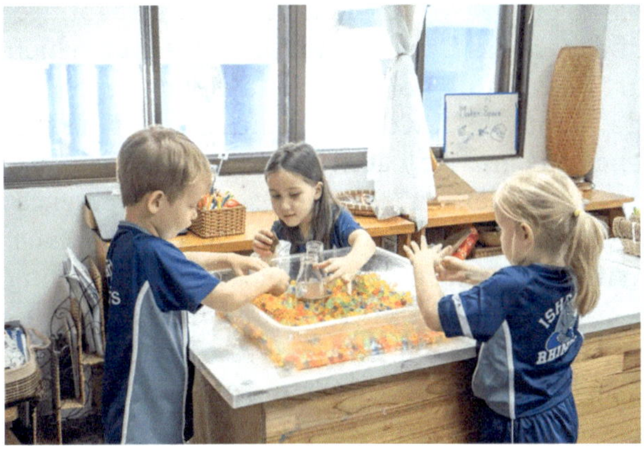

**Figure 2.8.** Young children engage in a hands-on sensory activity involving colorful beads, fostering cognitive development and collaborative learning in a classroom maker space.

*Source:* https://www.ishcmc.com/wp-content/uploads/sites/20/2024/09/cognitive-development-in-early-childhood-ishcmc-1.png.

For instance, observations have been made that kids with MS, although exhibiting fewer motor impairments, exhibit cognitive impairments that do not manifest until late stages of disease progression, affecting attention and memory functions (Tarantino et al., 2024). Similarly, kids with cyanotic CHD also exhibit profound impairments in cognitive function as evidenced by lower scores in tests of early learning compared to their acyanotic counterparts (Gunawijaya et al., 2020). These findings underscore the importance of early intervention and continued support in order to facilitate cognitive development of children with developmental challenges, thereby enhancing their school life as well as overall well-being throughout life (Figure 2.8).

### 2.2.1. Overview of Cognitive Development Theories

Understanding cognitive development theories is at the core of pediatric growth and development because cognitive development theories provide insight into how children learn, develop problem-solving abilities, and process emotions. Among the most well-known theories is Piaget's theory of cognitive development, which defines distinct stages that children pass through so that researchers and practitioners can craft education experiences. Similarly, Vygotsky's sociocultural theory is concerned with social interactions and cultural context in the manner cognitive abilities are acquired, pointing out that learning is extremely social and collective. Both theorists emphasize the importance of developmentally appropriate practices in the school context. In addition, recent evidence emphasizes neuropsychological testing for identifying cognitive challenges among children since, in research examining such tools in Southeast Asia, namely Vietnam (Ashley et al., 2024), the matter is addressed. In addition, information on the influence of disorders like adenotonsillar hypertrophy on children's cognitive abilities also justifies comprehensive approaches to children's health (Zagury-Orly et al., 2024).

## 2.2.2. Piaget's Stages of Cognitive Development

It is important to understand Piaget's stages of cognitive development in order to understand how children learn and adjust to their environment during the years of peak pediatric development. Piaget established four stages: the sensorimotor, preoperational, concrete operational, and formal operational stages, each with unique cognitive abilities that evolve according to age. Throughout the sensorimotor stage, infants acquire information regarding the world by means of sensory experiences and motor behaviors, which lay down the foundation for more complex thinking. When they move into the preoperational stage, children start using symbols and words, but their thinking remains egocentric.

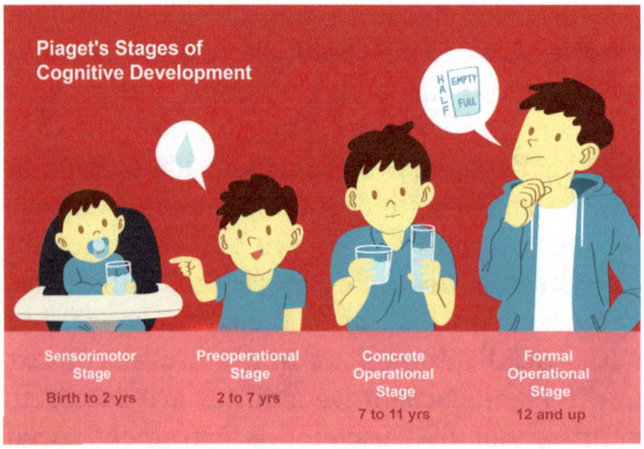


**Figure 2.9.** Piaget's stages of cognitive development.

*Source:* https://i.pinimg.com/originals/c4/fb/10/c4fb102ddb54b1d706cfef0205f88d0d.png.

Subsequent processing stages promote additional rational thought processes and the ability to understand abstract concepts, which play a critical role in practical uses. Laying out these stages illuminates how pedagogical practice, such as play learning referred to by Heidecker et al. (2021), can enhance early cognitive capacities of childhood, specifically in environments that support learning diversities, such as for students with traumatic experiences as discussed by Minuci et al. (2019) (Figure 2.9).

## 2.2.3. Role of Play in Cognitive Growth

Play is essentially necessary for the growth of the mind during childhood because it offers opportunities for children to try out, investigate, and make sense of the world. Through various forms of play, including pretend play, building play, and role-play, children learn to develop critical thinking and problem-solving abilities. For instance, imaginative play results in children fantasizing, which enhances creativity and expands their ability to look at things from others' perspectives. In addition, social play provides necessary interaction through which children learn to communicate, negotiate, and cooperate with each other, all of which are essential to emotional and cognitive development. Evidence indicates that formal and informal play activities result in enhanced academic performance and social competence, ultimately developing well-rounded individuals. With pediatricians and educators recognizing the significant contribution play makes in children's development, their recommendation is usually in favor of integrating play into learning environments as a means of promoting holistic development (Peacock et al., 2017; Jennifer et al., 2021).

## 2.2.4. Language Acquisition Milestones

Language acquisition milestones are key indicators of a child's intellectual and social development during the initial years of life. Children typically progress through several stages, beginning with six-month-old cooing, followed by eight-month-old babbling, and eventually speaking their first words at about one year of age. These milestones are not only significant in the measurement of linguistic abilities but also in understanding broader issues of development, specifically in deafness. The intersection of language development and deafness is significant; research indicates that bilingualism, as in sign language usage, can positively affect oral language in children with deafness or hearing loss, suggesting a more integrated approach to language acquisition (Farber et al., 2016). In addition, awareness of the emotional impact of a child's hearing loss on parents can also inform interventions, leading to improved educational and support approaches for parents (Grima et al., 2015).

### 2.2.5. Impact of Environment on Cognitive Skills

Environmental factors powerfully affect intellectual capabilities in childhood development and growth. Young exposure to enriched environments, variable experiences, stimulating interactions, and nutritious foods, powerfully shapes children's intellectual capabilities.

Conversely, poor environments, characterized by limited social interactions and a lack of stimulation, can disrupt intellectual development to cause long-term disability. Research points to the profound function of socio-economic status, where children who grow up in wealthier backgrounds get better educational facilities and care, eventually aiding their cognitive development in a positive manner. Further, stressors in the environment, such as family instability or socio-economic disadvantage, may lead to increased anxiety and reduced attention related abilities among children and reduce their cognitive potential. It is paramount that the caregivers and instructors give supportive learning settings founded on accessibility and creativity to actually bring about cognitive capabilities at such formative periods (Jennifer et al., 2021; Peter & Wittenberg, 2021) (Figure 2.10).

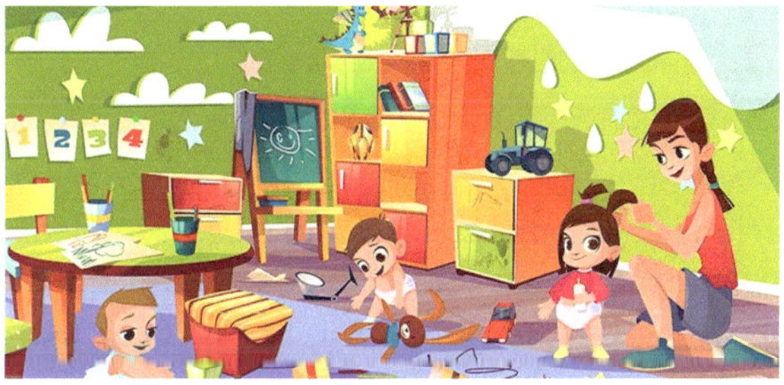

**Figure 2.10.** Impact of environment on cognitive skills.

*Source:* https://lead-academy.org/blog/wp-content/uploads/2023/01/Important-Environmental-Factors-That-Affect-Child-Development-5-1.webp.

### 2.2.6. Assessment of Cognitive Development

Assessment of early childhood cognitive development is crucial as it has long-term implications for educational and social success. Various studies indicate that growth indicators, such as weight-for-age z-scores and maternal education, correlate with subsequent measurement of cognitive functions.

For instance, children who demonstrated enhanced measures of growth and whose mothers had higher levels of education were more likely to test higher than average on standardized cognitive tests at age eight, showing how early life affects cognitive development (Kakwangire et al., 2024). Moreover, ergonomic and musculoskeletal health know-how helps contribute to cognitive ability since such training for parents translates into improved practices and increased knowledge, ensuring safe physical environments among children, hence helping their physical and cognitive development

(Hegazy et al., 2024). Such implications are important in highlighting integrative means in defining and enhancing cognitive capacity during critical stages of growth.

### 2.2.7. Common Cognitive Developmental Delays

Developmental cognitive delays manifest in various impairments in a child's ability to learn or process, which can have a profound impact on their overall direction of development. These include conditions like autism spectrum disorder and intellectual disabilities, which both impair a child's learning and social interaction abilities. Evidence argues that conditions such as premature birth are well-documented to raise the risk for intellectual delays, and it is therefore crucial to have close monitoring and intervention strategies to improve intellectual capacities. For instance, Masita et al. (2024) demonstrate that children who are born prematurely are susceptible to medical conditions that may result in intellectual delays and the need for early medical and developmental intervention. Also, the inadequacies in such critical nutrients as Vitamin B12 have been identified as reversible determinants that exacerbate cognitive impairments. These are corrected through precise early intervention for maximum cognitive benefit and enhancing pediatric growth and development more broadly, as documented by Pratiksha et al. (2024).

### 2.2.8. Importance of Early Childhood Education

The significance of early education in children's pediatric growth and development cannot be overemphasized since it forms the foundation for a lifetime of education and health. It is in early life that children experience rapid cognitive, emotional, and social development, and learning contexts must thus ensure secure and responsive relationships. As indicated by N/A (2010), the establishment of early childhood policies that ensure safe and supportive physical environments and healthy nutrition can promote lifelong health and the prevention of diseases. Moreover, the application of community-based strategies to build early learning systems in poor neighborhoods can significantly contribute to the development of children. The data provided by Bruner et al. (2007) reflect the necessity to integrate services with activities in a neighborhood and to build a diverse early education workforce. Both these factors emphasize the need for early childhood education to build the whole child and to give all children an equal opportunity (Figure 2.11).

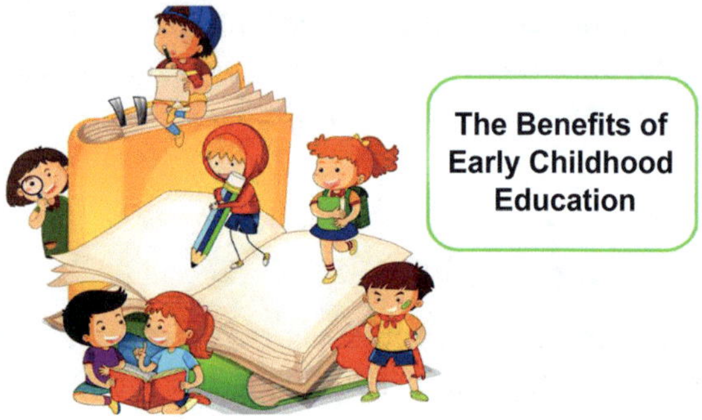


**Figure 2.11.** Importance of early childhood education.

*Source:* The significance of early childhood education in pediatric growth.

### 2.2.9. Technology's Influence on Cognitive Development

Technology plays a pivotal role in shaping cognitive development among children and youth in the current society. With an increasing number of digital devices, children and youth are exposed to an assortment of learning devices and settings that develop problem-solving skills and critical thinking. Nevertheless, the effect of this technology is two-pronged; while digital platforms can enable learning growth, over-reliance on virtual interaction can drain out face-to-face interaction abilities, thereby potentially hindering social growth. Furthermore, participation in structured activities, e.g., youth sport, accentuates the balance of technology use and physical activity. Statistics indicate that there are approximately 47 million youth who participate in sporting programs, which not only contribute to physical health but also team spirit and discipline (Duda et al., 2005). Technological advancements have even accelerated the dissemination of learning programs so that they are accessible and participation, as seen in disseminating new paradigms in health care (Bradley et al., 2004). Hence, identification of this two-way influence is crucial to good pediatric development and growth.

## Test Your Knowledge

1. Name any two stages of Piaget's cognitive development theory and mention one key feature of each.
2. What are two common signs of cognitive developmental delay in toddlers?

## 2.3. Social and Emotional Development

**Learning Outcome**

1. Definition of social and emotional development;
2. Attachment theory and its significance;
3. Development of self-regulation skills;
4. Role of family in social development;
5. Peer relationships and their impact;
6. Emotional milestones in early childhood;
7. Effects of trauma on emotional development;
8. Importance of social skills training;
9. Cultural influences on social development.

The social and emotional growth of a child plays an important part in shaping their future interactions, self-concept, and overall mental health. Important milestones typically encompass the acquisition of self-regulatory abilities, emotional expression, and social interaction, which can be assessed through developmental scales. These scales assess behaviors such as curiosity, sensory reactivity, and language development, all of which indicate the integration of cognitive and emotional development (Handargule et al., 2024). Moreover, the impact of chronic diseases, for example, inflammatory bowel disease (IBD), can exacerbate struggles in social and emotional realms, thus reinforcing negative body image and incompetent sentiments in involved children (Andreea et al., 2023). As children move through developmental stages, early identification and supportive treatments for social and emotional needs may enhance resilience and lead to better psychosocial outcomes, leading to their overall pediatric growth and development (Figure 2.12).

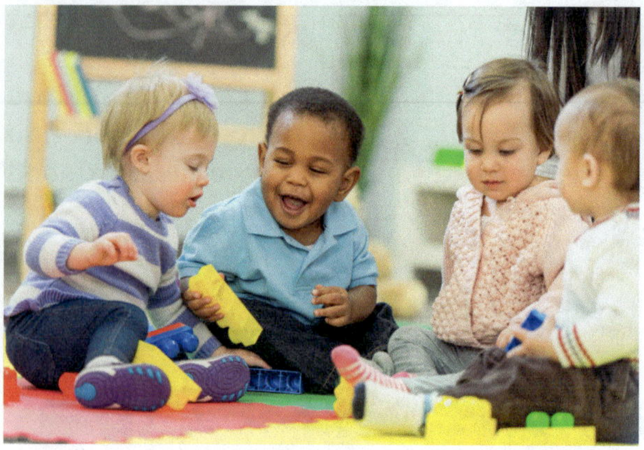

**Figure 2.12.** Toddlers play collaboratively with building blocks in an early childhood setting, supporting social interaction and fine motor development.

*Source:* https://childhoodconnections.ca/wp-content/uploads/2020/12/141016-editorial.jpg.

### 2.3.1. Definition of Social and Emotional Development

Social and emotional development is the most critical in pediatric development, reflecting how children manage and regulate their feelings, create relationships, and comprehend the social world. The multi-dimensional process involves the ability to create attachments, express emotions, and comprehend empathy, all of which are required for building resiliency and adaptive social skills.

Interestingly, early investment in supportive settings has been shown to have long-term payoffs far into the future; e.g., Campbell et al. indicate that wide-reaching interventions early in life can enhance adult socio-economic functioning and health (Frances et al., 2014). Furthermore, conclusions drawn from randomized controlled trials cite established emotional learning frameworks as having a positive influence on children's social relationships and educational outcomes (Bradley et al., 2004). Thus, social and emotional development is not only an extra aspect of child development but is also an integral part of it that has ramifications in many facets of a child's life and future.

### 2.3.2. Attachment Theory and Its Significance

The importance of attachment theory to the development and growth of children lies in its profoundly meaningful implications for social and emotional well-being. According to the theory, early infant-caregiver interactions form the foundation for subsequent relationship quality and psychological adjustment overall. Securely attached children are linked to resilience that allows them to cope with adversity more successfully, while insecurely attached children are at risk for anxiety and conduct problems. Research indicates that maternal health behaviors like prenatal care use are important in the establishment of these attachments. Specifically, Allen et al. (2005) suggest that prenatal care-influenced maternal-infant interaction is a determining factor in developmental outcomes, such as risk of failure to thrive. Additionally, Templeton et al. (2013) emphasizes adaptive plasticity in the development of adolescents exposed to family stress, since it demonstrates attachment influences are time-varying and carry over to subsequent life stages. Hence, learning about attachment theory becomes imperative for the purpose of fostering healthy child growth trajectories.

### 2.3.3. Development of Self-Regulation Skills

The acquisition of self-regulation skills is a critical part of child growth and development that affects children's effective management of emotions, behavior, and social relations. Experiences during early childhood greatly influence self-regulation because children acquire skills to deal with their surroundings and react to diverse stimuli. A good and nurturing environment supports the growth of such skills, so that children can learn to control impulses and emotions, very important for their academic as well as social success. It is seen through research that such children with good self-regulation have better cognitive abilities as well as better peer relationships, both of which are very crucial aspects of their overall development. Behavioral strategy and parent-child interaction-based interventions can also enhance self-regulation skills further, fostering resilience against adversity in later stages of life (Dennis et al., 2017; Jennifer et al., 2021). Therefore, emphasizing the acquisition of self-regulation skills in early childhood can have long-term benefits throughout a child's lifespan trajectory (Figure 2.13).

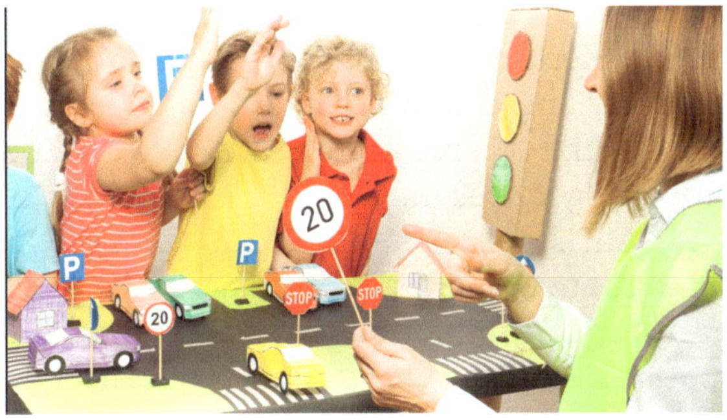


**Figure 2.13.** Development of self-regulation skills.

*Source:* https://www.whizkidz.com.au/wp-content/uploads/2024/02/Whiz-Kidz-Self-Regulation-scaled.jpg.

## 2.3.4. Role of Family in Social Development

The role of the family in socialization is undoubtedly central, as it involves the principal context through which children learn and develop social norms. Kids learn behavior and morals from their first interactions with caregivers, which mold their identities and social relationships. According to Meng (2024), family education basically establishes the character traits children develop before they enter wider social environments. Secondly, parents are very much involved in the modeling of relationship patterns and communication, which may be imitated by children. As they move through complex social situations, the first lessons learned in the home environment significantly shape their ability to form relationships outside the home. Besides, effective family planning, as by Juliannisa et al. (2023) underscores the necessity of purposeful support in education and finances to empower the family to establish conducive development and growth environments. Consequently, a well-adjusted family arrangement not only enables personal development but also improves an adjusted society.

## 2.3.5. Peer Relationships and Their Impact

The dynamic nature of early childhood peer relationships is one prominent factor that affects a lot of aspects of child development and growth. Through peer interactions, children not only learn social skills but also get exposed to various perspectives, which can affect their emotional and cognitive development. Through peers, children gain insight into complicated social situations, encouraging resilience and adaptability. Furthermore, positive relationships with peers can facilitate lower levels of stress and improved emotional well-being, while negative ones can contribute to increased anxiety as well as loneliness. This is particularly important in children who have a specific medical condition, such as Chiari malformation, whereby positive peer support might minimize some of the emotional impacts associated with their diagnosis (Matthew et al., 2024). In addition, economic stability and resource access can support children in developing and sustaining healthy peer relationships, supporting the interlinkage among social and economic determinants of pediatric development (Okeowo et al., 2024).

### 2.3.6. Emotional Milestones in Early Childhood

Emotional milestones in early childhood are most vital to children's overall development, dictating the potential for emotional coping with social relationships and forming healthy relationships. This is the time when more complex emotions such as empathy, guilt, and pride are formed, a child's awareness of his or her own and others' emotions. Research illustrates that children begin to recognize and respond to caregivers' and others' affective signals, laying the groundwork for social competence and emotion regulation (Grima et al., 2015). Moreover, intervention and programming aimed at augmenting emotional abilities can effectively enhance school readiness, especially in those in home-based daycare settings, who can have unique challenges compared to classmates in formal schooling environments (Peters & Wittenberg, 2021). Thus, creating emotional development in the early years is paramount to setting children up for success both academically and personally (Figure 2.14).

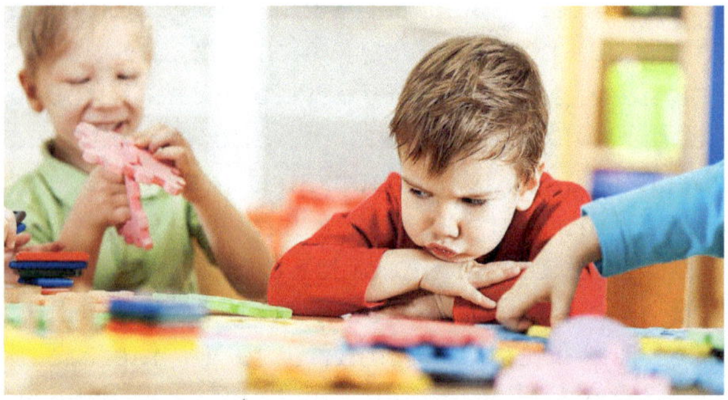

**Figure 2.14.** A young child appears frustrated during playtime, highlighting the importance of supporting social-emotional wellness and self-regulation in early childhood settings.

*Source:* https://blog.schoolspecialty.com/wp-content/uploads/2023/02/social-emotional-wellness-GettyImages-185096653-1200x624.jpg.

### 2.3.7. Effects of Trauma on Emotional Development

The literature on trauma and its impact on emotional development in children is vast and wide-ranging, affecting not only the immediate response, but also long-term mental well-being. Trauma, such as domestic violence or family conflict, can lead to heightened stress, depression, and behavior difficulties in children, altering their ability to form secure attachment and manage emotions. As they struggle with issues of trauma, children will likely develop maladaptive coping strategies and become increasingly susceptible to future mental health problems. Importantly, trauma can hinder a child's capacity to empathize and engage with others, diminishing emotional intelligence. Research highlights the fact that exposure to violence in direct or indirect terms can increase adverse effects on emotional development, which are experienced more strongly in vulnerable groups, and thereby generate dysfunction-reinforcing cycles in families (Ferrara et al., 2021; Christopher et al., 2022). Recognition and treatment of these traumas at an early age are equally important in ensuring healthier emotional and developmental trajectories for the impacted children.

### 2.3.8. Importance of Social Skills Training

Among child growth and development, acquiring social skills is among the most imperative components influencing a child's health and school performance. Social skills training equips children with the critical skills to communicate effectively, resolve conflicts, and empathize, enabling them to navigate complex social settings. As highlighted in recent discussions of psychosocial skills, these variables are fundamental in shaping the interactions and learning experiences of a child, particularly during those initial years of goal orientation and attitude development (Voitova et al., 2025).

Further, evidence highlights the potential of emotional intelligence in framing an improved learning experience, suggesting that the development of interpersonal competencies can yield strong, responsive learners (Banga, 2024). Thus, through social skills training, investing not only creates amiable peer relationships but also forms a fundamental framework that promotes the child's all-around growth and ultimately his/her capacity to adjust in different environments (Figure 2.15).

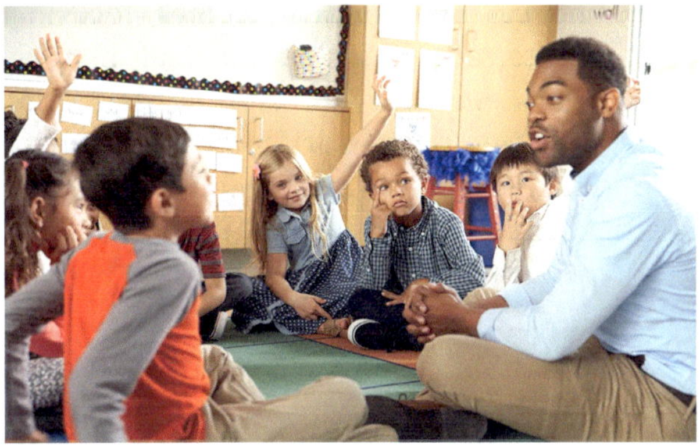

**Figure 2.15.** The acquisition of social skills stands as a critical component influencing a child's overall well-being and academic success.

*Source:* https://360behavioralhealth.com/wp-content/uploads/2018/11/skills.jpg.webp.

### 2.3.9. Cultural Influences on Social Development

Social forces have a strong impact on social development in child development, as children learn how to move around them and internalize social norms. The family is one of the socializing forces that pass culture-dependent values, thus influencing children's behavior and relationships. For instance, children in collectivistic cultures would develop strong interdependent relations, while children who are brought up in individualistic cultures would emphasize individual achievement and autonomy. Besides, variations in social inclination to diversity, particularly in gender assignments, emphasize the importance of culture in children's construction of identity and social roles. As noted in current studies, nontypical genitalia clinical presentations emphasize the importance of having a multi-disciplinary approach that is culturally responsive, hence promoting informed support from the family and individualized management plans (Ahmed et al., 2017). Additionally, the problems related to Pediatric Feeding Disorders underscore the need for cultural considerations in treatment planning to address different needs and facilitate effective interventions (Goday et al., 2019).

## Test Your Knowledge

1. What is the significance of secure attachment in early childhood, and how does it influence the development of self-regulation skills?
2. How can peer relationships support emotional development, and what is one common effect of early childhood trauma on emotional health?

## 2.4. Behavioral Development

**Learning Outcome**

1. Understanding typical behavioral patterns;
2. Role of parenting styles in behavior;
3. Common behavioral issues in children;
4. Strategies for positive behavior reinforcement;
5. Impact of screen time on behavior;
6. Behavioral assessments and interventions;
7. Importance of consistency in discipline;
8. Role of schools in behavioral development;
9. Long-term effects of childhood behavior.

Development of pediatric patients' behavior is a multifaceted process that is a product of many internal and external variables. Such development is significant insofar as it shapes a child's ability to deal with his or her surroundings, form relationships, and navigate social milieus.

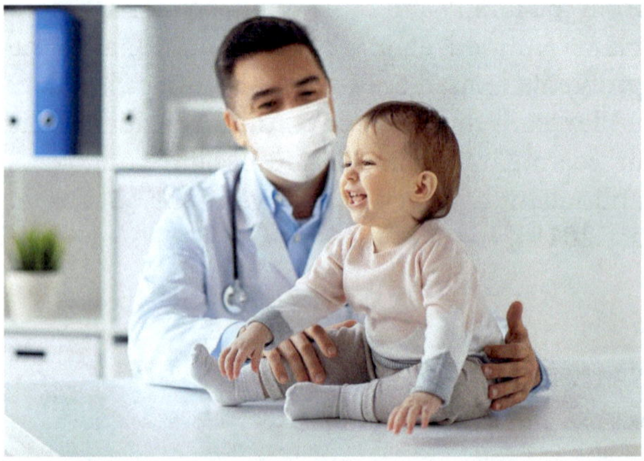

**Figure 2.16.** A pediatrician gently supports a smiling infant during a wellness check, illustrating the importance of compassionate care in early childhood health.

*Source:* https://dam.northwell.edu/m/2a9e881ac54ede9e/Drupal-web_AS_382989609.jpg.

Significant developments of behavior, such as the ability to communicate, show emotion, and play, are measures of the child's general development. Furthermore, psychosocial aspects should also be a point of concern; those who struggle with emotional regulation or social skills might need targeted interventions to help their developmental trajectory. Clinical evidence indicates that a notable percentage of cancer survivors have identifiable psychosocial needs that demand targeted attention (Kimberly et al., 2016). Such high-level care addresses not only the physiological aspect of health but also enhances behavioral outcomes, focusing on the interface between medical history and developmental development. Thus, understanding these variables is essential to optimizing pediatric care and supporting healthy behavioral development (Figure 2.16).

### 2.4.1. Understanding Typical Behavioral Patterns

A clear understanding of general behavioral trends is crucial in children's growth and development, as these trends reflect the complex interaction between maturation and external influences. Research has demonstrated that motor skill acquisition, such as stepping, exhibits remarkable plasticity in infants, with neurological development and sensory exposure shaping behavioral outcomes (Lee et al., 2015). Furthermore, interventions like animal-assisted therapy (AAT) have gained increasing attention for their ability to enhance socio-emotional well-being in children, highlighting how targeted therapeutic approaches can positively influence developmental trajectories (Verdeyen et al., 2024). By recognizing these typical behavioral functions, caregivers and healthcare professionals are better positioned to support optimal development and address challenges that may arise during critical developmental windows. Such insights encourage evidence-based interventions that foster enabling environments, ultimately promoting healthier outcomes in pediatric populations.

### 2.4.2. Role of Parenting Styles in Behavior

Parenting styles significantly contribute to the behavioral development of children, influencing their psychological adjustment and social skills. Warm and consistent parenting, as characteristic of authoritative parenting, has been associated with positive behaviors such as self-regulation and social competence that are predictive of resilience for children. Authoritarian parenting will tend to yield a more violent climate and lead to increased anxiety and potential behavioral difficulties in children. Also, the permissive style, while loving, can result in poor impulse control and issues with authority. There is indication that these parenting approaches not only impact short-term behavior repercussions, but also long-term effects on health and development, such as the prevalence of conditions such as pediatric obesity (Dennis et al., 2017). Therefore, appreciating these dynamics is central to advancing healthy child development interventions, not only to treat behavioral outcomes but to address the wide range of pediatric health management (McCrory et al., 2013).

### 2.4.3. Common Behavioral Issues in Children

Behavioral issues among children have a tendency to emerge as significant issues within the realm of pediatric growth and development. Issues can happen in a variety of forms, such as hyperactivity, worry, and issues with social interaction, which are influenced by environmental and biological processes. For instance, research indicates that children with mothers who have chronic conditions, such as chronic kidney disease, have increased possibilities of having externalizing behavioral problems, suggesting a child behavior and maternal health interaction (Banerjee et al., 2010). Similarly, studies of parenting practices indicate that mothers of children with congenital heart disease tend to exhibit higher levels of vigilance, which influences the emotional development and children's behavior (Carey et al., 2002). In light of these findings, determining the etiology of behavioral challenges can be used to inform intervention strategies. Through support of supportive environments and minimizing parental stress, healthcare professionals can help alleviate the adverse outcomes of such challenges on children's development and, in the long run, promote healthier developmental pathways (Figure 2.17).

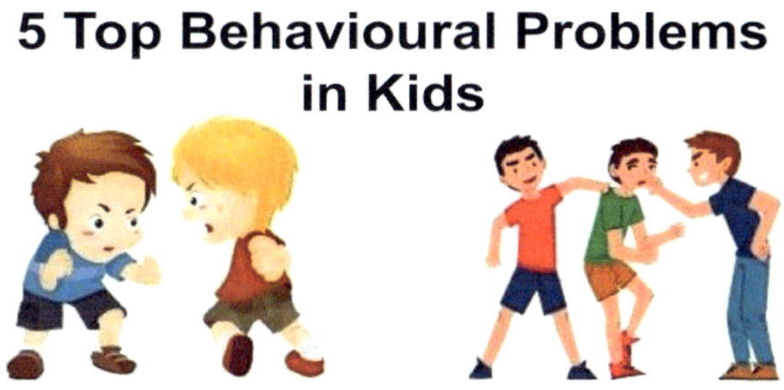


**Figure 2.17.** Common behavioral issues in children.

*Source:* https://www.theblogchatter.com/uploads/blogrolls/thumb/1617331021_behavior.jpg.

### 2.4.4. Strategies for Positive Behavior Reinforcement

In regard to pediatric growth and development, the implementation of effective positive behavior reinforcement strategies is essential in the development of healthy habits in children. A widespread successful approach involves the implementation of systematic reward systems that reinforce desired behaviors, thereby rewarding good behavior through immediate acknowledgement. For instance, theories of behavior change have indicated the importance of matched intervention that resonates with children's individual needs, as evidenced in existing literature synthesizing models of health behavior change for children and families (Sahota et al., 2010). Additionally, such programs aimed at specific groups, such as parents with children with autism spectrum disorder, prove the efficiency of parent-based interventions in the establishment of good behaviors such as increased physical activity and improved dietary habits (Boutelle et al., 2019). By integrating these measures into pediatric health care, specialists can maximize kids' activity and interest and, therefore, their general development.

### 2.4.5. Impact of Screen Time on Behavior

An increasing reliance on screens among children has raised significant questions regarding their influence on behavior as well as development overall. Research shows that excessive screen use can create adverse effects on behavior, including shorter attention span, higher aggression, and more social isolation. These impacts can disrupt significant aspects of pediatric growth, as children require physical contact and active play in order to grow healthily on an emotional and social level. Besides, an obesogenic environment with excessive screen exposure has been associated with sedentary behaviors that negatively impact physical health, like obesity, as illustrated in recent reviews (Fruh et al., 2021). Moreover, the impact of screen time on mental health is also more obvious, as found in research that indicates the symptoms of depression and anxiety are linked to high usage rates (Damsky, 2021). Therefore, other developmental activities that promote good behavioral practices among children have to be balanced with screen time.

### 2.4.6. Behavioral Assessments and Interventions

In the context of children's growth and development, behavioral assessments and interventions become crucial to the comprehension and facilitation of children's general well-being. By incorporating preventive intervention within primary care, integrated behavioral health preventive (IBH-P) interventions are able to improve parenting habits, particularly for low-income families, to provide healthy mother-infant interaction during times of susceptible development (Robert et al., 2024).

Aside from that, the employment of digital behavioral dietary interventions (DBDIs) offers new avenues for intervening upon child and adolescent dietary behavior with opportunities for driving behavioral change across technology platforms (Zoë et al., 2024). Such evaluations not only identify where interventions might be most helpful but also provide caregivers with education and skills to support better child development. Hence, IBH-P and DBDIs both emphasize the importance of theory-informed interventions, which are individually customized, ultimately contributing to improved health outcomes and developmental trajectories in children (Figure 2.18).

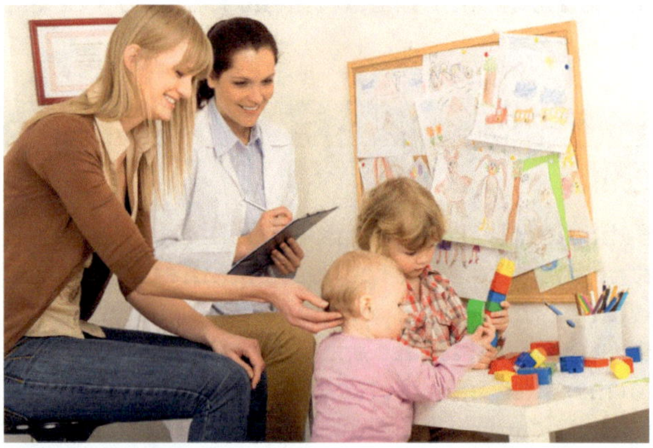

**Figure 2.18.** The behavioral assessments and interventions play a critical role in understanding and enhancing children's overall well-being.

*Source:* https://superkidsaba.com/wp-content/uploads/2020/06/ABA-Assessments-Crystal-Kids-Center-1024x682.jpg.

## 2.4.7. Importance of Consistency in Discipline

The importance of consistency in discipline cannot be overstated with reference to pediatric growth and development. A consistent pattern of disciplinary action provides children with a framework within which they are able to interpret the consequences of their actions, creating a sense of security and predictability essential for their emotional growth. Literature indicates that inconsistency in discipline has the ability to bring more stress to parents, which ultimately translates to their ability to manage children's behavior (Wang et al., 2019). Further, disciplinary variation among parents results in ambiguity in children and contributes to the escalation of behavioral issues as well as reduced self-regulation ability. Parents, particularly those with socio-demographic issues, have only added issues to deal with, which is the complexity of constant discipline. Grasping these dynamics is important, as caregivers' experiences play an important role in shaping parenting practices and, in turn, the developmental trajectory of children (Carlson et al., 2020). Thus, focusing on consistency in discipline is essential to raise healthy, well-adjusted children.

## 2.4.8. Role of Schools in Behavioral Development

Schools are instrumental in fostering the behavior of children, as places not only for academic success but also as sites for the establishment of social skills and emotional resilience. Through the provision of organized interaction time and exposure to diverse groups of peers, schools establish essential competencies such as working together, understanding others, and dealing with conflict. Emphasizing resilience and healthy development within educational frameworks is essential; radical changes within school environments can significantly enhance academic achievement as well as social accommodation for students (Nicoll et al., 2014). Schools also contribute to the general development of children by tackling issues related to health that impact their ability to learn effectively, such as dental health. Embracing educational programs that promote oral health and awareness can lead to better overall health outcomes, thereby optimizing children's participation in schools (Drengler et al., 2005). Schools thus have a determining role in shaping the developmental and behavioral trajectories of adolescents, maximizing their potential for fulfillment.

## 2.4.9. Long-Term Effects of Childhood Behavior

The long-term consequences of childhood behavior greatly influence the health and psychosocial development of individuals throughout life.

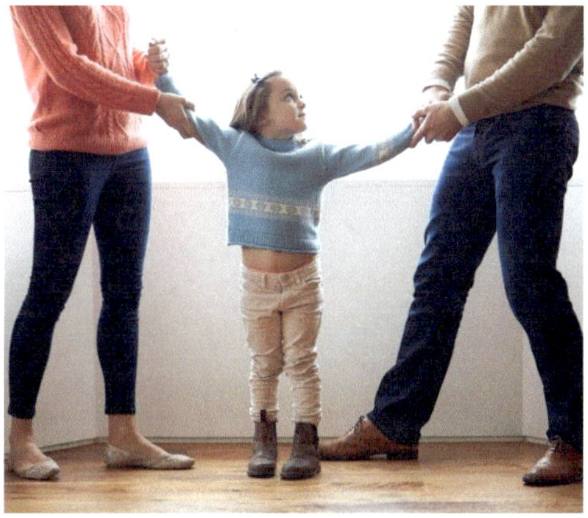

**Figure 2.19.** A young girl stands between two adults pulling her in opposite directions, symbolizing the emotional impact of parental conflict or divorce on children.

*Source:* https://integrativelifecenter.com/wp-content/uploads/2021/08/Little-girl-being-pulled-in-two-directions-by-her-parents-going-through-a-divorce.jpg.

Early experience, such as exposure to supportive settings and caring relationships, is important in establishing resilience and emotional well-being. Particularly, habits developed in childhood will go a long way to affect health-related quality of life (HRQOL) in the future, e.g., when one has survived childhood cancer, e.g., children who have retinoblastoma, where late complications can include visual impairment and psychological distress, hence affecting a diminished HRQOL compared to their counterparts (Belson et al., 2020). In this case, the early childhood policy frameworks for sustaining resilient and responsive relationships are crucial in offering a sound platform for health promotion and disease prevention (Sahota et al., 2010). These interventions are essential in offsetting the damaging long-term impacts of early maladaptive behaviors and developing constructive pathways of development in children (Figure 2.19).

## Test Your Knowledge

1. What are two common behavioral issues in children, and how can positive reinforcement be used to address them?
2. How can early childhood behavioral patterns impact emotional and social development in later life?

## SUMMARY

The nuances of children's growth and development underscore the critical importance of early detection and timely intervention in all developmental concerns. Developmental screenings play a pivotal role by enabling the early identification of challenges that may hinder a child's progress; hence, the use of multiple validated tools is indispensable for professionals in this field (Drotar et al., 2008). Moreover, the profound psychological and emotional impact of certain diagnoses—such as hearing loss—on parents highlights the necessity of robust support systems tailored to their unique experiences (Grima et al., 2015). These insights not only deepen understanding of child development but also reinforce the need for coordinated interventions among healthcare providers, educators, and families to create environments that maximize developmental potential. By prioritizing early intervention and strengthening parental support, stakeholders can substantially improve outcomes for children with developmental challenges, thereby shaping a healthier future generation.

The intricate interdependence of pediatric growth and development is further highlighted by the multidimensional challenges arising from both physical health and neurodevelopmental processes. Traumatic brain injury (TBI), for instance, disrupts neurological maturation during critical developmental stages, with post-injury outcomes only partly explained by injury severity (Dennis et al., 2017). Similarly, the aftermath of critical care experiences, such as pediatric intensive care unit (PICU) stays, complicates recovery trajectories for both children and their families. Evidence indicates that survivors often face enduring physical, emotional, and social difficulties long after hospital discharge, underscoring the necessity for comprehensive assessments to identify those at greatest risk (Coad et al., 2020). Together, these findings emphasize the urgency of addressing the multiple, interconnected factors influencing pediatric growth and development. Only by acknowledging this complexity can clinicians provide holistic, evidence-based care that ensures optimal recovery and long-term developmental success for children facing health challenges.

## KEY TERMS FROM THIS CHAPTER

- Adolescence
- Chronic conditions
- Cognitive advancements
- Congenital heart disease (CHD)
- Emotional skills
- Genetic influences
- Minerals
- Nutritional intake
- Body mass index (BMI)
- Chronic health
- Cognitive skills
- Emotional growth
- Fostering optimal development
- Infancy
- Multiple sclerosis (MS)
- Pediatric growth

## CRITICAL THINKING QUESTIONS

1. **What is the primary factor influencing a child's growth and development?**
   a. Genetic inheritance
   b. Parental income
   c. Number of siblings
   d. Favorite food
2. **At what age does a child typically start to walk independently?**
   a. 6 months
   b. 12 months
   c. 18 months
   d. 24 months
3. **Which of the following is an example of fine motor development?**
   a. Running
   b. Jumping
   c. Holding a crayon
   d. Climbing stairs
4. **What is the primary developmental task of infancy according to Erik Erikson?**
   a. Trust vs. Mistrust
   b. Autonomy vs. Shame and Doubt
   c. Initiative vs. Guilt
   d. Industry vs. Inferiority
5. **Which of the following is a characteristic of cognitive development in early childhood?**
   a. Ability to solve algebra problems
   b. Egocentric thinking
   c. Understanding abstract concepts
   d. Full emotional regulation

### Short Answer Questions

1. When should a child start walking independently?
2. What is the average head circumference at birth?
3. What is the first developmental milestone lost in developmental regression?
4. Which growth parameter is most sensitive to nutritional status?
5. Which theorist proposed the stages of cognitive development in children?

### *Answers to Critical Thinking Questions*

1. (a) 2. (b) 3. (c) 4. (a) 5. (b)

# REFERENCES


1. Alex, A. M., Botteron, K., et al. (2024). A global multicohort study to map subcortical brain development and cognition in infancy and early childhood. https://core.ac.uk/download/604217781.pdf (accessed on 16th June 2025).
2. Alharbi, R. A., Arfaj, Y., Alshehri, E. M., & Alkhaldi, M. A. (2024). Thyroid hormone resistance (positive THRB gene), child case study. *Saudi Journal of Medicine*. https://www.semanticscholar.org/paper/cc787db86b70adeaac0a345adf775bfa7a1d30e8 (accessed on 16th June 2025).
3. Allen, C. L. (2005). Prenatal care utilization as a predictor of failure to thrive. https://core.ac.uk/download/480679801.pdf (accessed on 16th June 2025).
4. Gupta, N., Lustig, R. H., Chao, C., Vittinghoff, E., Andrews, H., & Leu, C. S. (2018). Thiopurines are negatively associated with anthropometric parameters in pediatric Crohn's disease. *World journal of gastroenterology*, *24*(18), 2036–2046. https://doi.org/10.3748/wjg.v24.i18.2036 (accessed on 16th June 2025).
5. Dennis, E. L., Faskowitz, J., Rashid, F., Babikian, T., Mink, R., Babbitt, C., Johnson, J., Giza, C. C., Jahanshad, N., Thompson, P. M., & Asarnow, R. F. (2017). Diverging volumetric trajectories following pediatric traumatic brain injury. *NeuroImage. Clinical*, *15*, 125–135. https://doi.org/10.1016/j.nicl.2017.03.014(accessed on 16th June 2025).
6. Banerjee, I., Barnes, J., Powis, S., Shevlin, M., et al. (2010). Health outcomes of children born to mothers with chronic kidney disease: A pilot study. https://core.ac.uk/download/5687.pdf (accessed on 16th June 2025).
7. Belknap, R., Clayton-Jones, D. L., Haglund, K., Schaefer, R., et al. (2016). Spirituality and religiosity in adolescents living with sickle cell disease. https://core.ac.uk/download/213077574.pdf (accessed on 16th June 2025).
8. Belson, P. J., Brecht, M. L., Eastwood, J. A., Hays, R., et al. (2020). A review of literature on health-related quality of life of retinoblastoma survivors. https://core.ac.uk/download/286729013.pdf (accessed on 16th June 2025).
9. Goday, P. S., Huh, S. Y., Silverman, A., Lukens, C. T., Dodrill, P., Cohen, S. S., Delaney, A. L., Feuling, M. B., Noel, R. J., Gisel, E., Kenzer, A., Kessler, D. B., Kraus de Camargo, O., Browne, J., & Phalen, J. A. (2019). Pediatric Feeding Disorder: Consensus Definition and Conceptual Framework. *Journal of pediatric gastroenterology and nutrition*, *68*(1), 124–129. https://doi.org/10.1097/MPG.0000000000002188(accessed on 16th June 2025).
10. Bruner, C., et al. (2007). Village Building and School Readiness: Closing Opportunity Gaps in a Diverse Society. State Early Childhood Policy Technical Assistance Network: Des Moines, Iowa.(accessed on 16th June 2025).
11. Carey, L. K., Fox, R. A., & Nicholson, B. C. (2002). Maternal factors related to parenting young children with congenital heart disease. https://core.ac.uk/download/213077045.pdf (accessed on 16th June 2025).
12. Carlson, M. M. (2020). A qualitative analysis of caregiver goals for urban children with and without asthma. https://core.ac.uk/download/323474194.pdf (accessed on 16th June 2025).
13. Coheley, L. M., Hill Gallant, K. M., Kindler, J. M., Laing, E. M., et al. (2018). Whole egg consumption and cortical bone in healthy children. https://core.ac.uk/download/228066155.pdf (accessed on 16th June 2025).

14. Dean, M. L., Fields, R., & Fritz, H. (2018). Got caries? Breast milk and early childhood caries? https://core.ac.uk/download/215483270.pdf (accessed on 16th June 2025).

15. Drengler, L. (2005). Evaluation of an oral health training program for school nurses. https://core.ac.uk/download/223074297.pdf (accessed on 16th June 2025).

16. Drotar, D., Dworkin, P., & Stancin, T. (2008). Pediatric developmental screening: Understanding and selecting screening instruments. https://core.ac.uk/download/71353748.pdf (accessed on 16th June 2025).

17. Duda, J. L., & Ntoumanis, N. (2005). After-school sport for children: Implications of a task-involving motivational climate. https://core.ac.uk/download/pdf/19118.pdf (accessed on 16th June 2025).

18. Eldridge, S., Chan, C., Campbell, M. J., Bond, C., Hopewell, S., Thabane, L., & Lancaster, G. (2016). CONSORT 2010 statement: Extension to randomized pilot and feasibility trials. *Pilot and Feasibility Studies, 2.* https://doi.org/10.1186/s40814-016-0105-8 (accessed on 16th June 2025).

19. Falkner, B. (2018). The childhood role in development of primary hypertension. https://core.ac.uk/download/213445721.pdf (accessed on 16th June 2025).

20. Farber, S. (2016). Early exposure to both sign and spoken language for children who are deaf or hard of hearing: Might it help spoken language development? https://core.ac.uk/download/212866357.pdf (accessed on 16th June 2025).

21. Tarantino, S., Proietti Checchi, M., Papetti, L., Monte, G., Ferilli, M. A. N., & Valeriani, M. (2024). Neuropsychological performances, quality of life, and psychological issues in pediatric onset multiple sclerosis: a narrative review. *Neurological sciences : official journal of the Italian Neurological Society and of the Italian Society of Clinical Neurophysiology, 45*(5), 1913–1930. https://doi.org/10.1007/s10072-023-07281-y (accessed on 16th June 2025).

22. Köhler, S., Gargano, M., Matentzoglu, N., Carmody, L., Lewis-Smith, D., Vasilevsky, N., Daniš, D., et al. (2020). The Human Phenotype Ontology in 2021. *Nucleic Acids Research, 49*, D1207–D1217. https://doi.org/10.1093/nar/gkaa1043 (accessed on 16th June 2025).

23. Lee, D. K., Teulier, C., & Ulrich, B. D. (2015). Early gait development in human infants: Plasticity and clinical applications. https://deepblue.lib.umich.edu/bitstream/2027.42/111276/1/dev21291.pdf (accessed on 16th June 2025).

24. Bradley, E. H., Webster, T. R., Baker, D., Schlesinger, M., Inouye, S. K., Barth, M. C., Lapane, K. L., Lipson, D., Stone, R., & Koren, M. J. (2004). Translating research into practice: speeding the adoption of innovative health care programs. *Issue brief (Commonwealth Fund)*, (724), 1–12.(accessed on 16th June 2025).

25. Lopez-Cepero, A., Moore Simas, T. A., Nobel, L., Rosal, M., et al. (2017). Trajectories of weight for length growth for infants during the first year of life. https://core.ac.uk/download/213106847.pdf (accessed on 16th June 2025).

26. McAllister, J. W., Popp, J., & Antonelli, R. (2009). Making care coordination a critical component of the pediatric health system: A multidisciplinary framework. https://core.ac.uk/download/71352885.pdf (accessed on 16th June 2025).

27. Miller, S., Naccache, S. N., Samayoa, E., Messacar, K., Arevalo, S., Federman, S., Stryke, D., et al. (2019). Laboratory validation of a clinical metagenomic sequencing assay for pathogen

detection in cerebrospinal fluid. *Genome Research, 29*, 831–842. https://doi.org/10.1101/gr.238170.118 (accessed on 16th June 2025).

28. Julie. Cooper; Cynthia. Alendy; Lisa. Simpson; Gunther Christina. Murphy(2008). *Childhood Obesity: The Role of Health Policy*. Child Policy Research Center, University of Cincinnati; Robert Wood Johnson Foundation. https://core.ac.uk/download/71342400.pdf (accessed on 16th June 2025).
29. Nicoll, W. G. (2014). *Developing Transformative Schools: A Resilience-Focused Paradigm for Education*. https://core.ac.uk/download/46603629.pdf (accessed on 16th June 2025).
30. Patel, R. (2015). Pediatric nurse practitioner home visitation is associated with a decrease in home care and healthcare utilization errors in high-risk infants. https://core.ac.uk/download/129532636.pdf (accessed on 16th June 2025).
31. Peters, Malea and Wittenberg, Shelby, "Improving School Readiness in Home-Based Care Settings" (2021). *Occupational Therapy Capstones*. 480. https://commons.und.edu/ot-grad/480(accessed on 16th June 2025).
32. Sahota, P and Wordley, J and Woodward, J (2010) Literature Review - Health behaviour change models and approaches for families and young people to support HEAT 3: Child Healthy Weight Programmes. Project Report. NHS Health Scotland. (accessed on 16th June 2025).
33. Templeton, A., Arquitt, A. B., Migliano, A. B., Pesonen, A. K., Parent, A. S., Bogin, B., Campbell, B., et al. (2013). Evo-devo of human adolescence: Beyond disease models of early puberty. https://core.ac.uk/download/18528095.pdf (accessed on 16th June 2025).
34. Thai, A. M., Lowenstein, D., Rejeski, D., & Ching, D. (2009). *Game Changer: Investing in Digital Play to Advance Children's Learning and Health*. https://core.ac.uk/download/71351412.pdf (accessed on 16th June 2025).
35. Voitova, T., Bernhofs, V., & Müllensiefen, D. (2025). The influence of psychosocial skills on the development of musical abilities: Cross-sectional results from secondary school pupils in Latvia. *Gifted Child Quarterly*. https://www.semanticscholar.org/paper/330191a7568beb5226bbffec7939332b7ab15624 (accessed on 16th June 2025).
36. Wang, Q. (2019). Mothers' perceptions of stress, parenting self-efficacy, and permissive and inconsistent discipline: Insights from China, Japan, and the United States. https://core.ac.uk/download/287621736.pdf (accessed on 16th June 2025).
37. Wani, P., & Anand, R. (2024). Unraveling the physiology of taste sensation in newborns: Mechanisms, development, and clinical implications. *European Journal of Medical and Health Sciences*. https://www.semanticscholar.org/paper/0e6a7584cd9a0a77275c2ca8fddf0918c445d182 (accessed on 16th June 2025).
38. Witchel, S. F., Oberfield, S. E., Rosenfield, R. L., Codner, E., Bonny, A. E., Ibáñez, L., Peña, A. S., et al. (2015). The diagnosis of polycystic ovary syndrome during adolescence. *Hormone Research in Pediatrics, 83*, 376–389. https://doi.org/10.1159/000375530 (accessed on 16th June 2025).

# PEDIATRIC NUTRITION

# 3

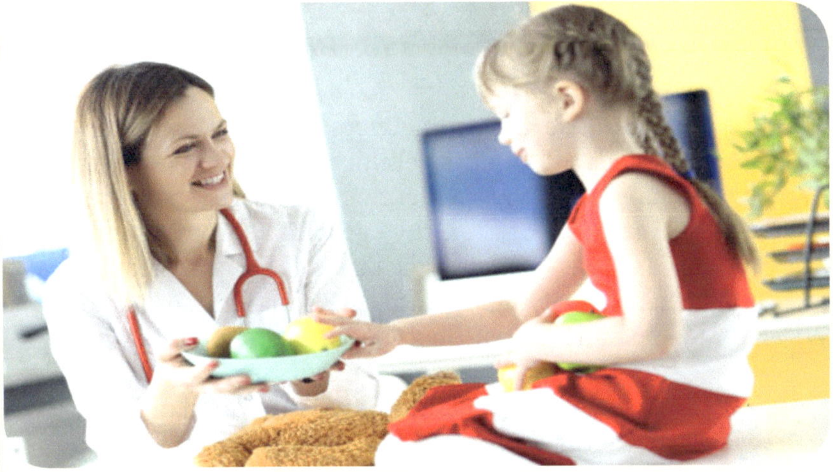

## LEARNING OBJECTIVES

**After studying this chapter, you will be able to:**

1. Understand the nutritional requirements by age group;
2. List the common nutritional deficiencies in children;
3. Define the role of breastfeeding;
4. Give an introduction of solid foods;
5. Focus on the impact of nutrition on child development;
6. List the addressing pediatric obesity.

## Introduction

Children's nutrition plays a crucial role in controlling the unique dietary needs of infants, adolescents, and children. It is not only what one consumes but also when it is introduced and how. Nutrition between birth and adolescence lays the foundation for well-being, influencing physical health, cognition, and mood. The nutritional requirements of children are quite different from those of adults; for example, they require more of certain nutrients about their body size. A balanced diet containing a high proportion of carbohydrates, proteins, fats, vitamins, and minerals is needed to aid rapid growth and development characteristic of children and adolescence. Moreover, the development of healthful eating habits, food likes and dislikes, and an improvement in the body's relationship with food have long-term implications for health. Introduction of solids is a pivotal milestone with both advantages and disadvantages in the nutrition of children. Typically, around six months of age, this phase needs to be approached with careful planning to ensure optimal nutrient intake without intolerance. It is also during this stage that kids can develop preferences, and exposure to a variety of flavors and textures is essential. Research indicates that early exposure to a variety of foods may reduce food aversions in adulthood. Caregivers need to remain vigilant for potential allergens and the risk of choking hazards while creating an environment for food exploration and appreciation. Parents and caregivers have a vital role in providing healthy options as well as educating healthy food, which form the pillars of a child's relationship with food for the rest of their life. As children progress through different stages of development, their requirements for nutrients vary, requiring ongoing evaluation and reevaluation of nutritional strategies. Adolescents, on their part, undergo drastic physical transformations and increased energy demands, all of which are met by diet.

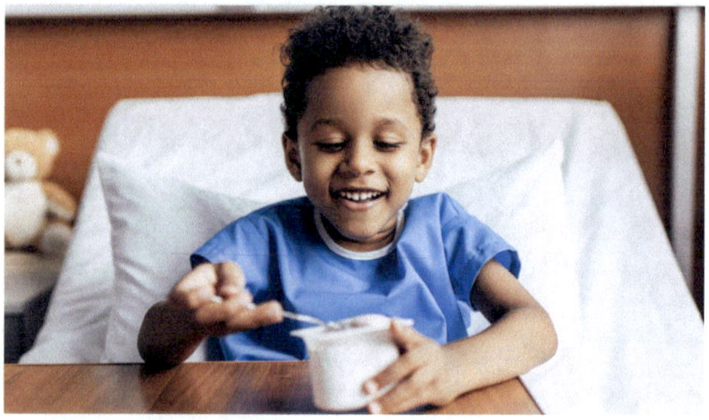

**Figure 3.1.** The pediatric nutrition.

*Source:* https://external-content.duckduckgo.com/iu/?u=https%3A%2F%2Fnyulangone.org%2Ffiles%2Fpediatric-patient-eating-yogurt-inline.jpg&f=1&nofb=1&ipt=c075b3e56d8de563a6072ef56658ea9e8fe7e0494bef8d12e442989a658085ba&ipo=images.

Their onset usually coincides with the process of peer influence and social forces that can influence eating behavior, and therefore, it is particularly vital to encourage healthy eating habits. Comprehensive education regarding the importance of well-balanced meals, restraint in the quantity of food intake, and the risk of excessive consumption of processed foods is vital. Operating on the psychological and social dimensions of eating, children can be assisted in managing challenges such as body image and disordered eating behavior. Establishing an environment that focuses on healthy food choices and positive eating experiences, caregivers can profoundly impact their child's long-term health and nutrition literacy, setting them up for a lifetime of wellness (Figure 3.1).

## Definition and Importance of Pediatric Nutrition

Pediatric nutrition encompasses the dietary needs of infants, children, and adolescents, applying the principles of nutrition in the interest of healthy growth, development, and well-being. It is beyond the provision of enough food; it entails an understanding of specific nutritional needs at various stages of childhood, based on age, sex, and health status. Child nutrition lays the foundation for a lifetime of healthy eating, ideally reducing the risk of future chronic disease. As a core aspect of pediatric medicine, effective nutrition interventions can directly impact developmental milestones, brainpower, and immune function in children to help them achieve their full physical and intellectual potential. The importance of pediatric nutrition can be reinforced further through the central position it occupies in the management of particular medical issues, such as pediatric feeding disorders. Issues like feeding disorders need specialist nutritional measures to help children who might otherwise have a problem swallowing adequate nutrients due to medical or behavioral reasons. The necessity for action in the treatment of these disorders is evident; the focus on improving care and well-being in children with pediatric feeding disorder requiring tube feeding confirms, for instance, there is an urgent need for regular data collection and multidisciplinary intervention (Dadich et al., 2021). Through such interventions, medical professionals are able to prevent long-term consequences of poor nutrition, educate and improve eating patterns and resilience in vulnerable pediatric populations. Additionally, the socio-economic background to pediatric nutrition cannot be disregarded, as children's eating habits are highly influenced by parental behavior. Experimental economics studies have shown how parental altruism has a direct effect on the nutritional intake of a child, establishing a familial connection with increased risk of obesity (Ballenger et al., 2025). Such dynamics imply that interventions need to address both the provision of information to parents and the promotion of healthy eating among children. By understanding and solving the family environment that affects eating habits, healthcare professionals can develop programs that not only enhance pediatric diet but can also facilitate families to adopt sustainable practices leading to healthier generations.

## Overview of Nutritional Needs in Children

In understanding the nutritional needs of children, one must consider the various stages of development and growth that significantly influence food needs. In early childhood, i.e., between birth and five years of age, the child has intense physical as well as intellectual growth. All this development necessitates a greater intake of fundamental nutrients like proteins, vitamins, and minerals in order to facilitate milestones in growth. Iron, calcium, and vitamin D are particularly crucial at this stage because these nutrients play a role in making bones strong and supporting immune function. And establishing healthy eating habits early in life provides a solid foundation for optimal nutrition throughout life, which reduces the risk of developing chronic diseases later in life. Therefore, the diet of children has to be approached in a holistic way with regard to the quantity and quality of food consumed. Children grow up and develop into adolescence, and their nutritional needs alter due to the physiological changes that take place, like higher energy demands and onset of puberty. Teenagers tend to require an amplified caloric burden for sustaining their growth spurts and active lifestyle. Micronutrient demands also become increasingly essential at this time, with particular reference to iron and calcium for the promotion of bone growth as well as to facilitate menstruation in females. These nutrients' dietary intake should be a priority, as their lack of availability can have implications for health in the development of anemia and reduced bone strength.

Inadequate meeting of these nutritional demands can have long-term effects on general bodily health and well-being. Subsequently, the promotion of equal meals with a combination of food groups becomes a necessity to respond to adolescents' unique nutritional requirements. More intricate feeding issues like pediatric feeding disorders (PFDs) and dysphagia can significantly interfere with the nutritional intake of children, leading to potential malnutrition and impairment in growth. PFDs, which are characterized by impaired oral intake affecting age-linked feeding, have etiologies that are multifactorial with medical, psychosocial, and developmental factors (Goday et al., 2019). Research has indicated that dysphagic children often do not attain caloric needs, with research indicating that nearly 40% are unable to achieve their total energy expenditure (Herrador-López et al., 2024). This indicates the necessity of personalized and multidisciplinary management to address the specific needs of such children, with interventions such as speech therapy and nutritional rehabilitation being some of the options. These individualized strategies not only work to enhance caloric intake but also enhance broader dietary acceptability and, in turn, contribute to improved quality of life and health outcomes for the compromised children (Figure 3.2).

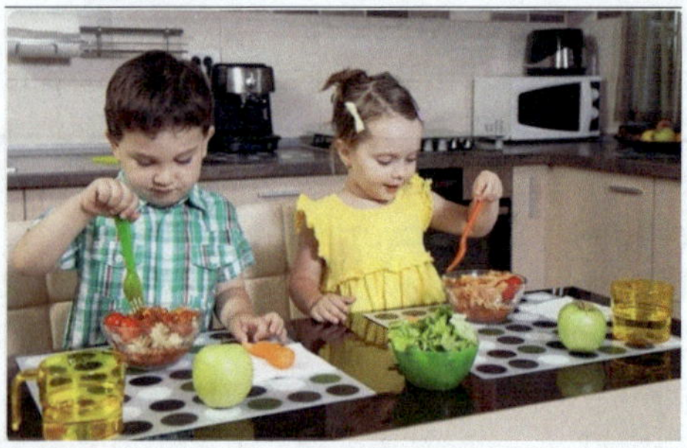

**Figure 3.2.** Two young children eat a nutritious meal together at a kitchen table, reinforcing healthy eating habits and independence in early childhood.

*Source:* https://d2jx2rerrg6sh3.cloudfront.net/image-handler/picture/2018/6/shutterstock_144310366.jpg.

## *Role of Pediatricians and Nutritionists in Child Health*

The collective role of pediatricians and nutritionists in the health of children is brought to the fore by their coordinated interventions to secure the best support for development and growth in childhood. Pediatricians are often the first to identify children's illnesses, taking total-person histories including physical health, developmental screening, and nutrition needs. Their education equips them with the capability to recognize symptoms of nutritional deficiencies and obesity and hence enable early interventions which can prevent chronic diseases. Pediatricians are also capable of offering special dietary advice based on a child's specific needs so that families become empowered with information in order to make informed decisions regarding their child's diet. This cooperation between pediatricians and parents creates a supportive environment that focuses on the health of the child and allows for proper eating habits early in life, setting the stage for a lifetime of good decision-making. Among the enormous responsibilities pediatricians have to offer, nutritionists possess the singular experience that is vital in addressing child-specific nutritional needs. Such experts possess extensive information regarding the type of nutrition needed at various periods in childhood. They provide individualized meal planning and counseling that is specially crafted to meet the specific nutritional needs of children. For instance, they can assist families in managing conditions such as food allergy or intolerance, which are increasingly common in pediatric populations. Nutritionists also play a key role in public health interventions that target healthy eating in children and adolescents in schools and communities and therefore in the child health agenda in general. By collaboration with pediatricians, nutritionists can strengthen nutrition education and treatment so that children not only gain through proper nutrition but also through medical care, which benefits their cognitive and physical growth. Effective training of healthcare professionals in nutrition is key to enhancing the health outcomes of children, particularly in the wake of challenges posed by under nutrition and obesity. Recent studies have indicated that in-service nutrition training has a significant effect on health workers' knowledge and skills concerning the management of nutrition, particularly pediatrics. Nutrition training improves the competence of healthcare professionals, such as pediatricians, to screen and correct malnutrition at an early stage. In one of the studies, 18 out of 25 were found to have noted significant nutrition knowledge improvement among health workers following training, where the effectiveness of the programs was shown (Sunguya et al., 2013). Additionally, in settings like the Special Supplemental Food Program for Women, Infants, and Children (WIC), increased confidence in dental practice in health is said to be linked with better child health outcomes. Therefore, the integration of focused nutrition education into healthcare education is vital to creating a collective strategy for pediatric nutrition that eventually leads to healthier childhood development and well-being (Cooper et al., 2008).

## 3.1. Nutritional Requirements by Age Group

**Learning Outcome**

1. Infants (0–12 months);
2. Toddlers (1–3 years);
3. School-age children (4–12 years).

Children's dietary requirements evolve significantly with age to accommodate their respective phases of growth and physiological needs. Newborns, for example, dependent predominantly on breast milk or formula for nutrient intake, provide them with the requisite macro-nutrients and micro-nutrients for growth. Though they transition to solid foods at six months of age, the introduction of iron-rich foods is crucial to avoid anemia, which is extremely prevalent in light of the maternal stores of iron that are lost. In the meantime, the role of breastfeeding remains of utmost significance in this context, given that scientific evidence indicates that breast milk prevents necrotizing enterocolitis (NEC) in preterm infants (Courtney et al., 2020). Caregivers need to adhere to instructions on the advancement of feeding to ensure a gradual transfer from liquid to solid diet and nutritionally adequate to respond to the high rates of growth at this age. Toddlers and preschool children also possess different nutrient problems concerning tasting a greater variety of food when forming preferences and taste. This is the time when nutritional deficiency risk can be high unless a well-balanced diet is maintained. Nutrients like calcium, which is vital for bone development, and vitamins A, C, and D, for overall health, are extremely crucial at this time. Whole cereals, fruits, and vegetables must take priority to ensure adequate fiber. Furthermore, enteral feeding may be applied in cases where normal feeding is insufficient, emphasizing the importance of safe and accurate delivery methods in both hospital and home settings (King et al., 2014). Parents and caregivers play a crucial role in managing quantities and educating healthy eating patterns, eventually shaping long-term nutritional habits as children learn to make food choices independently. As the children transition to school days and adolescence, their need for nutrition becomes increasingly important, related to more physical activity and growth spurts.

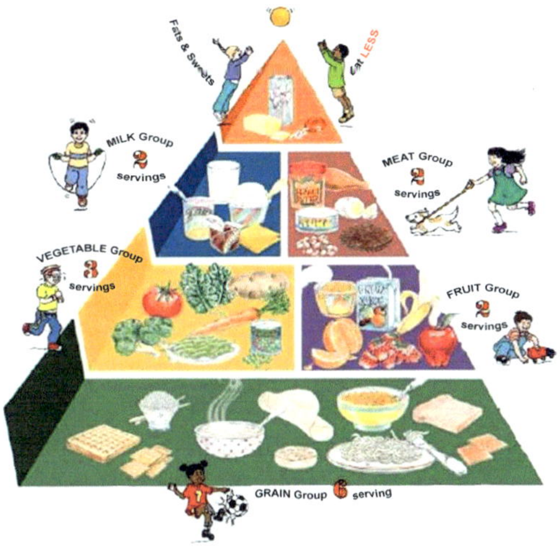


**Figure 3.3.** The nutritional requirements of children vary significantly across different age groups.

*Source:* https://farmveda.in/cdn/shop/articles/nutrir-req-2048x2048_1200x630.webp?v=1678524815.

The body's nutritional requirements shift to meet these modifications through increased amounts of protein, vitamins, and minerals. Adolescents have a peak growth rate, necessitating a significant increase in caloric consumption, particularly in protein and calcium for muscle development and bone growth. Furthermore, the increasing prevalence of nutrition problems, such as obesity and eating disorders, emphasizes the necessity of informing people about healthy food habits. Such educational interventions need to consider media and peer influence on food behaviors with the aim of establishing a healthy relationship with food that prioritizes health and wellness. Monitoring nutritional intake during these early years is critical to prevent long-term health issues that would compromise the basis of pediatric nutrition for optimal and certain development and growth (Figure 3.3).

### 3.1.1. Infants (0–12 Months)

The first year of life is the most important time for establishing a basis for wholesome growth and development in pediatric nutrition. During this time, infants grow and develop very quickly, and they require an optimum balance of macro-nutrients and micro-nutrients to enable physical and mental growth. Breast milk remains the optimal method of feeding babies under six months, as it consists of essential fatty acids, immunoglobulins, and enzymes that not only nourish but also support the infant's immune system. The arrangement of breast milk also adapts to accommodate the evolving needs of the developing baby, a dynamic that highlights its singular standing among baby feeding routines. According to various studies highlighted in pediatric literature, adequate infant feeding during this critical period is linked with improved health outcomes in subsequent years, impacting obesity levels, cognitive abilities, and global health as evident in trends observed in pediatrics (Bernasconi et al., 2019). With the arrival of babies to solid foods at six months, the introduction of complementary foods must adhere to dietary guidelines for nutritional adequacy. Caregivers must take a thoughtful step in introducing diverse food groups while gauging against infants' natural developmental readiness. Iron-containing foods such as fortified breakfast cereals and meat puree become increasingly important, given the increased physiological requirement for iron in infants at this age. The Early Childhood Nutrition and Anemia Prevention Project (ECNAPP) has developed a great understanding of the effectiveness of nutritional intervention, particularly in those groups where deficiency is prevalent. By promoting iron-rich diets and heightened maternal knowledge about infant feeding, such programs have been shown to minimize nutritional deficiency and enhance healthier results among vulnerable groups (Aquino D).

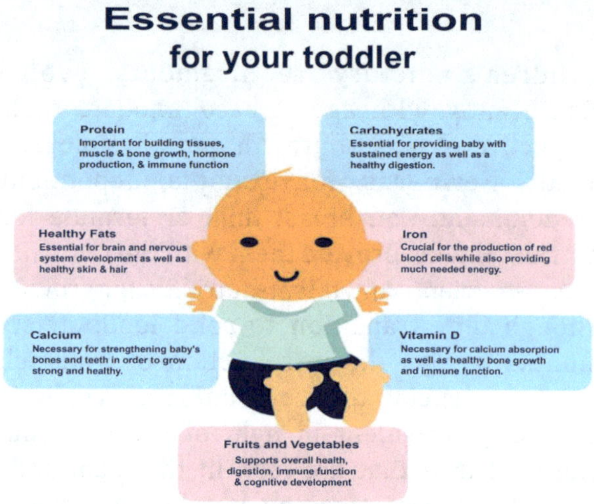


**Figure 3.4.** Essential nutrition for infants and toddlers.

*Source:* https://cdn.shopify.com/s/files/1/0523/3469/0479/files/essential-nutrition-for-your-toddler-en_600x600.png?v=1692006609.

The careful planning of nutrition at this phase catalyzes developing nutritious consumption habits throughout later childhood. The supplementation of micro-nutrients plays a critical role during the first year of life, where deficiencies have been associated with long-term health implications. Pediatric caregivers and providers must be vigilant in monitoring an infant's diet for deficiencies that result from poor feeding practices or limited variation of diet. Significantly, it has been noted through evidence that community programs aimed at nutrition education, as well as enhanced availability of healthy sources of food, play an important role. For instance, information from recent findings in infant nutrition in pediatrics invokes an appeal to concerted measures in meeting demand and supply of healthy infant nutrition across diverse settings (Bernasconi et al., 2019). In addition, cultural practices and dietary preferences are an imperative in the development of public health interventions. Thus, an integrated approach to infant feeding is vital, not just for the short-term health, but also for setting the stage for healthy nutrition throughout life (Figure 3.4).

### 3.1.2. Toddlers (1–3 Years)

Children between 1 and 3 years old are toddlers and have nutritional requirements characterized by high development and growth and thus require increased attention in feeding processes. During this time, children would usually transition from milk to diversified solid foods, and caregivers should hence provide a balanced intake of essential nutrients. The nutritional focus should include a healthy consumption of proteins, fats, vitamins, and minerals to support physical and mental growth. Secondly, exposure to diversity in food textures and tastes during infancy lays a basis for improved eating habits in the long run. Therefore, caregivers need to promote a healthy meal environment, prioritizing the importance of sharing meals together as a family while serving healthy foods. As independent children, toddlers develop eating habits through increasingly prominent parental modeling of good behavior. Socio-cultural influence in toddlers' nutrition cannot be overestimated, particularly in the case of immigrant families. Research has established that caregivers of varying backgrounds are likely to experience difficulties in interpreting the subtleties of nutrition and feeding behavior in a new environment. Specific interventions for immigrant families, such as the First Foods curriculum, have proven effective in mitigating such challenges by enhancing caregivers' knowledge of pediatric nutrition and proper feeding at various levels. Such curricula only address issues such as child development, food safety, and healthy living, which are important in instilling healthy feeding practices. Through the empowerment of caregivers, the potential for healthier eating habits in toddlers within such groups exists, promoting healthier growth trends in conjunction with the alleviation of food security. Additionally, these education interventions serve to fill gaps within culturally specific nutritional practices and knowledge, delivering whole-family support to immigrants. Beyond immediate access issues related to food consumption, the nexus between nutrition and developmental needs, such as malnutrition, is vital to address. Especially among some populations, for example, cerebral palsy, malnutrition is capable of quite significantly hampering developmental milestones and overall welfare. There is a high prevalence of malnutrition among them, most often due to feeding problems as well as socio-demographic restrictions. Nutrition among this group thus requires unique interventions consisting of dietary management and supportive feeding techniques. For young children with developmental disabilities, a well-structured approach to nutrition can guarantee better results by minimizing the risk of malnourishment, thus guaranteeing that their development and growth are attained. A multi-faceted approach with education, community support, and individualized care is of primary importance in the promotion of ideal pediatric nutrition and feeding habits in all the kids, regardless of their problems.

### 3.1.3. School-Age Children (4–12 Years)

School children, typically aged between 4 and 12 years, undergo a very rapid growth and development process, during which their nutrition becomes extremely significant. This period of development is characterized by increased physical activity and varying nutritional demands as kids develop from preschool to school age. Supplying school-going children with a nutritionally adequate diet that is rich in adequate amounts of macro-nutrients and micro-nutrients is essential to sustain their energy levels and enhance cognitive function. Nutritional consumption at this stage of development can have long-term effects on health, like the likelihood of contracting diseases like diabetes and obesity. Hence, medical doctors and caregivers must encourage healthy food consumption, reinforcing the necessity of properly planned meals with a variety of food types. Obesity is one of the principal public health concerns among school children and requires strict surveillance of food and lifestyle. Subsequent studies revealed that such environmental factors as healthy diet access and parental involvement in nutrition education are crucial to the establishment of children's dietary patterns. The interaction between these factors was also focused on a study that established parental nutritional knowledge had a significantly strong relationship with overweight prevalence among preschool children. Exactly, the study highlighted that children whose parents possessed greater dietary knowledge had a better-quality diet and therefore reduced their chances of becoming obese. Secondly, understanding how factors such as fast food consumption fit into the determinants of childhood obesity is essential in developing the correct prevention interventions for this group (Anas et al., 2014). Therefore, educating parents on nutrition is a critical step to reverse childhood obesity. Early taste preferences and long-term eating habits have also been associated, placing a focus on feeding in preschool years. Evidence has shown that early preference by children for fruits and vegetables (FV) is a strong predictor of their food habits in later life. Systematic review of dietary observation found that children who preferred FV in their early years exhibited higher consumption rates later in life, directly affecting their overall health outcomes. Furthermore, the level of education of mothers as well as socio-economic status play a significant role in affecting children's diets and food intakes. In particular, higher levels of maternal education have been linked to children's eating healthier foods, that is, encouraging consumption of FV in the early stages will avert risks of obesity and encourage better lifestyle habits (Adamson et al., 2016). Hence, the formation of food liking early in life is crucial for instilling healthy food habits in life (Figure 3.5).

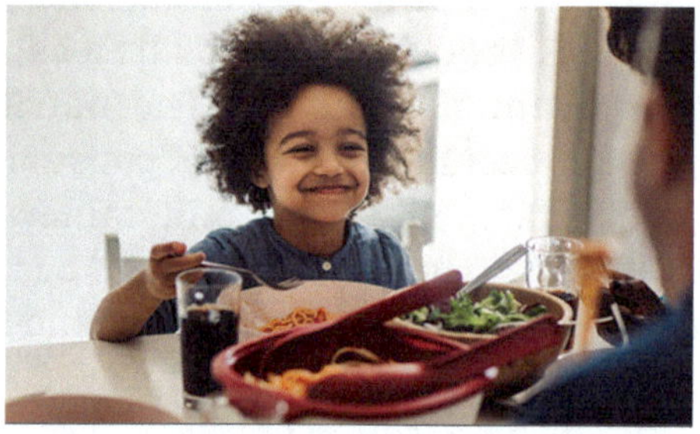

**Figure 3.5.** A smiling child enjoys a balanced meal with family, promoting healthy nutrition and positive mealtime experiences in childhood.

*Source:* https://www.hopkinsmedicine.org/-/media/images/health/_-images-to-be-filed/schoolaged-nutrition.jpg.

## Test Your Knowledge

1. What are the primary nutritional needs of infants (0–12 months), and how do these differ from those of toddlers (1–3 years)?
2. How do the nutritional requirements of school-age children (4–12 years) support their growth and development during this stage?

## 3.2. Common Nutritional Deficiencies in Children

**Learning Outcome**

1. Iron deficiency anemia;
2. Vitamin D deficiency;
3. Calcium deficiency.

Nutritional deficiencies in children are prevalent and normally not detected, potentially resulting in serious health conditions lasting into adulthood. Iron deficiency is one of the most widespread deficiencies and is capable of producing anemia, as well as preventing mental and physical development. Iron is crucial in the synthesis of hemoglobin, the oxygen carrier within the blood. Tiredness, irritability, and compromised immune systems can occur in children with low iron levels. To combat this deficiency, caregivers must incorporate iron-rich foods such as lean meats, beans, and fortified cereals into the child's diet. Further awareness of signs of deficiency and regular health check-ups can go a long way to enable early interventions that are most crucial for holistic growth and development. Vitamin D deficiency is another extreme issue in children in regions with low sunlight exposure. The vitamin is also responsible for the absorption of calcium and bone building and, directly, children's growth and vulnerability to diseases like osteoporosis. A lack of adequate vitamin D will cause rickets, a disease of soft and weakened bones. Supplementation might be required in children during periods of scant sunlight or in areas where food consumption is lacking, particularly in vegetarian and vegan children. Moreover, the caregivers must be briefed on the need to include sources of vitamin D, such as fortified milk and fish, in their child's diet program so that they have ample supplies and healthy bone growth is ensured. Certain medical conditions also add to the risk of nutritional deficiency among children, necessitating special dietary management. For instance, cerebral palsy can develop problems with both control of muscles and swallowing, which can limit diet and result in problems such as vitamin deficiency. This not only affects growth but also leads to more generalized health issues, including dental health and impaired immune function. It is important that medical practitioners evaluate these children via a multidisciplinary process, as research has indicated that effectively resolving their unique feeding problems can significantly enhance their quality of life and overall health. With the addition of knowledge from the proposed framework to child feeding disorders, it is feasible to have a holistic approach, thus highlighting individualized nutrition programs and ongoing caregiver counseling (Cannon et al., 2018; Goday et al., 2019) (Figure 3.6).

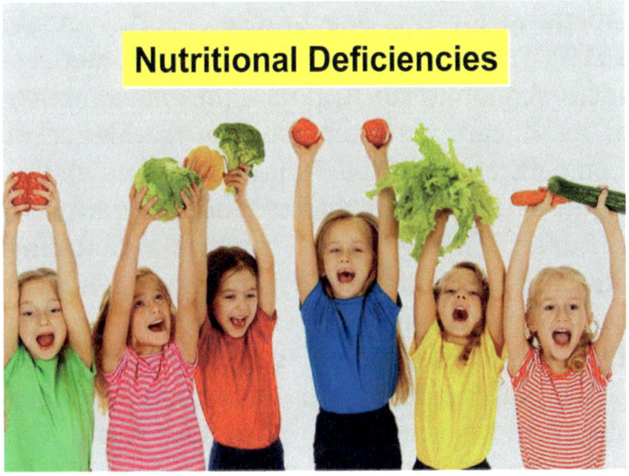


**Figure 3.6.** Nutritional deficiencies in children.

*Source:* https://images.onlymyhealth.com/imported/images/2021/August/11_Aug_2021/NutritionalDeficiency_big2.jpg.

### 3.2.1. Iron Deficiency Anemia

Iron deficiency anemia (IDA) is a significant health issue in pediatric nutrition and feeding. IDA results from having insufficient iron in the body for the production of adequate amounts of hemoglobin, leading to low oxygen transport in the blood. Five-year-olds and younger are at higher risk due to their rapid growth rate and high nutritional demands. A diet deficient in iron-containing foods may result in retardation of development, cognitive impairment, and susceptibility to infections. Awareness and dietary improvement programs at the public health level play a critical role in controlling IDA as part of an overall pediatric nutrition strategy. Supplementation with iron-fortified foods and supplements, wherever necessary, is a critical control measure in this prevalent nutritional disorder among vulnerable populations. Experience indicates that iron deficiency anemia affects tens of millions of children across the globe, with the prevalence being much larger in developing nations. For instance, a study indicated that an astonishing 64.6% of African preschool children suffer from anemia, with the outcome contributing to increased child mortality for this age bracket (Goday et al., 2019). The conditions of poor dietary practices, socio-economic constraints, and unavailability of healthcare can increase the prevalence of iron deficiency anemia. Malnutrition contributes significantly to morbidity and mortality in children throughout the world, including Ghana, as manifested by the prevalence of various micronutrient deficiencies, like iron. Targeted interventions, such as community health interventions and education campaigns about the importance of dietary iron, are key components in the prevention of IDA in children. Effective treatment of iron deficiency anemia in pediatric populations can often be accomplished by a multidisciplinary approach, including healthcare providers, nutritionists, and community leaders. The majority of children who come to health facilities with anemia have had chronic nutritional deficiencies, resulting in multifactorial health issues that complicate the treatment. Ensuring that a complete care plan serves to cope with the complications appropriately, such as nutritional counseling, supplementation, and the provision of appropriate medical treatment. Regular monitoring and quality assurance of medicine supply chains in health facilities must also be conducted to facilitate successful, timely and sufficient treatment outcomes among the affected children. With the application of far-reaching management practices, the occurrence of iron deficiency anemia is minimized and overall results for child health are improved in the event of nutritional deficiency (Figure 3.7).

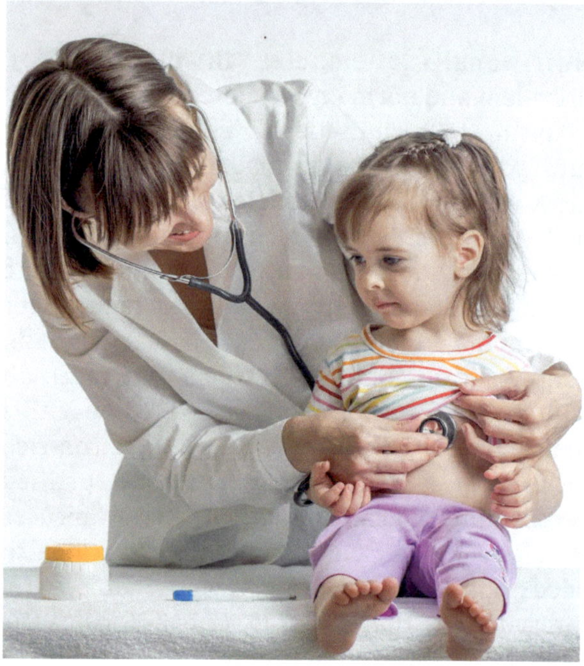

**Figure 3.7.** Iron-deficiency anemia.

*Source:* https://www.momjunction.com/wp-content/uploads/2014/09/Iron-Deficiency-Anemia-In-Toddlers.jpg.webp.

### 3.2.2. Vitamin D Deficiency

Vitamin D deficiency is also a cause of concern in pediatrics, given its role as a required component in bone metabolism and overall metabolic processes in the pediatric population. As nutritional guidelines evolve, the fact that the majority of North American children possess ominous levels of vitamin D below the sufficiency level supports the need for evaluation and treatment. Epidemiological data suggest that 65% to 70% of children older than one year lack proper vitamin D levels, a public health policy issue that is alarming as far as children's feeding habits are concerned. Inadequate exposure to sunlight and absence of food sources typically exacerbate this deficiency, so it is necessary to rethink how vitamin D is integrated into pediatric dietary guidelines, especially in the period of formative growth. The implications of a deficiency of vitamin D are not limited to bone health but are increasingly linked with other respiratory complications, which can be disabling in young patients. Literature indicates that a deficiency of vitamin D is linked with a high risk of upper respiratory tract infection (URTI) and hospitalization due to asthma in children.

These conditions not only equate to increased healthcare costs but also drastically impact the quality of life for families and children affected. The controversy over pediatric nutrition must then include strategies that aim to detect and compensate for deficiencies that predispose children to respiratory infection. Research into successful dietary interventions and supplementation would significantly reduce the incidence of URTIs and associated complications, further establishing the function of vitamin D in childhood health. Emerging evidence identifies the potential for targeted vitamin D supplementation in overcoming the pathological effects of deficiency in children. A recent pragmatic randomized trial also intends to compare high-dose versus standard-dose vitamin D supplementation on asthma exacerbations and URTIs frequency in preschool children. This kind of research not only aims to establish optimal doses but also the impact of vitamin D supplementation on overall child health outcomes. By bridging the prevention-diet behavior connection gap, these research studies open up an era of evidence-based pediatric nutrition that can potentially contribute significantly to vitamin D deficiency-related morbidity reduction. Eventually, the practice of specific health policies following rigorous clinical evidence can trigger health trajectories for children according to prevailing pediatric nutrition standards (Birken et al., 2014) (Figure 3.8).

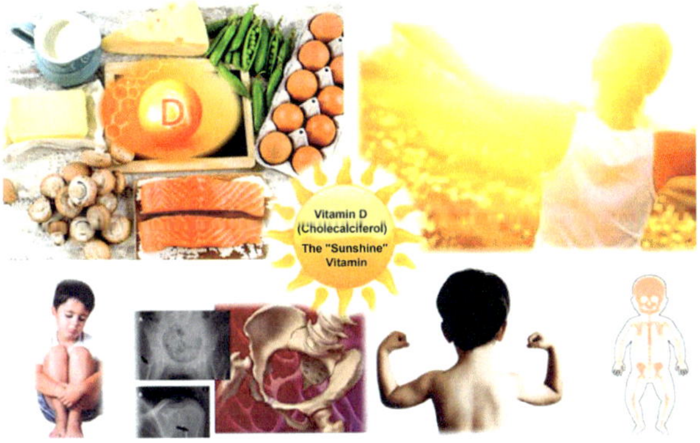


**Figure 3.8.** Vitamin D deficiency has emerged as a significant concern in the context of pediatric nutrition.

*Source:* https://editor4.babynama.com/wp-content/uploads/2024/04/vitamin-d-deficiency-in-children.webp.

## 3.2.3. Calcium Deficiency

Calcium deficiency poses a very risky condition to the pediatric group, and it may result in long-term health problems. Adequate calcium intake during childhood and adolescence is necessary because it facilitates bone and tooth development and other physiological processes. The prevalence of calcium deficiency among children has been brought about by a number of eating habits. Increased consumption of fortified beverages, such as energy and sports drinks, generally equates to decreased intake of essential nutrients, such as calcium. These beverages, aggressively promoted to teenagers, are often laden with high levels of sugars and artificial components rather than nutrient-dense substitutes and encourage imbalanced meals that cannot supply the adequate calcium needed for the day. Because diet habits are set early in life, deficiency of calcium treatment is most essential to prevent other health issues in later life, i.e., osteoporosis or oral problems. Factors contributing to calcium deficiency among children are multifaceted and are compounded further by a lack of awareness about healthy foods. Parents would unwittingly prioritize modern, calcium-enriched drinks over traditional calcium-rich foods like dairy products, leafy greens, and fortified cereals. This trend of highly marketed beverages creates a disconnect between nutrition education and food marketing within families. Despite alternatives, such as plant milk substitutes, not all provide adequate levels of calcium, often requiring supplements. Moreover, pediatric health care providers must educate families about the importance of calcium not only for bone formation but also for its role in muscles, as well as overall health. Solutions to such issues require concerted effort by many healthcare practitioners, parents, and teachers in an effort to enhance the access and understanding of healthy food among children. Aside from dietary practices, determinants of calcium status include the interaction between vitamin D and calcium. Vitamin D plays a crucial role in the body in several ways to facilitate the absorption of calcium; hence, vitamin D deficiency also contributes to exacerbating the effects of low calcium levels.

Recent studies have shown that many children, particularly those with some health issues, are prone to vitamin D deficiency, coupled with the generally prevailing problem of calcium deficiency in children (Burnham et al., 2011). This reliance calls for a general approach against nutritional deficits through balanced diets supplemented with both vitamin D and calcium. Encouraging outdoor activities that trigger natural vitamin D synthesis, along with education about well-balanced dietary habits, can encourage healthier practices. Ultimately, the resolution of both calcium and vitamin D deficiency problems through informed dietary maneuvers and individualized nutritional recommendations will be of primary significance in overcoming these problems in pediatric nutrition and feeding (Figure 3.9).

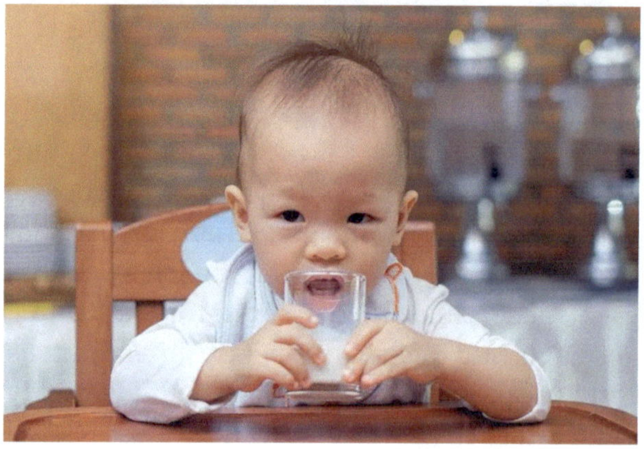

**Figure 3.9.** A baby drinks milk from a glass while seated in a highchair, supporting early childhood nutrition and calcium intake for healthy growth and development.

*Source:* https://cdn.cdnparenting.com/articles/2018/01/16143251/Calcium-deficiency-in-babies.webp.

## Test Your Knowledge

1. Which vitamin deficiency is most commonly associated with rickets in children?
2. Why is vitamin D important for calcium absorption in the body?

## 3.3. The Role of Breastfeeding

**Learning Outcome**

1. Benefits of breastfeeding for infants;
2. Recommended duration of breastfeeding;
3. Challenges and Solutions for Breastfeeding Mothers

Breastfeeding is a cornerstone of infant nutrition, providing essential nutrients and protective factors that are fundamental to healthy growth and development. The World Health Organization identifies breastfeeding as the optimal method of infant feeding due to its profound benefits for both infants and mothers. Breast milk offers an ideal balance of proteins, fats, vitamins, and antibodies that not only strengthen the infant's immune system but also protect against infections and reduce the risk of chronic diseases later in life. Despite these well-documented advantages, breastfeeding rates in many regions remain below established public health targets, such as those outlined in the Healthy People 2010 goals. For example, Arkansas and several other states continue to report initiation and continuation rates below the national average, underscoring the need for targeted interventions that support and empower mothers in their breastfeeding practices (Smith et al., 2010).Initiation and continuance of breastfeeding can be decided by various factors, including the attitude of the mother, the method of delivery, and support from healthcare. Research has uncovered strong associations of rates of breastfeeding with factors such as the mother's first feeding preference, type of delivery, and interval since birth until initiation of breastfeeding. Mothers, for instance, who are given skin-to-skin contact during delivery are likely to begin breastfeeding, while those receiving formula supplementation are generally dissuaded from exclusive breastfeeding. An awareness of the dynamics between these relationships informs healthcare provider practice, particularly that of nurses, who have a key role in advising new mothers. Training nurses to be more aware and assertive in support of breastfeeding can result in hospital discharge rates of breastfeeding, which will serve as a foundation for ongoing breastfeeding at home (Smith et al., 2010). Breastfeeding also influences long-term health, namely obesity, in childhood. Breastfeeding duration has been associated with infant healthy weight gain, demonstrating its protective role against overweight and later obesity.

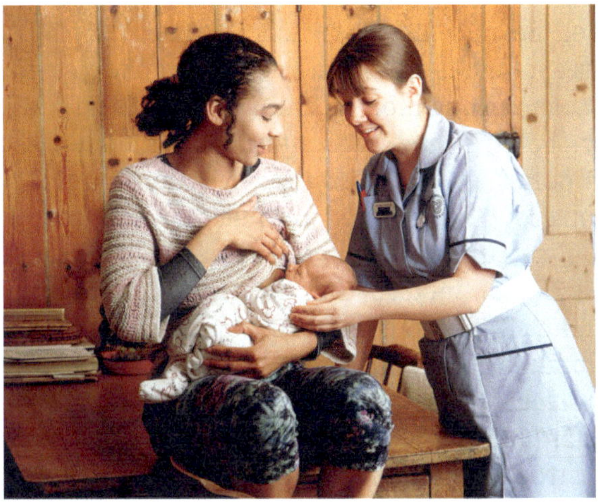

**Figure 3.10.** The role of breastfeeding.

*Source:* https://external-content.duckduckgo.com/iu/?u=https%3A%2F%2Fimages.fineartamerica.com%2Fimages-medium-large-5%2Fmidwife-helps-mother-to-establish-breastfeeding-ruth-jenkinsonmidirsscience-photo-library.jpg&f=1&nofb=1&ipt=b607a6365114ffd9ebcd9338eed86081913c532571a610ec1a5026dc53da2c7a&ipo=images.

High correlations between maternal factors and overweight rates, such as nutrition knowledge and duration of breastfeeding, were found in a study among preschool children. Specifically, the greater duration of breastfeeding for children led to lower overweight risks when parents' weight was adjusted for. This suggests that improving mothers' knowledge of nutrition and the benefits of breastfeeding could be pivotal to preventing obesity in early childhood. By underlining the central role of breastfeeding in pediatric nutrition and its long-term impact on children's health, healthcare practitioners can equip families with the resources necessary to promote healthier weight development from birth to later childhood (Figure 3.10).

### 3.3.1. Benefits of Breastfeeding for Infants

Breastfeeding gives a world of benefits to infants well beyond mere nourishment. To start with, breast milk is specifically formulated to provide maximum nutrition, including the precise balance of proteins, fats, carbohydrates, vitamins, and minerals an infant requires in order to develop and grow. This tailored formula cannot be readily replicated by formula, which may lack the same biological factors that initiate physical and mental development. Additionally, breast milk contains high levels of antibodies and bio active molecules that boost the immune system of an infant, reducing the risk of infections, such as gastroenteritis and respiratory infections. As can be observed from studies by the World Health Organization, such immunological benefits have far-reaching implications for the health of adults, which emphasizes how breastfeeding is a central component of pediatric nutrition (Smith et al., 2010).

In addition, the psychosocial advantages of breastfeeding ensure the overall well-being of infants. Simply breastfeeding contributes to building a good mother-child relationship that provides emotional security and attachment. This feeling of emotional attachment might play a pivotal role in the infants' brains in terms of future developmental implications. Breastfeeding also fosters responsive parenting practices since mothers are more attuned to infants' needs and cues when they are breastfeeding. Additionally, studies show that breastfed infants are less anxious and more sociable compared to formula-fed infants. Therefore, breastfeeding promotion not only contributes to physical health but also fosters emotional and social development, hence enriching the overall pediatric nutrition system (Montalto et al., 2002). The ultimate impact of increased breastfeeding on society in the long run should not be underestimated. With increasing proof of its benefit to the health of infants and mothers, public health has increasingly emphasized promoting breastfeeding as routine in society.

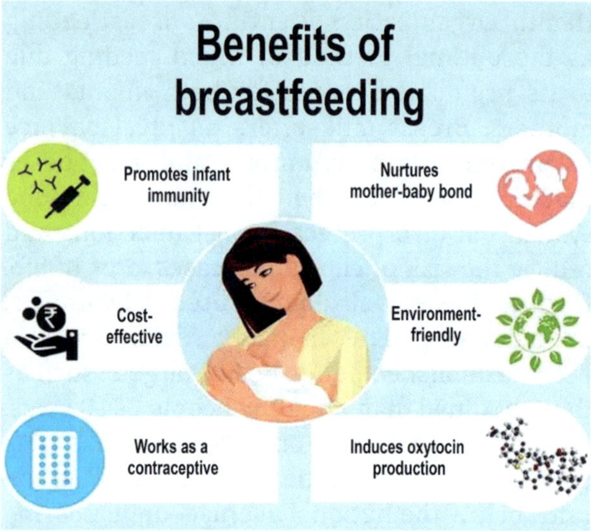


**Figure 3.11.** Benefits of breastfeeding for infants.

*Source:* https://femina.wwmindia.com/content/2018/aug/info1533210087.jpg.

Higher rates of breastfeeding can mean reduced healthcare costs associated with infant illness and can also reduce burdens on the healthcare system. In addition, bridging the gaps in breastfeeding rates, particularly where the rates are extremely low, can contribute to increased health equity. To address these challenges, coordinated action like improved education for parents and caregivers, flexibility in the workplace, and community support initiatives is essential. By embracing comprehensive strategies to promote and protect breastfeeding, society stands to gain considerably in both immediate health benefits to babies and long-term health benefits for future generations (Smith et al., 2010) (Figure 3.11).

### 3.3.2. Recommended Duration of Breastfeeding

Breastfeeding has been accepted worldwide as a fundamental component of child feeding, with overwhelming empirical evidence attesting to its universal health benefits among infants and mothers. Exclusively promoting breastfeeding in the first six months, supplemented by continued breastfeeding along with appropriate complementary foods to two years or beyond, is advocated by bodies like the World Health Organization. This is a recommendation on the grounds that breast milk offers essential nutrients and antibodies that favor healthy development and growth and enhance immune function. Various studies have indicated that babies who are exclusively breastfed during this critical period have less risk of acute infections, obesity, and chronic diseases in later life, such as asthma and ear infections. These remarks underscore the paramount importance of maintaining adherence to norms of breastfeeding length as a fundamental element of pediatric health policy, particularly for public health programs aimed at promoting levels of breastfeeding among diverse populations. The impact of maternal influences on breastfeeding length cannot be minimized, especially in the context of socioeconomic inequalities that routinely erode compliance with prescribed norms. Research has established maternal pre-pregnancy body mass index (BMI), pregnancy weight gain, and education to be critical determinants of breastfeeding practices. For instance, children of mothers with higher pre-pregnancy BMI or women who gain excess weight during pregnancy are at a higher risk of developing obesity, showing the interplay between child nutrition and maternal behavior. Also, it has been established that longer periods of breastfeeding are linked with decreased childhood obesity levels, thus putting emphasis on the need for targeted support for mothers, especially among poor communities. Reducing maternal weight-associated behavior through counseling can assist in supporting more compliance and awareness of appropriate duration of breastfeeding, confirming breastfeeding as a protective agent against early childhood obesity (Garnier-Villarreal et al., 2019). Despite the apparent advantages associated with breastfeeding, the United States demonstrates alarming disparities in breastfeeding prevalence and durations among racial and ethnic groups.

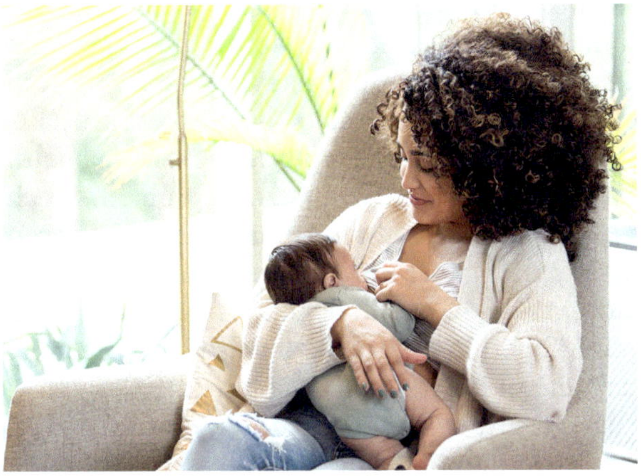

**Figure 3.12.** A mother breastfeeds her infant in a calm, supportive environment, highlighting the importance of maternal bonding and optimal infant nutrition.

*Source:* https://www.themotherbabycenter.org/assets/img/breastfeeding_fb.png.

Evidence indicates that minority women, particularly those of lower income, often face severe barriers to initiating and maintaining breastfeeding, resulting in exacerbation of nutritional inequalities. Effective interventions must place priority on education, providing access to resources, and developing an awareness of the benefits of breastfeeding following the neonatal period. By establishing an environment that fosters favorable practices, such as workplace accommodations for breastfeeding women and community outreach programs tailored for culturally diverse populations, physicians can ensure adherence to recommended breastfeeding durations. Hence, this combined strategy not only improves the health of mothers but also helps in developing healthier babies, thereby reducing the transmission of obesity and other health disparities among children in such groups (Coker et al., 2020) (Figure 3.12).

### 3.3.3. Challenges and Solutions for Breastfeeding Mothers

Mothers' breastfeeding experience may be complicated by a multitude of problems that discourage them from achieving their expected breastfeeding results. Major among these are pain, stigma, and a lack of proper support from health care professionals. For instance, problems such as difficulty latching or painful engorgement can lead to early cessation of breastfeeding, which hides its infant health benefits. Additionally, the general public's attitudes toward breastfeeding can deter mothers from breastfeeding altogether. Public attitudes also call for more education and training of healthcare professionals, as they play a crucial role in offering advice and addressing these issues. By ensuring an enabling environment, women are more likely to look for help, ultimately leading to sustainability and the duration of breastfeeding. In addressing these problems, some efficient interventions have been discovered that can greatly benefit breastfeeding mothers. One such effective strategy is through the use of peer support schemes that connect experienced breastfeeding mothers with problem mothers. This model has been discovered to facilitate knowledge transfer and emotional assistance, thereby increasing the confidence of mothers. Further, community-based education can educate the public on breastfeeding, making breastfeeding common and acceptable. A good example of an interesting case is the ECNAPP in remote Aboriginal communities of Australia that demonstrates an overall strategy to maternal and child nutrition, i.e., supportive breastfeeding through peer counseling and nutrition education at a community level (Goday et al., 2019). These programs not only empower women but also ensure overall acceptance of breastfeeding in society. Besides, availability of resource persons such as lactation consultants and community health services is required in overcoming breastfeeding obstacles. Maternity homes and health facilities can adopt care models that prioritize breastfeeding support, where new mothers are given hands-on assistance soon after giving birth. For instance, maternity care programs that integrate breastfeeding education with prenatal and postnatal care can render maternal care more effective (Cook et al., 2009). These generic approaches have the potential to enhance the process of breastfeeding by directly confronting individual problems and providing solutions according to individual needs. Ultimately, a culture of breastfeeding through effective support channels and material accessibility is necessary to uphold pediatric nutrition and empower mothers to overcome effectively the individuality of breastfeeding.

## Test Your Knowledge

1. What are two key benefits of breastfeeding for infants?
2. What is the recommended duration for exclusive breastfeeding, and name one common challenge breastfeeding mothers may face?

## 3.4. Introduction of Solid Foods

**Learning Outcome**

1. Guidelines for introducing solids;
2. Common first foods and their nutritional value;
3. Signs of readiness for solid foods.

The introduction of solids is a decisive milestone in pediatric diet that structures the growth and development of a child. Often recommended at six months, this process not only adds much-needed nutrients that enhance breast milk or formula but also ensures the learning of healthy eating habits. While feeding the baby, the caregivers are also encouraged to offer a variety of different foods so the babies are exposed to lots of varied flavors and textures, which can limit fussy eating later on. Also, these foods must be nutrient-dense, as they constitute much of a child's physical and intellectual foundation. Both strategic food selection and food ordering are significant contributions to minimizing the risk of allergic reactions, especially laying the groundwork for good eating habits throughout one's lifetime. The initiation of solid foods must be handled with an awareness of cultural and personal family patterns. Various immigrant groups possess varying nutritional histories, which require special education programs adapted to address unique needs and preferences. For example, recent research has found that community-level curricula, including the First Foods program, successfully enhanced caregivers' knowledge and behavior concerning child feeding practices among immigrant families. These classes provide critical information on food safety, healthy eating, and developmental milestones and ultimately create a supportive environment for parents and children alike during this transition. By identifying and integrating a range of cultural food and healthcare habits, clinicians can enhance the effectiveness of nutritional education interventions in producing optimal feeding outcomes among diverse populations. There is evidence that indicates early feeding habits have long-term effects, not just for nutrition but also for the prevention of allergy. A study that had looked into infant dietary habits found a positive correlation between breastfeeding and increased instances of nut allergies, and early exposure to a variety of foods has been suggested to confer protective effects against these allergies. In pediatric nutrition, caregivers have to be cautious while introducing solid food by being on the lookout for potential allergens while promoting diversity in a child's diet. This strategy is consistent with best practice in promoting thoughtful introduction and monitoring of new foods, as a method of enhancing children's acceptance of a wide range of nutrition. With increasingly profound insight into the relationship between early feeding patterns and subsequent health, it serves to support the worth of evidence-based and thoughtful action in bringing about solid food introduction, as a foundation for a lifetime of nutritional well-being (Figure 3.13).

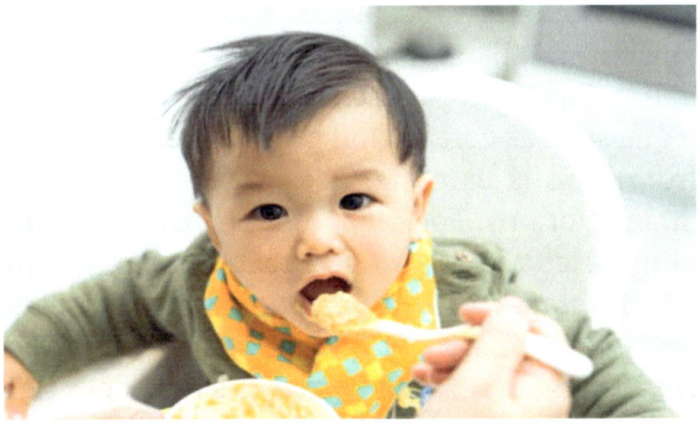

**Figure 3.13.** A baby is spoon-fed soft food while seated in a highchair, representing the transition to solid foods and the development of healthy eating habits in infancy.

*Source:* https://annapolispediatrics.com/sites/default/files/2021-01/AdobeStock_134897673-1-800x533.jpeg.

### 3.4.1. Guidelines for Introducing Solids

The introduction of solid foods into an infant's diet marks a significant milestone in his or her growth and development. Pediatric guidelines are usually that parents introduce this at six months of age when babies present readiness signs such as sitting with support removed, interest in food, and loss of the tongue-thrust reflex. The timing of when to introduce solids is crucial because it can have long-term consequences on nutritional well-being and the risk of developing allergies. Current systematic reviews indicate that introducing solid foods, particularly allergens, at 4 to 6 months is beneficial, in that waiting for their introduction will not lower the risk of allergy but raise it instead (Dipasquale et al., 2019). Thus, establishing the right time is a function of proper balancing of each infant's readiness and nutritional needs. Timing being a secondary issue, the choice of foods introduced during this period is crucial for the proper acquisition of healthy eating habits. The recommended approach is to initiate with single-grain cereals or fruit and vegetable purees and introduce new foods in small amounts to gauge tolerance and liking. Caregivers must focus on iron-fortified foods such as cereals and pureed meats, as iron from food is essential in the development of infants' brains. For older infants, the addition of a variety of flavors and textures can aid in the development of their palate and accept a variety of foods in the long term. It must be ensured that the introduction of solids does not replace breast milk and formula, which are still the principal sources of nutrition until the age of 12 months. Breastfeeding, particularly, has been noted to be associated with numerous health benefits, and continued support of breastfeeding must remain a priority within this transition period (Dipasquale et al., 2019). Moreover, it is important to understand the relation between the introduction of solid foods and allergenic risk in pediatric practice. In accordance with the current evidence, introducing supposedly allergenic foods like eggs and peanuts at the age of 4–6 months reduces allergy risk, particularly for children with a family history of allergy. Pediatricians are responsible for enlightening parents about these guidelines, counseling on the diversity of foods, and referring infants at high risk to be consulted by allergy specialists. A tailored feeding plan based on the infant's family history of allergies and developmental readiness is necessary. This adaptive approach, based on available evidence, ensures optimized nutritional needs at this critical phase and lessens potential allergic effects, thereby providing a favorable environment for appropriate development and growth in early life (Larson et al., 2016).

### 3.4.2. Common First Foods and Their Nutritional Value

Infant solid feeding is a turning point in pediatrics because it is important in establishing good eating habits. Iron-fortified cereal, pureed fruits and vegetables, and small amounts of meats are common first foods. These foods, such as sweet potatoes and applesauce, provide more than essential vitamins and minerals but also expose an infant to a variety of tastes. Iron-fortified cereals are particularly crucial as they offer babies the iron necessary for the growth and development of the brain. Presenting these foods at the optimal stage of development, typically around six months, offers babies a balanced diet that aids in their fast growth at this time, setting them up for healthy eating for the rest of their lives. Cultural influences also make major contributions to establishing the first foods among different populations. For a parent who is an immigrant, adaptation of traditional foods to meet nutritional standards can enhance food adherence and offer familiar flavors that promote acceptance. For instance, in the majority of cultures, rice and lentils, the staple foods of most cuisines, can serve as initial foods, providing carbohydrates and protein for infant growth. Educational interventions, such as the First Foods curriculum highlighted in literature, are found to be effective in improving parents' knowledge regarding appropriate first foods and their nutritional value in children. In most instances, educational interventions aim to bridge knowledge gaps among immigrant populations by emphasizing healthy foods that are acceptable within culture while placing emphasis on nutritional sufficiency (Dawson-Hahn et al., 2019).

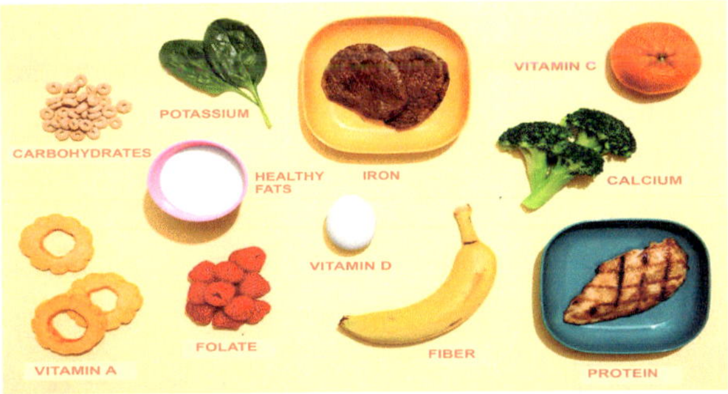


**Figure 3.14.** Common first foods and their nutritional value.

*Source:* https://www.parents.com/thmb/Sab5A1D5IqINfuHit4sv8wfVXjs=/1500x0/filters:no_upscale():max_bytes(150000):strip_icc()/Parents-PRT-must-eat-nutrients-Jordan-Provost-hero-055-2a412c23ec9a4168ba8f04675bd5a5aa.jpg.

Dietary status within children's groups can be very varied by gender and socioeconomic status, and this adds to the picture in pediatrics and nutrition. Studies have identified differences between boys and girls in food intake and lifestyle patterns, with boys often reported to have increased rates of overweight and obesity. This is attributed to dietary lifestyle and access to unhealthy meals, since boys tend to indulge in energy-dense foods as opposed to healthy meals. Moreover, unbalanced diets rich in processed food are likely to fuel such trends, thus pointing towards the need for appropriate nutritional education regarding balanced dietary habits (Andronache et al., 2018). To address these inequalities, the solution must come in the form of multiple ways, such as community involvement and specific educational interventions that foster awareness of shared first foods and nutritional advantages to ensure a healthier future for all children (Figure 3.14).

### 3.4.3. Signs of Readiness for Solid Foods

The introduction of solid foods into an infant's diet is a significant event in pediatric nutrition that should be approached seriously with respect to readiness cues. Typically, around six months old, readiness can be assessed through the demonstration of several clues from the child. Significant clues are sitting with minimal support, having mastery over overhead movement, and showing curiosity about food behavior through reaching out or leaning forward when offered. These changes in the physical body mean that the infant's digestive system is developed enough to include solid foods, which is crucial for nutrient intake and growth. Delaying solids until after six months can lead to nutritional deficiencies because infants require larger amounts of iron and other nutrients that are not necessarily found in breast milk or formula in sufficient quantities. This makes these physical signs of readiness so critical in pediatric nutrition. Also, behavioral signs such as the child's reaction to food can assist caregivers in making informed timing decisions regarding the introduction of solid foods. Infants show natural interest in food by watching as the family members eat or demonstrating fascination with the discovery of new textures and flavors. It is essential to differentiate between hunger cues and mere curiosity, as this will enable the caregiver to provide foods appropriate for the child's age at the appropriate time. Inappropriately introducing solids too early, for example, has the possibility of creating issues in the formation of a healthy eating pattern later in life, as the infant will have developed a tolerance for sweeter or more highly processed diets. Education of caregivers about these signs, especially in multiculturally diverse patient populations where differences in cultural practice may influence feeding, is central to the promotion of healthy eating behaviors and prevention of obesity-related morbidity beginning in infancy, as reported by Mecklenburg (2022). Emotional readiness on the child's part is also an important consideration in addition to behavioral and physical signs. Infants must also have some comfort and predisposition to experiment with new foods, facilitated by positive meal experiences with caregivers. Setting up a pleasant feeding atmosphere, where the child feels safe enough to refuse or accept a variety of foods, promotes healthy eating behaviors. This is particularly important in immigrant populations, since cultural feelings about feeding habits may be quite different from those in the general community. Tailored nutrition education programs, such as the First Foods caregiver training curriculum for immigrant caregivers, could enhance infant feeding developmental milestone knowledge and enhance confidence in infant nutrition care. Framing instruction on readiness cues and social-cultural feeding environments, caregivers could best foster healthy eating behaviors that are associated with long-term health, which aligns with targets outlined by Dawson-Hahn et al. (2019).

### Test Your Knowledge

1. What are two signs that a baby is ready to start eating solid foods?
2. Name one common first solid food and explain its nutritional benefit.

## 3.5. Impact of Nutrition on Child Development

**Learning Outcome**

1. Physical growth and development;
2. Cognitive development and learning;
3. Emotional and social development.

Nutrition is an essential component that determines child development, impacting not just physical growth but also cognitive ability. Good nutrition is especially vital at times of important growth, particularly early childhood, when foundations for healthy adult health and development are established. Protein, vitamin, and mineral deficiencies can lead to stunted growth, weakened immune systems, and intellectual disability. For instance, malnutrition can adversely affect neurodevelopment with a possibility of lifetime learning disabilities and behavioral issues. The interaction of nutrition and developmental milestones highlights the necessity for particular nutritional interventions that adapt to the specific demands of pediatric populations. It is crucial to realize these dynamics to promote optimal growth trajectories and resistance to various health problems, so that each child is given an opportunity to develop optimally in their early life. Additionally, pediatric feeding disorders (PFDs) have the potential to complicate the child nutrition landscape, exposing the intricacies of providing proper dietary intake. PFDs are a continuum of conditions that limit oral intake to the age-appropriate level, possibly due to medical, nutritional, feeding skill, or psychosocial dysfunction. The inability to come up with a widely accepted definition for such disorders confirms the need for an integrated solution that considers all factors affecting children's feeding behaviors and nutrition status. New studies suggest that a critical analysis of the multifaceted nature of PFDs can be more effective in intervention by identifying functional deficits that can hamper successful feeding. Such global strategies not only address bodily health but also are primarily responsible for psychosocial development, creating a partnership in care for the multifaceted needs of children with feeding disorders, this being expressed in interfacing between medical and developmental paradigms in pediatrics (Goday et al., 2019). Beyond the home setting, in such locations as pediatric intensive care units, the challenges of providing perfect nutrition to critically ill children are evident.

It seems that a majority of pediatric patients receive delayed enteral nutrition (EN) progression, as per studies, and that this may interfere with the healing and growth of these children. Particularly, congenital heart defect patients may have more hours of fasting and deteriorated nutrient intake compared to controls, reflecting differences in nutritional support practice between clinical environments. The results emphasize the optimization of enteral feeding over other forms of fluid delivery to effectively achieve nutritional goals. By giving proper and timely nutritional care, clinicians can significantly influence patient outcomes, thus creating more favorable developmental trajectories and enhanced quality of life in critically ill children (Slater et al., 2014) (Figure 3.15).

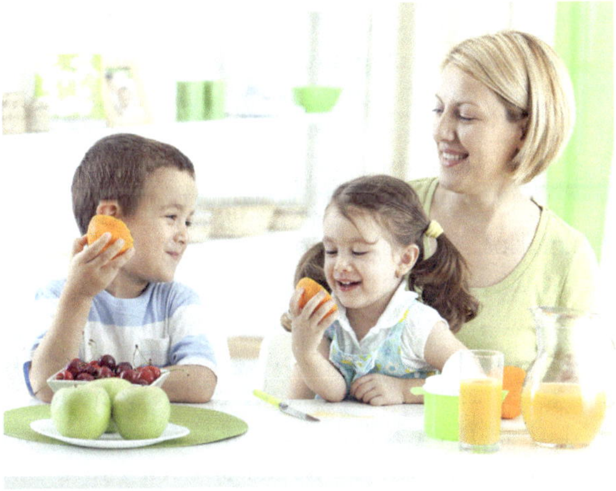

**Figure 3.15.** Impact of nutrition on child development.

*Source:* https://novakdjokovicfoundation.org/wp-content/uploads/2016/09/children-eating-healthy-nutrition.jpg.

### 3.5.1. Physical Growth and Development

Knowing about children's physical growth and development is significant, especially as it applies to infant feeding patterns and pediatric nutrition. During the first few years of life, children experience a great deal of height and weight increase, positioning them for future overall health. Nutrition plays a critical role in this process because it allows for the proper nutrients that are needed for physical and mental growth. A well-balanced diet rich in macro-nutrients like carbohydrates, proteins, and fats and micro-nutrients is essential during these initial years of development. Furthermore, variations in growth rates are governed by genes, environment, and economic and social status, requiring individualized nutritional assessments for maximum growth. Shortfalls in nutritional supply can lead to adverse growth outcomes, impacting not only physical stature but also psychosocial functioning. Infancy and early childhood eating habits significantly affect long-term development and health conditions. Pediatric Feeding Disorders (PFDs) are a critical area of concern that is characterized by non-age-appropriate oral intake that is impaired. The disorders can occur as a result of intricate factors like medical, psychosocial, and feeding skill-related conditions, which are associated with nutritional problems. The International Classification of Functioning of the World Health Organization provides a model for conceptualizing PFDs and, importantly, identifying the necessity for global assessment and intervention. Treatment of the functional limitations in such disorders, with interventions tailored to the unique needs of each child, can be undertaken by health care providers. Hence, effective feeding disorder management is crucial to promote healthy growth patterns and a better quality of life for these children (Goday et al., 2019). In later childhood and adolescence, the growth patterns alter, typically in concurrence with the occurrence of developmental milestones such as puberty. Nutritional demands rise at this stage, requiring increasing caloric and nutrient uptake to facilitate the augmented physical growth characteristic of growth spurts. Coexistent with this are rising rates of health conditions precipitated by lifestyle issues, such as pediatric obesity and type II diabetes, and the necessity for vigilant nutritional education and intervention (Foering et al., 2018). Parents and caregivers accompany them in their role as the food intake is set by them and dietary habits for healthy living are introduced. Public health interventions to enhance balanced nutrition and physical activity are instrumental in the prevention of chronic diseases, therefore guaranteeing that the children not only achieve their growth potential but also develop into healthy adults capable of performing in the environment where they are.

### 3.5.2. Cognitive Development and Learning

Early childhood cognitive development is primarily influenced by a series of factors, one of which is downright essential: diet. An adequate diet provides the platform for brain growth and function, particularly at the critical stages of life. Macro-nutrients such as omega-3 fatty acids, vitamins, minerals, and proteins are important in various cognitive processes, including memory, attention, and problem-solving capacity. During this period, children's brains undergo rapid synaptic and neuronal growth, which is compromised when the diet is not sufficient. Therefore, a diet that is rich in nutrients supports the formation of good brain architecture and enhances cognitive processes, ultimately affecting learning. Children who are nutrition-deficient may present with impairments in learning and delayed milestones in cognitive development, highlighting the necessity of pediatric nutrition in learning and cognitive development. Intrauterine growth restriction (IUGR) further complicates the interaction of nutrition and cognitive development. IUGR newborns develop severe neurodevelopmental issues, which are attributed to poor nutrition during fetal growth. The literature reports that IUGR has been attributed to white matter and neuronal injury in the neonatal brain, influencing cognitive function in later life. Specifically, variations in the GABA receptor expression in the brains of IUGR infants can be largely accountable for cognitive disabilities. As noted in earlier studies, GABA receptors play a key role in neurodevelopment and dysfunctional GABAnergic systems may be accountable for cognitive disabilities recurrently observed in IUGR populations (Bjorkman et al., 2017). Thus, intervention in nutritional factors during pregnancy and early infancy is of utmost importance to counteract these risks and optimize cognitive development. To promote effective cognitive development in children, interventions must give high priority to nutrition in different stages of growth. Pediatric nutrition must not just ensure minimum dietary requirements but also improve the quality of nutrients to better facilitate cognitive functions. Early identification and treatment for high-risk individuals, for example, with a history of IUGR, can be key to ensuring the best possible brain health and cognitive development. Investing in parent education on the importance of nutrient-dense diets can empower parents to make informed decisions that shape their children's developmental trajectory. In addition, healthcare professionals must be educated in the role of nutrition in cognitive development so that they are able to facilitate policies supportive of better maternal and child nutrition (Bjorkman et al., 2017). Ultimately, an integrated approach to pediatric nutrition can result in spectacular improvement in cognitive learning outcomes (Figure 3.16).

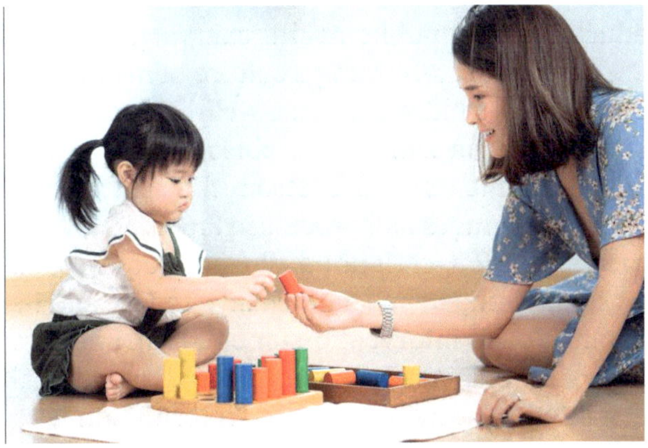

**Figure 3.16.** Cognitive development and learning.

*Source:* https://childdevelopmentinfo.com/wp-content/uploads/2022/03/cognitive-development-min-scaled.jpg.

### 3.5.3. Emotional and Social Development

Children's social and emotional growth is highly interlinked with their feeding behavior and nutrition. The early experiences of children towards food have an enormous impact on shaping the emotional well-being as well as the social interaction of a child. If children are exposed to responsive and secure relationships during meals, they are likely to have a positive relationship with food. A caregiving environment promotes the sense of safety and belonging, which are a high priority for emotional health. Therefore, the emotional feeding environment cannot be overlooked in the diet of children since meals could be a source of social encounter and development.

Furthermore, when children experience positive feeding interactions, they can better regulate social situations and develop peer relationships, which further enhance their emotional resilience. The concept of Pediatric Feeding Disorder (PFD) addresses the medical, nutritional, psychosocial, and feeding skill domains that impair a child's ability to eat in an age-appropriate manner. Dyssynchrony in any of these domains can lead to emotional and social impairment. For instance, children with eating difficulties or restrictive eating can become isolated at mealtime, and this can lead to self-esteem problems or shame among peers. Intervening in these multi-faceted issues requires a holistic approach as outlined in the proposed definition of PFD that underscores the importance of addressing various areas that impact feeding.

Merging this multi-faceted perspective with intervention and treatment plans implies that practitioners can provide services to children by not only addressing physical feeding issues but also emotional and social needs (Goday et al., 2019). In order to further highlight the interrelation between nutrition and emotional development, early childhood policies should endeavor to create contexts that promote nurturing relationships and proper nutritional practices. This calls for grounding stable and responsive caregiving within feeding environments as well as ensuring access to healthful food. Such an approach has a far-reaching effect on children's lifetime health and increased social competence. As noted, supportive and safe environments along with healthy diets are essential in ensuring all-around development of the child (Goday et al., 2019). Through the acknowledgment of the central role emotional and social factors have in childhood eating and nutrition, caregivers and medical professionals can help develop healthier, well-adjusted children to thrive in every aspect of their lives.

## Test Your Knowledge

1. How does good nutrition support a child's physical growth and development?
2. Name one-way proper nutrition can influence a child's cognitive or emotional development.

## 3.6. Addressing Pediatric Obesity

**Learning Outcome**

1. Causes and risk factors of pediatric obesity;
2. Strategies for prevention and management;
3. Role of family and community in promoting healthy habits.

Childhood obesity necessitates a multi-component intervention comprising effective food behavior and awareness of the socio-environmental determinants of children's diet. In the past decades, the prevalence of obesity among children has increased sharply, primarily because of greater consumption of energy-dense foods and reduced physical activity. To curb this increase, health professionals and policy makers have persistently advocated the creation of healthy eating-promoting environments. This calls for not only educating parents about nutrition choices but also enacting community-level initiatives, such as school-based nutrition education and public health campaigns. These are aimed at establishing a culture of health that encourages children to make well-balanced food choices rich in fruits, vegetables, whole grains, and lean meats and restrict their intake of sugary beverages and processed foods. Following the debate on childhood obesity requires an understanding of behavior change theory and its application to intervention for children. Effective interventions need to embrace psychological insight into motivation and habit formation with practical resources for families to develop better eating habits. Psychological factors have been consistently recommended by agencies such as NICE and SIGN, highlighting their crucial role in successful weight management among children. Nevertheless, a commissioned review by NHS Health Scotland indicates inadequate evidence on the effectiveness of some behavior techniques. Such inadequacy implies an immediate need for research to establish which intervention would work best, as well as recommendations on what skills and competencies are necessary for healthcare practitioners in guiding childhood obesity intervention programs towards improved health outcomes in populations. Additionally, there has to be collaboration between multiple stakeholders for developing sustainable solutions towards fighting pediatric obesity. Policymakers, educators, parents, and health professionals must collaborate in developing and implementing health weight intervention programs that address the multifaceted needs of populations. The establishment of the CPRC and the NICHQ Childhood Obesity Action Network was a milestone in forging cooperation and sharing of effective practices at national conferences, such as the Second Childhood Obesity Congress in Miami in 2008. Promoting community engagement in such initiatives not only helps tailor interventions to local nuances but also establishes collective responsibility between institutions and families in shaping children's well-being. While we strive to achieve remarkable reductions in childhood obesity, it is critical that we put these collaborative strategies into action while monitoring their effectiveness continuously, building the foundation for healthier generations (Figure 3.17).

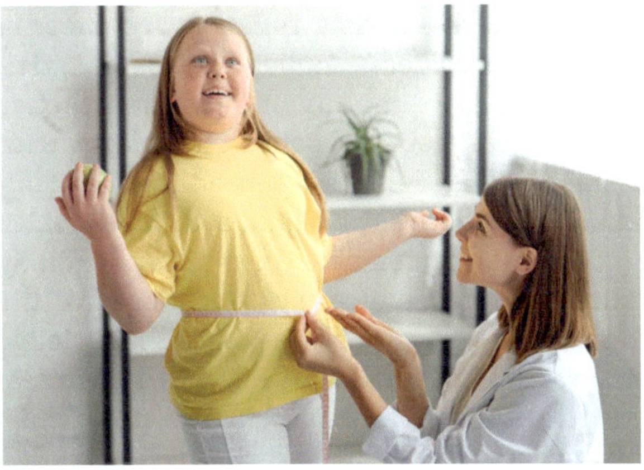

**Figure 3.17.** A healthcare professional measures a smiling child's waist circumference as part of a wellness assessment, emphasizing the importance of healthy lifestyle habits and positive body image.

*Source:* https://www.thuas.com/sites/hhs/files/2022-10/HI-project-overgewicht.jpg.

### 3.6.1. Causes and Risk Factors of Pediatric Obesity

Pediatric obesity has a multifactorial etiology that includes a spectrum of genetic, environmental, and behavior-related causes. Among these, diet-related causes are the prime reason for obesity, with increased reliance on carbohydrate-rich and lipid-rich foods increasing calorie excess. Additionally, the ready accessibility of fast foods enables one to avail oneself of poor meals with too low an intake of nutrients required for growth and development. This trend is often further exacerbated by socioeconomic status because lower-income families may not have access to affordable, quality food and nutrition education. The combination of these eating habits with the built environment, such as neighborhoods with insufficient safe spaces for physical activity, contributes to the risk. Understanding these causes is essential to designing effective interventions against pediatric obesity, particularly in building supportive environments for healthier habits and active living. Psychosocial issues also contribute significantly to obesity in children. Children who are distressed or come from dysfunctional families tend to use eating as a coping mechanism, and they end up overeating or consuming unhealthy foods. Also, the role of media cannot be underestimated because children are constantly bombarded with advertisements for unhealthy foods and inactivity, such as sitting down and watching television. This interaction results in a vicious cycle in which increased intake of energy-dense foods and decreased physical activity promote excess weight gain. Furthermore, family relationships and parenting style can create or diminish risk factors for obesity. For instance, inadequate parental monitoring of eating habits can lead to unrestricted access to unhealthy food. These psychosocial components are important for the application of family-centered approaches in pediatric nutrition to promote enhanced habits. Finally, pediatric feeding disorders (PFDs) also pose serious problems in managing obesity. PFDs are a group of disorders in which children experience compromised oral intake that compromises their nutritional status and leads to heightened risk for the development of obesity due to maladaptive eating patterns. PFDs have a complex interplay of medical, psychosocial, and skill-based determinants that not only control appetite but also the ability to consume a suitable diet. More understanding of PFDs is needed since early treatment is necessary to prevent the associated nutritional issues that lead to obesity. Through a comprehensive approach that considers the medical, dietetic, and psychosocial needs of the child, health practitioners can come up with customized ways that suitably address obesity in children with feeding problems. Management of these issues holistically emphasizes the need for inter-disciplinary interventions in pediatric feeding and nutrition, therefore promoting healthy outcomes in vulnerable populations (Bernasconi et al., 2019; Goday et al., 2019).

### 3.6.2. Strategies for Prevention and Management

Effective prevention and management of pediatric nutritional complications are crucial factors in ensuring healthy development and reducing the risk of complications. One particular area of concern here is feeding to prevent illnesses like necrotizing enterocolitis (NEC), most commonly occurring in preterm infants. It has been proven through evidence that breast milk is the only proven method of substantially reducing the incidence of NEC, further supporting its significance in the neonatal diet. Although timing and method of introduction of feeds may have some effect, late feed initiation and slow advancement have not been demonstrated to have any specific benefit in preventing NEC. Consequently, further research must be conducted to determine optimal feeding regimes, particularly for neonates born at less than 28 weeks' gestation, who have a greater risk for NEC (Courtney et al., 2020). Such practices need to be confronted directly to establish effective clinical guidelines for children's nutrition. Other than breastfeeding, innovative community-based programs are of paramount importance in treating children's nutritional deficiencies. The Early Childhood Nutrition and Anemia Prevention Project (ECNAPP) demonstrates the significance of multi-component interventions, including miicronutrientsupplementation and peer counseling, especially in underprivileged communities. Working in other areas of Australia, the program demonstrated that with advocacy for nutrition and aid, children's health could be significantly improved. Evaluations of ECNAPP indicated improved knowledge regarding infant feeding behavior and reduction in anemia rates, the latter being one of the contributing issues among Aboriginal populations. These findings emphasize the importance of culturally sensitive interventions and a collaborative effort to enhance nutritional care, reaffirming that community empowerment is critical to effective pediatric nutritional management (Goday et al., 2019). Lastly, pediatric nutrition problems must be addressed as a collaborative effort of healthcare providers, families, and communities. For effective management, healthcare practitioners need to consult regularly with families in developing customized feeding plans, taking into account a child's unique health needs and circumstances. Incorporating family education into medical practice can have the ability to empower parents with the knowledge they require to properly deal with nutritional complications. There is also the possibility, through collaborative work, to determine biomarkers of intestinal recovery in the case of NEC, thus permitting reintroduction of feeds based on patient-specific improvement. By facilitating a synergistic relationship between families and health professionals, pediatric nutrition interventions can be improved, resulting in improved health outcomes and a sound foundation for health throughout life in children (Figure 3.18).

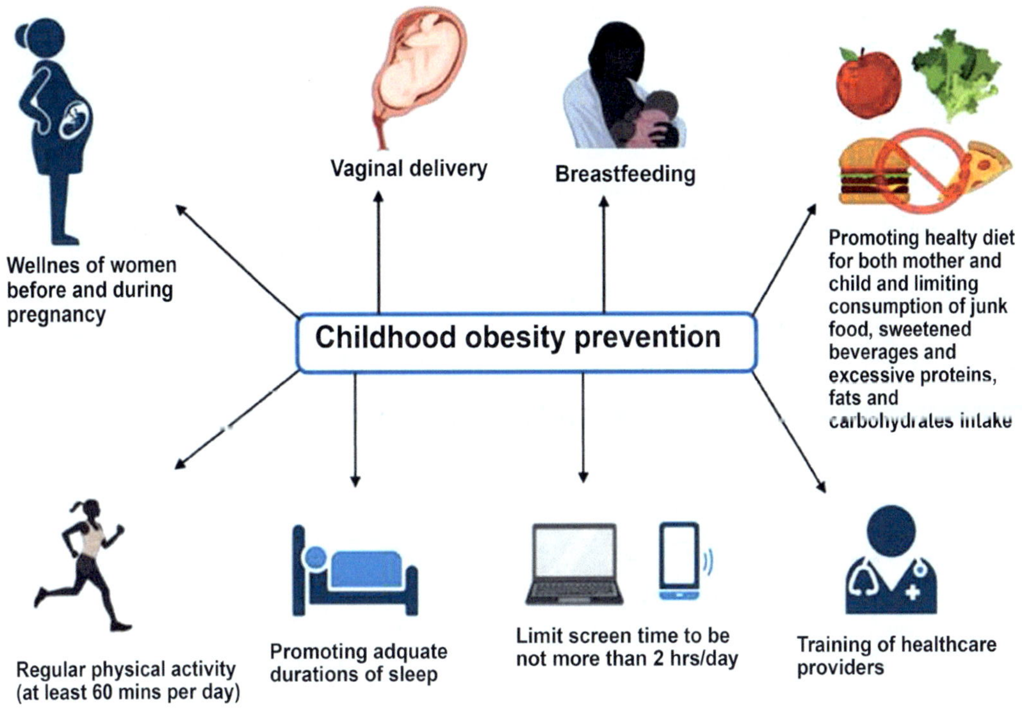


**Figure 3.18.** Risk factors, clinical consequences, prevention, and treatment of childhood obesity.

Source: Shaban Mohamed, M. A., AbouKhatwa, M. M., Saifullah, A. A., Hareez Syahmi, M., Mosaad, M., Elrggal, M. E., Dehele, I. S., & Elnaem, M. H. (2022). Risk Factors, Clinical Consequences, Prevention, and Treatment of Childhood Obesity. *Children*, *9*(12), 1975. https://doi.org/10.3390/children9121975

### 3.6.3. Role of Family and Community in Promoting Healthy Habits

Family and community environments have a big influence on instilling healthy habits in children. Families are the first unit from which children learn their physical lifestyle and diet. Mothers have been proven to be key in instilling eating and exercise behaviors, shaping the lifestyle choices of their children (Porter et al., 2017). This is why it is significant that parents play a role in creating a framework of nutrition and exercise that encourages healthier outcomes for children. When parents themselves are engaged in health-promoting habits, then children are more likely to follow suit and develop these habits themselves, establishing a cycle of healthy living. Therefore, it is vital to empower parents with the information and tools to emulate these habits in order to instill healthy habits throughout the lifespan of their children. The community is instrumental in promoting pediatric nutrition and healthy eating habits. Social networks and local organizations can help families by providing them with access to resources such as exercise programs, cooking programs, and healthy foods. Successful community interventions involving schools, health centers, and recreation centers are essential in creating environments that promote healthier lifestyles. For example, studies have revealed that coordinated school programs that include nutrition education along with physical activity can impact the attitudes of children toward healthier habits (Goday et al., 2019). Through forging partnerships between community agencies and families, children can benefit from needed support, guidance, and encouragement, thus enhancing their potential to adopt healthier habits. Additionally, family and community partnerships are essential to address public health problems, such as childhood obesity. Where communities are aware of the prevalence of unhealthful behaviors, they can formulate targeted public health education programs that have significance concerning cultural behaviors and customs. For instance, large variations in activity and eating patterns between and across ethnic groups underscore the need for education programs that are culturally sensitized to engage families effectively (Porter et al., 2017). Public health practitioners are able to align interventions with assets present in communities and so allowing children to make better choices and enable families to take control of their well-being. Hence, the symbiotic relationship between the community and family interventions plays a critical role in developing long-term healthy behavior among children to provide long-term health dividends that persist into adult life.

## Test Your Knowledge

1. What are two common causes or risk factors of pediatric obesity?
2. How can families and communities help prevent or manage pediatric obesity?

## SUMMARY

The magnitude of quality pediatric nutrition and feeding patterns cannot be overstated, since they determine health and development in childhood and throughout life. Nutrition at critical growth periods influences not only bodily health but intellectual and emotional growth in children as well. Long-term programs such as home visiting programs for high-risk families emphasize the priority of personalized nutritional guidance with consideration of varied family environments and requirements. By engaging parents as part of the decision-making process for nutrition strategies, programs are more likely to achieve positive outcomes. The fact that evidence-based strategies prove this assertion warrants that an integrated strategy has higher compliance with dietary recommendations and improved well-being. Reviews of literature also present evidence that the mode of delivery of nutritional care and education has a significant influence over their efficacy. Literature on home visiting programs is such that the relational processes between service providers and families can enhance or detract from outcomes. Partner-based involvement is central, illustrated through CCCH's reviews of the literature, which indicate that process-related aspects of service delivery are as important as the content being transmitted. When carers are empowered and appreciated, they are likely to embrace recommended nutritional practice, thus healthy eating by the children in the long term. Finally, novel education schemes such as FEED Safe in Zambia emphasize the global need for extensive access to nutritional education by all families, especially those with children who have disabilities. These programs not only provide caregivers with foundational knowledge but also enable a learning culture where the caregivers can exchange ideas and practices. This collaborative model of learning empowers the caregivers and provides them with the skill sets necessary to address the nutritional requirements of their children adequately. Addressing pediatric nutrition using holistic and integrated approaches ensures that all children are provided with an opportunity to excel and provide a benchmark for upcoming generations in a pluralistic cultural context.

In pediatric nutrition, there is a need to comprehend the mechanisms and implications of feeding to ensure proper growth and development in children. Nutrition support is particularly critical following medical interventions such as hematopoietic stem cell transplantation (HSCT), where children experience profound side effects such as anorexia and nausea. These side effects restrain oral consumption and even lead to malnutrition, necessitating the administration of nutrition support to prevent these complications. Previously, parenteral nutrition (PN) was the preferred approach; however, more recent studies are advocating the use of enteral nutrition (EN) as a major player. EN has been seen to possess potential benefits in reducing complications such as acute graft-versus-host disease (aGVHD) as well as improving platelet engraftment, showing signs of change in the practice of nutritional care of children undergoing HSCT (Evans et al., 2019). Additionally, nutritional screening is a key element in pediatric practice because it ensures early identification of at-risk children for malnutrition. Understanding the disproportionate burden of childhood obesity and the heterogeneity of nutritional needs across the life span is essential for healthcare providers. Proper balance among nutrients can act as a buffer against both undernutrition and obesity risks, thus ensuring that the dietary intake of children aligns with their developmental needs. Embracing good meal planning and accommodation of varied nutritional requirements and limitations is essential, especially in multiracial groups. This way, not just the physical health is guaranteed but also psychological well-being in kids, and nutrition is an important aspect of total pediatric management (Coxall et al., 2008). Of additional significance is the fact that pediatric nutrition needs to take into consideration the unique challenge posed by pediatric disease and its treatment, such as HSCT. The intersection of disease and nutrition necessitates targeted dietary therapy that meets the child's physiological and psychological needs. Not only can the nutritional quality, but the delivery route as well, impact the result of recovery and general pediatric health. Current literature highlights the importance of recognizing that both EN and PN constitute nutritional intervention, though the subtle effects and potential complications inherent in their delivery necessitate ongoing study. This covers not only the effectiveness of different nutritional interventions but also their effects on post-treatment survival and quality of life in children, enabling more tailored treatment of children's nutrition (Evans et al., 2019).

## KEY TERMS FROM THIS CHAPTER

- Breastfeeding
- Dysphagia
- Macronutrients
- Micronutrients
- Nutrition management
- Pediatric nutrition
- Public health strategies
- Cognitive function
- Health professionals
- Malnutrition
- Necrotizing enterocolitis (NEC)
- Pediatric feeding disorders (PFDs)
- Promote optimal growth
- Undernutrition

## CRITICAL THINKING QUESTIONS

1. **Which nutrient is essential for brain development in infants?**
   a. Vitamin C
   b. Iron
   c. Fiber
   d. Sodium
2. **At what age is it generally recommended to introduce solid foods to an infant's diet?**
   a. 2 months
   b. 4–6 months
   c. 9–12 months
   d. 1 year
3. **Which of the following is the best source of nutrition for newborns?**
   a. Cow's milk
   b. Breast milk or infant formula
   c. Fruit juices
   d. Solid baby food
4. **Which vitamin is crucial for calcium absorption and bone development in children?**
   a. Vitamin A
   b. Vitamin D
   c. Vitamin K
   d. Vitamin B12
5. **Which feeding practice is recommended to reduce the risk of choking in young children?**
   a. Allowing children to eat while playing
   b. Giving large pieces of food
   c. Encouraging slow, supervised eating
   d. Letting children eat while lying down

### Short Answer Questions

1. What are the key nutritional needs for infants, toddlers, school-aged children, and adolescents?
2. How does breastfeeding compare to formula feeding in terms of nutritional benefits?
3. What are the recommended caloric and protein intake levels for different pediatric age groups?
4. What are the signs and symptoms of malnutrition in children?
5. How can a balanced diet help in a child's growth and development?

### *Answers to Critical Thinking Questions*

1. (b) 2. (b) 3. (b) 4. (b) 5. (c)

## REFERENCES


1. Adamson, A., Fletcher, S., Jones, A., Parkinson, K., et al. (2016). Tracking of toddler fruit and vegetable preferences to intake and adiposity later in childhood. https://core.ac.uk/download/161100869.pdf (accessed on 16th June 2025).
2. Andronache, L. F., Arsene, A., Badiu, C. D., Ditu, M., et al. (2018). Dietary habits and lifestyle in school-aged children from Bucharest, Romania. https://core.ac.uk/download/216808125.pdf (accessed on 16th June 2025).
3. Aquino, D. (2025). Early childhood nutrition and anemia prevention project: Summary report June 2013. https://core.ac.uk/download/pdf/30675892.pdf (accessed on 16th June 2025).
4. Becker, C., Crawford, P. B., & Pirotin, S. (2014). Looking beyond the marketing claims of new beverages: Health risks of consuming sports drinks, energy drinks, fortified waters, and other flavored beverages. https://core.ac.uk/download/75778515.pdf (accessed on 16th June 2025).
5. Bjorkman, S. T., Colditz, P. B., Kalanjati, V. P., Miller, S., et al. (2017). GABAA receptor expression and white matter disruption in intrauterine growth restricted piglets. https://core.ac.uk/download/83983517.pdf (accessed on 16th June 2025).
6. Goday, P. S., Huh, S. Y., Silverman, A., Lukens, C. T., Dodrill, P., Cohen, S. S., Delaney, A. L., Feuling, M. B., Noel, R. J., Gisel, E., Kenzer, A., Kessler, D. B., Kraus de Camargo, O., Browne, J., & Phalen, J. A. (2019). Pediatric Feeding Disorder: Consensus Definition and Conceptual Framework. *Journal of pediatric gastroenterology and nutrition*, *68*(1), 124–129. https://doi.org/10.1097/MPG.0000000000002188(accessed on 16th June 2025).
7. Burnham, J. M., & von Scheven, E. (2011). Vitamin D supplementation in the pediatric rheumatology clinic. https://core.ac.uk/download/323072035.pdf (accessed on 16th June 2025).
8. Cannon, K. R., Ryan, B., & Stowe, M. (2018). Consideration for care for your patient with cerebral palsy. https://core.ac.uk/download/215483266.pdf (accessed on 16th June 2025).
9. Ciszek, K., Ding, P., Kljakovic, M., Paton, K., et al. (2015). Infant feeding practices and nut allergy over time in Australian school entrant children. https://core.ac.uk/download/156621000.pdf (accessed on 16th June 2025).
10. Coker, S. (2020). Determining racial and ethnic disparities in breastfeeding in the United States. https://core.ac.uk/download/322958902.pdf (accessed on 16th June 2025).
11. Cook, A., & Palmer, L. (2009). Providing maternity care to the underserved: A comparative case study of three maternity care models serving women in Washington, D.C. https://core.ac.uk/download/71348405.pdf (accessed on 16th June 2025).
12. Dipasquale, V., Serra, G., Corsello, G., & Romano, C. (2020). Standard and Specialized Infant Formulas in Europe: Making, Marketing, and Health Outcomes. *Nutrition in clinical practice : official publication of the American Society for Parenteral and Enteral Nutrition*, *35*(2), 273–281. https://doi.org/10.1002/ncp.10261 (accessed on 16th June 2025).
13. Courtney, C. M., Ou, J., Steinberger, A. E., Tecos, M., et al. (2020). Nutrition in necrotizing enterocolitis and following intestinal resection. https://core.ac.uk/download/287888117.pdf (accessed on 16th June 2025).

14. Coxall, K., Dawes, E., Forsyth, E., Lloyd, M., et al. (2008). Applying the key principles of nutrition to nursing practice. https://core.ac.uk/download/4145815.pdf (accessed on 16th June 2025).

15. Dadich, A., Disher-Quill, K., Elliot, C., Frederiksen, A., et al. (2021). Pediatric tube-feeding: An agenda for care improvement and research. https://opus.lib.uts.edu.au/bitstream/10453/151380/2/Binder2.pdf (accessed on 16th June 2025).

16. Darby, M. L., Fuller, L. A., Stull, S. C., Tolle, S., et al. (2014). Oral health promotion: Knowledge, confidence, and practices in preventing early-severe childhood caries of Virginia WIC program personnel. https://core.ac.uk/download/217284850.pdf (accessed on 16th June 2025).

17. Dawson-Hahn, E. E., Farmer, B., et al. (2019). First Foods Nutrition Curriculum for New Immigrant Families: A pilot study. https://core.ac.uk/download/228022797.pdf (accessed on 16th June 2025).

18. Dimitrov, L., Dzhogova, M., Eubova, S., Hristanova, D., et al. (2023). Comprehensive review of assessment tools for nutrition and feeding practices in early childhood: Applications, strengths, and limitations. https://core.ac.uk/download/616882122.pdf (accessed on 16th June 2025).

19. Evans, J. C., Hirani, S. P., & Needle, J. J. (2019). Nutritional and Post-Transplantation Outcomes of Enteral versus Parenteral Nutrition in Pediatric Hematopoietic Stem Cell Transplantation: A Systematic Review of Randomized and Nonrandomized Studies. *Biology of blood and marrow transplantation : journal of the American Society for Blood and Marrow Transplantation*, *25*(8), e252–e259. https://doi.org/10.1016/j.bbmt.2019.02.023(accessed on 16th June 2025).

20. Fairchild, K. S. (2021). FEED Safe: Functional Eating Education for family caregivers of children with disabilities in Lusaka, Zambia. https://core.ac.uk/download/519800744.pdf (accessed on 16th June 2025).

21. Foering, A. (2018). Pediatric type II diabetes mellitus: Examining the upward trend. https://core.ac.uk/download/158970346.pdf (accessed on 16th June 2025).

22. Garnier-Villarreal, M., Ohlendorf, J. M., & Robinson, K. M. (2019). The impact of maternal BMI, gestational weight gain, and breastfeeding on early childhood weight: Analysis of a statewide WIC dataset. https://core.ac.uk/download/286544060.pdf (accessed on 16th June 2025).

23. Griffin, S., Hardeman, W., Kinmonth, A. L., Lakshman, R., et al. (2014). Using the Medical Research Council framework for the development and evaluation of complex interventions in a theory-based infant feeding intervention to prevent childhood obesity: The baby milk intervention and trial. https://core.ac.uk/download/41990954.pdf (accessed on 16th June 2025).

24. Larson, K., McLaughlin, J., Stonehouse, M., Young, B., & Haglund, K. (2017). Introducing Allergenic Food into Infants' Diets: Systematic Review. *MCN. The American journal of maternal child nursing*, *42*(2), 72–80. https://doi.org/10.1097/NMC.0000000000000313(accessed on 16th June 2025).

25. Herrador-López, M., Martin-Masot, R., Navas-López, V. M., Ortiz Pérez, M., et al. (2024). Nutritional issues in children with dysphagia. https://core.ac.uk/download/621567739.pdf (accessed on 16th June 2025).

26. Ibrahim, K. (2022). Prevalence of anemia and factors affecting its management strategies among children below five years at Mityana general hospital, Mityana district. A cross-sectional study. https://core.ac.uk/download/552646462.pdf (accessed on 16th June 2025).

27. Sunguya, B. F., Poudel, K. C., Mlunde, L. B., Urassa, D. P., Yasuoka, J., & Jimba, M. (2013). Nutrition training improves health workers' nutrition knowledge and competence to manage child undernutrition: a systematic review. *Frontiers in public health*, *1*, 37. https://doi.org/10.3389/fpubh.2013.00037(accessed on 16th June 2025).

28. Jones, L. D. (2006). Minority adolescents at risk for obesity: Health behaviors and perceptions. https://core.ac.uk/download/223074309.pdf (accessed on 16th June 2025).

29. King, L., & White, H. (2014). Enteral feeding pumps: Efficacy, safety, and patient acceptability. https://core.ac.uk/download/29018498.pdf (accessed on 16th June 2025).

30. McDonald, M., Sanjeevan, S., & Moore, T. G. (2025). Evidence-based service modules for a sustained home visiting program. https://core.ac.uk/download/pdf/30672643.pdf (accessed on 16th June 2025).

31. Mecklenburg, C. (2022). Childhood obesity prevention: Infant nutrition and feeding education. https://core.ac.uk/download/596994611.pdf (accessed on 16th June 2025).

32. Julie. Cooper; Cynthia. Alendy; Lisa. Simpson; Gunther Christina. Murphy(2008). *Childhood Obesity: The Role of Health Policy*. Child Policy Research Center, University of Cincinnati; Robert Wood Johnson Foundation. https://core.ac.uk/download/71342400.pdf(accessed on 16th June 2025).

33. Porter, L. S. (2017). Family eating and physical activity practices among African American, Filipino American, and Hispanic American families: Implications for developing obesity prevention programs. https://digitalscholarship.unlv.edu/cgi/viewcontent.cgi?article=1027&context=apin (accessed on 16th June 2025).

34. Slater, A., Rousseau, A. F., Lambe, C., Young, D., Health, D. O., Rogers, E. J., Gentles, E., et al. (2014). An evaluation of enteral nutrition practices and nutritional provision in children during the entire length of stay in critical care. https://core.ac.uk/download/20480255.pdf (accessed on 16th June 2025).

35. Smith, M. (2010). Factors influencing breastfeeding in a hospital setting. https://core.ac.uk/download/84120010.pdf (accessed on 16th June 2025).

# IMMUNIZATION AND PREVENTIVE CARE

# 4

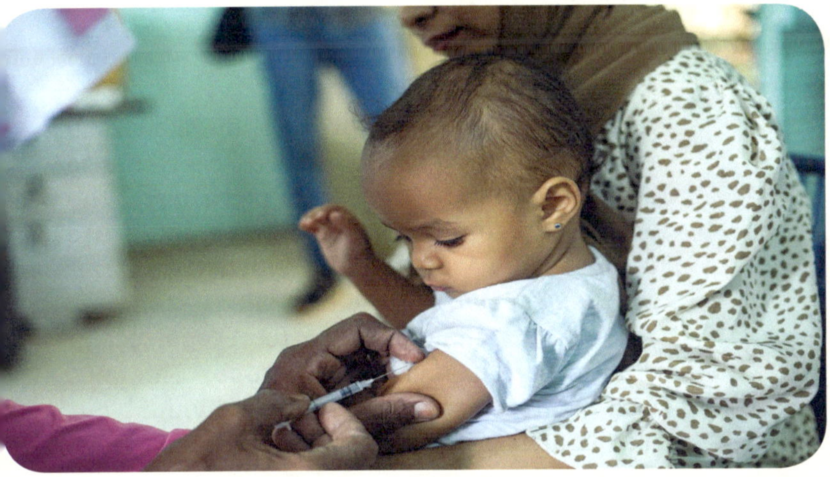

### LEARNING OBJECTIVES

**After studying this chapter, you will be able to:**

1. Discuss the historical context of immunization;
2. Explain the types of vaccines;
3. Define benefits of immunization;
4. Know challenges in immunization;
5. Focus on preventive care beyond immunization;
6. Understand policy and legislation.

## Introduction

The scope of immunization and preventative treatment encompasses an important collection of mechanisms intended to safeguard individual and collective health. Preventative treatment, via the vaccine among other controls, helps to greatly limit infectious disease spread. Community health education programs play a central role in this regard, empowering people with the facts they require regarding preventative behavior, from the necessity for vaccination to a healthful lifestyle. For instance, a study highlighted how well-planned community health education significantly enhanced participants' knowledge about preventive health and practices, with considerable improvement in such behaviors as hand washing and health monitoring. These findings underscore the significance of including health education in preventive care as educated individuals are best positioned to implement interventions that protect not just their health but also that of their communities (Akbar et al., 2025). Immunization is a cornerstone of public health, tremendously preventing morbidity and mortality from preventable diseases. BCG vaccination against tuberculosis is among the oldest and most common vaccinations, targeting high-risk groups. Its application is crucial in the prevention of severe clinical forms of tuberculosis, particularly where rates are high, such as in areas like the Pomoravlje District. The effectiveness of vaccine campaigns may be realized through statistical research that indicates high rates of coverage, including coverage rates for the Pomoravlje District, which were consistently more than 95%. Such data demonstrates the success of national immunization policy, confirming ongoing support for vaccination programs as part of an integrated public health policy (Jovanovi et al., 2023).

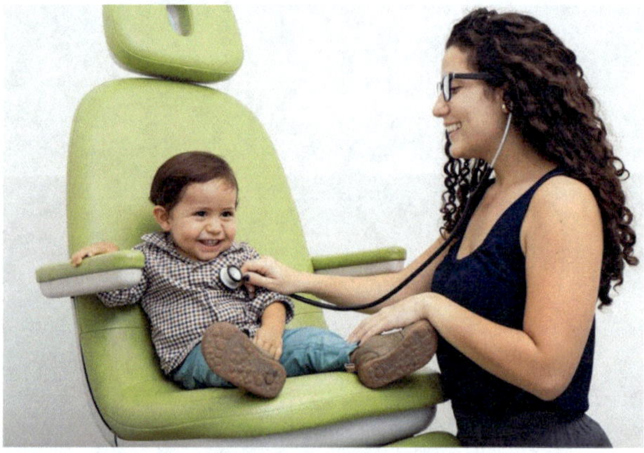

**Figure 4.1.** A smiling toddler sits comfortably during a preventive checkup as a healthcare provider uses a stethoscope, illustrating a positive pediatric care experience.

*Source:* https://alegriahealthbronx.com/wp-content/uploads/2025/01/Preventive-Pediatric-Care.jpg.

Lastly, the overlap between immunization and preventive care demonstrates the multidimensional character of interventions in public health. It is not just necessary to encourage vaccination but also to encourage education regarding the overall importance of preventive measures. It encompasses encouraging healthy lifestyle choices that might even limit the incidence of diseases further. With the integration of educational programs with robust vaccination programs, health systems can significantly improve the health outcomes of a population. Continual evaluation of such programs also serves to fine-tune strategies so that they remain sensitive to changing health problems. The vow to immunization and preventive care thus emerges as both a public health requirement and a civic responsibility (Akbar et al., 2025) (Figure 4.1).

## Definition of Immunization

Immunization is the process by which an individual becomes immune or resistant to an infectious disease, usually through the administration of a vaccine. Vaccines are composed of weakened or killed pathogens, or their specific proteins, which stimulate the body's immune system to recognize and eliminate the invading microbe. This not only protects the vaccinated individual but also contributes to herd immunity, a broader community protection that shields those who cannot be vaccinated for medical reasons. The importance of immunization in public health cannot be overstated, as it prevents outbreaks, reduces transmission of vaccine-preventable diseases, and lowers healthcare costs. As Patel et al. (2020) emphasize, immunization is central to preventive care, playing a critical role in maintaining population health and supporting sustainable healthcare systems.. For instance, massive vaccination drives for diseases such as smallpox, polio, and measles have resulted in their eradication or substantial suppression. These kinds of programs work on achieving the threshold level of vaccine coverage so that there is a mechanism of herd immunity that protects those who are not immunized due to health issues. Such programs require planning and implementation with a solid public health infrastructure, often supported by huge health databases. Denmark's population-based system of medical databases is a case in point since meticulous record-keeping can contribute to enhanced epidemiological research and effective immunization campaigns, as seen with their universal health care system and registries, as stated by Sanders et al. (2018). Furthermore, immunization is not merely the delivery of vaccines, but also an entire approach to disease prevention through education, access to health care and continuous observation of the vaccine effect. Healthcare professionals have a key part to play in explaining to patients the benefits and potential risks of vaccines, debunking misconceptions, and keeping scrupulously to vaccination timetables. The integration of immunization into preventive care structures highlights the interconnectedness of individual health choices and public health outcomes. Effective immunization practice significantly impacts morbidity and mortality prevention from infectious diseases, thereby re-emphasizing its core position among preventive care interventions and its applicability as a collective commitment between individuals and health care systems.

## Importance of Preventive Care

Preventive care is the foundation of public health and plays an enormous role in preventing disease and improving overall well-being. Emphasis on that which is done to avoid the development of disease gives individuals a sense of well-being and lowers medical costs. Community health education programs, for instance, are very effective at promoting awareness about preventive actions. Research showed that structured educational interventions can play a huge role in improving the participants' knowledge and practices regarding hygiene, nutrition, exercise, and immunization. Post-intervention results revealed remarkable improvements in health-related behaviors such as hand washing and regular health monitoring, attributing the success to preventive education as the key in achieving healthier communities (Akbar et al., 2025). Essentially, the promotion of preventive care not only empowers individuals via education but also creates a ripple effect that can lead to improved public health outcomes. The value of preventive care goes beyond mere health education; it encompasses timely screenings and immunizations that are critical for early detection and intervention. For example, childhood vision screening, as proposed by the US Preventive Services Task Force, is key in identifying such disorders as amblyopia before it causes permanent harm. The screenings, now more extensively implemented, have reported drastic increases in detection rates between 2015 and 2022, showing the effect of systematic preventive interventions in enhancing child health (Stults et al., 2024). The results are clear: detecting early through screening not only ensures better health results for individuals but also lightens healthcare burdens on society in the long term. Prevention of disease through organized care reduces the need for more costly and extensive treatments later on, showing that investing in preventive care pays high dividends. Additionally, preventive care contributes to being part of a broader public health effort to try to address healthcare disparities between various populations. Including equitable access to preventive services can substantially benefit underrepresented groups, whose rates of vaccination and health screening always lag behind. For instance, studies indicate that specific racial and ethnic groups experience discrepancies in screening as well as treatment, providing evidence for targeted interventions aimed at bridging these gaps (Stults et al., 2024). Accessibility and culturally relevant community health education programs are crucial in ensuring that all people can access preventive care. This enables a more holistic healthcare system, prioritizing not just individual health but also community awareness and action towards health. Lastly, preventive care is not only an individual choice; it is also a social necessity that advances equity and resistance to prevalent health disorders (Figure 4.2).

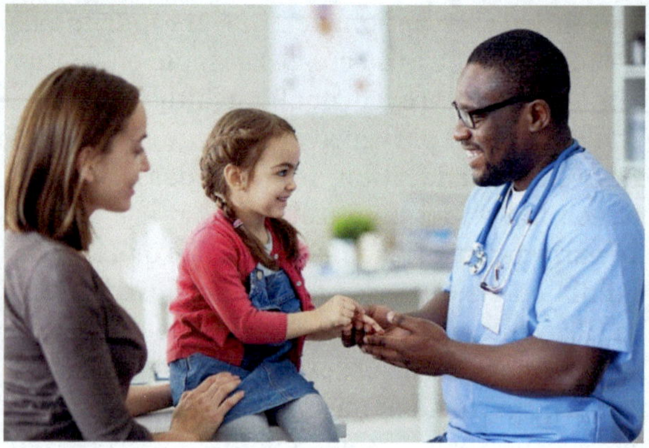

**Figure 4.2.** Preventive care serves as the cornerstone of public health.

*Source:* https://www.emeraldpediatricandfamilyclinic.com/wp-content/uploads/preventative-medical-care-2201.jpg.

## 4.1. Historical Context of Immunization

**Learning Outcome**

1. Early methods of disease prevention;
2. Development of vaccines;
3. Impact of immunization on public health.

The history of immunization captures an in-depth evolution from the early methods of preventing disease to the sophisticated schemes of vaccination in the contemporary era. The procedure began with variolation during the 16th century, where material gathered from the lesions of smallpox was intentionally injected into healthy individuals in an attempt to elicit immunity. This crude procedure laid the ground for the work of Edward Jenner in 1796, as he initiated the smallpox vaccine using cowpox. Jenner's discovery not only provided compelling evidence of the body's ability to become immune but also opened the door to the general acceptability of vaccination as a scientific means of public health. As immunological knowledge expanded, the development of vaccines for diseases such as diphtheria, tetanus, and pertussis further transformed the field of preventive care, resulting in the dramatic decline of infectious diseases in the 20th century. As the 20th century rolled on, vaccine development and mass application became a major force in propelling public health initiatives. Global momentum toward immunization was further spurred with the introduction of national vaccination programs, particularly in the post-World War II era when infectious illnesses were the leading cause of death. Anti-polio campaigns in the U.S. and deratification on a global basis against smallpox demonstrate how immunization emerged as a cornerstone of preventive health care. The collaborative effort between governments, health authorities, and communities played a key role in driving these initiatives forward. In addition, the success of vaccines highlighted the importance of herd immunity and collective responsibility towards the prevention of disease, fostering a robust public health system that would address the health matters in the decades to come. While unprecedented successes were attributed to immunization, the past trends also reveal strong public resistance and the rise of anti-vaccine ideologies. These mindsets tend to be based on several factors, such as misinformation, lack of faith in governmental healthcare programs, and fears regarding the safety and effectiveness of vaccines. Contemporary times have seen a revival of vaccine reluctance, which has public health implications as demonstrated by measles and other vaccine-preventable disease outbreaks in many areas. Identifying the history of immunization enables public health workers to come up with a strategy to counter misinformation as well as address concerns raised in the community. By doing this, they can reaffirm the importance of vaccines as discrete health interventions but also as part of a grand system of preventive care aimed at safeguarding the health of the community, thereby advancing the general purpose of public health and well-being (Papanicolas et al., 2018).

### 4.1.1. Early Methods of Disease Prevention

The past of disease prevention has been closely connected with the development of community health practice and information dissemination regarding infectious diseases. Disease prevention in the past mainly entailed quarantines that were used to repress outbreaks by separating ill individuals from the rest of the population. For instance, during the bubonic plague, towns quarantined ships and travelers entering the town, effectively restricting the disease's spread. These measures set the stage for modern conceptions of public health containment. These initial interventions also emphasized cooperation between communities and adherence to public health regulations, which remain relevant today in the management of outbreaks. By examining historical means like quarantine, one can gain a further understanding of current practices towards epidemics, which testify to the enduring utility of preventive measures in upholding public health. Besides quarantine, early immunization methods represent a turning point towards the prevention of disease. Variolation for smallpox in ancient China and subsequently in the Ottoman Empire entailed the use of smallpox sore material to create immunity. The practice, though primitive, demonstrated an early appreciation for the principles of vaccination before Edward Jenner's more organized method in the late 18$^{th}$ century. Jenner's development of the smallpox vaccine led to large-scale vaccination campaigns and indirectly to the eradication of the disease in the 20$^{th}$ century. Such early immunization procedures not only reflect the scientific inquiry into mechanisms of disease but also the potential of preventive interventions to hinder epidemics, lending evidence for ongoing research and development of preventive care today. The disease prevention landscape also shifted with developments in medical science, namely with the emergence of new monoclonal antibodies (mAbs) and pathogen-specific vaccines. An example is research on long-acting monoclonal antibodies for viruses such as respiratory syncytial virus (RSV), highlighting how early preventive interventions have led to contemporary day strategies to cover both active and passive immunization. These advances not only enhance immunity but also allow for targeted intervention with which the susceptible groups, such as infants and the elderly, can be targeted. As seen in recent studies, combining mAbs with traditional vaccines can drastically limit disease morbidity and mortality and show the continued legacy of initial preventative practices in developing successful immunization protocols. As there is more complexity in public health practice, history continues to play its role in offering context to current practices and future trends in preventive medicine and immunization (Figure 4.3).

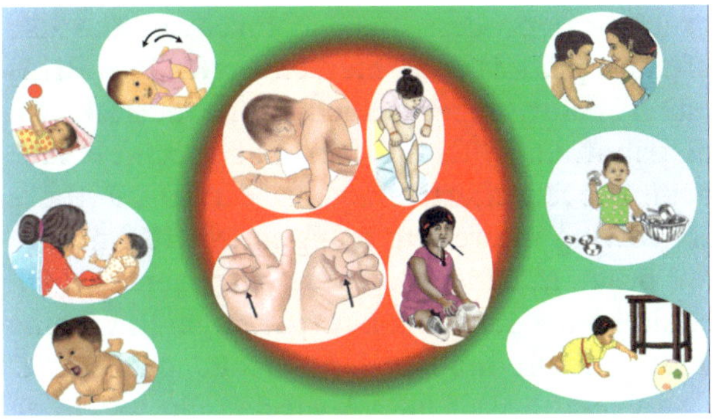

**Figure 4.3.** Early methods of disease prevention.

*Source:* https://blk-pediatric-practice.com/wp-content/uploads/2022/10/mcp.jpg.

### 4.1.2. Development of Vaccines

Vaccine development is a cornerstone in preventive medicine and immunization, significantly slowing morbidity and mortality from infectious diseases. Vaccines stimulate the immune system to recognize and combat pathogens, thereby conferring immunity without the individual being sick with the disease itself. Over the past century, the science of vaccine research has advanced fast because of advances in biotechnology, genomics, and knowledge about the workings of the immune system. An example is how quickly the mRNA vaccines were developed during the COVID-19 pandemic, highlighting how new science techniques rapidly bring about the production of vaccines to combat dangers in real time. This agile process has established a new benchmark for vaccine development and research, demonstrating the potential of accelerated responses to global health crises without sacrificing safety and efficacy in immunization programs (Hu et al., 2020). In today's era of rapid technological advancements, the integration of artificial intelligence and machine learning into vaccine development processes presents promising avenues towards higher efficiency and predictability. Such platforms are able to examine vast data sets, identify potential antigens, and even predict immunogenic responses, thus making the preclinical process easier. Moreover, the use of such platforms as messenger RNA (mRNA) has revolutionized vaccine production and distribution. With the fact that vaccines have been proven effective against COVID-19, there is growing interest in using mRNA technology for other infectious disease pathogens, which could be the start of a new paradigm in vaccine development models for various pathogens. The versatility of mRNA vaccines in targeting multiple varieties underscores the imperative to innovate in the search for efficient preventive care interventions and reinforces the imperative for continued investment in research and development (Patel et al., 2020). Equitable access and global cooperation are central to the success of vaccine development and roll-out. The global response to the COVID-19 pandemic highlighted vaccine access inequalities, underscoring the need for actions that ensure the immunization of all population segments. Initiatives such as COVAX, aiming to advance equitable access to vaccines in low- and middle-income countries, are steps toward bridge-building to offset such imbalances. Also, public health campaigns that enlighten communities about the importance of vaccinations can dispel myths and deter vaccine hesitancy, something vital in achieving herd immunity and preventing outbreaks. With improving vaccine development, the government, non-profit, and private sectors will have to collaborate to enhance the resilience of public health infrastructures globally, such that all populations are enriched by advances in immunization and preventive care (Hu et al., 2020).

### 4.1.3. Impact of Immunization on Public Health

Immunization exerts a profound and lasting impact on health, extending well beyond the individual to entire populations. As vaccination coverage rises, the incidence of vaccine-preventable diseases declines dramatically, reducing both morbidity and mortality while alleviating the economic strain on healthcare systems. High levels of coverage also establish herd immunity, protecting vulnerable groups who cannot be vaccinated for medical reasons. Historical successes—such as the eradication of smallpox and the dramatic reduction in polio cases—demonstrate the transformative potential of coordinated immunization efforts. Beyond the health benefits, the economic return on investment in vaccination campaigns underscores their central role in public health, reinforcing the need for sustained support and funding (Gillian et al., 2016).Yet, despite these achievements, vaccine hesitancy remains a formidable challenge. Concerns about vaccine safety and necessity often rooted in misinformation, cultural beliefs, or personal experiences continue to undermine coverage rates. Left unaddressed, such skepticism risks reversing decades of progress by enabling the resurgence of once-controlled diseases. Public health authorities must actively confront hesitancy through education, outreach, and transparent communication that rebuild trust and highlights the proven safety and efficacy of vaccines (Ève et al., 2013).Equally critical is the recognition of immunization's cost-effectiveness in modern healthcare. As systems face mounting pressure to deliver high-value care, rigorous cost-effectiveness analyses provide vital evidence for policymakers. The guidance of the Second Panel on Cost-Effectiveness in Health and Medicine emphasizes evaluating both healthcare and societal perspectives to fully capture immunization's benefits—not only in health outcomes but also in long-term economic savings from reduced disease burden. Demonstrating this dual value strengthens advocacy for ongoing investment and firmly establishes immunization as a cornerstone of preventive medicine and public health strategy (Gillian et al., 2016).

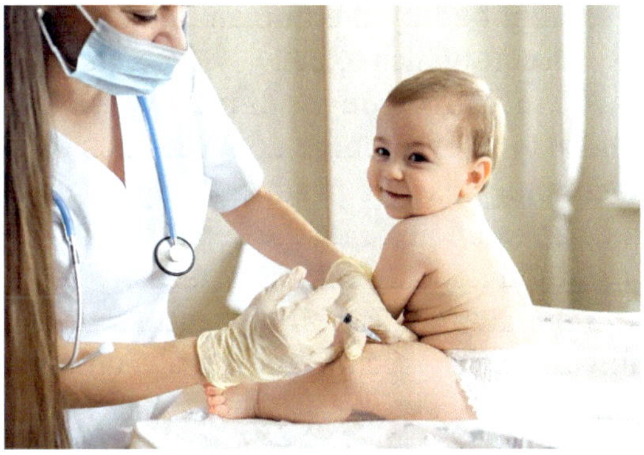

**Figure 4.4.** A healthcare professional administers a vaccination to a smiling infant, emphasizing the role of immunization in promoting early childhood health and disease prevention.

*Source:* https://health-e.in/wp-content/uploads/2023/05/Newborn-Baby-Vaccination.webp.

## Test Your Knowledge

1. 1. What was one early method used to prevent infectious diseases before modern vaccines?
2. How has the development of vaccines impacted public health over time?

## 4.2. Types of Vaccines

**Learning Outcome**

1. Live attenuated vaccines;
2. Inactivated vaccines;
3. mRNA vaccines.

Vaccine development has revolutionized public health by offering various ways to prevent infectious diseases. The primary types of vaccines are live-attenuated, inactivated, subunit, recombinant, and messenger RNA (mRNA) vaccines. Live-attenuated vaccines use attenuated strains of the causative organism to produce a robust immune response without causing the disease itself. Examples of these include the measles, mumps, and rubella (MMR) vaccine. Alternatively, inactivated vaccines are constituted by killed microorganisms, conferring immunity in possibly immunocompromised patients. Poliovirus vaccine is a classic example of this category, keeping one safe from poliomyelitis with the help of a non-infectious vaccine. All of these have a certain role to fulfill in immunization schedules, fitting the nature of the causative agents they are targeting and the population to which they are being given. Subunit vaccines disrupt the pathogen into small pieces of immunogenic matter, usually proteins or polysaccharides, which cause an immune reaction without risk of inducing disease. It is best exemplified by the human papillomavirus (HPV) vaccine, which effectively protects against a few cancers through immunity to some strains of viruses. Recombinant vaccines involve biotechnology used to produce antigens in a lab setting, an example being the hepatitis B vaccine. This method not only enhances security but also allows the administration of multiple antigens within a single vaccine, ultimately enhancing efficacy.

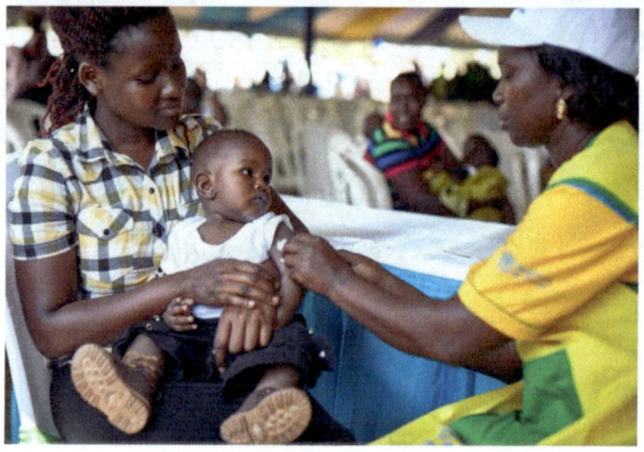

**Figure 4.5.** The development of vaccines has revolutionized public health.

*Source:* https://cdn.who.int/media/images/default-source/global-malaria-program-(gmp)/photostory/malaria-vaccine-one-year-on/malaria-vaccine-first-babies-7.tmb-1920v.jpg?sfvrsn=b50a6434_11.

The differences between vaccines demonstrate the innovative tactics utilized in creating successful immunizations against diverse pathogens. Messenger RNA (mRNA) vaccines are a significant advancement in vaccine technology using genetic material to cause cells to produce viral proteins, which triggers an immune response. The Pfizer-BioNTech and Moderna COVID-19 vaccines are excellent examples of this technology. These have proven to be quick in development but with high efficacies, transforming the field of vaccine distribution in response to new infectious outbreaks. The versatility of mRNA platforms also allows quicker modification to adapt to viral mutations, an important feature in the context of ongoing pandemics. This range of vaccines distinguishes the focal role of immunization in preventive medicine and hence reduces the incidence of infectious diseases and contributes to global health security (Figure 4.5).

### 4.2.1. Live Attenuated Vaccines

The development and application of live attenuated vaccines represent a significant milestone in the field of immunization and preventive medicine. Live attenuated vaccines use a weakened type of the infectious agent, which has the potential to cause strong immunity without disease. The advantages of live attenuated vaccines are their ability to cause long-term immunity and to generate both humoral and cellular immunity. Their effects are particularly noteworthy in the control of viral infections, such as measles, mumps, and rubella, whose occurrence has been reduced significantly worldwide. Since they mimic a natural infection, live attenuated vaccines can prime the immune system to recognize and respond to subsequent attacks by the true pathogen, underscoring their role in public health policy aimed at eliminating infectious diseases. A prime example of innovation in the area of live attenuated vaccines is the creation of the chikungunya vaccine using baculovirus display technology. The new platform facilitates display of the envelope proteins of the chikungunya virus, E1 and E2, on the baculovirus surface. Experiments demonstrate that immunization using this recombinant vaccine induces high-level antibody responses and T-cell immunity, which completely protects against the chikungunya virus in preclinical models. These developments indicate that live attenuated vaccines can be developed through current biotechnology, offering effective and safe protection against emerging pathogens. Successful deployment of such vaccines demonstrates the potential for rapid adaptation towards disease prevention against diseases that have potentially serious consequences for global health, as with increased cases of chikungunya in the Americas, which highlights the necessity for effective vaccines to mitigate socio-economic impacts (Caillava et al., 2024). Furthermore, live attenuated vaccine application goes beyond traditional viral illnesses, as seen with groundbreaking efforts in the war against Japanese encephalitis. With the major risk in endemic areas and among travelers, Japanese encephalitis has been managed through the application of live attenuated vaccines for vaccination. Despite diminished rates of occurrence in vaccinated populations, awareness and uptake remain problems, with acceptance diverging broadly among travelers globally. This underscores the necessity of medical professionals to develop an understanding of the benefits and safety of vaccinations. The efficacy of the live attenuated Japanese encephalitis vaccine, among other immunization strategies, further supports the importance of large-scale preventive care practices in limiting infectious disease risks, ultimately fostering better public health results and protection of susceptible populations (Asawapaithulsert et al., 2023).

### 4.2.2. Inactivated Vaccines

Inactivated vaccines have been a crucial component of immunization campaigns because they can induce effective immunity without the associated risks of the live pathogens. The manufacture of these vaccines requires the killing or inactivation of the virus or the bacterium responsible for causing the disease so that it cannot replicate or cause disease in the vaccinee. This aspect makes inactivated vaccines particularly useful for individuals with compromised immune systems because they have minimal risk when compared to live attenuated vaccines. The previous success of inactivated vaccines against diseases such as polio and hepatitis A says a lot about their usefulness in the prevention of infectious diseases and the significance of their application in public health programs aimed at the achievement of herd immunity and eradication of disease (Connors et al., 2021). The manufacture of inactivated vaccines has presented difficulties, particularly balancing safety and immunogenicity. Researchers must ensure that inactivation preserves the structural conformation of the pathogens to enable the immune system to recognize and respond favorably. The application of vaccine technology, including the incorporation of adjuvants, has provided additional boosts to the immune response elicited by inactivated vaccines.

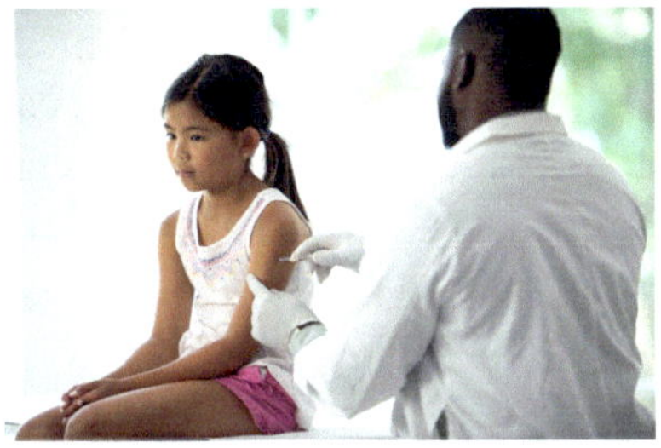

**Figure 4.6.** A healthcare provider prepares to administer a vaccine to a young girl, underscoring the importance of routine immunizations in childhood disease prevention.

*Source:* https://cdn.britannica.com/45/148345-050-D33104D8/nurse-patient-vaccination.jpg.

However, there remain questions regarding protection duration and the need for booster doses. Strong clinical trials must assess these safety factors and confirm the long-term effectiveness of inactivated vaccines, specifically for newly emerging causes of disease such as SARS-CoV-2 (Dong et al., 2020). In the current vaccine development world, inactivated vaccines are being compared to new technologies such as mRNA and viral vector vaccines to determine how well they react against COVID-19. With the growing demand for vaccination drives becoming the agenda of countries, one must be aware of what inactivated vaccines have to offer. They can be a crucial element in global immunization programs, especially where access to developed vaccine technology is weak. Furthermore, by having inactivated vaccine platforms at the center of attention, health authorities can prepare for potential future pandemic risks. Continued research and investment in inactivated vaccine technology will also work to harvest new solutions for current and emerging infectious diseases, justifying their value in immunization and preventive medicine (Connors et al., 2021) (Figure 4.6).

### 4.2.3. mRNA Vaccines

The discovery of mRNA vaccines has revolutionized the science of immunization and preventive medicine, particularly in response to the COVID-19 pandemic. Traditional vaccination methods typically involve the delivery of weakened or killed pathogens into the body, which causes the immune system to respond. mRNA vaccines do the opposite by utilizing a synthetic strand of messenger RNA that instructs cells to produce a harmless spike protein characteristic of the SARS-CoV-2 virus. The process conditions the immune system to recognize and battle the virus upon actual exposure, thereby activating the body's defense mechanism. The mechanism of action of mRNA technology is a shift towards quicker and more responsive vaccine generation, emphasizing the capacity of mRNA vaccines to successfully address emerging infectious diseases. Their efficacy, as attested in recent clinical trials, highlights their potential as a cornerstone of public health measures in infectious disease control, according to the global commitment to immunization programs (Dewan & Islam, 2022). Recent data on the efficacy of mRNA vaccines against COVID-19 reveal astounding figures that attest to their central role in preventive health care. Studies have shown that the fully vaccinated persons have significant protection, with up to 91.2% efficacy for the Pfizer-BioNTech vaccine and 98.1% efficacy for the Moderna vaccine against SARS-CoV-2 infection, as reported in some health assessments (Zheng et al., 2021). In addition, these vaccines have been highly effective against severe outcomes such as hospitalization and death, with projected protective efficacy estimates of 97% and higher against critical illness from COVID-19. These results not only further confirm the utility of vaccination in preventing disease but also clarify the public health implications more broadly. By significantly reducing disease transmission, mRNA vaccines are instrumental in achieving herd immunity, which is crucial for stopping the spread of the disease and safeguarding vulnerable populations. The use of mRNA vaccines also has important implications for the future of vaccine development and research. The platform used in mRNA technology is versatile; hence, it can be quickly tailored to create new or emerging strains of viruses, such as emerging SARS-CoV-2 variants. This flexibility is important in light of the accelerated genetic change seen in pathogens, with the implication being that vaccines must be able to engender strong and long-lasting immune responses as these changes occur. Also, research into how mRNA vaccines can be personalized may make them more effective while reducing side effects, with implications being that ongoing innovation in immunization technology is necessary. As global vaccination keeps moving forward, the experience from mRNA vaccines will play a central role in how preventive healthcare will evolve in the future and foster resilience to infectious diseases all over the world (Dewan & Islam, 2022).

## Test Your Knowledge

1. What is the main difference between live attenuated vaccines and inactivated vaccines?
2. How do mRNA vaccines work to protect the body from disease?

## 4.3. Benefits of Immunization

**Learning Outcome**

1. Individual health protection;
2. Community immunity (herd immunity);
3. Economic benefits of vaccination programs.

Immunization is one of the greatest success stories in public health and a cornerstone of preventive medicine. Through vaccination, we have witnessed a spectacular decline in the incidence of infectious diseases that once threatened populations. Polio, measles, and rubella are spectacularly less common due to mass immunization, leading to the near elimination of these diseases from a large part of the globe. This diminishment not only eliminates the direct disease burden from people but also helps to produce herd immunity, protecting those who cannot be vaccinated, for example, babies and people with weakened immune systems. The net impact of vaccination seems not just in improved health results but also in reduced healthcare costs for the prevention of preventable ailments, thereby enhancing community health on multiple dimensions. Further, the effects of immunization extend more widely to society than to individual health, with huge economic benefits to societies. Vaccines reduce the incidence of hospitalization and healthcare expenditure for infectious diseases, leading to vast savings to healthcare systems and families. To illustrate, the Centers for Disease Control and Prevention has projected that vaccinations in children alone save the United States over $70 billion in direct medical expenses and related societal costs within one year. In addition, immunization promotes a more stable workforce as healthier workers can participate more intensely in the economy. The connection between vaccine coverage and productivity emphasizes the central function that immunization performs in the realization of economic stability and growth, further indicating the utility of preventive care strategies as a priority within public health policy. The role that education and awareness play in maximizing the benefit of immunization cannot be overstated. Community education programs through public health that inform communities about the role, safety, and efficacy of vaccines significantly boost immunization coverage.

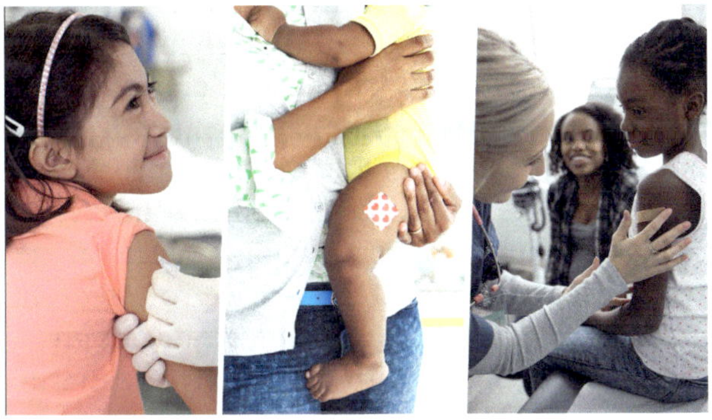

**Figure 4.7.** Immunization represents one of the most significant advancements in public health.

*Source:* https://www.fda.gov/files/Childhood-vaccines-03-1600x900.jpg.

Through outreach efforts, internet platforms, and partnerships with health professionals, individuals are equipped with information to make informed choices about their own health as well as the health of their family members. Patient education is just like preventive intervention in other areas of health, a good example being in dental clinics where preventive interventions such as fluoride therapies and regular check-ups are promoted (Rehab et al., 2024). The combined synergism of education and immunization has the potential to foster stronger health impacts, furthering initiatives toward higher vaccination coverage and effective control of infectious diseases among the population, just like AI-driven wearables improving chronic disease management through real-time tracking and targeted interventions (Kumar, 2024) (Figure 4.7).

### 4.3.1. Individual Health Protection

Personal protection of health is a basic guideline of public health activities, with particular mention of immunization and preventive medicine. Vaccination is one of the key measures for protecting individuals against vaccine-preventable diseases, which have an unfavorable impact particularly on high-risk groups like the elderly or chronically ill. For instance, patients who have severe underlying medical illnesses are at greater risk for serious outcomes of these illnesses. Implementing targeted immunization programs maximizes protection for the people while also benefiting the health of the community by restraining disease spread (Odone et al., 2024). High-risk groups often also require special vaccination strategies given their respective health needs. Through the realization of these limitations and prioritizing vaccination, public health organizations can effectively maximize individual and population health levels. The growing world life expectancy calls for renewed focus on health literacy and awareness, particularly among the elderly. With the number of geriatric people on the increase in society, they must be well equipped with the health challenges that they may face, including diabetes and hypertension. Evidence indicates that while the majority of older individuals are cognizant of the most prevalent illnesses, there remains very little awareness of less transparent conditions—e.g., cognitive impairment and depression (Majumdar et al., 2017). This gap in knowledge highlights the necessity for holistic health literacy interventions among the elderly, particularly regarding the importance of immunization to avoid susceptibility to infections. By raising awareness on immunization, health care providers are able to empower older adults to embrace practices of proactively protecting their health and well-being. The incorporation of preventive care within routineHealth checks are a key strategy in promoting personal health protection. Regular checkups and consultations allow healthcare providers to detect potential health risks early, enabling timely interventions that improve long-term outcomes. For example, routine immunization provided during health visits significantly reduces the incidence of infectious diseases, particularly among vulnerable populations. Results from local assessments in the Lombardy region show that while some hospitals can introduce the use of vaccines within health facilities, inconsistency continues to define coverage and access to high-risk populations (Odone et al., 2024). Therefore, it is essential to develop harmonized efforts among healthcare facilities, stakeholders, and policymakers to unify immunization practices. In doing so, health systems can allow that preventive care becomes irretrievably integrated into patient care, ultimately leading to a more safeguarded and stronger population.

### 4.3.2. Community Immunity (Herd Immunity)

Community immunity, or herd immunity as it is otherwise termed, plays a vital role in public health in that it protects populations from infectious diseases. This occurs when a large proportion of a population is immune to a disease, either through vaccination or through already having had the disease and thereby curbing the opportunity for disease spread. The concept is essential in sustaining outbreaks of diseases such as measles, mumps, and rubella, which need a high rate of vaccination coverage to protect individuals who are unable to be vaccinated, such as those with certain medical conditions and infants. Studies have shown that the achievement of herd immunity not only safeguards susceptible populations but also leads to the eventual decline of disease rates in populations, citing the importance of community effort in vaccination programs (Woodland, 2015). The most effective method of achieving herd immunity is through vaccination. Through the administration of vaccines to people, they are given immunity to some pathogens without having to experience the otherwise severe effects of the disease itself. For example, the introduction of the measles, mumps, and rubella (MMR) vaccine in the US has resulted in a substantial decrease in the incidence of these three diseases by over 99% since its introduction. However, the return of measles in areas where vaccination levels have decreased demonstrates the volatility of herd immunity, where rates of vaccination decrease below a threshold, typically around 95% for measles, by which time quickly, outbreaks become quickly evident, threatening both the vaccinated and unvaccinated community (Woodland, 2015). This serves to underscore the imperative for sustained public health efforts in maintaining high rates of vaccination as the foundation for prophylactic care.

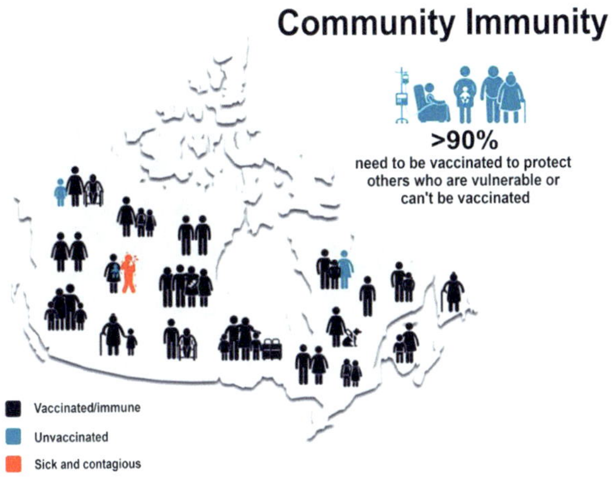


**Figure 4.8.** Community immunity, commonly referred to as herd immunity.

*Source:* https://ecampusontario.pressbooks.pub/app/uploads/sites/483/2019/06/Community-Immunity.jpeg.

In addition to preventing individual illness, herd immunity also prevents the overall social impacts of infectious diseases, including healthcare costs and economic productivity. Herd-control diseases reduce hospitalizations and health costs for families and the overall health systems. For instance, the public health burden of bacterial meningitis in under-immunized populations still remains a high-priority public health issue, particularly in Sub-Saharan Africa, since an outbreak has devastating impacts on communities due to the contagious nature of such pathogens as *Neisseria meningitidis*. Hence, intense vaccination drives not only encourage population immunity against disease epidemics as well as economic stability of hit regions by lowering illness burdens for the population as well as the healthcare system. Hence, the synergic effort towards gaining and maintaining herd immunity is essential towards enhancing public health outcomes and ensuring long-term societal health (Figure 4.8).

### 4.3.3. Economic Benefits of Vaccination Programs

Vaccination initiatives are an investment that carries serious economic returns that exceed public health gains, building social and economic resilience. Economically, vaccination campaigns can reduce healthcare systems' costs of diseases that otherwise would lead to costly treatments and hospitalizations. Each dollar spent on immunization could yield around $44 in returns, according to the World Health Organization's estimates, highlighting the preventive care value proposition. Population immunity through vaccination not only reduces the short-term expense of outbreak control but also compensates for broader socio-economic impacts associated with lost productivity, as healthy populations are more productive and have more to offer the economy. Thus, vaccination programs are a prudent long-term investment in the economic and sustainability of healthcare spending. Also, vaccination programs help provide economic returns through enhanced public productivity. Healthy workers will be likely to remain in employment, minimize sick leave, and continue to perform community roles. The economic advantage also benefits parents who are able to manage work-life more conveniently because widespread immunity minimizes the likelihood that children will fall ill and inject stress into home and work life. As the Advisory Committee on Immunization Practices observes, adult immunization is equally critical in order to maintain workforce health and consequently, economic stability across most industries. This connection between economic performance and health raises the rationale for why vaccination programs constitute a high-priority field to maintain the economy strong and less vulnerable to the types of fluctuations infectious diseases would induce. In addition to direct savings in the area of healthcare and improvements in productivity, immunization programs can bring longer-term economic benefits through the promotion of broader social equity agendas. Public health measures like immunization programs are capable of influencing the determinants of health extensively and thus assist in narrowing socioeconomic inequalities in health. Through immunization of disadvantaged groups, populations can benefit from collective immunity, which leads to reduced disease prevalence among vulnerable groups. This comprehensive public health approach is in line with economic planning that promotes equity and, as a consequence, induces economic growth. In line with evidence derived from population-based health databases, such as those of Denmark, the correlation of high vaccination coverage with improved health outcomes further confirms the thesis that strong immunization not only serves to preserve public health but also fortifies the economic infrastructure upon which individuals and communities exist (Sanders et al., 2016).

## Test Your Knowledge

1. How does immunization protect individual health?
2. What is herd immunity, and why is it important for communities?

## 4.4. Challenges in Immunization

**Learning Outcome**

1. Vaccine hesitancy and misinformation;
2. Access to vaccines in underserved populations;
3. Global disparities in vaccination rates.

The vaccine environment is plagued by a multitude of challenges that greatly hinder effective vaccination campaigns. Vaccine hesitancy, in which people are reluctant or refuse to get vaccinated when vaccines are readily available, is perhaps the most pressing challenge. It is primarily due to misinformation, cultural preferences, and lack of trust in health systems, leading to low vaccine coverage. The recent increases in the diseases such as pertussis (whooping cough) result from waning immunity and inadequate coverage with immunizations. Increasing incidence rates in certain groups indicate towards the necessity to take determinants of hesitancy seriously and restore confidence in immunization among people. Through the application of focused education campaigns and community outreach programs, health organizations can attempt to counteract misinformation and ensure a culture of acceptance for immunization as a central component of preventive medicine. Logistical and infrastructural limitations also contribute to the challenges inherent in immunization programs, particularly in resource-poor environments. In settings of conflict, poverty, or inadequate healthcare infrastructure, the delivery of vaccines may be practically impossible. The logistical challenge of reaching isolated populations, as well as supply chain issues and the shortage of adequate healthcare personnel, pose deep challenges to vaccination rate optimization.

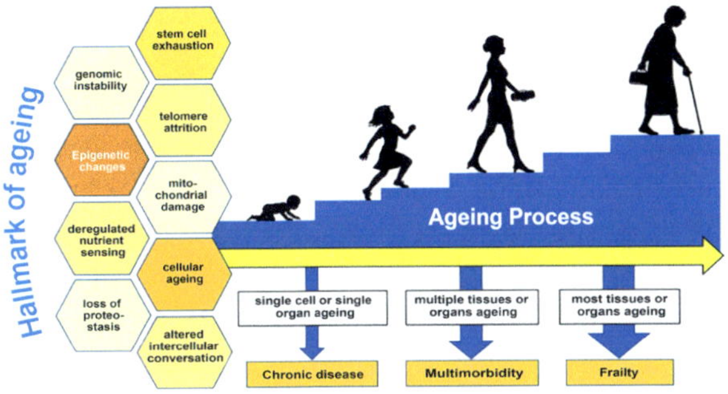


**Figure 4.9.** The landscape of immunization is fraught with multiple challenges that significantly hinder effective vaccination programs.

*Source:* https://www.mdpi.com/pathophysiology/pathophysiology-30-00014/article_deploy/html/images/pathophysiology-30-00014-g001.png.

In humanitarian settings, survival need is most frequently a greater need than preventive intervention, including immunization. Incentivized methodologies, such as those contained within studies, have been determined to offer worth in terms of increased vaccination rates as they bring attention to satisfying near-term needs of target groups. Community-based strategies are crucial to ensuring that immunization programs are not just effective but also sustainable in the long term. Besides logistical issues, the quality and supply of available vaccines also present significant barriers. While acellular vaccines have been useful with respect to safety, they have decreased immunity after some time and need booster injections to maintain effectiveness. The emergence of antibiotic-resistant disease strains like Bordetella pertussis underscored the loopholes of current vaccine formulations, prompting scientists to explore next-generation vaccines that are more protective and offer longer immunity. In addition, ethical issues in developing and distributing vaccines raise questions about equity and access. Fixing these intricate immunization challenges requires an integrated approach with innovative science and effective policy implementation. Strengthening global immunization policies is critical in encouraging people's health and well-being and in reducing the burden of preventable disease (Figure 4.9).

## 4.4.1. Vaccine Hesitancy and Misinformation

Vaccine hesitancy is a multifaceted factor that severely undermines endeavors toward the achievement of the highest level of immunization coverage. Vaccine hesitancy is particularly common where false information circulates, raising issues about the safety and effectiveness of vaccines. In countries on the African continent, for instance, despite the fact that vaccines are one of the most cost-effective public health measures, social, economic, and cultural barriers result in low immunization coverage. The majority of city residents are exposed to a barrage of disinformation that causes them to question the integrity of health care systems and immunization methods. Additionally, the poor are further disenfranchised since they might not be able to access credible health data and cannot afford the underlying costs of vaccine access. Overcoming such challenges is essential to the sustained use of immunization as a central aspect of preventive health care, particularly in vulnerable populations (Oluwaseyifunmi et al., 2025). The COVID-19 pandemic further escalated vaccine hesitancy, highlighting public perception gaps and actual vaccination rates among healthcare workers (HCWs). While a sizable majority of these HCWs from Nnamdi Azikiwe University Teaching Hospital said they knew of COVID-19 vaccines, uptake was correspondingly critically low. This reflected a serious mismatch between perception and practice. Misconceptions regarding vaccine safety and efficacy were the impetus for this resistance, with the majority of HCWs protesting on the grounds of concern regarding safety and general lack of trust in institutions that produced the vaccines. Unexpectedly, the incentives for vaccination, such as civic duty and fear of COVID-19, were also controlled by these cross-cutting barriers. The need for interventions that, while soothing the fears of healthcare providers, also maximize public confidence in immunization programs as a prime preventive care strategy (Umenweke et al., 2025). In the battle against vaccine resistance, a concerted action has to be taken to de-mystify myths that surround public awareness. Firstly, effective public health communication measures have to be initiated so as to establish transparency in vaccine development processes, thereby gaining community trust. Anti-myths education campaigns can erase vaccine myths based on robust evidence-based communication, tailored to plural social groups. In addition, the strength of healthcare workers and community leaders can be harnessed in order to disseminate accurate information and allay fear. Solving underlying issues in terms of health equity and access to care is also essential, as marginal communities are more likely to experience compounded vulnerabilities. Lastly, an integrated approach that entails public education, community engagement, and systemic change will be essential in countering vaccine hesitancy and ensuring successful immunization drives as part of proactive preventive care (Oluwaseyifunmi et al., 2025).

### 4.4.2. Access to Vaccines in Underserved Populations

Vaccine accessibility remains a problem for vulnerable populations, particularly among low-income countries where healthcare infrastructure is plagued by huge operational difficulties. The United Nations Sustainable Development Goals emphasize the importance of providing equal access to healthcare, which translates to the fact that immunization must not be an elixir for the wealthy. As per a recent study, 51% of youngsters in these countries have incomplete basic vaccinations, which points towards the disparity in vaccination coverage. Notably, geography has identified hotspots in Nigeria, Chad, Cameroon, and Niger where the rate of immunization is woefully low, demonstrating the effect of site-based socioeconomic factors on access to healthcare. These findings highlight the pressing need for targeted intervention programs that aim to promote immunization coverage in such targeted locations to improve public health outcomes among vulnerable children based on evidence derived from Demographic and Health Surveys conducted across 48 nations (Getnet et al., 2025). New interventions are essential to break the barriers that impede access to vaccines among disadvantaged groups. The pandemic of COVID-19, for instance, pushed the then-existing issues into focus, calling for innovative outreach efforts right away. A case in point was the application of Drive-Through Vaccine Clinics that were aimed at dispelling parental anxiety over contracting COVID-19 while making vaccination accessible. The initiative proved successful, providing 745 vaccines to 415 patients in a brief waiting time of five minutes on average, thus providing an operational model for improving access. The upvoting also suggests that alternative methods of vaccine delivery will become crucial in maintaining the continuation of immunization activities during pandemics. Through the augmentation of such innovative practices, healthcare providers can reach out effectively, taking advantage of disadvantaged populations with required preventive care in the face of structural obstacles (Sowmya et al., 2021). In the assessment of vaccine access, it is apparent that different methods must be leveraged in addressing individual and population-level challenges. Obstacles such as food insecurity, maternal and child health disparities, and the accessibility of healthcare facilities can significantly affect vaccination coverage.

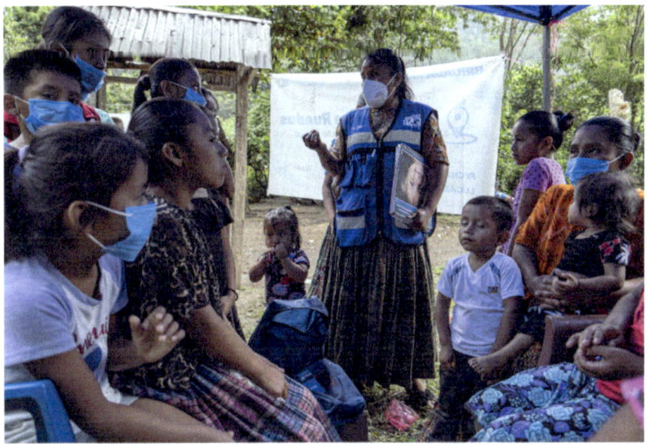

**Figure 4.10.** Access to vaccines remains a critical challenge for underserved populations.

*Source:* https://cdn.who.int/media/images/default-source/results-report/2023-eob/country-impact-stories/img_012---educadora-de-brigada-_-comunidad-corralpec-_-senahu--alta-verapaz-(1).jpg?sfvrsn=658b2b5a_3.

Public awareness interventions aimed at individuals' knowledge of the importance of vaccination, particularly through health information dissemination mechanisms and community education, are extremely critical in all targeted hot spots. Increased antenatal contacts, insurance coverage, and greater exposure of the community to health media information can contribute to creating an educated public for vaccine acceptance. As emphasized in research studies identifying individual and community-level factors in vaccine coverage, the presence of an overarching strategy encompassing these parameters will be able to increase immunization coverage among marginalized groups to a significant extent. These efforts will not only assist in improving public health but also facilitate the realization of larger objectives articulated by international health initiatives (Getnet et al., 2025) (Figure 4.10).

### 4.4.3. Global Disparities in Vaccination Rates

During the past several decades, the global vaccination map has uncovered widespread disparities that reflect underlying socio-economic gaps. Vaccines are a cornerstone of public health, providing efficient protection against infectious diseases, but access to vaccinations is not uniformly spread between countries. Wealthy nations tend to have success in achieving more than 90% immunization levels with well-established health care systems and public health infrastructures. By contrast, low-income nations typically encounter multifaceted obstacles like scarce healthcare infrastructure, lack of trained personnel, and limited financial assets. These disparities are exacerbated by the COVID-19 pandemic that gravely challenged the healthcare infrastructure, relegating focus to and suspending routine immunization programs. As outlined by McClung et al. (2020), such worldwide inequalities not only have resultant health consequences but also broader societal consequences that are designed to further complicate the pursuit of health equity and broader societal stability. The weight of such disparities is most obviously evident when examining the targeted groups that are affected by low vaccination rates, including children and minority groups. Routine immunization is also required to prevent infections like measles, which has recurred in areas with poor vaccination coverage. Remoteness of location, cultural reasons, and lack of information are compounded setbacks that undermine vaccination campaigns. Also, disadvantaged groups are more vulnerable to vaccine-preventable infections due to structural inequalities. The Advisory Committee on Immunization Practices emphasizes the necessity for policies of equitable distribution and access in emergencies like the COVID-19 pandemic, as exemplified by McClung et al. (2020). Removing these barriers is important to public health around the globe, as marginal improvements in vaccination rates would have important impacts on disease prevention and community resilience. Initiatives to mitigate global imbalances in the vaccination rate need to be pursued jointly by different stakeholders, including governments, agencies, and societies. Collective action is needed to develop useful vaccination schemes and help ensure access to the vaccine for the neediest. Organizations like GAVI, the Vaccine Alliance, aim to enhance vaccination availability in underprivileged regions by providing funds and technical assistance. These global partnerships are of central importance to the creation of sustainable healthcare systems that will endure the coming public health challenges. In addition, public health education programs are needed to eliminate false information and inform communities with accurate information about the benefits of immunization. As the spotlight is on, prompt and culturally appropriate communication steps are central to limiting hesitancy and encouraging acceptance of vaccines, ultimately resulting in a healthier global population and better public health opportunities.

### Test Your Knowledge

1. What is vaccine hesitancy, and how can misinformation contribute to it?
2. Name one challenge related to vaccine access in underserved populations.

## 4.5. Preventive Care Beyond Immunization

**Learning Outcome**

1. Regular health screenings;
2. Lifestyle modifications for disease prevention;
3. Role of healthcare providers in preventive care.

Preventive care is a concept that extends much wider than immunization to encompass a broad range of interventions for enhancing individual and community health. Preventive care encompasses general health screening, nutrition guidance, and lifestyle instruction to reduce the likelihood of chronic disease. Community health education programs have been proven to enhance knowledge about preventive practices among urban communities. For example, an organized program substantially improved the awareness of participants regarding hygiene, diet, and exercise, indicating the importance of available health education for enhancing public participation in preventive services. Such preventive measures can lead to fewer instances of preventable illnesses and improve public health in general, pointing towards the necessity of incorporating educational elements with immunization activities (Akbar et al., 2025). In discussing preventive care, it is important to discuss the specific needs of high-risk populations that are bound to have challenges in accessing essential health care services. These populations are prone to having aggregated health risks that not only make them more susceptible to infections but also necessitate specially crafted preventive interventions. Hospital-based immunization programs for high-risk populations have been suggested as an intervention to allow these individuals to access the proper vaccinations. In regions like Lombardy, Italy, assessments show that certain hospitals effectively deliver vaccines through formal clinical pathways, which reflects the shift towards overall care systems incorporating immunization and other prevention approaches. By targeting high-risk groups, health systems can both improve individual health results and the health of populations by means of herd immunity and reduced disease spread (Odone et al., 2024).

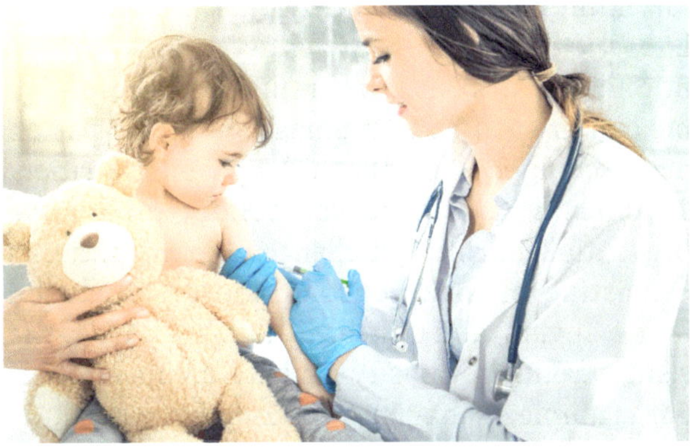

**Figure 4.11.** A healthcare provider administers a vaccine to a toddler, illustrating a supportive approach to pediatric immunization.

*Source:* https://centromedicoabc.com/storage/2023/01/vacunacion-ninos.jpg.

Also, the public health policy and healthcare provision system implications of preventive care strategies will need a multidisciplinary approach. Policymakers will need to recognize the importance of creating a culture of prevention that fosters both immunization programs and overall health initiatives. Strategies such as rewarding routine health screenings, encouraging healthy lifestyle change, and building community resources will create a synergistic effect, maximizing the impact of preventive care to its optimum level. As research continues to illustrate the substantial benefits of properly designed health education programs and targeted interventions, it is now more apparent that preventive care has to be an all-encompassing approach. Through intervention in the various factors of health, including mental, emotional, and physical well-being, society can produce healthier populations and ultimately stem healthcare costs associated with treating chronic diseases (Akbar et al., 2025) (Figure 4.11).

### 4.5.1. Regular Health Screenings

Regular health screenings are part of the regimen of immunization and preventive medicine, a major way by which future health issues can be identified before they become severe. The screenings are meant to identify sicknesses at an early point, before there is any noticeable symptom, something that is particularly applicable in cases of diseases such as hypertension, diabetes, and certain forms of cancer. For instance, regular screening can lead to the early detection of cervical cancer by Pap smears or breast cancer by mammograms and thus enhance survival rates of such conditions. Periodic health screening also strengthens an overall profile of patient health, allowing medical providers to tailor immunization dates and preventive interventions, as necessary. Consequently, through the inclusion of regular screenings in health care, the public is made capable of participating in proactive actions of guaranteeing their own well-being and health, fostering an active stance towards involvement in one's own health care. The impact of routine health screenings on the economy is fundamentally applicable, since the earlier diagnosis is made, the more typically health care costs are minimized in the future. Early identification of health issues can prevent the need for extensive therapies, hospital stays, and other expenses linked with advanced disease stages. For instance, the cost of serious infections such as typhoid can be staggering, with high costs related to hospitalization and treatment complications. Studies have proven that preventive interventions, including regular screenings and vaccinations, not only produce improved health outcomes but also considerable cost reductions in terms of both individuals and the healthcare system.

These findings emphasize the need to make regular health screenings a priority of public health policy, particularly within resource-limited environments where the cost of healthcare is prohibitively expensive. Bhattacharyya et al. (2024) highlight the degree to which indefensible routines, when deployed in native environments, can have a beneficial impact on accessibility and efficiency in healthcare. To this end, the merit of routine health screening is advanced by promoting public knowledge of vaccine-preventable diseases in communities. A complete understanding of one's health status may promote greater compliance with immunization schedules, thus enhancing community immunity and reducing infectious disease rates.

The interlink between regular checks and immunization coverage can be particularly important in the battle against myths about vaccine efficacy, which has picked up pace in recent years. Efforts in health education to dispel these myths will be assisted by relying on regular health checks as a core element and hence encouraging individuals to collaborate more with their health workers. Preventive care, as Yawn et al. (2021) point out, does not only include vaccinations but also regular checks that indicate to patients what their weaknesses in terms of health are and that they require recommended preventive measures. Periodic health checks, thus, play the role of a bridge, connecting individual health literacy with public health objectives, ultimately making community health resilience stronger.

### 4.5.2. Lifestyle Modifications for Disease Prevention

Lifestyle modification is crucial in disease prevention, particularly in the control of chronic ailments prevalent in the modern world. By adopting regular exercise, a balanced diet, and stress control, an individual can effortlessly lower his or her predisposition to ailments such as diabetes and cardiovascular disease. Engaging in at least 150 minutes of moderate exercise weekly not only strengthens the cardiovascular system but also increases metabolic processes, thereby lowering the risk for diseases like Type 2 diabetes. Also, consumption of a balanced diet consisting of whole foods, vegetables, and fruits has been seen to be rich in nutrients required for immune function and general well-being. Lifestyle change emphasizes active engagement in one's own health and reinforces preventive measures such as immunization, making it an overarching method of health upkeep. Nutrition, specifically, is a core component of disease prevention and lifestyle changes. Dietary patterns consisting of high consumption of processed foods, sugars, and unhealthy fats are part of the rising trend in obesity and its comorbidities. For example, managing Type 2 diabetes mellitus (T2DM) properly is not only drug-dependent, but also on the type of food one consumes for regulating blood glucose levels. A well-drawn meal plan with low glycemic index foods can stabilize insulin levels and prevent spikes in blood sugar, which are critical for individuals at risk of developing diabetes. As highlighted by the rhetoric of excess death caused by serious mental illness, the interaction of complex interventions that aim at changing health behavior is important to achieve better health. Incorporating nutrition education into public health programs is also likely to enhance the effectiveness of such measures in immunization and preventive care. Social determinants of health also control the efficacy of lifestyle modification for the prevention of disease. Socioeconomic status, education level, and the presence of healthcare facilities can facilitate or prevent individuals from adopting healthier lifestyle options. Societies that enjoy strong support systems possess facilities like fitness clubs, parks, and nutrition counseling that promote healthier lifestyles for their people. Those with scant resources to access such facilities might find themselves unable to institute necessary changes. Since interventions aim to maximize health equity, integration of community-level approaches to address environmental barriers is crucial. The intervention's multi-dimensional approach in the literature sustains a multi-level intervention, in recognition of the fact that individual behavior is interwoven with other social and environmental factors (Nancy et al., 2017). Therefore, community support systems development is significant not only for change of lifestyle but also for achieving the maximum effect from preventive care efforts, such as immunization drives, which eventually aim to reduce disease burden (Figure 4.12).

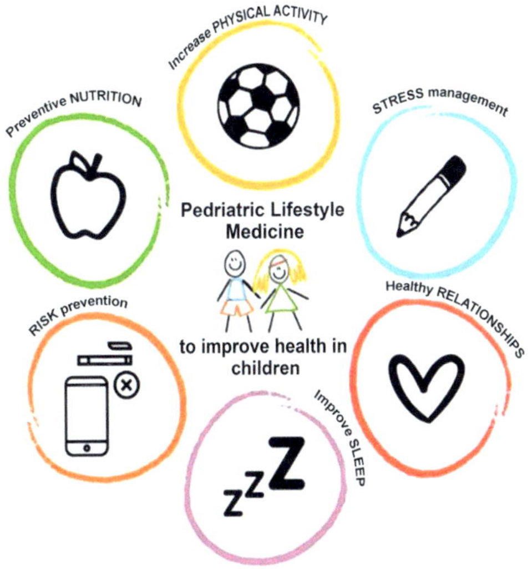


**Figure 4.12.** Lifestyle modifications play a critical role in disease prevention.

*Source:* https://www.mdpi.com/children/children-12-00304/article_deploy/html/images/children-12-00304-g001.png.

### 4.5.3. Role of Healthcare Providers in Preventive Care

Medical practitioners take a key role in preventive care, specifically with immunization. Their role does not stop at mere administration of vaccines; they play an active part in educating patients on the importance of immunization in preventing infectious illnesses. Healthcare practitioners are able to overcome vaccine resistance and myths that plague populations through communication and trust. For instance, they can debunk common myths regarding vaccine effectiveness and safety, which is crucial, considering that the dissemination of misinformation online is speeding up. As illustrated in recent literature, patient understanding and compliance with vaccination programs are significantly eased by healthcare workers' capacity to convey accurate health facts (Jain et al., 2024). Thus, as educated advocates of immunization, healthcare professionals contribute not just to the health of a single patient, but to the overall public health. In addition to communication, healthcare providers are integral components of the preventive care infrastructure in the form of systematic screening and risk assessment. Through identification of patients at risk for specific preventable conditions, providers can tailor immunization regimens that address individual health needs. For instance, studies have shown that a lack of knowledge on the part of healthcare personnel about some immunizations, such as against rabies, can lead to inadequate patient care (Ahmed et al., 2020). This underscores the need for continuous education among healthcare personnel, thus making them current with knowledge on preventive interventions. Additionally, by proactively advocating vaccinations based on standardized guidelines, health care professionals contribute to herd immunity that benefits all, especially those who are immunocompromised and unable to be vaccinated. Collaboration between healthcare professionals is another important ingredient for effective preventive care. Multidisciplinary teams consisting of physicians, nurses, pharmacists, and public health professionals work synergistically to maximize vaccination efforts in communities. This collaborative approach not only enhances the accessibility of immunization services but also allows integrated patient education. For instance, capitalizing on the expertise of various healthcare roles, organizations can implement community outreach programs that counter systemic barriers to vaccine distribution, e.g., transportation and affordability concerns. As noted in current studies, interdisciplinary collaboration has proven to be effective in raising awareness and increasing vaccination rates within underserved populations (Jain et al., 2024). Ultimately, the role of healthcare providers in preventive care is multifaceted, involving education, individualized care, and teamwork to ensure the optimal health of communities.

## Test Your Knowledge

1. How do lifestyle modifications contribute to disease prevention?
2. What role do healthcare providers play in promoting preventive care?

## 4.6. Policy and Legislation

**Learning Outcome**

1. Government mandates for vaccinations;
2. Role of public health organizations;
3. Ethical considerations in immunization policies.

The landscape of preventive and immunization services is constantly shaped by the laws and policies in the field of public health. Effective policy frameworks are required for the successful implementation of vaccination programs, which not only keep the person healthy but also the community healthy as well through herd immunity. Policies must also facilitate equal access to vaccines so that the poorer sections of society are given the necessary inputs so they can access immunization programs. Denmark, for instance, with its powerful health care system, characterized by thorough record-keeping and overall coverage, is the model for other countries as they strive to enhance their policy of immunization. There is a balancing act between comprehensive health care and preventive interventions that guarantees that the occurrence of vaccine-preventable diseases is significantly decreased, and an amendment in the form of legislative support is warranted in fostering a health-sensitive population (Sanders et al., 2016). Law also plays a significant role in shaping social attitudes and social practice in relation to immunization. Immunization requirements, particularly within the school system, can help speed up rising vaccination rates and lower infectious disease outbreak rates. These laws must be balanced against respect for individual choice and cultural beliefs, however, to engender public compliance and trust. In the past few years, various jurisdictions have seen heated debates on such legislation, primarily driven by misinformation regarding the safety of vaccines. To facilitate well-informed decision-making, it is essential to develop brief, evidence-based guidelines that communicate the benefits and drawback of vaccination. Policies must also offer exemptions but maintain an emphasis on the collective responsibility of maintaining public health standards. Constant interaction between policymakers and stakeholders is required to effectively deal with such controversial matters (Nancy et al., 2017).

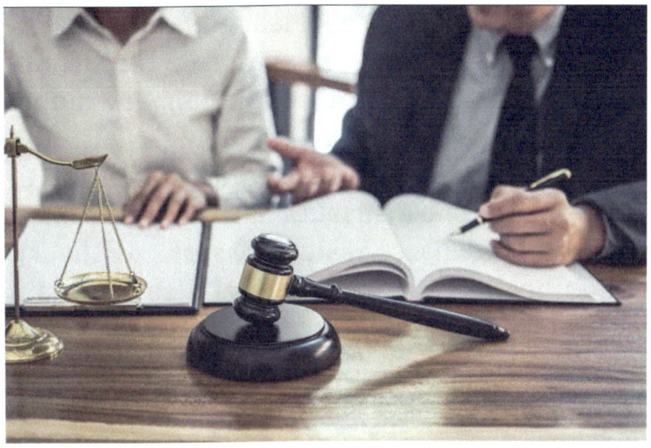

**Figure 4.13.** Policy and legislation.

*Source:* https://www.childprotectioncompany.com/wp-content/uploads/2022/11/Legislation-for-safeguarding-feature-pic.png.

In addition, integrating holistic health strategies within policy is able to control greater public health challenges, for example, those that the disadvantaged populations encounter. For example, individuals with severe mental disorders are usually exposed to dire health disparities that lead to a high death rate. Policies targeting such inequities not only improve access to immunization but also guarantee overall improvement in health outcomes. A model that addresses the individual, health system, and socio-environmental levels can be extremely helpful in developing effective programs and interventions. By providing policies with a comprehensive approach to health care, governments can implement interventions that reduce excess mortality and prioritize preventive care among various groups. Lastly, there is a need for laws to work towards building an integrated system where immunization protection and comprehensive health care are emphasized in order to ensure that nobody is left behind in the quest for better well-being (Nancy et al., 2017) (Figure 4.13).

### 4.6.1. Government Mandates for Vaccinations

The enforcement of government mandates for immunizations is an important aspect of public health policy and promoting community immunity. Through the enforcement of mandates for vaccinations, governments seek to safeguard vulnerable populations, such as those with compromised immune systems or those who cannot be vaccinated against certain diseases due to pre-existing conditions. As has been seen in most of the global health environments, such mandates have been successful in mitigating the spread of epidemic diseases and therefore reducing morbidity and mortality due to outbreaks. The necessity of such mandates becomes amply evident in the environments of communicable disease, where an extensive vaccination rate is required to provide herd immunity. Advocates argue that such policies not only ensure public health but also lead to economic benefits in the form of the avoidance of healthcare costs associated with disease treatment and hospitalization. Mandatory vaccination by the government, however, is normally faced with unyielding popular resistance, on the grounds of concerns over personal rights and personal liberty. Many people are concerned about the safety and efficacy of vaccines, perpetuated by misinformation usually communicated via social media sites like Facebook, YouTube, Twitter, et cetera.

This uncertainty could undermine confidence in health authorities and discourage vigorous immunization efforts. Furthermore, there is a complex debate about informed consent, in which ethical issues must be weighed against the needs of public health. As has been seen in countries with good health infrastructure, incorporating education in immunization activities can minimize public alarm and encourage compliance with government regulations. Thus, exploring the intersection of individual rights and community health gains is an enduring core concern as immunization policy responds to new health threats. To solidify immunization mandates, it is also necessary to implement and develop supporting programs that build trust and engagement across the community. Studies show that the incorporation of community-based health worker (CHW) programs into immunization initiatives can significantly increase outreach and education, resulting in increased compliance rates. Through relationship building at the community level, CHWs can demystify vaccines, deal with certain cultural concerns, and provide ongoing support during the vaccination process. As has been observed in many studies, the major features of successful CHW programs are local ownership, supportive supervision, and ongoing training in order to learn and adapt in harmony with local health dynamics. These efforts not only affirm the infrastructure necessary to enable vaccination mandates but also ensure that such mandates are grounded in a complete consideration of community values and needs, and that they promote a model for public health that is sustainable. The inclusion of community programs thus makes the ultimate effectiveness of vaccination efforts more consonant with measures of health equity and preventive care.

### 4.6.2. Role of Public Health Organizations

Public health organizations play a pivotal role in advocating for immunization and preventative care, acting as the anchor agencies that direct health programs within populations. Public health organizations not only assess healthcare needs but also develop strategic programs that are aimed at reducing healthcare access barriers. For instance, Blue Cross and Blue Shield of Minnesota Foundation's Growing Up Healthy program is a case in point of this role by focusing on vulnerable populations like immigrant communities and communities of color. By investing significant resources in increasing access to preventive medical and dental services, these organizations significantly reduce health disparities. Such initiatives are imperative in that they would guarantee that populations with high risks are given necessary immunizations and health screening, resulting in the overall healthy condition of the population. The model is multidimensional in that it highlights the intersection between targeted public health interventions and distributional health outcomes. In addition to direct healthcare service delivery, public health organizations are also the main vectors in disseminating information related to immunization and preventive measures. They leverage data analysis and community engagement in providing information to the public regarding the benefits of vaccination, along with preventive methods. Additionally, public health agencies integrating with electronic health record (EHR) systems is also a fine example of this role. Through the support of the proper use of EHRs, as illustrated in the Danish, New Zealand, and Swedish cases, public health agencies can enable complete sharing of information between medical practitioners, health authorities, and patients. The interlinking supports a more knowledgeable population, which is better equipped to make better health decisions through immediate access to up-to-date immunization histories and preventive health information. Such tech integration not only facilitates easier delivery of healthcare but also enhances patient engagement and compliance with vaccine cycles. Lastly, the activities of public health organizations also include advocacy and policy efforts at the local, state, and national levels to highlight the importance of immunization and preventive care. This advocacy is imperative in addressing legislative frameworks that govern public health programs, allowing for the influence of policies that allow for funding and resource allocation to vaccination programs. By advocating for evidence-based strategies, including the Growing Up Healthy program, public health agencies can successfully advocate for systemic changes that increase the eradication of health disparities. Furthermore, as they navigate issues of new health technology and adoption of practice, they provide knowledge-informed perspectives guiding policy discussions. These activities show the responsiveness of public health agencies in building a culture focused on preventive medicine and immunization that contributes towards healthier populations through equitable access to healthcare resources (Figure 4.14).

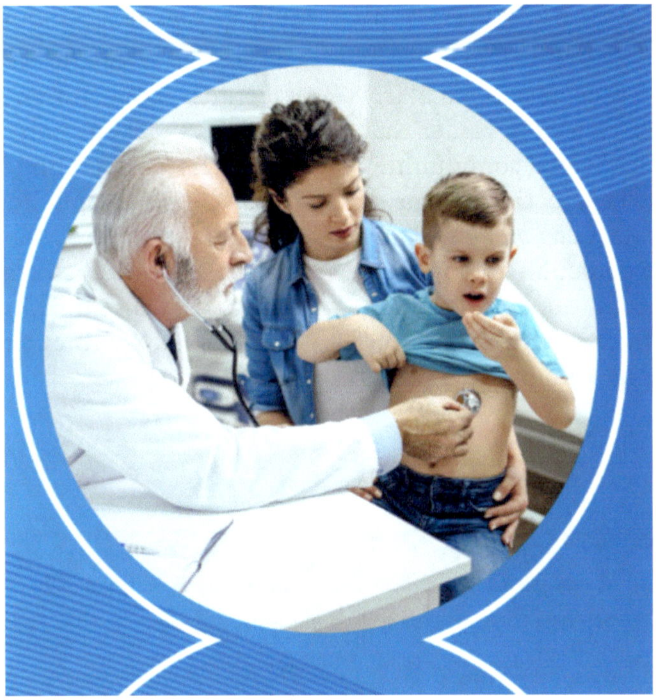

**Figure 4.14.** Role of public health organizations.

*Source:* https://media.licdn.com/dms/image/v2/D4D12AQEbAatVimyMfw/article-cover_image-shrink_720_1280/article-cover_image-shrink_720_1280/0/1690006990833?e=2147483647&v=beta&t=Zc3NkwVozYn57KsWAHTilTBxluDwkkCbdNhflNF1leI.

## 4.6.3. Ethical Considerations in Immunization Policies

The ethical considerations of immunization policies involve a rich array of factors that reflect social values, health equity, and public health requirements. In the particular context of vaccine administration, ethics like doing good and avoiding bad become of paramount importance. The ethical model not merely protects health care personnel and vulnerable populations but also identifies the greater interest of vaccination in the common good. For example, measures taken during the COVID-19 pandemic highlighted the need to deploy resources efficiently, a value reflecting commitment not only to individuals but also to public health outcomes. Ethical principles suggest that interventions required must be undertaken openly and inclusively, securing the interests of potentially marginalized communities, such as racial minorities, in these deliberations (Gadoth et al., 2021). Another important ethical component of immunization policies is promoting justice and minimizing health inequalities. The COVID-19 pandemic exposed pre-existing systemic disparities that disproportionately affected marginalized groups, referring to the glaring need for ethical guidance in vaccine distribution. The Advisory Committee on Immunization Practices (ACIP) has established ethical principles to ensure equitable distribution of vaccines, particularly when there are shortages. These are values that demand engagement with affected communities to ensure their voice is key in the design of policy frameworks. With its focus on justice, the framework facilitates the detection of loopholes hindering access to vaccinations, something crucial in fostering confidence and prompting better vaccination among vulnerable groups (McClung et al., 2020). Lastly, transparency is an essential element in ethical immunization policy practice. Building public trust is fundamental, particularly where the subject matter is vaccine refusal, which could be a result of historical injustices and disinformation. Open discussion of the benefits, risks, and processes of vaccine creation and dissemination encourages public wise decision-making. The transparent presentation of evidence-based rules and ongoing discourse with community leaders also favors the credibility of the antivaccination campaign. With the deployment of COVID-19 vaccines, government openness regarding decisions taken and the rationale behind prioritization grouping has played a critical role in assuaging the public's fears and trust in the immunization process (Gadoth et al., 2021). All these ethical considerations put together ensure that immunization policy is responsive to social need without compromising on health equity for all.

## Test Your Knowledge

1. What is the purpose of government mandates for vaccinations?
2. Name one ethical consideration involved in creating immunization policies.

## SUMMARY

The climax of the immunization and preventive healthcare research highlights the extreme importance that vaccination plays in a guaranteeing of public health. As is evidently illustrated in various case studies and reports, for example, those analyzing Sweden's COVID-19 plan, the effectiveness of immunization schemes has the potential to fundamentally alter the trajectory of infectious disease among populations. While there have been some criticisms of the Swedish model's voluntary policy on vaccination, it is an example of a larger trend in public health: the necessity for bespoke, and sometimes stricter, policies to protect vulnerable groups. In addition to serving as a shield against immediate health hazards, immunization also supports overall immunity, which can stem the spread of disease that threatens the population overall, primarily the elderly and those with weakened immune systems, as quoted in public health reports. Thus, investment in and attainment of successful immunization programs is central to securing long-term community well-being. Further, the review of access to next-generation vaccines, including HIV vaccines, finds that urgent public health infrastructure expansion is needed to maximize delivery mechanisms for vulnerable populations. Reports in collaboration with international health organizations indicate that without robust preparation and capacity for vaccine delivery, even breakthroughs in vaccine science may be unable to deliver their expected health impacts. The WHO and UNAIDS have put considerable focus on policy initiatives regarding delivery mechanisms to allow access to new vaccines on an equitable basis. Looking at the lessons of past vaccination campaigns and closing the gap in public health preparedness among countries, it is clearer than ever that immunization strategies need to be made adaptable to accommodate diverse community requirements without forgetting cost-effectiveness and feasibility concerns. In conclusion, the interface of immunization, preventive care, and public policy points to one stark reality: prevention is the solution in the battle against preventable diseases. The stark contrast in trends in health experienced in the various countries is at once an alarm and a call to action for public health officials and policymakers. The findings of case studies, for example, Sweden's pandemic response, criticized and research into the future supply of HIV vaccines, illustrate the complex system of the success of immunization. Critical analysis of these variables, such as community cooperation and adherence to vaccination programs, directs us in achieving safer futures. Finally, as global citizens, we must battle and invest in robust immunization systems that not only save our populations today but also prepare us to respond to challenges ahead, thereby creating a more resilient public health system.

Preventive care and immunization are significant in maintaining public health by actually preventing the spread of diseases and maintaining overall community health. A significant point is that vaccinations indeed reduce the incidence of infectious diseases such as measles, mumps, and rubella, lessening the complications and mortality rates from these ailments. In addition, by way of the acquisition of herd immunity, immunization offers protection to vulnerable people who are unable to be vaccinated due to medical conditions. Successful immunization programs, in this manner, safeguard not only a person's health but also the safety of the population at large, showing an essential investment in the prevention of disease and population health management. Economic considerations involved in immunization and preventive care are another essential consideration. Cost-effectiveness analysis is essential when evaluating the economic value of a disease versus the cost of a vaccine and preventive intervention. Stakeholders can make informed choices that support efficient utilization of resources within health care systems through the use of methodologies suggested by the Second Panel on Cost-Effectiveness in Health and Medicine

(Gillian et al., 2016). The benefit of these analyses extends beyond immediate health benefits; they also offer estimates of long-term savings in hospitalizations and treatment, further validating the economic rationale for mass immunization programs. The incorporation of mental health in the preventive care debate is also increasingly seen as a necessity. Patients with mental disorders have higher mortality rates, and this is an expansive area yet to be covered under the available preventive care services. The multilevel approach provided in recent studies suggests that there ought to be a firm framework that covers this issue thoroughly as far as individual, health system, and socio-environmental determinants are concerned (Nancy et al., 2017). By incorporating the teachings of comprehensive models that assess additional risk factors, stakeholders can develop multi-dimensional approaches to improving the health outcomes of individuals with mental illness so that preventive care addresses all essential dimensions of health and well-being.

## KEY TERMS FROM THIS CHAPTER

- Diphtheria
- Health monitoring
- Immunization
- Machine learning
- Population immunity
- Respiratory syncytial virus (RSV)
- Vaccine hesitancy
- Global health security
- Human papillomavirus (HPV)
- Infectious diseases
- Measles, mumps, and rubella (MMR)
- Public health
- Robust health
- Vaccine-preventable diseases

## CRITICAL THINKING QUESTIONS

**1. Which of the following vaccines is given at birth?**

a. DPT

b. Hepatitis B (first dose)

c. MMR

d. Varicella

**2. BCG vaccine is given to prevent:**

a. Hepatitis

b. Tuberculosis

c. Diphtheria

d. Measles

**3. The route of administration of the oral polio vaccine (OPV) is:**

a. Intramuscular

b. Subcutaneous

c. Intradermal

d. Oral

**4. Pentavalent vaccine protects against how many diseases?**

a. Three

b. Four

c. Five

d. Six

**5. The term "preventive pediatrics" includes all the following except:**

a. Immunization

b. Health education

c. Genetic counseling

d. Appendectomy

### Short Answer Questions

1. Define immunization. How does it help in disease prevention?
2. What is the difference between active and passive immunization?
3. Write a short note on the cold chain system in immunization.
4. What is the composition of the pentavalent vaccine and what diseases does it prevent?
5. Explain the concept of herd immunity.
6. What is preventive pediatrics? Name its three components.
7. What are the contraindications to live vaccines in children?
8. What is the importance of immunization cards in pediatric care?

### *Answers to Critical Thinking Questions*

1. (b) 2. (b) 3. (d) 4. (c) 5. (d)

## REFERENCES

1. Barth-Jones, R., & Hutubessy, R. (2007). Access-capacity and cost-effectiveness for future HIV vaccines. https://www.semanticscholar.org/paper/69a2b5ad07688907305e5f8f8710d44d3de565f3 (accessed on 16th June 2025).
2. Chaudhury, A., Duvoor, C., Dendi, V. S., Kraleti, S., Chada, A., Ravilla, R., Marco, A., et al. (2017). Clinical review of antidiabetic drugs: Implications for type 2 diabetes mellitus management. *Frontiers in Endocrinology, 8*. https://doi.org/10.3389/fendo.2017.00006 (accessed on 16th June 2025).
3. Connors, M., Graham, B. S., Lane, H. C., & Fauci, A. S. (2021). SARS-CoV-2 vaccines: Much accomplished, much to learn. *Annals of Internal Medicine, 174*, 687–690. https://doi.org/10.7326/m21-0111 (accessed on 16th June 2025).
4. Dewan, S. M. R., & Islam, M. R. (2022). Increasing reinfections and decreasing effectiveness of COVID-19 vaccines urge the need for vaccine customization. *Annals of Medicine and Surgery, 84*. https://doi.org/10.1016/j.amsu.2022.104961 (accessed on 16th June 2025).
5. Dong, Y., Dai, T., Wei, Y., Zhang, L., Zheng, M., & Zhou, F. (2020). A systematic review of SARS-CoV-2 vaccine candidates. *Signal Transduction and Targeted Therapy, 5*. https://doi.org/10.1038/s41392-020-00352-y (accessed on 16th June 2025).
6. Gadoth, A., Halbrook, M., Martin-Blais, R., Gray, A., Tobin, N. H., Ferbas, K. G., Aldrovandi, G. M., et al. (2021). Cross-sectional assessment of COVID-19 vaccine acceptance among health care workers in Los Angeles. *Annals of Internal Medicine, 174*, 882–885. https://doi.org/10.7326/m20-7580 (accessed on 16th June 2025).
7. Gray, B. H., Johansen, I., Koch, S., & Bowden, T. (2011). Electronic health records: An international perspective on "meaningful use." https://core.ac.uk/download/71358067.pdf (accessed on 16th June 2025).
8. Jain, M., Sharma, P. K., Kamboj, K., & Shyam, A. (2024). The impact of social media on medical education and health-care communication. *Journal of Orthopedic Case Reports, 14*, 1–3. https://www.semanticscholar.org/paper/b9b5922328e2fd5143d1e3ebd84cc77faed07afd (accessed on 16th June 2025).
9. Kumar, M. (2024). AI-powered wearables for continuous patient monitoring: Improving chronic disease management and preventive care. *International Scientific Journal of Engineering and Management*. https://www.semanticscholar.org/paper/20a9787c32d764c57def6c95f188dc8dec7f9722 (accessed on 16th June 2025).
10. Leimkugel, J. (2007). Clonal waves of meningococcal and pneumococcal meningitis in a region of the meningitis belt of Sub-Saharan Africa. https://www.semanticscholar.org/paper/5c882b3d1e235b4ac83bf587ca318abb886f5b91 (accessed on 16th June 2025).
11. Papanicolas, I., Woskie, L., & Jha, A. K. (2018). Health care spending in the United States and other high-income countries. *JAMA, 319*, 1024–1024. https://doi.org/10.1001/jama.2018.1150 (accessed on 16th June 2025).
12. Patil, S. N., Kerby, K., Ramick, A., & Criddle, J. (2021). "Is that for here or to go?" Drive-through pediatric vaccine clinic as a novel approach during a global pandemic. *Disaster Medicine and Public Health Preparedness*. https://www.semanticscholar.org/paper/df3510673870eef00abde7db9c6880ff9dbe3102 (accessed on 16th June 2025).

13. Riccò, M., Abu-Raya, B., Icardi, G., Spoulou, V., Greenberg, D., Falup Pecurariu, O., Hung, I. F., et al. (2024). Respiratory syncytial virus: A WAidid consensus document on new preventive options. *Vaccines, 12*. https://www.semanticscholar.org/paper/797c12eeab923a74cc39a94614197c18d5754e3e (accessed on 16th June 2025).

14. Sanders, G. D., Neumann, P. J., Basu, A., Brock, D. W., Feeny, D., Krahn, M., Kuntz, K. M., et al. (2016). Recommendations for conduct, methodological practices, and reporting of cost-effectiveness analyses. *JAMA, 316*, 1093–1093. https://doi.org/10.1001/jama.2016.12195 (accessed on 16th June 2025).

15. Scott, K., Beckham, S. W., Gross, M., Pariyo, G., Rao, K. D., Cometto, G., & Perry, H. B. (2018). What do we know about community-based health worker programs? A systematic review of existing reviews on community health workers. *Human Resources for Health, 16*. https://doi.org/10.1186/s12960-018-0304-x (accessed on 16th June 2025).

16. Yawn, B., Make, D., Mannino, D., Martinez, F., & Han, M. (2021). Letter to editor regarding the OCEAN study [Letter]. *International Journal of Chronic Obstructive Pulmonary Disease, 16*, 2501–2502. https://www.semanticscholar.org/paper/3fc358478961ed8dbd2ae51f8c9d62451b48bdb2 (accessed on 16th June 2025).

# NEONATOLOGY: CARE OF THE NEWBORN

# 5

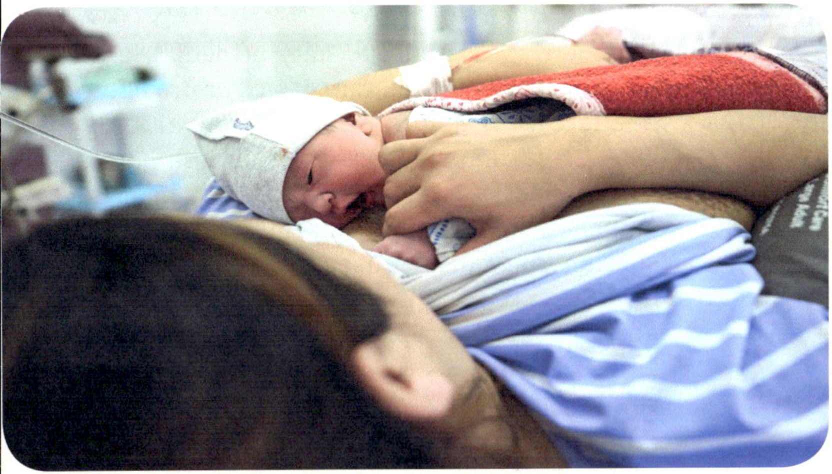

## LEARNING OBJECTIVES

**After studying this chapter, you will be able to:**

1. Explain the developmental stages of newborns;
2. List of discussed common neonatal conditions;
3. Focus on neonatal assessment and monitoring;
4. Discuss the nutritional needs of newborns;
5. Know the neonatal intensive care unit (NICU);
6. Learn about ethical considerations in neonatology.

## Introduction

Neonatology, a pediatric subspecialty, is concerned with the medical care of the newborn, especially the premature or ill babies requiring intensive medical attention. Neonatology encompasses a wide scope of topics, including life physiology in the neonate, normal pathologies in neonates, and care techniques to result in the optimal health outcome. Proper neonatal care is imperative, as neonatal death rates remain disproportionate in developing regions. The single most important aspect of neonatal care, such as early initiation of breastfeeding and cord care, matters for normal development in the early days of life. These practices, apart from enhancing survival, also lay the groundwork for lifelong health (Isac et al., 2025). An understanding of neonatology's nuances allows healthcare providers to meet the challenges of providing care to this at-risk patient population. A complete overview of neonatology also involves reviewing the determinants influencing newborn health and neonatal care practices, particularly among various cultures and socioeconomic backgrounds. For instance, in some rural areas, regional practices may lead to unsafe cord care or feeding patterns, which can significantly impair neonatal survival. In Bareilly district, studies have demonstrated that unsafe feeding and inappropriately initiated breastfeeding were more frequent in-home births, which underlines the significance of proper educational interventions (Islam et al., 2023). Addressing these disparities means strengthening the clinical competence of the healthcare providers as well as increasing the sensitivity of families regarding important newborn care practices.

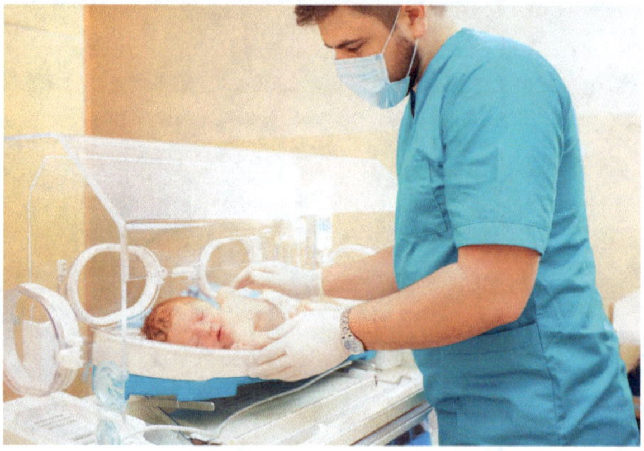

**Figure 5.1.** Neonatology, a subspecialty of pediatrics.

Source: https://www.apollocradle.com/backend/web/blog-images/1697608335shutterstock_414166414-scaled.jpg.webp.

Through the generation of a comprehensive understanding of such influences, healthcare systems can utilize targeted solutions to optimize neonatal health and reduce mortality. Finally, the role of healthcare systems in ensuring proper practice and information dissemination in neonatology cannot be exaggerated. Properly orienting healthcare staff with requisite skills and knowledge leads to improved optimal essential newborn care practice. Large variations in care based on the provider's skills have been noted, which accentuates the requirement of ongoing training and assessment of clinical competency (Isac et al., 2025). Further, including education of the family in neonatology may empower families and mothers since they are often the most immediate caregivers. By focusing on large-scale training of healthcare personnel and community awareness, neonatology can work towards achieving better outcomes in newborns, ultimately preventing the public health problem of neonatal mortality (Figure 5.1).

## Definition and Scope of Neonatology

Neonatology is a subspecialty of pediatricians and defines the overall care of sick or premature neonates. The definition of neonatology extends beyond standard care for well babies; it encompasses intricate features of neonatal pathology and physiology that must be treated by specialized medical procedures. Neonatologists have acquired the ability to manage intricate illnesses such as respiratory distress syndrome, an area that has seen tremendous growth in clinical practice through advancing guidelines (Webbe et al., 2019). By integrating evidence-based principles into their treatment protocols, neonatologists aim to optimize health outcomes for high-risk neonates, thus preventing potential future complications that stem from prematurity and congenital disorders. The neonatology specialty is comprehensive, with both acute and chronic disorders in neonates. It involves treating conditions ranging from sepsis, brain injury, and nutritional deficit that require multidisciplinary care. Recent consensus on neonatal core outcome sets names the main elements of health outcomes that are important to implement further research upon, so that clinical trials aim at issues most important to newborns and their families (Webbe et al., 2019). Stakeholder engagement focuses on outcome priority, capturing the need for an integrative approach in establishing what full neonatal care means. This collaboration between healthcare professionals, researchers, and families guarantees that the evolving practices in neonatology remain beneficial to all the stakeholders. With ongoing improvements in neonatology, new technologies and methods have a significant impact on neonatal management. For example, the management of respiratory distress syndrome has been greatly improved, with current practice guiding early use of surfactant therapy and non-invasive respiratory support therapy methods (David et al., 2019). These developments not only help enhance clinical outcomes but also help in avoiding the development of chronic lung disease in preterm infants. The dynamic nature of neonatology also involves constant education and revision of care protocols in response to ongoing research and clinical trials. This places neonatologists at the leading edge of care for neonates and allows them to apply the most up-to-date research to provide the optimal results for the most vulnerable patient group—infants (Figure 5.2).

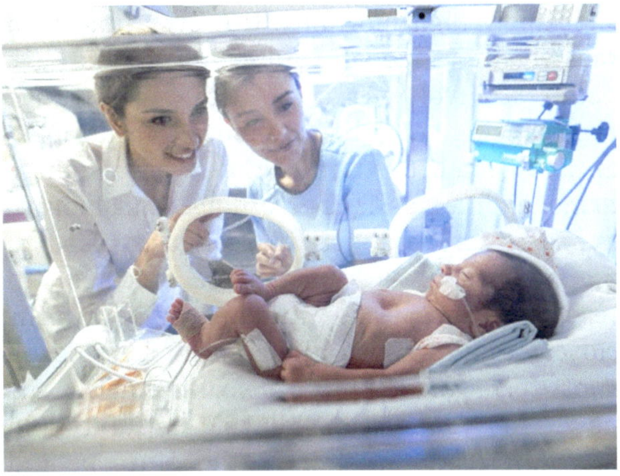

**Figure 5.2.** Definition and scope of neonatology.

Source: https://media.licdn.com/dms/image/v2/D4D12AQHp89dPFu85Zg/article-cover_image-shrink_720_1280/article-cover_image-shrink_720_1280/0/1655878789030?e=2147483647&v=beta&t=2f1P8WmNTF0sSSJygfaEbbC9Av40Q3Haeg7V9uzDuwM.

## Importance of Neonatal Care

Neonatal care is necessary for the health and well-being of babies, particularly those born prematurely or with illness. The first few hours of life are critical, as these are moments when babies are most vulnerable. Effective neonatal care involves a coordinated strategy that includes immediate medical care, observation, and infant care. Advances in medicine and technology have greatly improved outcomes for these vulnerable populations. These developments bring to the fore the importance of health systems relying on scientific evidence in guiding their neonatal services. As Ho et al. (2024) propose, decision-makers must navigate through the dangers of producing credible evidence in day-to-day neonatal practice, hence making the services tailored to specific needs without compromising the quality of care. Additionally, special units like the PANDA unit demonstrate the urgent importance of shared neonatal care. By encouraging an interdisciplinary approach among perinatal psychiatry, neonatology, and post-natal care, the units can provide comprehensive care to both mothers and infants. Such unification significantly enhances the quality of the care given during a most crucial phase of a child's life. The model not only addresses immediate physical welfare but also honors the interconnected factors influencing maternal mental health as well as infant growth. This combined framework enables early diagnostic screening and prompt intervention, which are critical in preventing adverse outcomes. As noted by Vitte et al. (2022), innovative interventions can lead to therapeutic as well as preventive interventions that are critical in promoting healthy mother-infant relations and abuse and neglect prevention. Lastly, the benefits of neonatal care extend to private health, reaching broader public health. High-quality neonatal care reduces infant mortality and long-term development issues that can arise as a result of early substandard care. Placement of high-level neonatal care, health systems are able to reduce future healthcare complications from chronic diseases that arose as a consequence of substandard initial treatment. The continued investment in neonatal care is a reflection of the societal investment in healthy life beginnings, including not just medical care but also creating supporting environments for families and newborns. The social value accorded to the care of infants cannot be overstated, as the article by Ho et al. (2024) has noted; decisions regarding screening and early interventions must be informed by this intrinsic value to achieve optimal health equity and access to services among diverse populations (Figure 5.3).

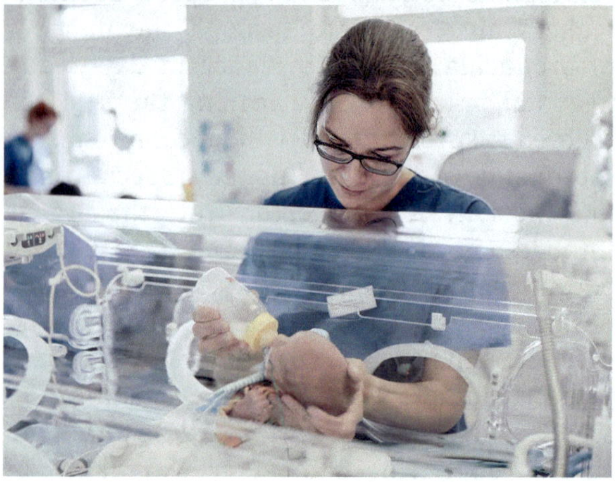

**Figure 5.3.** Neonatal care is imperative for ensuring the health and well-being of newborns.

Source: https://www.draeger.com/Media/Content/Content/neonatal-care-4-3-D-6667-2018.jpg.

## Overview of Neonatal Mortality and Morbidity Rates

When considering neonatal morbidity and mortality rates, one must recognize the massive impact of many medical advancements in reducing these rates, particularly in preterm infants. Neonatal mortality remains a significant global health issue, where preterm birth significantly contributes to it. Statistics indicate nearly 70% of neonatal deaths are due to prematurity, representing the urgency for specific interventions (Mortazavi et al., 2019). The recent years have witnessed a steady decrease in mortality rates due to improvements in neonatal intensive care units (NICUs), which improve the survival chances of extremely low birth weight infants. The early application of surfactant treatment, advances in neonatal imaging techniques, and enhanced monitoring practices have collectively transformed neonatal care, offering high-risk newborns a brighter future. But the unequal mortality rates among different areas provide evidence for the requirement of equal access to quality neonatal care to ensure that all newborns receive similar treatment. Mortality is generally preceded by morbidity in newborns, and this just adds to the problem. Respiratory distress syndrome (RDS), infection, and neurodevelopmental complications are prevalent among premature babies and tend to cause long-term health problems. The rate of occurrence between birth weight and neonatal outcome is particularly pertinent; e.g., infants weighing less than 700 grams experience shockingly high mortality. However, infants in the weight range of 1000–1500 grams have better survival with a significant percentage experiencing favorable outcomes (Mortazavi et al., 2019). In order for healthcare practitioners to modify interventions accordingly and improve neonatal care practice, these figures need to be understood. With ongoing developments in research, it is crucial to track morbidity patterns closely, as they have a significant bearing on short-term and long-term health courses for newborns. Along with knowing mortality and morbidity rates, examining the cause behind these events is crucial for improving neonatal care. Several studies highlight the importance of thorough data compilation to know more about the epidemiology of neonatal diseases and related factors. Variables like maternal age, prenatal access, and genetic factors contribute considerably to the impact on neonatal outcomes. In addition, acute kidney injury rates among neonates, especially in critically ill patients, highlight the importance of early identification and management strategies crucial to enhancing survival rates. With the intricacies that accompany neonatal care, sustained research and improvement of medical practice are necessary for effectively decreasing mortality and morbidity rates, ultimately ensuring a healthier future for neonates across different populations.

## 5.1. Developmental Stages of Newborns

**Learning Outcome**

1. Premature vs. full-term infants;
2. Physiological changes at birth;
3. Key milestones in the first month.

Newborn development phases are of critical significance from the neonatology viewpoint, as early stages of development have long-term implications for subsequent health. Newborns typically experience different developmental phases of physiological and neurological changes in the first weeks of life. During the first phase, also known as the neonatal period and continuing for as long as about 28 days postnatally, infants undergo a series of adjustments to external environments, including keeping their body temperature stable and physiological adjustments within the respiratory and circulatory systems.

Critical care during this stage is imperative because the healthcare workers must monitor the newborn for distress and developmental abnormalities, especially in high-risk populations, where complications can be more likely to develop (Kumar et al., 2024). Understanding these stages allows practitioners to conduct appropriate interventions and obtain optimal developmental outcomes for all newborns. The importance of environmental factors and access to healthcare in the neonatal period cannot be overstated, especially in light of recent findings demonstrating the striking role of situational stressors, such as military aggression, in shaping newborn health outcomes. For instance, studies have shown that crises can be linked to specific increases in low birth weights and increased incidence of congenital complications of health complications among newborn infants as a severe burden on neonatal healthcare systems (Antipkin et al., 2024). In areas experiencing instability, maternal health service breakdowns further complicate the trajectory of infant development, illustrating the interaction between environmental influences and biological development. This places in focus the importance of individually tailored interventions addressing the immediate medical issues as well as broader social determinants that influence health, encouraging holistic care strategies within neonatology that consider the special problems newborns face in varied environments. In addition, follow-up care for newborns as they transition beyond the early neonatal stage is necessary for ongoing development and monitoring. Once the first few weeks have passed, the practitioners need to continue screening for milestones of development, particularly sensory and motor skills milestones. This entails testing auditory and visual responses because underlying conditions in these areas can lead to significant developmental delay if not detected early. Current studies in support of newborn hearing screening (NHS) have shown that early intervention produces much better outcomes for language acquisition and overall quality of life in afflicted children (Kumar et al., 2024). By putting the identification of developmental delays first and ensuring their proper correction by using best practices in sophisticated care, neonatology can open doors to healthier futures. Lastly, the developmental stages of infants require an integrated, multidisciplinary approach that supports both short-term care needs and long-term growth (Figure 5.4).

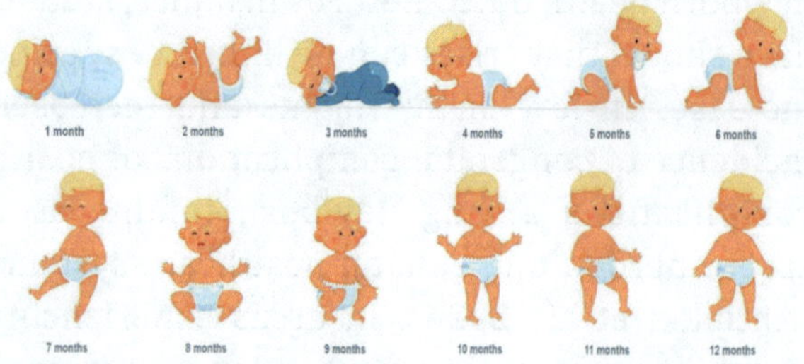


**Figure 5.4.** The developmental stages of newborns are critical in the context of neonatology.

*Source:* https://static.vecteezy.com/system/resources/previews/023/586/648/non_2x/baby-growth-stages-development-process-from-newborn-to-toddler-baby-milestones-timeline-sitting-crawling-standing-walking-illustration-vector.jpg.

### 5.1.1. Premature versus Full-Term Infants

In neonatology, the distinction between premature and full-term infants is of profound significance when it comes to treatment and states of health. Premature infants, by definition, are infants born before 37 weeks of gestation and suffer from extreme difficulties due to their underdeveloped systems, mainly lungs, which lead to greater respiratory-related complications. The lack of adequate development may necessitate interventions such as mechanical ventilation or oxygen therapy, rendering their postnatal care more complicated. Those born full-term at 39 to 41 weeks have sounder health profiles and require less aggressive medical care. This comparative review accentuates the necessity of certain care practices for the unique vulnerabilities of premature infants to plug gaps in their developmental and physiological milestones when placed against those of their full-term counterparts. The largest challenge to the care of premature infants is likely the risk of long-term developmental damage and chronic illness, particularly on the respiratory side. Studies have shown that premature infants are at significantly higher risk of developing pulmonary disease, such as bronchopulmonary dysplasia, which arises as a result of oxygen therapy and mechanical ventilation. Current research has shown that lung ultrasound (LUS) is much better at detecting edema and consolidations in the lungs of premature children compared to standard chest X-ray (CXR) scans. Specifically, studies indicate that LUS identified 45% of the cases with lung consolidations and CXR identified 19% of the cases with consolidations. Thus, employing advanced imaging techniques like LUS can revolutionize the approach to manage0ment of the recurrent health conditions in premature neonates by the neonatal care teams by enhancing the quality of the targeted interventions being delivered throughout their vulnerable developmental phase (Niu et al., 2024). Pre- and full-term infants need nutrition for the health of both groups, though opportunity and challenge are enormously disparate. Human milk is the gold standard of infant nutrition, critical to the development and growth of both groups. However, in the case of premature infants who often have to go through unique feeding protocols, the availability of donor human milk becomes crucial, especially when maternal milk is not available because of illnesses or maternal problems. The establishment of centers like the Donor Human Milk Bank has significant implications for the health of ill and premature full-term babies, as it allows these high-risk patients to be subjected to active biological agents that foster their nutritional needs. Such interventions are able to enhance growth velocities, immune capability, and potentially decrease the incidence of prematurity complications, strengthening the evidence base for coordinated, community-based care interventions in neonatology (Malachynska et al., 2025) (Figure 5.5).

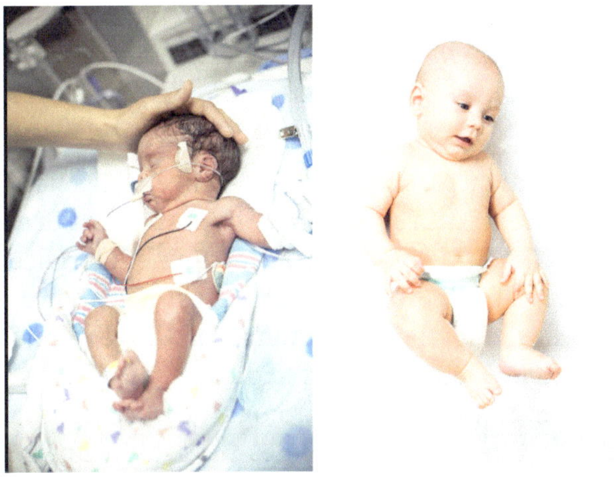

**Figure 5.5.** Premature versus full-term infants.

*Source:* https://cdn-wordpress-info.futurelearn.com/info/wp-content/uploads/4d3f4c9a-8d19-4a1f-905d-d3ddf58c3e11-768x578.jpg.

## 5.1.2. Physiological Changes at Birth

The moment of birth is a crucial juncture that encompasses numerous physiological changes, which are crucial to the adjustment of the neonate to extrauterine life. At the moment of birth, the neonate experiences a sudden shift from a placentally maintained environment with placental gas exchange to one that requires autonomous breathing. During this period, respiration begins, instigated by changes in environmental stimuli and cessation of the umbilical blood supply. The newborn's lungs are filled up for the first time, ventilating liquid with air, and surfactant, a byproduct produced within the lungs, begins to play a vital role in reducing surface tension and hence preventing alveolar collapse. All these processes highlight the need for immediate respiratory support; delay in this adjustment will lead to respiratory derangement, such as respiratory distress syndrome (RDS) (Zaigham et al., 2020). Cardiovascular adjustments are also crucial at this time. The circulatory system of the infant must rapidly adjust to increased constraints upon umbilical cord clamping. The ductus arteriosus, a significant fetal artery that allows bypassing of functional lungs by blood, closes, changing the hemodynamics of circulation to favor pulmonary circulation. The closure reconstitutes fetal circulation to a postnatal form to promote effective oxygenation through the lungs. Furthermore, the foramen ovale, which is fetal, also closes in response to elevated pressures within the left atrium as the final steps toward a fully functional neonatal heart are undertaken. Such cardiovascular system adaptations are highly dependent on maternal disease states, such as COVID-19, which has been associated with severe maternal morbidity and potential perinatal complications (Zaigham et al., 2020).

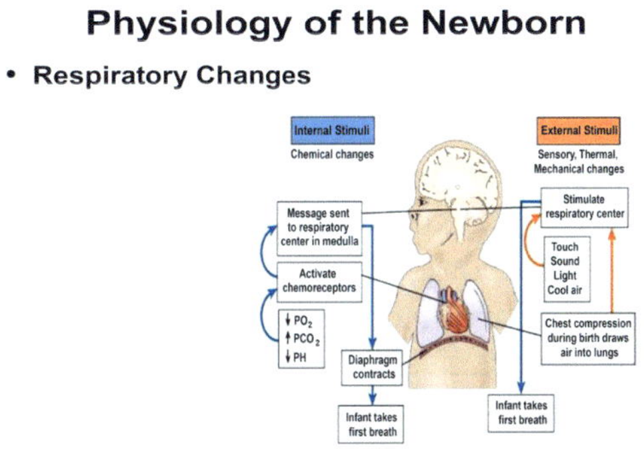


**Figure 5.6.** Physiological changes at birth.

*Source:* https://image4.slideserve.com/9193452/physiology-of-the-newborn-l.jpg.

It is important that there are such changes in newborn baby care, especially in those with prematurity or who have health risks. Thermoregulation is also another issue to be addressed immediately upon birth ,as infants are highly susceptible to hypothermia due to their comparatively large surface area compared to body mass. The loss of heat from the mother and the exposure to the air necessitates immediate and effective management of temperature. Newborns are unable to shiver and instead utilize non-shivering thermogenesis, which is metabolizing brown fat to produce heat. It is essential that normothermia is maintained, as hypothermia results in metabolic and cardiovascular instability and enhances further complications such as respiratory distress and hypoglycemia. Accordingly, healthcare workers must implement timely and appropriate interventions, including skin-to-skin contact with the mother to increase warmth and bonding, solidifying the importance of integral care while the infant acclimates to the new setting (David et al., 2019) (Figure 5.6).

### 5.1.3. Key Milestones in the First Month

The newborn's initial month of life is crucial for survival and healthy development, with several milestones. The month is characterized by rapid physiological adaptation, during which babies transition from intrauterine life to autonomous life outside the uterus. Prominent among these is the acquisition of proper respiratory function because newborns must adapt to ambient air and get into normal rhythms of breathing. Also of importance is the maintenance of body temperature since newborns have inadequate thermoregulatory skills and can develop hypothermia unless properly managed.

Monitoring of these essential signs is an imperative to ensure stability and readiness for subsequent phases of development, once again highlighting the experience of neonatal care as paramount in the management of this transition phase. The nutrition also assumes a definitive role during the first month of newborns, with feeding milestones determining attainment of maximal growth.

Regardless of whether breastfed or formula-fed, the baby requires adequate caloric nutrition to support their active growth and metabolic demands. Exclusive breastfeeding is highly recommended during this period because colostrum, the early milk secreted, offers critical immunological benefits. Second, the feeding lays the foundation for gastrointestinal function and the prevention of complications like necrotizing enterocolitis, particularly among premature babies.

With increasing frequency and effectiveness of more mature feedings by the newborn, practitioners must monitor feeding intolerance or signs of dehydration closely, further emphasizing the importance of diligent and skilled neonatal monitoring throughout this first month. Sensory and neurologic development in the first month also includes the establishment of developmental milestones, setting the stage for later achievements. Infants exhibit reflexive activities such as rooting and grasping, which illustrate their normal response to stimuli in their environment.

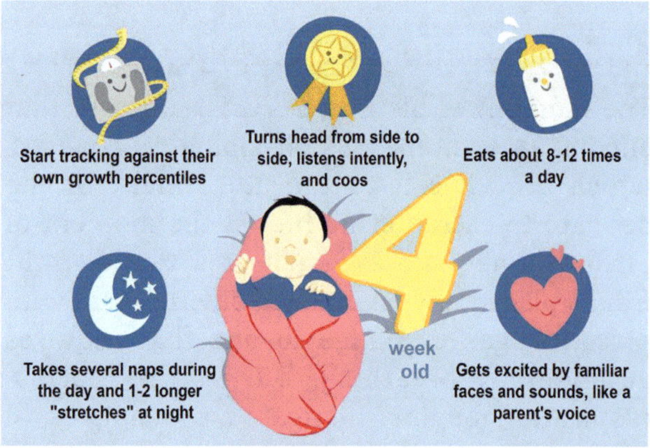


**Figure 5.7.** Key milestones in the first month.

*Source:* https://www.parents.com/thmb/9Fxb7677mKDk0L2D9lujYvIyFM0=/1500x0/filters:no_upscale():max_bytes(150000):strip_icc()/babys-first-year-04-6d7ad836f4894109b4a1ec58fe8cb30b.png.

Vision, although limited at birth, gets better due to the fact that infants can fixate on objects near them and differentiate between light and darkness. Auditory functions also become evident; infants start to respond to sound, pointing towards developmental progress. While caregivers create these sensory experiences through stimulation and interaction, they maintain the critical neural synapses that form the basis of cognitive growth. Understanding these early milestones is important for healthcare providers, as it informs practices of care that are intended to optimize newborns' transition into the world outside the uterus and supportive long-term health outcomes, corroborating what was found in more recent studies in neonatology (Morris et al., 2020) (Figure 5.7).

## Test Your Knowledge

1. What is one key difference between premature and full-term infants?
2. Discuss about important developmental milestones that newborns typically reach in the first month.

## 5.2. Common Neonatal Conditions

**Learning Outcome**

1. Respiratory distress syndrome;
2. Jaundice in newborns;
3. Infections and sepsis.

The management of common neonatal diseases is the core to the preservation of the health and well-being of newborns. Respiratory distress syndrome (RDS), jaundice, and infection are among the most prevalent of the neonatal diseases. RDS is particularly common in premature infants, with the lack of surfactant inducing compromised gas exchange and a heavy burden of morbidity. This syndrome needs supportive therapy and potential interventions such as the administration of exogenous surfactant to maximize pulmonary function. Jaundice is also frequently present due to high bilirubin from the immature liver function of the newborn. Jaundice will cause kernicterus if not treated properly, which will lead to permanent neurological injury. Thus, early identification and management of such conditions form a crucial component of neonatal care, emphasizing the role of a vigilant clinical approach by physicians. Another salient characteristic of neonatal care is the management of genetic disorders and malformations that may arise. It is thought that most of the newborns admitted to Neonatal Intensive Care Units (NICUs) have genetic disease or syndromic disorders that might not have been identified prenatally. The neonatologist must be aware of recognizing the disorders because early detection will lead to better outcomes in diseased infants. Genetic diagnosis will also result in more informed discussions with parents regarding prognosis and potential interventions (Serra et al., 2021). Practitioners require communication skills as presenting complex information regarding genetic diagnosis will significantly determine parental understanding and emotional response.

An effective conversation will promote beneficial family participation in the infant's long-term care. Lastly, the emotional and ethical dimensions of neonatal treatment cannot be overlooked. The impact of genetic diagnosis on family relationships and parental stress is significant, with more frequently than not, suboptimal communication strategies in breaking bad news (Serra et al., 2021). Neonatologists must walk through these delicate interactions with frankness and compassion because the initial message can significantly influence future parental satisfaction and engagement in their infant's care. Consensus among experts recommends best practice in delivering bad news, and the need for a formalized process that can enhance the overall experience for families. With effective communication and ethical standards at the forefront, healthcare professionals can improve the quality of care given to newborns with common neonatal conditions that ultimately lead to better health outcomes and emotional coping in families (Figure 5.8).

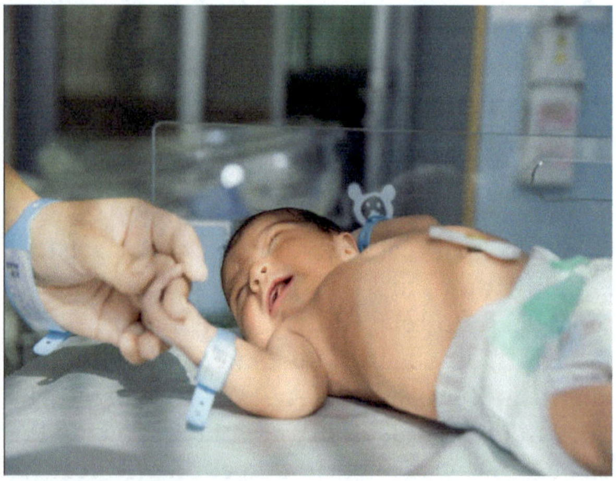

**Figure 5.8.** The management of common neonatal conditions.

*Source:* https://motherlandhospital.com/wp-content/uploads/2024/07/newborn-baby-neonatology-1.png.

### 5.2.1. Respiratory Distress Syndrome

Respiratory distress syndrome (RDS) is a severe neonatal complication, particularly in preterm infants with not yet developed lungs. RDS happens primarily due to surfactant deficiency, which decreases the surface tension within alveoli so that they will not collapse during exhalation. Clinical manifestations of RDS typically begin within hours after birth, and these include tachypnea, grunting, and cyanosis. Early and appropriate diagnosis is necessary because it determines the immediate respiratory supportive treatment, which can include supplemental oxygen, continuous positive airway pressure (CPAP), or mechanical ventilation. The Silverman-Andersen scale has been a critical tool in assessing the severity of RDS by providing a systematic method of evaluating newborn respiratory status, hence enabling clinicians to use interventions accordingly and ultimately enhance outcomes for this vulnerable population, as noted by Zavyalov et al. (2023). RDS management has significantly changed over the decades in accordance with transformations in neonatal care. Among these developments, the advent of antenatal corticosteroids has been a milestone intervention. The use of these steroids in high-risk mothers to accelerate fetal lung development significantly decreases the incidence and severity of RDS among preterm infants. Besides pharmacologic interventions, the quality of neonatal intensive care units (NICUs) has been instrumental because they employ advanced monitoring technology and provide specialized respiratory therapy. Ongoing monitoring of vital signs, including heart rate variability (HRV), can assist in identifying stress reactions and potential complications. Evidence suggests that the application of HRV can enhance clinical judgment by pre-empting RDS-related adverse events, thereby enhancing responsiveness to the infants' needs and improving the quality of care provided, as per Chiera et al. (2020). While stabilization and support are the most urgent concerns in the management of RDS, follow-up of affected infants over the long term reveals additional points to consider. Survivors of RDS are at high risk for subsequent development of several complications, including bronchopulmonary dysplasia (BPD) and other respiratory complications. The correlation of early respiratory distress with later disease necessitates multi-disciplinary follow-up on a routine basis to assess lung function and overall development. Besides, interdisciplinary collaboration among members of healthcare teams is crucial to ensure comprehensive care at various phases of the life of a newborn. Interdisciplinary collaboration is what drives research and unifies obstetric, neonatology, and pediatric departments' practices, which is crucial for heightened prevention and management measures of RDS, hence ultimately neonatal improvement as described by Chiera et al. (2020) and Zavyalov et al. (2023) (Figure 5.9).

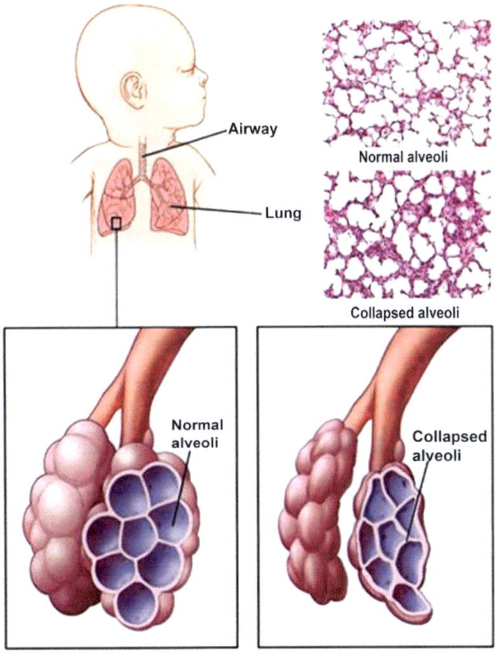


**Figure 5.9.** Respiratory distress syndrome.

*Source:* https://nursesrevisionuganda.com/wp-content/uploads/2023/01/infant-respiratory-distress-syndrome-842x1024.jpg.

## 5.2.2. Jaundice in Newborns

Jaundice in the newborn is a common neonatology finding with various causes and implications. Neonatal jaundice, characterized by skin and yellow sclera due to hyperbilirubinemia, affects a large percentage of newborns, particularly premature infants and those with conditions like hemolytic disease of new born. The biochemical pathway of bilirubin production, which comes primarily from the breakdown of red blood cells, may burden the immature liver of the neonate and lead to unconjugated hyperbilirubinemia. Bilirubin should be closely monitored because untreated jaundice, in turn, may lead to severe complications such as kernicterus, a bilirubin-induced brain injury. Thus, an understanding of pathophysiology and management of jaundice is essential in the provision of successful health outcomes among newborns. Jaundice is evaluated by careful clinical assessment, including measurement of total bilirubin levels, identification of the onset and timing of jaundice, and determination of risk factors such as maternal incompatibility of blood group or birth weight. For instance, in Down syndrome newborns, diagnoses must also include detailed evaluation of concomitant conditions that might complicate the clinical picture. In a study of medical issues in Down syndrome newborns, jaundice was noted as an established clinical indicator among other severe manifestations. Therefore, clinicians need to engage a multidisciplinary team consisting of pediatricians, neonatologists, and others to identify and treat jaundice correctly, considering the broader range of health conditions found in high-risk populations as highlighted in research in this field (Telman et al., 2022). Current studies have emphasized another mandatory aspect in treating jaundice, parents' health-seeking behavior driven by externalities. Specifically, the COVID-19 pandemic also presented unprecedented challenges to the timely admission of newborns with jaundice-related conditions. A study conducted at a tertiary care hospital documented a marked decline in admissions for jaundice during the period under the impact of COVID, citing a concerning trend where families will be reluctant to approach a medical intervention for fear or because of pandemic-imposed restrictions. Such decreases in healthcare use not only impacted the acute treatment of jaundice but also negatively impacted neonatal health outcomes, further underscoring the importance of continued education for parents on identifying jaundice symptoms and prompt medical care (Liu et al., 2022). The relationship between outside-of-the-clinic health crises and pediatric service necessitates continued research and development of neonatology practice to safeguard the health of neonates (Figure 5.10).

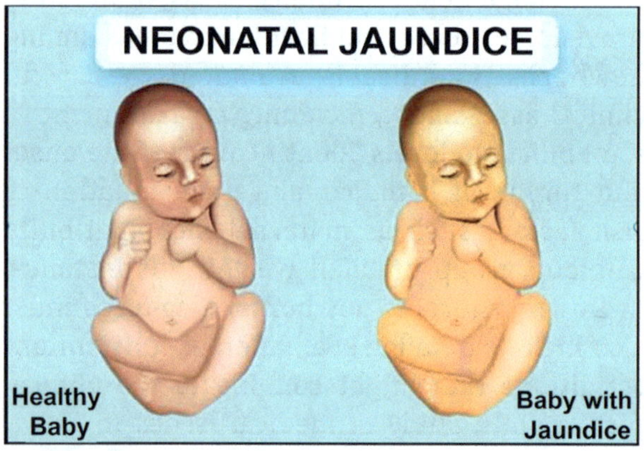


**Figure 5.10.** The incidence of jaundice in newborns.

*Source:* https://static.wixstatic.com/media/7196e0_e234a515a830489ba086b732fb360e3f~mv2.png/v1/fill/w_568,h_388,al_c,q_85,usm_0.66_1.00_0.01,enc_avif,quality_auto/7196e0_e234a515a830489ba086b732fb360e3f~mv2.png.

### 5.2.3. Infections and Sepsis

In neonatology, infection and sepsis are a seriously threatening factor to the health of newborns, particularly those that fall under the category of very low birth weight (VLBW) infants. These fragile neonates are at a higher risk of acquiring healthcare-associated infections (HAIs) that can actually hinder their recovery process significantly and increase mortality. A retrospective cohort study revealed that nearly 40% of VLBW babies in a Brazilian NICU were found to have HAIs and approximately 30% developed sepsis, indicating the direct connection between low birth weight and increased susceptibility to infection. In an interesting finding, sepsis was even more prevalent among individuals with weights under 750 g, further making managing processes within neonatal intensive care units (NICUs) complicated. These grim figures indicate the overwhelming need for infection control measures to limit HAIs' morbidity and improve outcomes among this vulnerable population (Caixeta et al., 2025). The pathogenic role of various pathogens in neonatal infection is multifaceted, with Gram-negative bacteria (GNB) and fungi constituting a considerable proportion of those diagnosed cases. Among the 456 cases of VLBW neonate infections, an impressive 30.3% were caused by GNB, with a smaller but concerning percentage by fungal causes. The growing trend of multidrug-resistant pathogens exacerbates the issue of controlling these infections effectively, further fueling the clinical challenge. Interestingly, the use of antifungal agents was the most significant predictor for infections, indicating that previous exposure to antimicrobial therapy could be one of the factors contributing to the resistance process. Moreover, infections not only prolong hospitalization stays but also significantly influence the survival of these high-risk neonates, highlighting the urgent necessity for targeted prevention and treatment strategies in NICUs (Caixeta et al., 2025). Struggles against neonatal infections have gained momentum with global initiatives in enhancing the quality of care for infants. The World Health Organization's initiative to roll out Standards to enhance the quality of care, particularly for the management of neonatal infections, aligns with country-level agendas such as Every Newborn Action Plan (ENAP). The plan seeks to reduce neonatal mortality through better total care. However, a systematic review of infection control guidelines in 90 ENAP countries revealed substantial inconsistencies with the implementation of WHO guidelines. While the majority of national guidelines addressed critical elements like clinical symptom assessment and antibiotic usage, considerable gaps persist in the full execution of best practice. Closing these gaps is fundamental to enhancing neonatal care, outcomes, and eventually the prevention of avoidable deaths due to infection and sepsis.

## Test Your Knowledge

1. What causes respiratory distress syndrome in newborns?
2. How is jaundice in newborns typically identified?

## 5.3. Neonatal Assessment and Monitoring

**Learning Outcome**

1. Apgar score and its significance;
2. Physical examination techniques;
3. Monitoring vital signs and growth.

In neonatology, neonatal monitoring and assessment are essential in keeping their health and well-being intact. Premature or complicated newborns require careful monitoring of their vital parameters like heart rate, breathing patterns, and oxygen saturation. Traditional monitoring methods sometimes prove to be invasive and distasteful to the baby. New contactless approaches such as imaging photoplethysmography have therefore emerged as a promising alternative. These methods have been very accurate in clinical practice, offering a non-invasive method of monitoring important signs. In minimizing pain, these advancements enable a more holistic neonatal care, where professionals can respond quickly to any variations without compromising the comfort of the babies (Svoboda et al., 2024). Secondly, understanding neurological infant development is crucial, particularly in infants who are preterm. The use of amplitude-integrated electroencephalography (aEEG) has gained more popularity as a valuable tool for the monitoring of brain function in neonates. The process of monitoring over a prolonged period not only assesses the acute brain function but also enables clinicians to identify patterns that give an indication of potential neurological injury or developmental delay. Particularly in preterm infants, aEEG assists in the diagnosis of conditions such as hypoxic-ischemic encephalopathy and seizure activity, thereby enabling therapeutic intervention. By comparing aEEG findings with gestational and postconceptional age, practitioners can tailor assessment, guided care decision-making on strategies that respect the infant's individual growth trajectory (Babintseva et al., 2024). Lastly, effective neonatal assessment and monitoring require a multidisciplinary approach that blends physiological and neurological examination. Care providers need to be responsive to indicators of distress or developmental problems, intervening correctly. The combination of cutting-edge monitoring techniques, such as non-contact measurement of vital signs and aEEG, has the potential to transform neonatal treatment. While the medical community strives to better the prognosis for fragile newborns, ongoing research and technological development are paramount. By following a systematic evaluation technique as a first priority, neonatologists can develop a favorable environment for healthy growth and development and ultimately improve infant survival and quality of life in high-risk situations (Babintseva et al., 2024; Svoboda et al., 2024) (Figure 5.11).

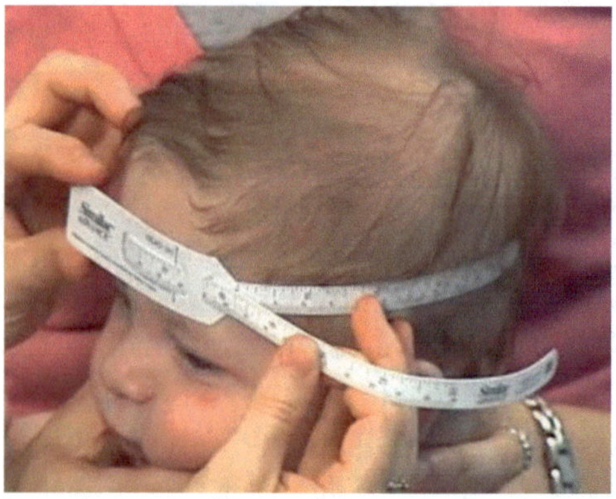

**Figure 5.11.** Neonatal assessment and monitoring.

*Source:* https://nurseslabs.com/wp-content/uploads/2017/10/measuring-infant-head-circumference-e1509217297607.jpg.

## 5.3.1. Apgar Score and Its Significance

Apgar score is a valuable instrument in neonatal practice that specifically assesses the newborn's health and viability at birth. The scoring system was developed by Dr. Virginia Apgar in 1952, which considers five categories: appearance, pulse, grimace response, activity, and respiration, with a zero to two score. The total score is from zero to ten, where higher scores indicate healthier status. This quick assessment allows medical practitioners to identify infants requiring emergency medical intervention, thereby facilitating timely and effective interventions. Crucially, the Apgar score not only facilitates the identification of immediate health and potential resuscitation requirements but also provides information on long-term developmental possibilities. Thus, awareness of the Apgar scores is paramount for pediatricians and nurses who are present at newborns because it directly affects clinical decisions and neonatal management. The Apgar score implications go beyond neonatal care, affecting other aspects of health and research. For instance, it has been established through research that a low Apgar score is associated with higher neonatal complications in the form of neurological disabilities and infant death, highlighting its role as a predictor of high-risk newborns. Additionally, some have been found to correlate with low Apgar scores, e.g., birth weight and duration of labor (Yeshambel et al., 2024). New evidence has highlighted the need to modify the use of the Apgar score among different populations, including specific breeds in veterinary practice, where modified tests for viability are essential (Veronesi et al., 2023). Such advanced awareness enables medical professionals to implement targeted interventions, enhance follow-up care, and ultimately optimize developmental outcomes in newborns identified as high-risk after their Apgar scores. Lastly, the Apgar score remains a cornerstone of neonatology, a testament to the core aim of achieving newborn health at life onset. In providing a unifying mechanism to gauge critical physiological parameters, it establishes a basis for immediate neonatal treatment recommendations. Furthermore, ongoing research in the Apgar score maintains its value and adaptability as physicians continue to explore its potential changes to suit a broad spectrum of populations. Knowledge of the limitations of the scores and numerous variables that affect their readings is a vital component for physicians who desire to enhance neonatal outcomes. With such a clear grasp of the Apgar score significance, medical practitioners can administer an even more individualized approach to neonatal treatment that is no less vital in facilitating the delivery of immediate intervention as well as ensuring the long-term health of the neonatal community.

### 5.3.2. Physical Examination Techniques

The physical examination techniques in neonatology play a critical role in achieving the optimal health and well-being of newborns. Systematic and thorough examination enables the identification of any potential issue that could affect an infant's development. General appearance, muscle tone, and respiratory effort observation are critical among other techniques. Initial assessment is the basis for assessing whether further clinical assessment is needed. The importance of early identification of health anomalies is emphasized in practice guidelines that promote extensive examinations that are intended to detect potential anomalies during the early period of a newborn's life. As proposed by Dewi et al. (2025), the assessment approaches are best performed in a stress-free environment that does not subject the infant and caregiver to additional stress, which results in a more accurate identification of the newborn's physical status. Critical signs like temperature, heart rate, and respiratory rate are part of routine physical examination and are important determinants of the newborn's health status. The physical examination should begin immediately after birth so that early intervention can be initiated as indicated. Physical examination maneuvers also involve a careful examination of the newborn's extremities, head, and skin, as these can reveal pathological findings. The evaluation should also include the evaluation of the Apgar score, and this initial evaluation tells us about the baby's ability to adapt to life outside the womb. The clinical evaluations contribute not only to the acute evaluation of the physiological parameters but also form the basis for further observation during the neonatal period. According to guidelines by Clare et al. (2024), practitioners need to possess the skill and knowledge required to effectively perform these examinations to provide the best standards of care for newborns. In addition, the incorporation of particular assessment methods, like ocular examination, is of critical importance within the neonatal assessment model. Ocular abnormality screening is a significant consideration, as early recognition of visual impairment can lead to better management and outcomes.

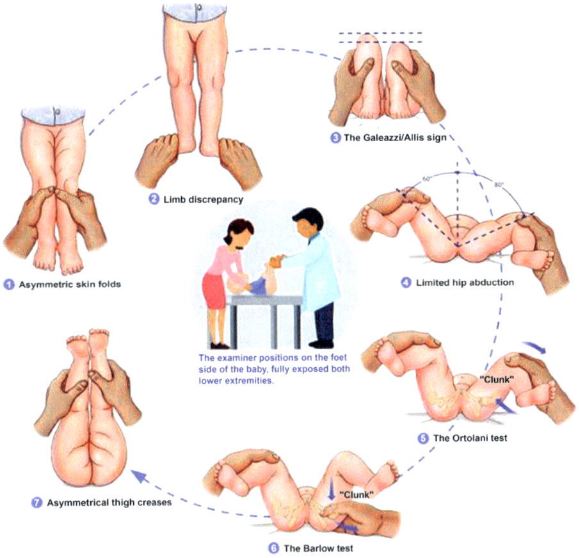


**Figure 5.12.** Physical examination techniques.

*Source:* https://www.researchgate.net/publication/361418562/figure/fig3/AS:11431281180708191@1691679409937/Physical-examination-methods-for-the-hip.png.

Screening is advisable despite some difficulties, as early recognition of ocular pathology will have a great impact on long-term development. Screening of ocular structures, movement, and red reflex forms an essential component of an assessment that can be performed without extensive cooperation from the infant. This concurs with best practice found by Clare et al. (2024), that improved, opportunistic examination methods enhance the efficiency and effectiveness of neonatal examinations. The intertwining of these physical examination procedures is needed to build a solid foundation within neonatal practice and promote the well-being of infants as they emerge into the world (Figure 5.12).

### 5.3.3. Monitoring Vital Signs and Growth

Growth monitoring and vital signs are an integral part of neonatal care as they provide useful information on the physiological status and overall health of infants. As neonates, particularly intensive care neonates, are liable to rapid changes in their condition, parameters such as heart rate, respiratory rate, oxygen saturation, and temperature must be monitored uninterruptedly. Latest monitoring technology, including heart rate variability (HRV) assessment, is becoming a significant aid in the quest. HRV, on the other hand, has proven to be a promising non-invasive tool to evaluate the level of stress in the infant and determine early signs of distress, pain, or evolving complications like respiratory distress syndrome or hyperbilirubinemia, allowing interventions in a timely fashion to enhance neonatal outcomes and lower the risk for severe illnesses like sepsis or necrotizing enterocolitis (Chiera et al., 2020). The integration of new bioinformatics- and machine learning-based monitoring systems can significantly enhance the ability for personalized neonatal health trajectory evaluation and prediction. With the processing of several key vital signs and historical health data, these systems can develop predictive models enabling healthcare providers to customize interventions more effectively. This feature is of most significance in neonatal treatment, where responses vary between subjects and dictate treatment modalities. In addition, incorporating innovative technology in monitoring vital signs and development not only optimizes acute care but also feeds into wider projects across neonatal departments to optimize information sharing between obstetricians, pediatricians, and neonatologists. As such, better communication ensures there is a more holistic approach to neonatal health surveillance and treatment (Chiera et al., 2020). Recent clinical trials indicate the promising possibility of new therapeutic interventions, such as mesenchymal stem cell (MSC) transplantation, in the management of neonates. Such interventions might need careful monitoring of vital signs to ensure efficacy and safety. A case in point is a clinical trial examining MSC transplantation in neonates with extreme intraventricular hemorrhage that yielded favorable results, including no mortality incidence during the study period. This type of monitoring has a double benefit: it not only ensures the short-term safety of infants who are being given innovative treatments but also contributes to the gathering of information that will direct future studies. By closely monitoring changes in vital signs and clinical parameters of such interventions, medical practitioners can refine existing guidelines and develop new approaches to improve care for high-risk newborn groups.

## Test Your Knowledge

1. What does the Apgar score assess in a newborn, and why is it important?
2. Name two vital signs commonly monitored in newborns during their first days of life.

## 5.4. Nutritional Needs of Newborns

**Learning Outcome**

1. Breastfeeding benefits and challenges;
2. Formula feeding guidelines;
3. Nutritional requirements for preterm infants.

The nutritional demands of newborns play a critical role in their growth and physiological health. Newborns require a specific composition of macro-nutrients, largely carbohydrates, proteins, and fats, and several micro-nutrients for growth acceleration in the early months of life. Human milk has been regarded numerous times as the ideal food for children, providing not just the essential fatty acids and immunoglobulins but also a unique blend of proteins that facilitate digestibility and absorption. Exclusive breastfeeding up to the age of six months is advocated by the World Health Organization to have the assurance that infants get the right nutrition since the milk readily adapts to address the evolving requirements of the growing baby. Understanding the requirements for such nutrients is essential in neonatal care since inappropriate nutrition can have long-term impacts on physical as well as intellectual growth (Philominal et al., 2017). Moreover, the nutritional requirements of low birth weight (LBW) infants are a further complicating factor in neonatal care. Such infants are likely to face challenges in meeting their energy and growth needs due to being smaller and at a greater risk of complications. Research has also indicated that targeted interventions, such as the implementation of feeding protocols, can enhance their nutritional status and aid in better growth outcomes. Methods of nesting, for instance, have been revealed to stabilize bio-physiological measures and facilitate increased sucking responses among LBW infants. This highlights the necessity for individualized feeding interventions that consider individual newborn conditions for LBW babies to receive enough supply of nutrients for healthy development and weight gain. Besides caloric provisions, the role of micro-nutrients such as vitamins and minerals cannot be overlooked when caring for newborns. Vitamin D has emerged as a critical element in the prevention of rickets and the achievement of peak bone density. Human milk contains essential nutrients, but may not fully provide vitamin D, which would need supplementation in some cases. Similarly, iron is quite crucial in the prevention of anemia, particularly in preterm infants who may have reduced iron stores. The interaction between nutrition and the microbiome is also a growing area of interest, with work indicating that gut microbiota during infancy can be modified by diet and potentially impact long-term health. Thus, understanding and control of the overall nutritional needs of neonates reinforce the fundamental tenets of neonatology and further optimize the care of this vulnerable group (Figure 5.13).

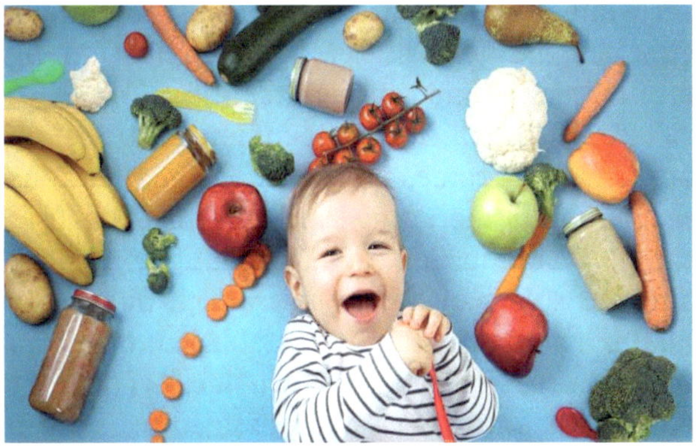

**Figure 5.13.** A smiling infant is surrounded by a colorful assortment of fruits, vegetables, and baby food, highlighting the importance of balanced nutrition in early childhood development.

*Source:* https://drabhaykumarpeds.com/wp-content/uploads/2022/03/infant-child-nutrition-doctor-in-begusarai.jpg.

### 5.4.1. Breastfeeding Benefits and Challenges

Breastfeeding is a cornerstone in the practice of neonatology that is extremely popular for its wide range of advantages to the infant and mother. The composition of human milk is specifically formulated to meet the dietary needs of infants, such as essential fatty acids, antibodies, and vitamins that play a critical role in the initial stages of development, particularly in preterm infants who are exposed to greater risks of complications. Research emphasizes that breastfeeding not only helps in optimal growth and development but also has a core role in reducing morbidity and mortality rates among high-risk newborn populations, especially those in Neonatal Intensive Care Units (NICUs). These health benefits underscore the necessity for health care professionals to accord a high priority and advocate for breastfeeding as a critical intervention in newborn care processes, particularly in light of evidence suggesting that early initiation of breastfeeding could potentially enhance the general health outcomes among mothers and infants significantly (Afreen et al., 2025). Despite the documented benefits, breastfeeding comes with a set of complications that young mothers may experience, especially in the NICU setting. Conditions like fatigue, anxiety, and the stress of having a preterm baby may hinder a mother's ability to establish and sustain milk expression. Moreover, a lack of proper education and care on breastfeeding within the NICU will delay the onset of breastfeeding, hindering the quantity of milk production. As an example, one study found that there were only 4% of the mothers who were offered instant teaching and demonstration of expressing breast milk, resulting in inadequate volumes of milk on critical feeding days (Afreen et al., 2025). These hindrances call for the implementation of targeted educational interventions and supportive approaches uniquely tailored to facilitate breastfeeding among preterm baby mothers, thus facilitating a more effective transition to exclusive breastfeeding where possible. The COVID-19 pandemic worsened the situation with breastfeeding programs, particularly in NICU settings, where visitation limitations promoted a separation of parents and newborns. This physical separation was disturbing because literature emphasizes the significance of early maternal engagement and bonding in promoting short- as well as long-term developmental potential in preterm infants. Furthermore, the emotional status of mothers is compromised by such separations, making breastfeeding activities more complicated. In response to these new obstacles, health care systems have had to innovate solutions such as telehealth visits and enhanced communication plans to keep parents connected with their infants. These adjustments not only facilitate constant education on correct breastfeeding technique but also enhance emotional support during a time of heightened separation anxiety, thus ensuring the general well-being of parent and child in these unprecedented times.

### 5.4.2. Formula Feeding Guidelines

In neonatal care, formula feeding guidelines are critical in ensuring that the infant receives adequate nutrition, particularly when breastfeeding is not possible or not acceptable. The guidelines provide the basis upon which medical practitioners can support families in making the right choice with regard to feeding the infant. They bring out the importance of selecting an appropriate formula that is in relation to the nutritional needs of the newborn based on parameters such as age, weight, and specific health considerations. In addition, the guidelines advocate for a process of progressive adjustment to formula feeding in such a way that infants are well adapted to the new form of nutrition while verifying any reaction or allergy. The rationale behind this is to promote optimal growth and development during the early days of life, which can determine long-term health. The administration process is a crucial component of formula feeding guidance that can have a large impact on an infant's experience with feeding. Parents are informed to be guided by health workers on the right method of preparation and storage of formula to minimize the risk of contamination and loss of nutrients. Also, paced bottle feeding and other styles of feeding should be employed to replicate breastfeeding to encourage breastfeeding mothers who might wish to supplement with formula, but not at the cost of their intimate mother-infant bond. Notably, where babies experience issues such as hypoglycemia, as highlighted in recent studies, health workers have been able to employ expressed breast milk as an alternative. This approach not only adheres to the principles established for safe feeding but also reaffirms the perception that formula feeding can coexist with maternal attempts at breastfeeding and has even been recorded in the effective management of different feeding challenges in clinical settings (Rollins, 2013). For optimal utilization of formula feeding, vigilant monitoring and education of parents are required. Health workers must be accessible to address matters pertaining to formula selection, feeding plans, and detecting signs of adequate nutrition. Check-ups are vital, particularly with infants requiring special care due to health complications or developmental issues. Continuous education and communication can empower parents, and they become an essential component in the nutritional process of their infants. Moreover, guidelines for formula feeding also need to be revised and updated in view of new evidence, to align with current knowledge and practice so that they reflect the best available evidence. The addition of these new guidelines to neonatal care standards indicates the need for flexibility in pediatric care so that each baby has the best possible beginning in life, regardless of their feeding pattern (Katarzyna et al., 2021) (Figure 5.14).

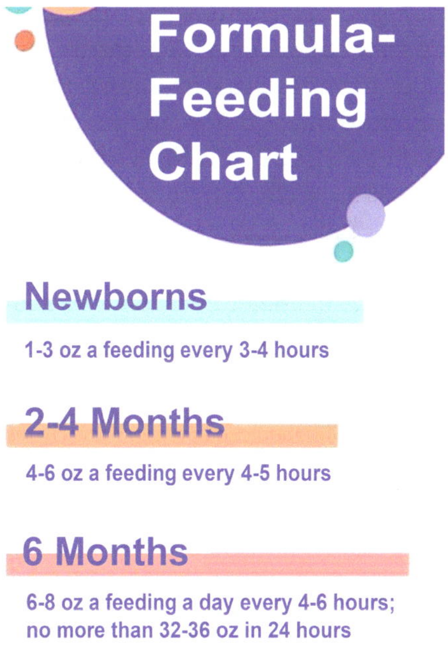


**Figure 5.14.** In the realm of neonatal care, formula feeding guidelines are critical in ensuring that infants receive adequate nutrition.

*Source:* https://images.agoramedia.com/wte3.0/gcms/formula-feeding-chart.gif?width=596.

## 5.4.3. Nutritional Requirements for Preterm Infants

The diet of preterm infants differs immensely from that of term infants owing to their underdeveloped body systems. Preterm babies have the tendency to be delivered before they can store adequate energy reserves and nutrients that facilitate rapid growth and development. Owing to this, extra care has to be taken regarding the composition of their diet, for instance, macro-nutrients such as proteins, fats, and carbohydrates. Protein, for example, is essential for the growth and repair of tissues, whereas fats are essential for brain development and energy. Carbohydrates, in addition, supply very important energy required for metabolic functions. The European Society of Pediatric Gastroenterology, Hepatology and Nutrition (ESPGHAN) emphasizes that preterm infants require higher amounts of these nutrients to support their unique growth patterns, suggesting continual nutrition assessment in order to accommodate changing needs as they develop (Nicholas et al., 2022). Preterm infants also have unique issues with nutrient absorption that necessitate individualized feeding strategies. Their poorly developed gastrointestinal tracts normally lack proper digestion and absorption of nutrients; hence enteral feeding measures are required to their nutritional care. Methods such as the fortification of the breast milk with added calories and nutrients are normally employed to provide them with the high demands. Fortification allows these preterm infants to receive sufficient energy, proteins, vitamins, and minerals necessary for normal development. Use of breast milk fortifiers, when used appropriately, can make a significant positive impact on the growth outcomes by supplementing the intrinsic nutrient deficiencies in preterm diets. Further, evidence is found that surveillance of weight gain, particularly with the change in weight Z-score ($\Delta$Z weight), is a critical determinant of nutrition adequacy and the progression of growth in these vulnerable populations (Chou et al., 2019). Apart from macronutrients, micronutrients are also of paramount significance in the nutritional requirements of preterm infants. Vitamins and minerals such as iron, calcium, and phosphorus are needed to avert the risks of developmental delay and long-term illness. Iron deficiency, for instance, is much more elevated among preterm infants and may lead to impaired cognitive and motor development. Close attention to micro-nutrients, often urgently required by dietary restriction and malabsorption that are common in such infants, is essential. That there is insufficient strong evidence for optimal levels of most micro-nutrients helps to emphasize the need for an agreement on guidelines so that preterm infants can be given appropriate supplementation to aid growth and overall health. Joint efforts, as espoused by ESPGHAN, seek to establish evidence-based guidelines to address these micronutrient needs comprehensively (Nicholas et al., 2022).

## Test Your Knowledge

1. What is one key benefit and one common challenge of breastfeeding newborns?
2. Why do preterm infants have different nutritional requirements compared to full-term infants?

# 5.5. Neonatal Intensive Care Unit (NICU)

**Learning Outcome**

1. Role and function of the NICU;
2. Common interventions and technologies used;
3. Family involvement in NICU care.

The Neonatal Intensive Care Unit (NICU) is a highly specialized environment that responds to the complex needs of critically ill newborns. Here, medical staff employ high-tech medical equipment and monitor vital signs, thus fully attending to premature and low-birth-weight newborns. NICU is an intervention area where infant mortality rates are significantly reduced by early and effective medical interventions. As the unit operates under firm guidelines to care for a range of acute conditions, it also concentrates on the family-based model, realizing the importance of patient involvement in the process of their infant's care. Evidence has confirmed that parent participation optimizes perceived safety in the care environment, with families being more likely to support healthcare staff who take their views into account (Karen et al., 2025). One of the numerous challenges that the NICU must contend with is handling common hematological conditions such as thrombocytopenia. Thrombocytopenia, or low platelet count, occurs in 18–35% of neonates who are admitted to intensive care, and at higher rates in instances of preterm delivery or low birth weight (Chawda et al., 2023). The condition is often a reflection of significant underlying morbidity, as the disease can be attributed to infections or complications associated with prematurity. Treatment depends on a multidisciplinary group of pediatric hematologists, nurses, and intensivists. By way of early intervention and regulation of platelet levels, the NICU team seeks to avoid complications and improve survival and health gains for affected infants, illustrating the value of specialist neonatal care in increasing post-NICU survival and health. The process of infant transfer of infants from the NICU to intermediate units or home is also a significant component of neonatal care. Evidence shows that parents and professionals consider safety while making these transfers as a vital element of good care (Karen et al., 2025). Perceived safety is affected by issues such as proper communication, transfer timing, and involvement of parents throughout the process. Attitudes among stakeholders vary significantly throughout the phases of transfer, indicating that routine protocols need to be established to facilitate safe and smooth transfers. By putting a strong focus on the meticulous assessment of both logistical and emotional issues in transitions, healthcare providers can maximize the overall quality of care delivered in the NICU and in subsequent transfers, ultimately enhancing outcomes for compromised newborns and their families (Figure 5.15).

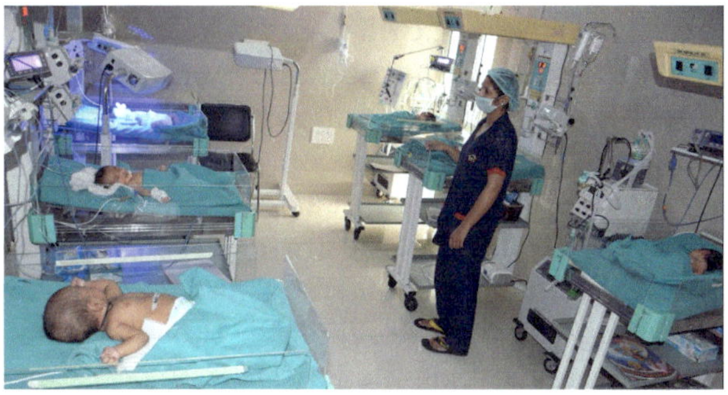

**Figure 5.15.** The neonatal intensive care unit (NICU).

*Source:* https://mimanihospital.com/wp-content/uploads/2017/02/mimani-nicu.jpg.

## 5.5.1. Role and Function of the NICU

The Neonatal Intensive Care Unit (NICU) serves an essential role in providing care to vulnerable newborns who require specialized medical intervention. Designed to care for premature infants as well as ill babies, the NICU applies advanced technologies and therapeutic regimens to address a wide variety of complications such as respiratory distress, infection, and congenital anomalies. The unit also attempts to provide a supportive environment not only for the affected babies but also for their families, thereby fostering an integrated neonatal care model. The NICU also has ongoing monitoring ability, which allows experts to track vital signs and detect abnormalities in real time, thereby enabling interventions in a timely manner that can greatly improve neonatal outcomes. One of the primary functions of the NICU is to ensure the preterm infant is properly nutritionally supported, which is crucial to their development and growth. Research has proven that a mother's own milk delivers necessary nutrients to the infant and significantly reduces the risk of acquiring complications such as necrotizing enterocolitis. There are, nonetheless, barriers that prevent the earlier initiation of breast milk expression in neonatal units. Interventions to increase maternal support and education in this region have been shown to effectively raise the rate of mothers who use early and frequent breast milk expression and thus support the availability of nutrition for preterm infants in the NICU. This mutualistic relationship between neonatal care and maternal health practice has a direct impact on the survival and long-term well-being of these at-risk infants, emphasizing the its role in maximizing outcomes by nutritional intervention (Afreen et al., 2024). The NICU is also a referral institution for diagnosis and treatment of hematologic complications such as thrombocytopenia that affect a significant number of neonates admitted. Thrombocytopenia is reportedly more common in preterm infants, and when it happens, early detection by routine laboratory tests can alert practitioners to potential complications to their health. Awareness of thrombopoiesis and thrombocytopenia conditions enhances the healthcare practitioners' ability within the NICU environment to make informed decisions regarding treatment modalities and interventions. This level of care affects augmented prognostic results and demonstrates the significant role the NICU plays in addressing neonatal health problems in general, successfully treating both the acute and prolonged demands of high-risk groups of newborns (Chawda et al., 2023).

### 5.5.2. Common Interventions and Technologies Used

Developments in neonatology have offered a range of interventions and technologies essential for maximizing outcomes among critically ill newborns. Among them, the use of continuous positive airway pressure (CPAP) has become irreplaceable in the care of respiratory distress, particularly in preterm infants. CPAP does this by establishing a uniform level of air pressure in the lungs, which allows for the preservation of alveolar patency and avoidance of lung collapse at the end of expiration. This non-invasive method significantly reduces the need for more invasive ventilation strategies with supplemental oxygenation and lower work of breathing. Also, the use of pulse oximetry makes continuous monitoring of oxygen saturation possible, and healthcare workers can modify interventions in real time based on real-time data. The integration of these technologies has revolutionized neonatal intensive care units (NICUs) as centers of modern medical care, significantly changing neonatal morbidity and mortality statistics. But another key neonatology intervention has been the evolution of thermoregulation techniques, which help maintain the newborns body temperature levelled. Newborn hypothermia, especially in preterm infants, could complicate the recovery and lead to catastrophic complications. Technologies such as incubators and radiant warmers provide controlled atmospheres that stabilize a newborns temperature throughout and shortly after birth. Incubators are particularly useful in very low birth weight infants, offering an insulated environment for temperature control with requisite monitoring and support on other physiological parameters. With emphasis on providing a suitable thermal condition, these interventions are critical to maintaining metabolic function and facilitating vulnerable newborns to gain weight and strength to support additional medical treatment (Kuchler et al., 2023).

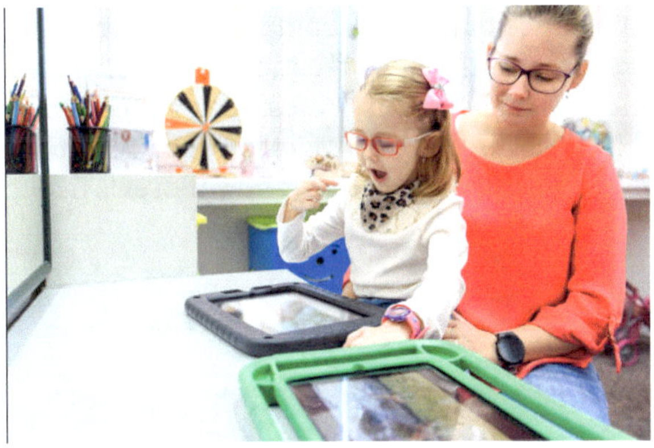

**Figure 5.16.** A young girl uses a digital tablet for communication with the support of a caregiver, illustrating assistive technology in speech and language development for children with special needs.

*Source:* https://media.istockphoto.com/id/1430043244/photo/non-verbal-girl-living-with-cerebral-palsy-learning-to-use-digital-tablet-device-to.jpg?s=612x612&w=0&k=20&c=hD3PUR0Fl0S34OwL6-1qcONCqKnHiQYr_rxEuBG6l7M=.

Thus, successful thermoregulation is a fundamental aspect of practice in the neonate that attests to the importance of technology in modern practice. Besides respiratory care and thermoregulation, intravenous (IV) nutrition is a quintessential intervention in neonatology. For preterm neonates who are unable to be fed orally, parenteral nutrition (PN) takes center stage in addressing their nutritional needs. This stage is the intravenous administration of required nutrients like proteins, carbohydrates, fats, vitamins, and minerals into the blood and subsequent normal growth and development in the event of oral feeding contraindication (Thissen et al., 2022). Technologies in the form of pumps for feeding are utilized in the process of weaning infants from enteral feeding, with precise delivery of the breast milk or formula and reduced risk of complications associated with feeding intolerance. The application of advanced nutrition delivery systems allows for precise monitoring of nutrient intake and weight increment, individualized for every individual infant, permitting optimization of patient outcomes safely while minimizing the risks of malnutrition (Figure 5.16).

## 5.5.3. Family Involvement in NICU Care

Involvement by the family in Neonatal Intensive Care Units (NICUs) is vital to both infants' clinical status and parents' emotional well-being. Parents are likely to experience a complex emotional backdrop when dealing with children's hospitalization, and their expectation of involvement is high. Evidence has shown that while parents report higher satisfaction levels concerning their NICU care involvement, they feel the need for better communication about their child's condition and greater involvement in medical decision-making (Thébaud et al., 2022). Enhancing these communication lines can lead to more empowered parents, which has been associated with better psychological health for parents as well as better developmental outcomes for preterm infants. Consequently, the healthcare providers have to identify and encourage such involvement positively. The process of creating family-centered care incorporates respect for family preferences and authority into NICU care in a day-to-day way. This empowerment enables parents to participate actively in the care of their child, up to the level of feeding, soothing, and being included in the medical consultations. There is evidence of parents' desires to take part in care and their experience of being overlooked or criticized by health professionals (Thébaud et al., 2022). The Newborn Individualized Care and Assessment Program (NIDCAP) is one model that provides excellent integration of parental involvement without compromising the medical needs of the infants. By creating an open environment of communication and cooperative practices, NICUs can assist families during this trying time more effectively. In addition, an awareness of the emotional needs of the entire family, including siblings, is necessary for comprehensive care in the NICU process. Bereavement support for siblings when a neonatal family member passes away remains insufficiently addressed, which demonstrates enormous gaps within the availability of particular resources. With the emotional challenges associated with NICU admissions, the inclusion of bereavement services in general family care has been crucial to mitigate long-term negative effects on siblings. Enhanced palliative care team support has been identified to improve the quality of information and education siblings receive, highlighting the importance of an all-encompassing approach in care interventions. By treating the whole family unit in NICUs, health professionals are capable of facilitating long-term emotional resilience, which is critical to parents' and children's health.

## Test Your Knowledge

1. What is the primary function of the NICU?
2. Name one common intervention or technology used in the NICU to support newborns.

## 5.6. Ethical Considerations in Neonatology

**Learning Outcome**

1. Decision-making in critical care situations;
2. End-of-life care and palliative options;
3. Informed consent and parental rights.

The ethical issues in neonatology are particularly subtle due to the vulnerable position of the patient population. Neonates, especially intensive care neonates, require individualized treatment that often consists of difficult decisions regarding their care and overall lifestyle. Physicians must weigh the potential benefits of interventions against the risks and harms they impose on the newborn. Informed consent is a part of good ethics practice, but the obtaining of consent from parents is not without its challenges, particularly where there are immediate decisions to be made. The scope of the implications of these decisions is significant because they have a considerable impact on both the newborn's health consequences and the psychological wellbeing of the family. The technology used in neonatal care creates additional ethical considerations. A major trend is the use of live video surveillance in neonatal units, with advantages of improved parental bonding and distant observation by clinicians. Wherever video is used, however, serious issues around privacy and data protection loom large. Staff and parents have demanded steps to ensure the appropriate application of these technologies. As highlighted in current studies, there is a shared understanding between professionals and parents that while video monitoring can enhance care and attachment, caution must be taken to prevent risks of consent issues and pressure it could place on carers (Bris et al., 2020). The second key ethical element entails the behavior of healthcare professionals in finding a balance between their duty of care to the baby and the one to their families.

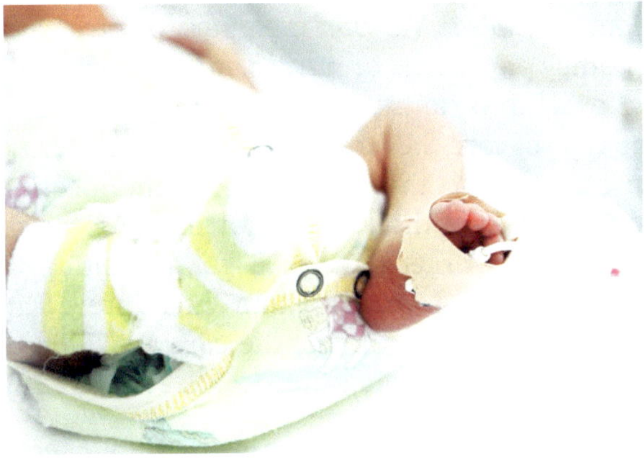

**Figure 5.17.** A newborn in a neonatal intensive care unit (NICU) is monitored using medical sensors on the foot, highlighting the critical care and technology used to support premature or medically fragile infants.

*Source:* https://journalofethics.ama-assn.org/sites/joedb/files/2018-09/shutterstock_455297464_0.jpg.

The infant's medical needs often call for treatment in a team setting, providing the potential for dispute among the different stakeholders' perspectives. For instance, problems might arise concerning how aggressive the treatment interventions need to be or when decisions regarding withdrawal of support need to be made. Evidence indicates that healthcare professionals realize the importance of engaging parents in decision-making but are also faced with the challenge of dealing with clashing perceptions of what is proper and suitable care for the baby (Bris et al., 2020). This is a reflection of the need for ongoing ethical training and consultancy in neonatology to impart the capacity to resolve problems wisely and compassionately (Figure 5.17).

### 5.6.1. Decision-Making in Critical Care Situations

In neonatology, decision-making in critical care situations is full of complexities demanding a combination of clinical expertise, ethical considerations, and effective communication. Neonatal caregivers are faced with emergent situations around the clock, such as stabilizing very preterm babies or babies with congenital defects. The nuances of making informed decisions in such situations often rest on rapid assessment of the clinical status of the infant, consideration of the potential benefit of the treatment, and anticipated quality of life outcomes. For instance, in cases of Down syndrome, clinicians must balance the newborn's acute medical needs against the long-term implications of their decisions for both the neonate and the family, emphasizing the need for comprehensive evaluation and counseling throughout the continuum of care (Marilyn et al., 2022). Ethical nuances also make decision-making in neonatal critical care challenging. Health care workers must walk the tightrope between professional advice and parental wishes, particularly where the stakes are high and results may not be guaranteed. For example, in congenital illness such as Down syndrome, heterogeneity of presentation complicates the work of health professionals to sit with parents and discuss prognosis, possible interventions, and care. There is also a need for a facilitative framework that allows clinicians to report their observations and findings to the clinical team and honor the values and priorities of the participating families. This not only ensures trust and understanding are fostered but also that decisions are made together with regard to the dignity of infants and parents alike (Mary et al., 2020). Also, multidisciplinary teams need to be incorporated for the purposes of enhancing decision-making processes within neonatal critical care environments. Such teams, including neonatologists, pediatric surgeons, nurses, and genetic counselors, provide a comprehensive approach to the treatment of complicated patients. With the shared diverse expertise of the teams, health practitioners ensure they always consider all angles of care for every infant. For example, when evaluating a newborn with Down syndrome, a team-based approach can provide a better overall picture of immediate medical management and long-term care choices on both clinical and psychosocial levels. This model of collaboration not only improves care coordination but also promotes overall family support, which is essential in neonatology, where decisions can truly influence short-term survival and long-term quality of life (Marilyn et al., 2022).

### 5.6.2. End-of-Life Care and Palliative Options

The practice of end-of-life care and palliative care in the area of neonatology is a delicate and multifaceted undertaking. Neonatologists tend to struggle with the difficult choices that accompany working with critically ill infants, especially those that are preterm or born with life-threatening illness. The advancement of medical technology has allowed for the rescue of some of the most vulnerable infants; however, the treatments themselves raise ethical issues regarding the quality of life and pain that the infants endure. A dialogue among the healthcare team, parents, and an effort to balance the technical potential of treatment with the emotional and ethical dimensions of the treatment is crucial. The nuance of collaborative decision-making stands forth in such circumstances, underscoring the need for open communication that respects parental values and the infant's global health and honors the limits of medical interventions. This is an authentic issue for healthcare professionals who practice in neonatal intensive care units (NICUs) with end-of-life care decisions. As stated, moral distress arises when health care professionals are caught between the goodness of a line of treatment that may not be in agreement with their professional values or one that will violate the family's will. In the NICU, where end-of-life care and periviable resuscitation are frequent issues of decision-making, there is a high likelihood of moral distress affecting the collaborative dynamic among the medical team members. Various members of the team, whether physicians or nurses, may undergo this suffering in various ways, ultimately influencing the type of care the patients receive. By fostering an atmosphere that has open communication and addressing the reasons for moral distress, healthcare workers are in a good position to manage the ethical dilemma encountered in practice, hence enhancing the care provided to neonates and their families (Mills et al., 2020).

The inclusion of proper palliative care interventions is imperative in the field of neonatology because it can contribute most importantly to improving the quality of life for both the baby and the family at difficult moments. Palliative care extends not just to the physical symptoms but to the emotional, psychological, and spiritual aspects as well. Once curative treatments are no longer an option or desired, palliative care can provide a model for families to make a decision on the most compassionate and appropriate action, tailored to their specific circumstances. The role of health professionals in communicating appropriate information to families about what options are available is also a crucial consideration. Providing parents with knowledge of the consequences of their decisions and honoring their autonomy leads to informed choices that uphold the infant's dignity. Therefore, incorporating palliative care principles allows families to actively engage in the care process and reduce the extreme complexities of end-of-life decision-making for their infants (Baumgartner et al., 2020) (Figure 5.18).

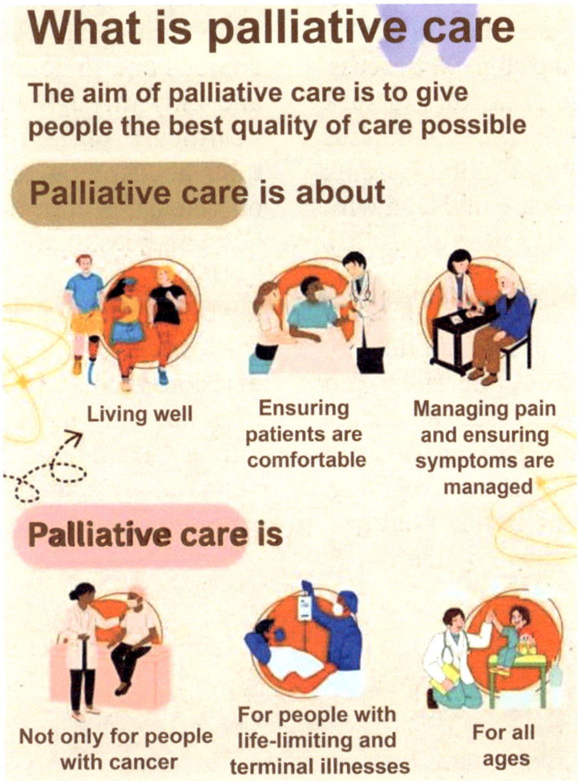


**Figure 5.18.** The provision of end-of-life care and palliative options within the field of neonatology.

*Source:* https://sc ontent.fdel11-4.fna.fbcdn.net/v/t39.30808-6/486539497_1091 85608965 4130_3106838729599124421_n.jpg?_nc_cat=105&ccb=1-7&_nc_sid=127cfc&_nc_ohc=Btzmp qWJFaUQ7kNvwGeWHVR&_nc_oc=Adk KwIkE-q1d3b P6 tVyVWLJnEljAChSQofqnXT65Wa hfUP1Qvr1nRaXwQod4ywn pBQGIpH2iF 2I7VTgN4hb8XC ce&_nc_zt=23&_nc_ht=sc ontent.fdel11-4.fna&_nc_gid=uAV205DZAXutG5EpTc2XAA &oh=00_AfJTN2JUzUtAIJJ98Fo_QPniL0EyfyzmbA4iahg 3L8RFWg&oe=68325C35.

## 5.6.3. Informed Consent and Parental Rights

The informed consent doctrine occupies a central role within the delicate balancing of parental rights and neonatal care. Decision-making regarding neonatal treatment within neonatology is often a complex ethical dilemma. When parents are trying to cope with the enormous responsibility of decision-making for their fragile new babies, there is a role that healthcare professionals can play in providing comprehensive information about the potential benefits, limitations, and meaning of the planned interventions. Parents as primary decision-makers must be well-educated to manage such intricacies, while autonomy is preserved and for the good of their child (Kelly et al., 2016). Clear communication between the parents and the neonatal team is crucial because it is where informed consent can be realized to the fullest to prevent miscommunication and build trust. In addition, the law that supports consent stipulates that consent be obtained from the parents before any intervention of the child by healthcare providers. It is crucial that nurses, often at the forefront of neonatal care, also remain directly engaged in the consent process. While it is typically the role of doctors to seek consent for intensive care treatments, nurses themselves have a sole role to guide parents through the intricate information involved with their infant's treatment (Alderson et al., 2006). This shared responsibility not only supports parents but also enriches the decision-making climate, promoting a partnership model. By initiating open dialogue about the risks and benefits of treatment options, nurses can enable parental anxiety reduction, bridging the gap between medical ethics and bedside caregiving. Ultimately, informed consent is not merely a legal technicality; it is the ethical obligation to promote parental involvement in neonatal care. As neonatal discharge and feeding decisions show, consent can be significantly enhanced by active communication and decision-sharing (Alderson et al., 2006). Parents will often be anxious and in doubt about their baby's status, and only through an enabling framework will healthcare professionals be able to address their needs. By placing the highest importance on releasing information in a straightforward but compassionate manner, practitioners can facilitate greater, more informed appreciation of the options available, systematically addressing the intricacies involved in high-stakes neonatal decision-making. Adherence to informed consent thus not only helps to uphold parental rights but also articulates the very ethical premises of neonatology, so that newborn care is conducted with respect, dignity, and sensitivity.

## Test Your Knowledge

1. Why is informed consent important in neonatal critical care decision-making?
2. What is one ethical challenge involved in providing end-of-life care for newborns?

## SUMMARY

It is important to determine the large differences that improvements in neonatal care practice make between outcomes for premature and severely ill newborns. As discussed by research determining the advantages of special training programs for medical staff, utilization of developmental supportive techniques can help bring a huge positive impact on both neonatal control of sleep as well as overall practice of healthcare. To illustrate, changing practice promoting respect for the sleep-wake cycle of the newborn has a clear connection to better developmental outcomes in this high-risk population (Faez et al., 2024). This highlights the importance of continued professional learning and the integration of evidence-based practice within neonatal intensive care units. In addition, the trends in the treatment of extremely premature infants highlight the importance of tailored interventions and the importance of collaboration among providers. Rising intervention and survival rates noted in studies across various centers indicate the delivery of quality care by uniform protocols (LoRe et al., 2024). Gradual changes over time in clinical practices illustrate that emergent treatments, such as the application of antenatal corticosteroids and enhanced resuscitation practices, cumulatively enhance the likelihood of survival of newborns delivered at 22 to 24 weeks of gestation. Such evidence increases the relevance of evidence-based practices in improving neonatal outcomes. Finally, the emerging body of evidence on determinants of the provision of neonatal care recognizes one critical imperative for equity of access to and delivery of healthcare. Race- and history-of-prior-birth differences require systematic consideration and response to ensure equal quality of care for birthing people and their infants. To eliminate such inequalities, apart from enhancing rates of survival, it also upholds the ethical responsibility of healthcare providers and facilities towards equitable practices of care. Thus, development of the specialty of neonatology depends on an integrative strategy with regard to training, uniform treatment, and dedication to achieving equal results for each newborn, in accordance with best practices for newborn care (LoRe et al., 2024).

In neonatology, the care of newborns encompasses various aspects vital to their healthy development. Among the primary areas of focus is early diagnosis and management of congenital diseases, with the case of congenital hypothyroidism (CH) being one. Latest advancements have led to the implementation of updated recommendations for diagnosing and treating CH, with particular stress laid on neonatal screening programs. As noted in the ENDO-European Reference Network initiative, these practice guidelines utilize a systematic review of existing literature to provide evidence-based recommendations that enhance the outcomes for affected infants. Such proactive measures allow for timely interventions, which are essential in mitigating the potential risks associated with delayed diagnosis, thus underscoring the critical role of organized screening programs in the neonatal care spectrum (Paul et al., 2020). Moreover, the interaction between maternal and neonatal outcomes cannot be belittled. The impact of disorders such as epilepsy during pregnancy demonstrates the thin line between fetal and maternal risk. The International League Against Epilepsy Task Force report states how seizures that are not controlled by medicine can put mother and baby at risk, which calls for a rethinking of the management of antiepileptic drugs during pregnancy. The review entails assessing the potential teratogenic effect on the developing fetus, resulting in serious congenital malformations and developmental challenges. Through the integration of past studies and experts' opinions, healthcare practitioners can optimize treatment methods pre-conception and during pregnancy, thereby improving neonatal treatment and outcomes (Torbjörn et al., 2019). Finally, the integration of evidence-based practices into neonatology not only improves short-term care but also lays the foundation for long-term health. The ongoing refinement of guidelines, be it in the management of congenital hypothyroidism or the treatment of maternal disease like epilepsy, suggests a focus on enhancing measures of neonatal health. By fostering collaborative initiatives among experts, as seen with ENDO-ERN and other organizations, the care provided to newborns becomes increasingly comprehensive and tailored to individual needs. Such collaborative approaches ensure that neonatology remains at the forefront of pediatric medicine, paving the way for healthier futures for newborns across various health conditions and challenges. It is a reflection of the growing realization of the intricacies involved in neonatal care.

## KEY TERMS FROM THIS CHAPTER

- Diphtheria
- Health monitoring
- Immunization
- Machine learning
- Population immunity
- Respiratory syncytial virus (RSV)
- Vaccine hesitancy
- Global health security
- Human papillomavirus (HPV)
- Infectious diseases
- Measles, mumps, and rubella (MMR)
- Public health
- Robust health
- Vaccine-preventable diseases

## CRITICAL THINKING QUESTIONS

1. **The neonatal period is defined as:**
   a. First 7 days of life
   b. First 14 days of life
   c. First 21 days of life
   d. First 28 days of life
2. **The most common cause of neonatal mortality in developing countries is:**
   a. Diarrhea
   b. Neonatal sepsis
   c. Birth asphyxia
   d. Prematurity and low birth weight
3. **The first immunization given at birth is:**
   a. DPT
   b. OPV
   c. BCG
   d. MMR
4. **What is the normal respiratory rate in a newborn?**
   a. 20–30 breaths per minute
   b. 30–40 breaths per minute
   c. 40–60 breaths per minute
   d. 60–80 breaths per minute
5. **Which reflex is normally present at birth?**
   a. Plantar reflex
   b. Moro reflex
   c. Babinski reflex
   d. Abdominal reflex

### Short Answer Questions

1. Define the neonatal period.
2. What is the Apgar score? What are its components?
3. What are the benefits of early initiation of breastfeeding?
4. Define low birth weight. What are its causes?
5. What is Kangaroo Mother Care (KMC)? State two benefits.
6. What is physiological jaundice? How does it differ from pathological jaundice?

### *Answers to Critical Thinking Questions*

1. (d) 2. (d) 3. (c) 4. (c) 5. (b)

## REFERENCES


1. Afreen, S., Mannan, M. A., Yasmin, F., Nasrin, U. T., & Akhter, S. (2025). Barriers to mother's own milk feeding for preterm newborns: Experience from a tertiary neonatal intensive care unit. *Asian Journal of Pediatric Research*. https://www.semanticscholar.org/paper/d603abc6c5fdedbb49998f635eb9a906e2f9f0a5 (accessed on 16th June 2025).
2. Afreen, S., Nasrin, U. T., Rahman, K. M., Jahan, I., Dey, S., Shahidullah, M., Chowdhury, R. M., et al. (2024). A quality improvement initiative to increase the supply of mother's own milk for preterm newborn admitted in neonatal intensive care unit of Bangabandhu Sheikh Mujib Medical University. *Journal of Neonatology, 38*, 88–97. https://www.semanticscholar.org/paper/7f14989b46dd829e7f015636443487090fab8c2d (accessed on 16th June 2025).
3. Ahn, S. Y., Chang, Y. S., Sung, S. I., & Park, W. S. (2018). Mesenchymal stem cells for severe intraventricular hemorrhage in preterm infants: Phase I dose-escalation clinical trial. *Stem Cells Translational Medicine, 7*, 847–856. https://doi.org/10.1002/sctm.17-0219 (accessed on 16th June 2025).
4. Alderson, P. (2006). Parents' consent to neonatal decisions about feeding and discharge. https://core.ac.uk/download/pdf/83447.pdf (accessed on 16th June 2025).
5. Anand Kumar, G., Kamalakannan, S. K., Asha, A., & Sudarsanan, H. (2024). Role of newborn hearing screening done over one year in a tertiary care hospital: A cross-sectional study. *Cureus, 16*. https://www.semanticscholar.org/paper/62d789e2f70472554eba1703a15e943917cba53d (accessed on 16th June 2025).
6. Baumgartner, H., De Backer, J., Babu-Narayan, S. V., Budts, W., Chessa, M., Diller, G. P., Lung, B., et al. (2020). 2020 ESC guidelines for the management of adult congenital heart disease. *European Heart Journal, 42*, 563–645. https://doi.org/10.1093/eurheartj/ehaa554 (accessed on 16th June 2025).
7. Bull, M. J., Trotter, T. L., Santoro, S. L., Christensen, C. K., & Grout, R. W. (2022). Health supervision for children and adolescents with Down syndrome. *Pediatrics, 149*. https://doi.org/10.1542/peds.2022-057010 (accessed on 16th June 2025).
8. Caporali, C., Pisoni, C., Naboni, L., Provenzi, L., & Orcesi, S. (2020). Challenges and opportunities for early intervention and neurodevelopmental follow-up in preterm infants during the COVID-19 pandemic. *Child, 47*, 140–141. https://www.semanticscholar.org/paper/03fff0d1c975b9831b1c68baf8f7aa012feeb7a2 (accessed on 16th June 2025).
9. Chiera, M., Cerritelli, F., Casini, A., Barsotti, N., Boschiero, D., Cavigioli, F., Corti, C., et al. (2020). Heart rate variability in the perinatal period: A critical and conceptual review. *Frontiers in Neuroscience, 14*. https://doi.org/10.3389/fnins.2020.561186 (accessed on 16th June 2025).
10. Chou, J. H., Roumiantsev, S., & Singh, R. (2019). Pedi Tools electronic growth chart calculators: Applications in clinical care, research, and quality improvement. *Journal of Medical Internet Research, 22*, e16204–e16204. https://doi.org/10.2196/16204 (accessed on 16th June 2025).
11. de Bijl-Marcus, K., Mossel, F., Ahaus, K., Pluut, B., Benders, M., Bruintjes, A., Buljac-Samardžić, M. (2025). The perception of safety regarding the transfer of infants from the neonatal intensive care unit to a level II neonatology department: A mixed-method cohort study using a Safety-II approach. *BMC Pediatrics, 25*. https://www.semanticscholar.org/paper/9c3e3232000853fcc39e9ae487a7d52ad62043c4 (accessed on 16th June 2025).

12. Dewi, W. C. M., & Hanum, S. M. F. (2025). Comprehensive midwifery care for Mrs. F through continuity of care. *Indonesian Journal on Health Science and Medicine*. https://www.semanticscholar.org/paper/32369e088c6c57949abf6c65752e6a8d29c0101e (accessed on 16th June 2025).

13. Embleton, N. D., Moltu, S. J., Lapillonne, A., van den Akker, C. H. P., Carnielli, V., Fusch, C., Gerasimidis, K., et al. (2022). Enteral nutrition in preterm infants (2022): A position paper from the ESPGHAN Committee on Nutrition and invited experts. *Journal of Pediatric Gastroenterology and Nutrition, 76*, 248–268. https://doi.org/10.1097/mpg.0000000000003642 (accessed on 16th June 2025).

14. Faez, N., Hmami, F., Boujraf, S., Kojmane, W., & Atmani, S. (2024). Practices for respecting the newborn's sleep-wake cycle: Interventional study in the neonatal intensive care unit. *Journal of Neurosciences in Rural Practice, 15*, 278–285. https://www.semanticscholar.org/paper/00e17e6d522b58c183e30b0cecc5487349c508cf (accessed on 16th June 2025).

15. Ho, V. H., Giguère, Y., & Reinharz, D. (2024). Economic rationality in decision-making regarding newborn screening: A case study in Quebec. *International Journal of Neonatal Screening, 10*. https://www.semanticscholar.org/paper/479211ac5ee3915d408421f9865ccf3267647dd8 (accessed on 16th June 2025).

16. Kelly, J., & Welch, E. (2016). Ethical decision-making regarding infant viability: A discussion. https://core.ac.uk/download/151161564.pdf (accessed on 16th June 2025).

17. Le Bris, A. L., Mazille-Orfanos, N., Simonot, P., Luherne, M., Flamant, C., Gascoin, G., Ó Laighin, G., et al. (2020). Parents' and healthcare professionals' perceptions of the use of live video recording in neonatal units: A focus group study. *Research Square (Research Square)*. https://doi.org/10.21203/rs.2.17226/v4 (accessed on 16th June 2025).

18. Liu, W., Yang, Q., Xu, Z., Hu, Y., Wang, Y., Liu, Z., Zhao, Q., et al. (2022). Impact of the COVID-19 pandemic on neonatal admissions in a tertiary children's hospital in southwest China: An interrupted time-series study. *PLoS ONE, 17*, e0262202–e0262202. https://doi.org/10.1371/journal.pone.0262202 (accessed on 16th June 2025).

19. LoRe, D., Groden, C. M., Schuh, A. R., Holmes, C., Ostilla, L., Vogel, M. M., Murray, P. D., Yamasato, K., Tonismae, T., Anani, U. E., Henner, N., Famuyide, M., Leuthner, S. R., Laventhal, N., Andrews, B. L., Tucker Edmonds, B. M., Brennan, K. G., Feltman, D. M., & INVESTIGATING NEONATAL DECISIONS FOR EXTREMELY EARLY DELIVERIES (INDEED) STUDY GROUP (2024). Variability of Care Practices for Extremely Early Deliveries. *Pediatrics, 154*(3), e2023065521. https://doi.org/10.1542/peds.2023-065521(accessed on 16th June 2025).

20. Morris, J., Brown, K., & Newnham, J. P. (2020). The Australian Preterm Birth Prevention Alliance. *Australian and New Zealand Journal of Obstetrics and Gynecology, 60*, 321–323. https://doi.org/10.1111/ajo.13171 (accessed on 16th June 2025).

21. Mortazavi, M., Abed, J., Abedini, Z., Karimi, Z., & Vafaee, A. (2019). Mortality and morbidity of neonates weighing less than 1500 grams, case study of Sarem Women's Hospital. *Sarem Journal of Reproductive Medicine*. https://www.semanticscholar.org/paper/442d0077d24ad9652e65c73c068fb340e79dabb4 (accessed on 16th June 2025).

22. Niu, L., Zhang, Z., Li, J., & Zhao, M. (2024). Efficacy of lung ultrasound vs chest X-ray in detecting lung consolidation and edema in premature infants in the NICU. *Medical Science Monitor: International Medical Journal of Experimental and Clinical Research, 30*, e944426-

1–e944426-7. https://www.semanticscholar.org/paper/840c220e55bb425a5613d43647d544f32fb5ac83 (accessed on 16th June 2025).

23. Renfrew, M. J., & Malata, A. (2020). Scaling up care by midwives must now be a global priority. *The Lancet Global Health, 9*, e2–e3. https://doi.org/10.1016/s2214-109x(20)30478-2 (accessed on 16th June 2025).
24. Rollins, K. (2013). There's nothing sweeter than mom's own milk. *Journal of Obstetric, Gynecologic, & Neonatal Nursing, 42*. https://www.semanticscholar.org/paper/bdd1109bd33e7a66c1135a3a1f8fda4264580e47 (accessed on 16th June 2025).
25. Svoboda, L., Sperrhake, J., Nisser, M., Taphorn, L., & Proquitté, H. (2024). Contactless assessment of heart rate in neonates within a clinical environment using imaging photoplethysmography. *Frontiers in Pediatrics, 12*. https://www.semanticscholar.org/paper/5cda1a1fe445b632faea098412defcd6a2e22728 (accessed on 16th June 2025).
26. Sweet, D. G., Carnielli, V., Greisen, G., Hallman, M., Özek, E., te Pas, A. B., Plavka, R., et al. (2019). European consensus guidelines on the management of respiratory distress syndrome–2019 update. *Neonatology, 115*, 432–450. https://doi.org/10.1159/000499361 (accessed on 16th June 2025).
27. Thissen, M., Estupiñán-Romero, F., Berna, E., Zeitlin, J., Farr, A., Vidal Benedé, M. J., et al. (2022). 2.N. Workshop: Improving perinatal health and reducing inequality: The value of European population comparisons. *The European Journal of Public Health, 32*. https://www.semanticscholar.org/paper/6c01ff6e03199ca3935b78c3c0665e83c849c659 (accessed on 16th June 2025).
28. Tillhof, K., Krawzak, K., Batza, J., & Feltman, D. (2021). Bereavement support for siblings after neonatal loss: An online survey of U.S. training centers. *American Journal of Perinatology, 41*, 1086–1093. https://www.semanticscholar.org/paper/f7a0adf0b4066abdf24c97702b033b35bc5499a3 (accessed on 16th June 2025).
29. Tomson, T., Battino, D., Bromley, R., Kochen, S., Meador, K. J., Pennell, P. B., & Thomas, S. V. (2019). Management of epilepsy in pregnancy: A report from the International League Against Epilepsy Task Force on Women and Pregnancy. *Epileptic Disorders, 21*, 497–517. https://doi.org/10.1684/epd.2019.1105 (accessed on 16th June 2025).
30. Veronesi, M., Bucci, R., Probo, M., Faustini, M., & Fusi, J. (2023). Apgar score for newborn dog viability assessment: Differences between English and French Bulldogs born via cesarean section. *Animals: An Open Access Journal from MDPI, 13*. https://www.semanticscholar.org/paper/580d2ad578ef91dd92d3383392f646415154ac61 (accessed on 16th June 2025).
31. Vitte, L., Hauguel, C., Benoit, V., Genet, M. C., Letot, J., Bruel, H., Delaunay, F., et al. (2022). Panda Unit, a mother-baby unit nested in a neonatal care service. *Frontiers in Psychiatry, 13*. https://www.semanticscholar.org/paper/f2fcfd6761bbbc97d8e426bea3ec2d2dbba712ef (accessed on 16th June 2025).
32. Webbe, J., Duffy, J. M. N., Afonso, E., Al-Muzaffar, I., Brunton, G., Greenough, A., Hall, N., et al. (2019). Core outcomes in neonatology: Development of a core outcome set for neonatal research. *Archives of Disease in Childhood Fetal & Neonatal, 105*, 425–431. https://doi.org/10.1136/archdischild-2019-317501 (accessed on 16th June 2025).

33. Wszolek, K. M., Chmaj-Wierzchowska, K., & Wilczak, M. (2021). Management of birth, postpartum care and breastfeeding–Polish recommendations and guidelines during SARS-CoV-2 pandemic. *Gynecologic Polska*. https://www.semanticscholar.org/paper/9a0cddc5d7afdb3ad880d13e4c2e727ba387c0f2 (accessed on 16th June 2025).

34. Zavyalov, O., Игнатко, И. В., Ilenko, L. I., & Пасечник, И. Н. (2023). The Silverman–Andersen scale in the assessment of respiratory distress syndrome in preterm infants: Clinical and prognostic significance. *Obstetrics Gynecology and Reproduction, 17*, 357–365. https://doi.org/10.17749/2313-7347/ob.gyn.rep.2023.403 (accessed on 16th June 2025).

# PEDIATRIC INFECTIOUS SKIN DISEASES

# 6

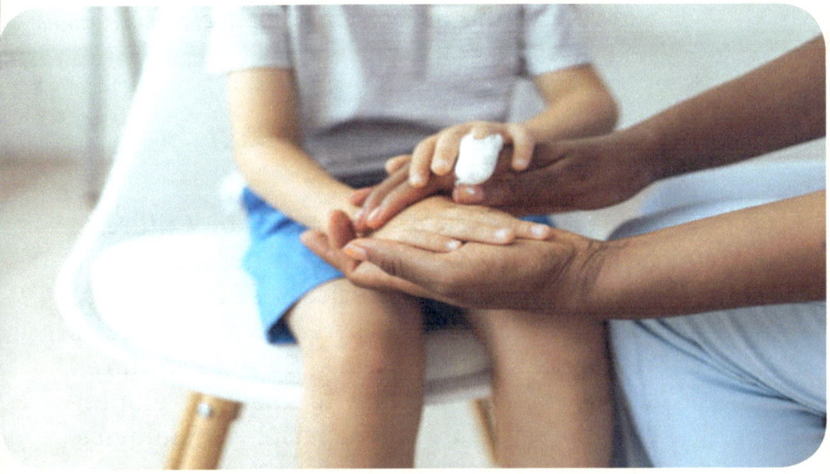

## LEARNING OBJECTIVES

**After studying this chapter, you will be able to:**

1. Discuss the common pediatric infectious skin diseases;
2. Explain the diagnosis and clinical evaluation;
3. Focus on treatment and management strategies;
4. Know prevention and public health implications.

## Introduction

The complex topography of pediatric infectious cutaneous disease presents tremendous challenges to caregivers, clinicians, and researchers alike. Pediatric infectious cutaneous diseases represent an enormous spectrum of infections by a wide range of pathogens, including bacteria, viruses, fungi, and parasites, with diverse clinical presentations and implications for treatment. The developing immune system of children, environmental exposure, and socioeconomic determinants are some of the factors that contribute to the vulnerability to such infections.

Additionally, skin illnesses in children often accentuate the necessity of premature diagnosis and treatment to avoid potential complications, such as secondary infection and scarring. Familiarity with the etiology, patterns of transmission, and clinical presentation of these diseases is necessary for effective prevention strategies and management. Since we are beginning to understand the intricacy of skin infections in children, it is evident that an integrated approach is warranted to improve infected children's health outcomes (Figure 6.1).

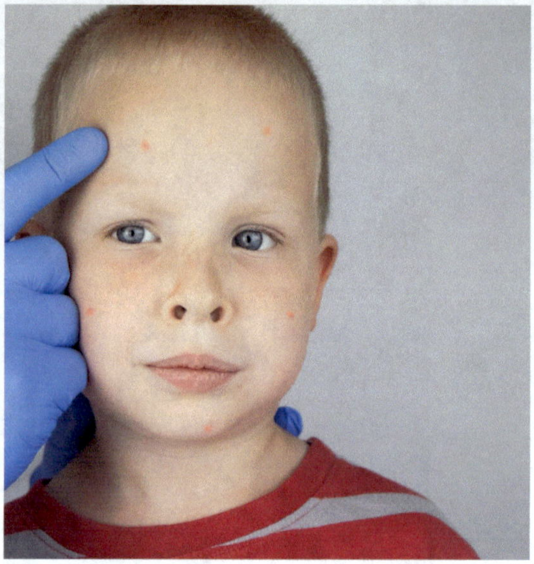

Figure 6.1. The complex landscape of pediatric infectious skin diseases presents significant challenges to healthcare providers.

Source: https://www.brynmawrdermatology.com/wp-content/uploads/Bryn-Mawr-Social-Media-3-1.jpg.

## Definition of Pediatric Infectious Skin Diseases

Pediatric infectious dermatoses encompass a range of diseases due to microbial pathogens targeting the child's skin specifically. They are most commonly caused by bacterial, viral, fungal, or parasitic infections with each of which causes distinct clinical manifestations. For instance, impetigo, a common bacterial infection, most commonly arises as a result of a break in the integrity of the skin, leading to characteristic crusting lesions. Viral infections such as herpes simplex present in the form of vesicular eruptions and constitute a considerable level of distress and complications among pediatric patients. Further, considering the widespread occurrence of drug-resistant pathogens, detection and treatment of such infections are extremely important to obtain favorable health outcomes among pediatric groups. To appropriately address the diagnosis and treatment complexities of these infections among children, there is a need for healthcare professionals to remain current with the epidemiology patterns and potential prevention practices of these infections among children (Andrade et al., 2011; Lamb et al., 2019). Prioritizing effective public health interventions will reduce the burden of pediatric infectious skin diseases.

## Importance of Studying Skin Diseases in Children

The significance of this study of children's skin disease extends beyond dermatological importance in that such diseases often serve as indicators of more widespread health problems and social determinants. Because children are so vulnerable due to their developing immune systems and special physiologies, early diagnosis and treatment are essential. For instance, a pediatric syphilis cohort study showed that 79.2% of the cases were followed by secondary skin lesions, which underscores the importance of identifying and treating such manifestations at an early stage to prevent further complications (Altcheh et al., 2021; Moscatelli et al., 2023). Furthermore, the household as well as environmental conditions among children, such as poor hygiene and crowding, enhance infectious skin disorders. With a clearer understanding of these intricate relationships, health care providers can execute specific interventions to address not only the immediate dermatologic conditions but also the socioeconomic determinants that shape pediatric health outcomes (Bertram et al., 2017). Ultimately, the study of skin disease in children encourages an interdisciplinary method of pediatric health care, increasing total well-being and quality of life.

## Overview of Common Infectious Skin Diseases

Infectious dermatoses are frequent in pediatric populations and cause a serious issue in clinical practice. Some examples are impetigo, resulting from a bacterial infection, and tinea, a fungal infection occurring in many forms, one of the most frequent being ringworm. Impetigo tends to occur as a highly contagious eruption in children, frequently in the face in the region surrounding the nose and mouth and should be treated early to prevent spread in schools or daycare settings. Similarly, tinea infections, including athlete's foot and corporis, thrive in moist environments and can easily transfer among children via activities like shared sports or swimming.

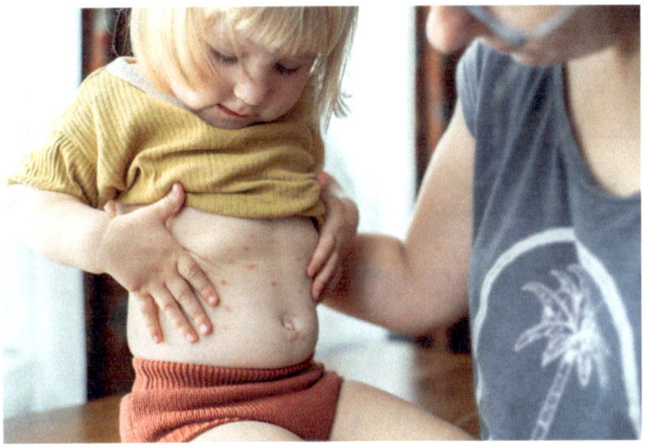

**Figure 6.2.** Infectious skin diseases are prevalent among pediatric populations.

*Source:* https://epidermatology.com.sg/wp-content/uploads/2023/08/epi-blog-common-paediatric-featured.jpg.

Additionally, viral infections, including herpes simplex and hand, foot, and mouth disease, contribute to the complexity of pediatric dermatologic health. It is important to know these typical conditions to effectively manage and prevent them, particularly in settings where kids with various backgrounds come together and share the same spaces (Lamb et al., 2019). It is a pediatricians work to be vigilant to detect, diagnose, and treat infectious diseases to safeguard children's health and welfare (Bernasconi et al., 2019) (Figure 6.2).

## Impact of These Diseases on Pediatric Health

The influence of pediatric infectious skin conditions goes far beyond physical manifestations, substantially impairing children's well-being and health. Impetigo and viral exanthems not only result in immediate threats to health in the form of secondary infection and systemic complications but also to psychological and social development. Visibly infected children become subject to stigmatization, developing anxiety or depression, while suffering from peer difficulties and self-esteem problems. Besides, tuberculosis (TB) prevalence in foreign-born children mirrors the public health challenges, as such children are disproportionately burdened with infectious diseases, carrying a higher burden in their early childhood years (Lamb et al., 2019). Care and intervention are thus crucial to undertake early, as neglecting these diseases could result in permanent morbidity and growth retardation. Thus, an utmost priority for pediatric health models should be caring for infectious skin conditions to provide broad health outcomes for children.

## Role of Pediatricians in Diagnosis and Treatment

Pediatricians are the most important individuals in the detection of infectious dermatological conditions at an early stage and effective treatment in the event of rising cases due to community-associated methicillin-resistant *Staphylococcus aureus* (CA-MRSA). Not only is their identification of clinical presentations of skin and soft-tissue infections (SSTIs) of significance, but their utilization of appropriate treatment methods, including incision and drainage (I&D), if necessitated, as recommended by current guidelines. However, some pediatricians are held back by impediments such as suboptimal training in procedural interventions and compromised access to contemporary epidemiologic information regarding SSTIs, which can fail to allow them to provide optimal care (Adam et al., 2009). Despite such adversity, pediatricians have an essential part to play in informing families about prevention methods and the handling of recurrent infections, emphasizing the value of continuous professional development and the sharing of treatment recommendations to enhance patient outcomes in pediatric infectious skin conditions (Mistry et al., 2017).

### *Brief Mention of Prevention Strategies*

Effective measures of prevention for infectious skin conditions among children are essential in controlling the spread and maintaining overall well-being among kids. Major steps include the implementation of effective hygiene practices, such as the constant washing of hands and avoiding sharing personal items, which can reduce the risk of infection from skin diseases like impetigo and tinea.

Immunization campaigns targeting specific pathogens of skin disease-causing diseases—e.g., the varicella vaccine to provide immunity against chickenpox—are a primary driving force in preventing children from infectious agents that tend to result in severe skin ailments. Moreover, sensitization of carers and parents regarding the signs and symptoms of widespread skin infections can assist with immediate medical treatment, reducing transmission rates among populations. The implementation of these interventions, coupled with education regarding the importance of personal hygiene and early treatment, significantly contributes to lessening the burden of infectious skin diseases in child populations (Mistry et al., 2017) (Figure 6.3).

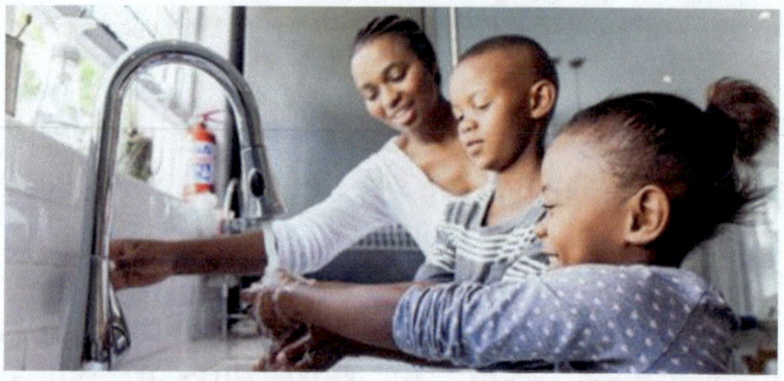

**Figure 6.3.** A mother helps her children wash their hands at a kitchen sink, promoting hygiene practices essential for preventing illness and supporting family health.

*Source:* https://www.healthychildren.org/SiteCollectionImagesArticleImages/family_washing_their_hands_together.jpg?RenditionID=3.

## 6.1. Common Pediatric Infectious Skin Diseases

**Learning Outcome**

1. Impetigo: Causes and symptoms;
2. Chickenpox: Transmission and prevention;
3. Hand, foot, and mouth disease: Overview;
4. Ringworm: Diagnosis and treatment;
5. Scabies: Symptoms and management;
6. Molluscum contagiosum: Characteristics;
7. Candidiasis: Risk factors in children;
8. Erysipelas: Clinical presentation;
9. Herpes simplex virus infections: Types and effects.

The increased prevalence of infectious cutaneous infections in the children's population necessitates a wide knowledge of their causations and implications for their health. Impetigo caused by *Staphylococcus aureus* and *Streptococcus pyogenes* appears as most infectious pustular lesions, particularly in children. Furthermore, other diseases such as tinea capitis and eczema herpeticum emphasize the danger of contact with fungal and viral pathogens, respectively.

Children's susceptibility to such infections is also augmented by immaturity of the immune system and extrinsic pressures like their proximity to each other in group settings, schools and playgrounds, where germs transmit easily. Additionally, with more and more children migrating from regions of higher incidence of such conditions, there are increasing public health concerns, particularly in the case of Texas, which also has a multicultural flow of refugees and immigrants (Lamb et al., 2019). Effective prevention measures, early detection, and management are critical to minimize the rate at which such infectious diseases affect the health of children (King et al., 2017).

### 6.1.1. Impetigo: Causes and Symptoms

Impetigo is a highly infectious bacterial skin disease that is prevalent in most young children and caused primarily by *Staphylococcus aureus* and *Streptococcus pyogenes*. Impetigo typically occurs after a cutaneous breach of the skin caused by minor injuries, bites, or existing cutaneous infections that provide access to the bacteria.

Clinically, impetigo is characterized by characteristic lesions that evolve from vesicles to honey-colored crusted lesions, which are often found on the arms, face, and legs. They are accompanied by mild itchiness and inflammation, but the presence of systemic signs such as fever may be seen in some cases. Notably, the condition is very contagious in communal settings, particularly in summer when the children spend more time outdoors and skin injury is more likely (Bendo et al., 2019). Early identification and management are important to prevent complications and transmission, highlighting the need for awareness by caregivers and medical practitioners in managing this infectious cutaneous disorder (Al-Wabel et al., 2020).

### 6.1.2. Chickenpox: Transmission and Prevention

Understanding the transmission and prevention of chickenpox is important in order to manage the extremely contagious viral disease. Chickenpox, caused by the varicella-zoster virus, is transmitted primarily through the airborne mode by way of coughing or sneezing by an infected person, as well as through direct contact with the fluid from the rash blister. As its extremely infectious nature causes its spread to quickly rise, especially in schools or daycare centers, outbreaks can rapidly increase.

Prevention includes immunization, which has reduced the incidence of chickenpox considerably in the majority of countries, including Belgium, with studies highlighting a heavy burden of varicella infection complication-related hospitalization (cumulative incidence of 29.5 per 105 person-years) during the pre-universal vaccination era (Belgian Group for Varicella, 2016). By promoting vaccination and imposing public health measures, the transmission of this disease can be restricted, safeguarding vulnerable groups as well as minimizing healthcare costs associated with dealing with extreme situations (Figure 6.4).

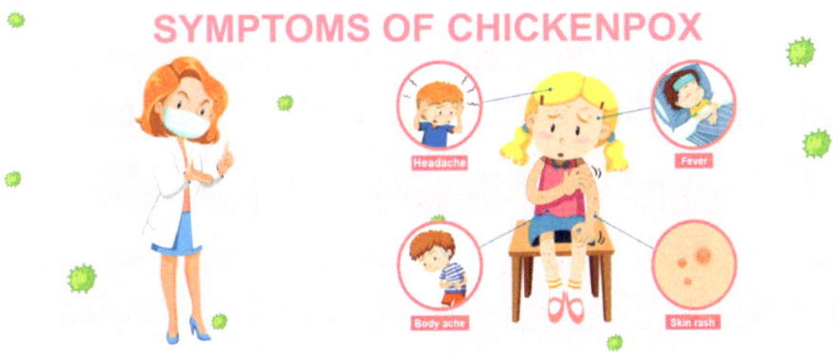


**Figure 6.4.** Chickenpox: Transmission and prevention.

*Source:* https://pathkindwebsiteprod.blob.core.windows.net/websiteprod/uploads/blogs/June-2.png.

### 6.1.3. Hand, Foot, and Mouth Disease: Overview

Hand, foot, and mouth disease (HFMD) is a common childhood infection characterized by fever and a typical rash on the hands, feet, and mouth produced by human enteroviruses, including enterovirus 71 (EV-71) and coxsackieviruses.

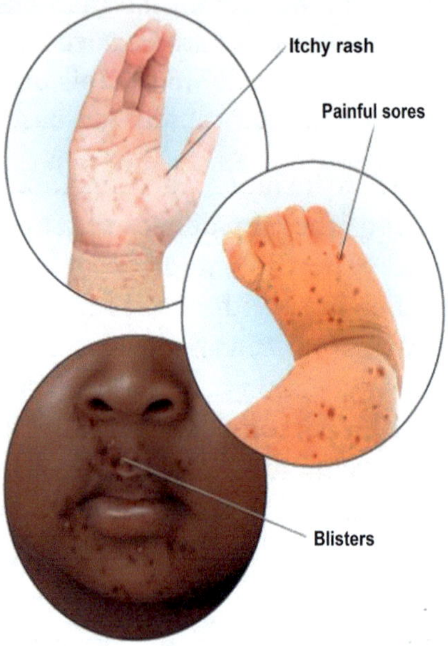


**Figure 6.5.** Hand, foot, and mouth disease can cause an itchy rash, painful sores, and blisters.

*Source:* https://my.clevelandclinic.org/health/diseases/11129-hand-foot-and-mouth-disease.

Notably, the disease is predominantly transmitted through feco-oral transmissions in the developing world, while respiratory droplets are a mere carrier for transmission in the developed world, as an indicator of dynamic patterns influenced by environmental determinants (Lau et al., 2010). Underreporting ensues due to the indolent nature of HFMD; severe complications can nonetheless present, particularly in the Asia Pacific region, with EV-71 being linked to neurological and cardiopulmonary complications. Systematic monitoring of HFMD and its epidemiological features is warranted, as advancement towards the development of a vaccine is still inhibited by the virus genetic heterogeneity and evolution (Lau et al., 2010). An understanding of these processes is crucial in order to enhance appropriate management and public health interventions for this infectious cutaneous disease in children (Figure 6.5).

### 6.1.4. Ringworm: Diagnosis and Treatment

Ringworm, or dermatophytosis, is a significant problem in childhood infectious dermatological infection, particularly among school children. Diagnosis is typically established on clinical examination and confirmation by fungal culture since studies indicate high dermatophyte infection prevalence, including tinea pedis and tinea capitis, particularly among children (Komba & Mgonda, 2010). Effective treatment typically entails local antifungal drugs like clotrimazole or terbinafine for less severe cases, with systemic antifungals being necessary for severe or resistant cases (Bipin et al., 2022). The administration of complementary treatments like homeopathy and herbal medicines has also been questioned through anecdotal evidence, implying effectiveness in some cases to necessitate further studies into their use alongside conventional treatments. Finally, timely intervention and appropriate management protocols are necessary for the prevention of the influence of ringworm on affected children since unmanaged cases lead to recurring infections and the build-up of the burden of the skin disease among children.

### 6.1.5. Scabies: Symptoms and Management

Scabies is a leading pediatric infectious dermatosis caused by *Sarcoptes scabiei* mite with intense pruritus and typical rash that often progresses to secondary bacterial infection. In children, it presents in the form of erythematous papules and burrows in intertriginous areas, i.e., between the armpits and fingers. Treatment of scabies is primarily topical scabicides, i.e., permethrin, or systemic drugs such as ivermectin in widespread cases or epidemics. Preventive measures are crucial due to the high transmissibility of mites through direct skin-to-skin contact. Effective measures of control include the Identify-Isolate-Inform (3I) Tool, through which healthcare workers can quickly identify those infected, isolate them to prevent further transmission, and inform public health authorities as necessary (Al-Wabel et al., 2020). Thus, timely detection and effective treatment are essential in controlling scabies in pediatric populations and minimizing its public health impact (Figure 6.6).

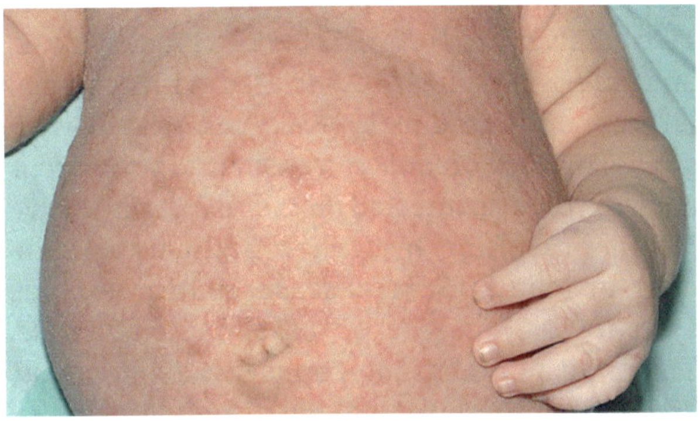

**Figure 6.6.** An infant's abdomen shows a widespread rash associated with scabies, a contagious skin condition caused by mites, highlighting the need for early diagnosis and treatment.

Source: https://my.clevelandclinic.org/-/scassets/images/org/health/articles/4567-scabies.

## 6.1.6. Molluscum Contagiosum: Characteristics

Molluscum contagiosum (MC) is a viral skin infection that mainly occurs in children, which is characterized by painless, umbilicated papules on the skin. This extremely prevalent condition, owing to its being self-limiting, can lead to significant discomfort and psychosocial morbidity due to its obvious appearance; thus, most pediatric patients must endure prolonged periods of visible lesions (Bhatia et al., 2023). The virus, being in the poxvirus group, is extremely opportunistic in immunocompromised patients, exacerbating the infection as well as risks (Bhatia et al., 2023). The traditional watch-and-wait strategy has been employed, which ends up prolonging both infection as well as peer-to-peer transmission (Bhatia et al., 2023). Therefore, active treatment is required not only to expedite resolution but also to reduce the psychological impact on affected children (Bhatia et al., 2023). Thus, understanding the nature and management of MC is of prime importance in the successful treatment of children in pediatric practice.

## 6.1.7. Candidiasis: Risk Factors in Children

Candidiasis, most commonly caused by Candida albicans, is a severe threat to pediatric patients, particularly those with predisposing conditions that compromise their immune status. Pediatric patients in hospital admission, particularly children in the pediatric intensive care unit and on therapy for malignancies, are at high risk of this fungal infection. Research indicates that invasive candidiasis is much more prevalent in children than invasive aspergillosis, suggesting underlying predisposition based on their clinical status (Burgos et al., 2012). Characteristics like the administration of antibiotics for more than a long duration, which disrupts normal flora, and the employment of catheters or surgery only serve to raise the risk of infection. The new epidemic trend in non-albicans species calls for more careful observation and particular prophylactic interventions in at-risk pediatric groups (Burgos et al., 2012). Thus, it is crucial to be aware of these risk factors to offer proper prevention of candidiasis in children, reducing associated morbidity and potential sequelae of long-term health effects.

## 6.1.8. Erysipelas: Clinical Presentation

Erysipelas, an infectious cutaneous disease primarily caused by *Streptococcus pyogenes*, has unequivocal clinical manifestations that can be utilized for diagnosis, particularly among children. The condition normally appears as a well-demarcated erythematous skin lesion with associated swelling, heat, and tenderness (Martinez et al., 2020).

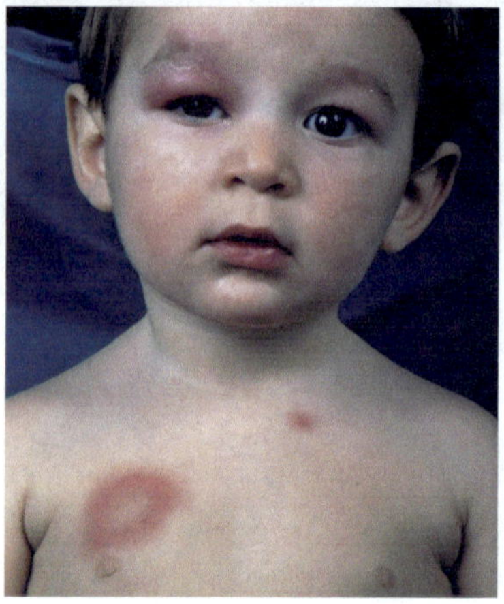

**Figure 6.7.** Erysipelas: Clinical presentation.

*Source:* https://www.researchgate.net/profile/Luisa-Lunardon/publication/6811355/figure/fig2/AS:352247646048259@1460993791888/An-erysipelas-like-lesion-on-the-upper-eyelid-and-a-lesion-mimicking-fixed-drug-eruption.png.

Affected areas also have systemic signs of fever and chills that complicate pre-existing health conditions. In kids, the lower limbs and face are common sites of infection from insect bites or skin breaks, and thus observation is crucial, with immediate treatment. Other comorbidities can influence disease severity, such that a prior evaluation of the overall status of health is required before formulation of treatment plans. Accordingly, information regarding erysipelas' clinical presentation is important for proper management and the prevention of complications in children (Bookstaver et al., 2018) (Figure 6.7).

## 6.1.9. Herpes Simplex Virus Infections: Types and Effects

Herpes simplex virus (HSV) infections are a significant problem among infant infectious dermatologic conditions because they can lead to serious complications in neonates and children. Two species of HSV exist: HSV-1 and HSV-2, and HSV-1 is typically associated with orofacial lesions and HSV-2 is typically associated with genital disease. Neonatal transmission can occur at birth when an infected mother is bearing active lesions, resulting in such conditions as skin, eyes, or mouth (SEM) disease, central nervous system (CNS) disease, or disseminated disease. The impact of these infections can be immense, given their association with high morbidity and mortality in infants. Interventions such as acyclovir have greatly improved outcomes, particularly when initiated early, minimizing both acute and long-term development issues prevalent in the infected neonates (Shehata et al., 2022). Nevertheless, close monitoring for complications remains the hallmark of the holistic treatment of HSV infections (Brador, 2019).

## Test Your Knowledge

1. What are the common causes and symptoms of impetigo in children?
2. How does erysipelas typically present in pediatric patients?

## 6.2. Diagnosis and Clinical Evaluation

**Learning Outcome**

1. Importance of accurate diagnosis;
2. Common diagnostic methods;
3. Role of medical history in diagnosis;
4. Physical examination techniques;
5. Laboratory tests and their significance;
6. Differential diagnosis considerations;
7. Challenges in diagnosing skin diseases in children;
8. Use of imaging studies in complex cases;
9. Referral to specialists when necessary.

Pediatric infectious cutaneous disease diagnosis and clinical evaluation are an interdisciplinary process involving patient history, physical examination, and selective advanced imaging when appropriate. An attentive history of presenting complaints such as rashes, lesions, or systemic symptoms forms the basis for evaluation of the potential infectious organism. For cases where traditional means of diagnosis may be inadequate, point-of-care ultrasound (POCUS) is now an invaluable addition, particularly in low-resource settings. While primarily known for applications in severe infectious diseases, POCUS protocols like focused assessment with sonography for HIV-associated tuberculosis (FASH) could indirectly affect dermatologic evaluations by drawing attention to systemic infections manifesting cutaneously (Abdalla et al., 2015). Secondarily, interprofessional practice promotes accurate diagnosis, which provides pediatric patients with timely and effective treatment interventions relevant to their individual needs (King et al., 2017). Through a multidimensional approach to diagnostic strategy, practitioners are better positioned to navigate the complexities of pediatric cutaneous infections.

### 6.2.1. Importance of Accurate Diagnosis

Accurate diagnosis of infectious diseases of the skin in children is required for effective treatment and control as incorrect diagnosis can lead to improper therapies and unfavorable health effects. The nature of skin disease in children typically requires careful differentiation of many etiologies, including bacterial, viral, fungal, and parasitic infections. Failure to identify the proper cause may result in delays in timely treatment or misuse of antibiotics, which may result in resistance issues, as indicated by low involvement of emergency departments in antimicrobial stewardship programs (ASPs) for optimal usage of antibiotics in children's settings (Mistry et al., 2017). Additionally, correct diagnosis has a direct consequence on public health policy, particularly in the case of illnesses such as tuberculosis that may occur in uncommon forms among children (Seddon et al., 2014). It is therefore imperative to enhance diagnostic ability among practitioners to be capable of responding in a timely and effective manner to infectious skin disease among children.

### 6.2.2. Common Diagnostic Methods

For infectious cutaneous diseases of children, prompt and accurate diagnosis is essential to ensure proper treatment and management. Routinely, diagnosis is carried out through elaborate clinical examination, where clinicians assess the patient's history and conduct physical examinations to identify characteristic skin features. Besides clinical assessment, laboratory investigations, such as skin cultures and polymerase chain reaction (PCR) analysis, are also important to determine facts regarding the microbial etiology of the infection. Dermoscopy is now a non-invasive imaging modality which aids in visualizing lesions of the skin, enhancing diagnostic accuracy through derivation of dermatological processes. Point-of-care ultrasound (POCUS) is also being used more and more because its inclusion in diagnosing skin abscess or cellulitis can help in reducing diagnosis time in resource-constrained settings, making it particularly relevant in children (Abdalla et al., 2015). Together, these diagnostic techniques ultimately enhance the treatment of children's infectious skin disorders and yield improved health outcomes (Figure 6.8).

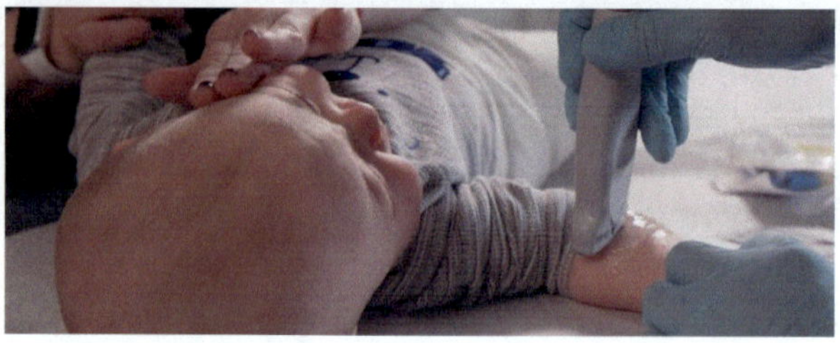

**Figure 6.8.** A medical professional performs an ultrasound scan on an infant's arm, demonstrating the use of noninvasive imaging techniques in pediatric diagnostics.

*Source:* https://healthcare-in-europe.com/media/story_section_image/2791/image-01-paediatric-ultrasound.jpg.

## 6.2.3. Role of Medical History in Diagnosis

Medical history serves the most significant function in the diagnosis of pediatric infectious skin disease as it provides extremely valuable information about a child's underlying health and exposures. Detailed medical history can illuminate previous infections, chronic medical conditions, and environmental exposures that may cause certain dermatoses. In addition, evaluation of family medical history assists in identifying inherited skin disorders or susceptibility to certain infections, thus guiding clinicians towards an accurate diagnosis. For instance, dermatological manifestations through viral infections can be akin to other illnesses, thus understanding patients' recent illnesses or immunizations becomes imperative to rule out appropriately. Also, travel history will determine endemic pathogen exposure, which is also crucial in the context of globalization since infectious diseases may also transcend geographical borders (Abdalla et al., 2015). As such, a critical examination of medical history is also crucial for clinicians to create a good plan of treatment for pediatric patients suffering from infectious skin ailments.

## 6.2.4. Physical Examination Techniques

An orderly approach to physical examination techniques is crucial in the effective diagnosis of pediatric infectious skin diseases because it enables clinicians to identify the significant signs correctly. It begins with a correct history and a visual examination of the skin, where morphology, distribution, and associated symptoms are scrutinized.

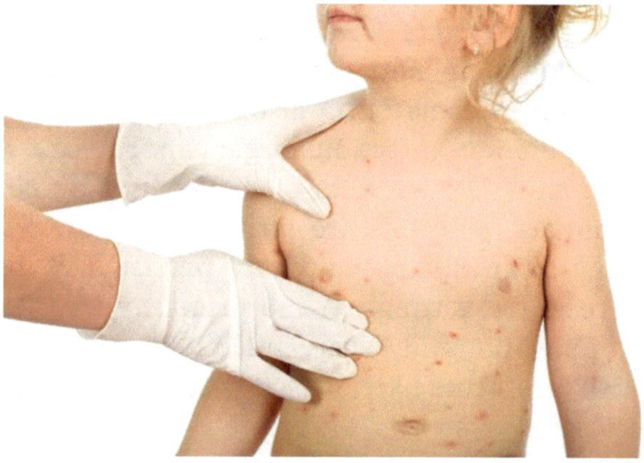

**Figure 6.9.** A systematic approach to physical examination techniques.

*Source:* https://static6.depositphotos.com/1140262/641/i/450/depositphotos_6411111-stock-photo-kid-with-small-pox-consulted.jpg.

Erythema, vesicles, or papules provide valuable information about potential infections. Mouth examination is also relevant; systemically occurring lesions could affect the diagnosis. Palpation of lymph nodes to check for inflammation can indicate systemic involvement in an extraoral assessment, so the diagnostic process is narrowed down. Employment of such technology as point-of-care ultrasound (POCUS) can also enhance evaluation further, especially in resource-constrained environments where there is no access to traditional imaging, enabling timely intervention and effective practice management of such vulnerable populations (Abdalla et al., 2015; Burgess et al., 2017). Ultimately, comprehensive physical examination techniques form the basis for effective diagnosis and treatment of these dermatological conditions (Figure 6.9).

## 6.2.5. Laboratory Tests and Their Significance

Laboratory studies play a crucial role in the diagnosis and management of pediatric infectious dermatoses, with relevant information influencing clinical decision-making.

For instance, skin biopsies can be employed to confirm specific pathogens and inflammatory patterns that lead clinicians to differentiate among various dermatoses, e.g., bacterial infection or cutaneous manifestations of systemic disease. Further, serological tests can identify underlying infections such as Mycobacterium tuberculosis infection, which is of extremely high prevalence among children in certain regions, as evidenced by a study reporting a 6.4% weighted prevalence of tuberculin skin test positivity among Philippine children (Leining et al., 2019). The timely performance of these tests not only aids in early diagnosis but also allows for targeted treatment regimens, ultimately reducing the risk of transmission and improving outcomes in patients. Thus, complete knowledge of laboratory tests enhances overall management of pediatric patients with infectious skin diseases in focus, highlighting their central position in clinical practice.

## 6.2.6. Differential Diagnosis Considerations

In diagnosing infectious skin diseases of children, differential diagnosis considerations are critical in creating an effective treatment regimen. The doctor must distinguish between myriad diseases whose presentation overlaps but differ significantly with regard to their etiology as well as their treatment. For instance, infectious diseases such as impetigo, candidiasis, and tinea corporis share overlapping presentations and thus need close examination of the patient's history, presentation, and, where necessary, laboratory findings. Systemic diseases, such as morphea or local scleroderma, although often non-infectious, can mimic some infectious cutaneous rashes in their inflammatory phase, necessitating discriminative examination so as not to be misdiagnosed (Ardeleanu et al., 2020). Hence, an integrative strategy consisting of a meticulous clinical examination, possibly supplemented by imaging techniques in low-resource settings, allows for more accurate diagnosis of children's cutaneous diseases, facilitating timely and appropriate intervention (Abdalla et al., 2015). This approach brings to the fore the significance of differential diagnosis in pediatric dermatology.

## 6.2.7. Challenges in Diagnosing Skin Diseases in Children

Diagnosis of skin diseases in children presents a challenging series of challenges, primarily because of the unique presentation of child dermatoses and the age-related status of young patients. Clinical presentation in pediatric patients may be significantly different from that in adults, leading to potential misdiagnosis. For example, illnesses such as scabies can have abnormal presentation, which hinders identification, especially because successful diagnosis is often dependent on the integration of clinical suspicion, history of the patient, and contact tracing (Slape et al., 2021). Also, the endemic nature of cacogenic diseases such as tuberculosis among kids makes things complicated since diagnostic techniques fail to work when fewer bacilli are present in children's samples, highlighting an imperative need for improved methods (Browning et al., 2017). Therefore, the infectivity of the aforementioned skin disorders and the inadequacy of available diagnostic machines make it necessary to address detection as well as management in an interdisciplinary context among this vulnerable group (Figure 6.10).

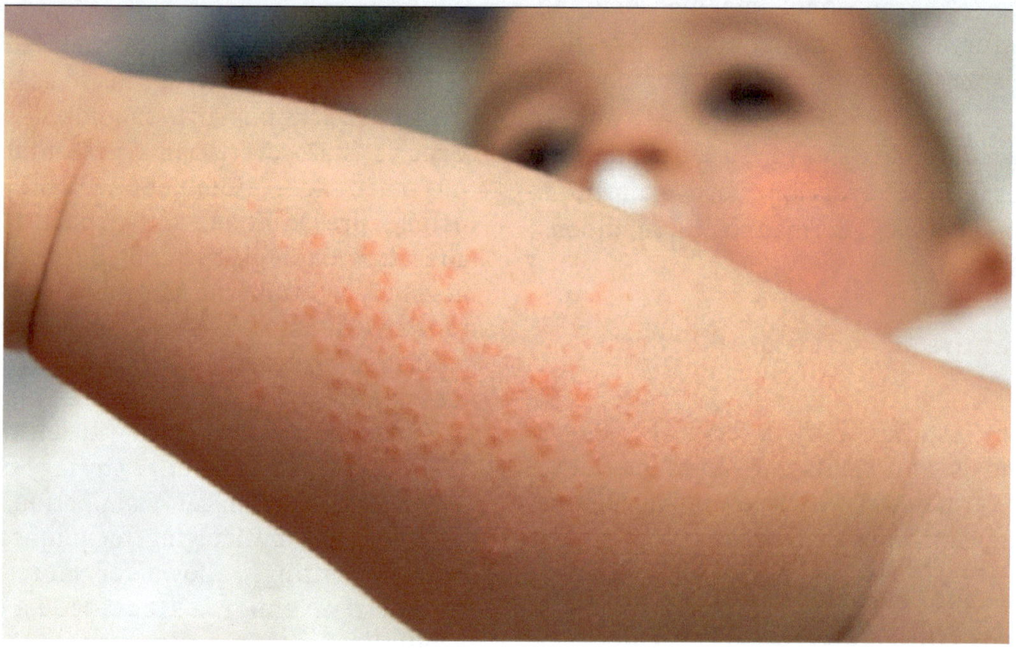

**Figure 6.10.** A close-up of a baby's arm shows a red, bumpy rash, commonly indicative of a skin condition such as eczema or heat rash, emphasizing the need for dermatological care in infants.

*Source:* https://www.parisadermatology.com/backend/blog/1716553455.png.

## 6.2.8. Use of Imaging Studies in Complex Cases

Imaging modalities have changed diagnostic strategies for skin infections in children, particularly in the complicated presentations where clinical examination may be inadequate. With the aid of modalities such as ultrasonography, magnetic resonance imaging (MRI), and computed tomography (CT), a comprehensive imaging of the underlying tissues can be done, and the detection of abscesses, soft tissue extension, and involvement of adjacent organs can be realized. In cases where simple observation fails to provide unequivocal results, these studies can reveal hidden infections or disease and ultimately guide specific therapeutic interventions. For instance, in cases where there is suspicion of deeper infection or involvement of anatomical structure, imaging can define the extent of infection and guide decision-making about surgical treatment or additional medical therapy. As imaging technology continues to improve, the ability to rapidly and accurately diagnose complex cases will improve, enhancing the outcomes for infected children with skin disease (Bertram et al., 2017).

### 6.2.9. Referral to Specialists When Necessary

Efficient management of pediatric infectious cutaneous disease often involves referral to specialists, particularly for cases that are outside general practice or have unusual features. The complexity of these diseases, e.g., those that include resistant organisms or require complicated treatment, underscores specialist intervention. For instance, pediatric dermatologists have the capacity to distinguish between common rashes and severe skin infections that may necessitate immediate treatment. Also, the utilization of diagnostic decision support software has the potential to improve referral accuracy because it assists the general practitioners in filtering the cases requiring specialist treatment. The applications have been shown to contain fewer diagnostic errors among physicians, making appropriate referrals more likely (Balu et al., 2016). Finally, early referral not only enhances the outcome of the patient but also promotes integral care, which guarantees children receive the focused treatment they need to cure their infectious skin illnesses efficiently.

## Test Your Knowledge

1. What is the importance of taking a thorough medical history in the diagnosis of skin diseases?
2. What are two common challenges in diagnosing skin diseases in children?

## 6.3. Treatment and Management Strategies

**Learning Outcome**

1. Overview of treatment options;
2. Topical treatments: Types and applications;
3. Oral medications: Indications and usage;
4. Role of antibiotics in treatment;
5. Importance of adherence to treatment plans;
6. Management of complications;
7. Supportive care and symptom relief;
7. Education for parents and caregivers;
8. Follow-up care and monitoring.

Timely and appropriate interventions are the key to proper treatment and care of infectious skin conditions among children. The first step is accurate diagnosis because it differentiates between bacterial, viral, and fungal infections, each calling for different therapeutic results. For bacterial infections like impetigo, topical and systemic antimicrobials are administered, while antiviral drugs are reserved for infections like herpes simplex virus infection. Besides that, antimicrobial stewardship programs (ASPs) in pediatric facilities can enhance the use of antibiotics by adding clinical decision support tools to electronic health records to guide optimal prescribing decisions (Mistry et al., 2017). Additional complementary actions are informing caregivers on appropriate wound care and hygiene practices to prevent secondary infections. Awareness of the potential complications, such as reactive arthritis following antibiotic therapy for Clostridium difficile infections, further highlights the need for a targeted management approach in this high-risk patient group (Derinkuyu et al., 2018) (Figure 6.11).

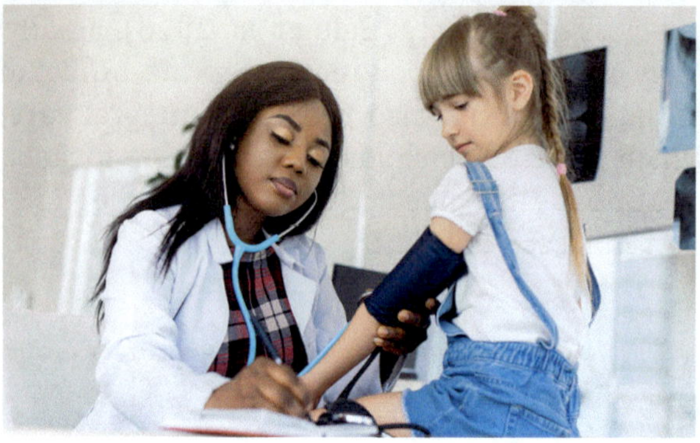

**Figure 6.11.** Effective treatment and management strategies for pediatric infectious skin diseases.

*Source:* https://nortonhealthcareprovider.com/wp-content/uploads/pediatric-hypertension_web.jpg.

## 6.3.1. Overview of Treatment Options

In infectious skin diseases in pediatrics, management is a multidimensional approach to manage various conditions with fewer complications. Antimicrobial therapy in the form of topical and systemic antibiotics is the prime treatment for bacterial infections like impetigo and cellulitis, while antifungal medications are utilized for tinea infections (Abdulhadi et al., 2023). More recent modalities, including the application of high-potency topical steroids and phototherapy, have been useful in controlling inflammatory skin diseases that may be accompanied by secondary infections, e.g., localized scleroderma (Ardeleanu et al., 2020). Moreover, the identification of prebiotics and probiotics indicates that there is a greater understanding of the microbiological environment in infection prevention (Abdulhadi et al., 2023). Vaccination remains a key preventive measure against certain viral infections that will complicate skin disease, and it reaffirms the role of the healthcare provider to remain current with evolving treatment strategies and preventive measures in pediatric practice. Overall, a treatment plan must be tailored to every patient in order to produce optimal results.

## 6.3.2. Topical Treatments: Types and Applications

Topical treatments are among the mainstays in the management of most pediatric infectious skin diseases, and they offer the advantage of localized treatment with the reduction of systemic side effects. Molluscum contagiosum is a prime example; it is primarily managed with topical agents like cantharidin, which is the only FDA-approved agent for this common viral infection (Bhatia et al., 2023).

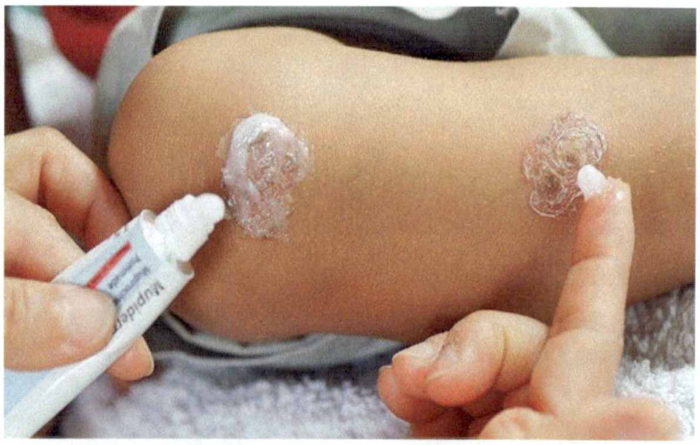

**Figure 6.12.** An adult applies medicated ointment to a child's skin lesions, showing treatment for impetigo, a common and highly contagious bacterial skin infection in children.

*Source:* https://images.everydayhealth.com/images/skin-beauty/impetigo/impetigo-treatment-and-therapy-rm-722x406.jpg.

In addition, new options like potassium hydroxide (KOH) solutions have emerged in clinical trials with the promise of providing effective therapy without the surgical invasion of removal (Cruz et al., 2011). Such approaches highlight the necessity of individualized treatment protocols that address the patient's specific conditions and presentation. Topical therapy not only permits the treatment of lesions but also addresses the psychological impacts that accompany symptomatic skin infections that are visible, thus enhancing the well-being of pediatric patients as a whole. As research advances, the destiny of topical therapies can shift, with advanced treatments that are more effective and better tolerated by children (Figure 6.12).

### 6.3.3. Oral Medications: Indications and Usage

In pediatric infectious cutaneous illness, the oral drug should be used appropriately for cure and healing. Oral antibiotics such as amoxicillin-clavulanate are commonly used for conditions like impetigo and cellulitis, in which appropriate management is critical in order to avoid complications and hasten recovery. Oral antifungals may also be employed in the treatment of dermatophyte infections, such as tinea capitis, where large dermatological manifestations are seen.

The practice of oral therapy must be grounded in responsible diagnostic workup and understanding of microbial susceptibility to prevent abuse, possibly leading to side effects and antimicrobial resistance. For instance, knowledge of body weight and proper dosing is essential, particularly in the pediatric population, to ensure optimal achievement of therapy with the lowest risk of toxicity. Thus, careful thought about presentation and correct administration are of utmost importance in the management of these common but important problems in children.

### 6.3.4. Role of Antibiotics in Treatment

Antibiotics form the core of the management of infective skin conditions in children, notably bacterial infections such as impetigo and cellulitis, which are common in children. The emergence of antibiotic-resistant organisms such as methicillin-resistant *Staphylococcus aureus* (MRSA) makes management challenging and necessitates careful selection of antimicrobial agents. Studies have indicated that awareness of local rates of resistant strain prevalence is required in order to develop effective interventions against such infection (Buttner et al., 2012). Moreover, the implementation of antimicrobial stewardship programs (ASPs) in pediatric facilities will optimize antibiotic use such that children are treated appropriately with diminished risk related to resistance (Mistry et al., 2017). Through the emphasis on the need for directed antibiotic treatment and ongoing resistance pattern monitoring, clinicians are able to maximize outcomes in children who are suffering from infective cutaneous disease, ultimately achieving enhanced clinical efficacy and safety in this vulnerable population.

### 6.3.5. Importance of Adherence to Treatment Plans

Compliance with treatment is necessary in the treatment of pediatric infectious skin illnesses because it significantly influences disease outcomes as well as overall patient health. When patient children strictly follow treatment protocols, the probabilities of effective clearance of the disease rise, thereby reducing the chances of complications such as secondary infection or chronic illness of the skin. Moreover, consistent compliance maintains antimicrobial stewardship principles with the objectives of optimizing the use of antibiotics as well as avoiding resistance. Evidence has shown that compliance not only improves clinical outcomes but also families' awareness of the importance of adhering to treatment guidelines, leading to better long-term health practices. For instance, approaches that embed clinical decision support in electronic health records can facilitate compliance by providing timely reminders and educational messages. Ultimately, having an effective system for compliance can significantly improve health outcomes for kids with infectious skin infections and promote a culture of preventive care within the healthcare facility (Figure 6.13).

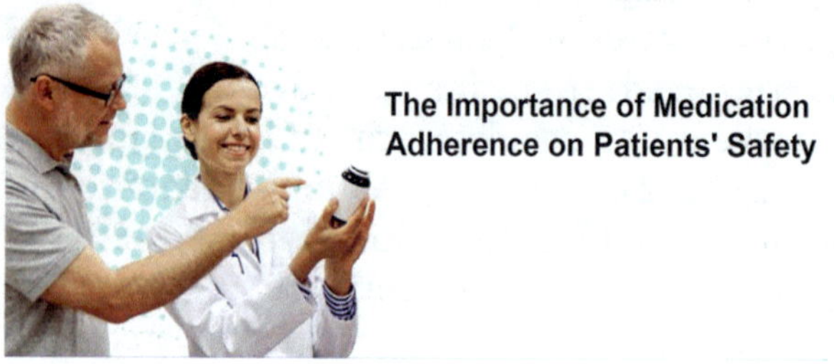


**Figure 6.13.** Importance of adherence to treatment plans.

*Source:* https://media.licdn.com/dms/image/v2/D4E12AQGoXfsIeDQsXw/article-cover_image-shrink_720_1280/article-cover_image-shrink_720_1280/0/1721577427295?e=2147483647&v=beta&t=ZxPKHCD7BlWC4_c8oH6dq4tIUP0PNbQ60DYjJZiT978.

## 6.3.6. Management of Complications

Treatment of complications following infectious skin disease in children must involve a polyfunctional approach addressing both immediate treatment and prolonged care methods. A successful intervention can begin with accurate diagnosis and timely initiation of effective antimicrobial therapy, which can moderate severe complications such as cellulitis or abscess. Furthermore, the integration of point-of-care ultrasound (POCUS) has proved to have an immense capacity for enhancing diagnostic accuracy and treatment planning in such a case, particularly in resource-poor environments where traditional imaging is not feasible (Abdalla et al., 2015). Besides, education of caregivers and health workers on the detection and handling of complications is necessary in avoiding delays in diagnosis as well as clinical outcomes. Continuous advancements in pediatric care, as noted by recent publications, emphasize the necessity of revised treatment regimens for the enhancement of better care for patients and reduced overall infectious cutaneous disease burden in pediatrics (Bernasconi et al., 2019).

## 6.3.7. Supportive Care and Symptom Relief

Good symptom relief and supportive care are key in the management of infectious skin conditions in kids because they play a vital role in making the child feel much better while undergoing treatment.

They typically form a multidisciplinary approach, which includes pharmacological management such as the use of topical corticosteroids to reduce inflammation and antibiotics to prevent secondary infections, as well as non-pharmacological measures including good skin care and fluid hydration. Educational interventions are essential, equipping caregivers with education regarding the necessity of monitoring signs and symptoms and the need for preventive care in preventing complications. Psychosocial support also cannot be overlooked since anxiety and distress issues can be provoked by skin signs (Abramovitz et al., 2006). Understanding the complexities of diseases like COVID-19, where oral presentation may be present, further highlights the need to exercise vigilance in supportive care in addressing both physical and psychological consequences of skin infections in children (Abbasi et al., 2023). Ultimately, symptomatic relief on an individual basis will play a part in overall treatment success and the well-being of infected children, aiding in their recovery and restoring normalcy in life.

### 6.3.8. Education for Parents and Caregivers

Caregiver and parent education plays a crucial role in the treatment of pediatric infectious skin disease, as infectious skin disease can have a significant impact on the quality of a child's life and family functioning. Effective caregiver education must include direct information about disease management that potentially increases self-efficacy and alleviates anxiety. Data indicate that the utilization of structured resources, i.e., written Eczema Action Plans (EAPs), has the capability of empowering caregivers in the management of their child's condition (Sena et al., 2019).

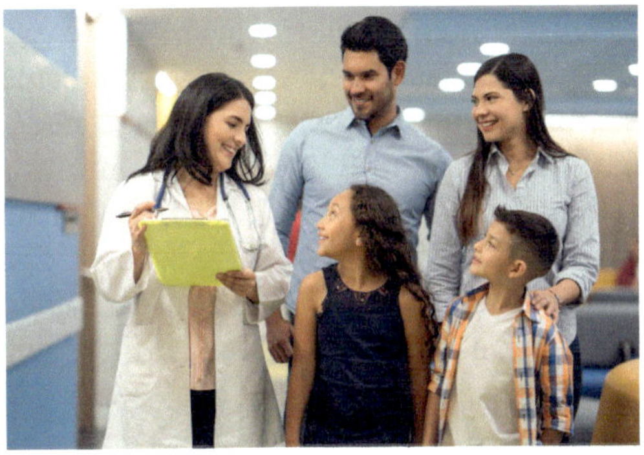

**Figure 6.14.** Education for parents and caregivers plays a crucial role in managing pediatric infectious skin diseases.

*Source:* https://www.dpcedcenter.org/wp-content/uploads/2021/05/Female-pediatrician-talking-to-her-sweet-patient-while-brother-and-parents-listen-to-them-all-smiling-960073228_2123x1416.jpeg.

Such plans provide concrete guidance on controlling atopic dermatitis, thus decreasing eczema severity by approximately 65% through enhanced caregiver adherence to treatment regimens. Furthermore, wide-ranging educational interventions must incorporate training in how to create safe and caring environments, healthy diet, and responsive relationships that are all central to preventing skin diseases from emerging or deteriorating (Mistry et al., 2017). Not only do these programs offer caregivers relevant information, but they also establish a supportive environment for enduring health outcomes (Figure 6.14).

### 6.3.9. Follow-Up Care and Monitoring

Regular follow-up care and monitoring are crucial in pediatric infectious skin disease management to ensure maximum patient outcomes and prevent complications. Monitoring helps health practitioners evaluate if the treatment given is effective, screen for potential side effects, and determine early recurrence of infection. Moreover, systematic follow-up visits provide opportunities for parent education regarding skin care management, hygiene, and treatment regimens, thereby promoting team-based care. Evidence indicates that antimicrobial stewardship programs (ASPs), although primarily focused on inpatient settings, can also prove beneficial to outpatient settings, particularly in emergency departments (ED), where they can optimize the utilization of antibiotics among children with skin infections (Mistry et al., 2017). This integration also complements monitoring activities by equipping medical personnel with clinical decision support systems to guide treatment, thereby ensuring that children receive proper and timely follow-up care (Abdalla et al., 2015).

## Test Your Knowledge

1. What are the main types of topical treatments used for skin diseases, and how are they applied?
2. How do antibiotics and supportive care contribute to the treatment and symptom relief of skin conditions?

## 6.4. Prevention and Public Health Implications

**Learning Outcome**

1. Importance of vaccination in prevention;
2. Hygiene practices to reduce transmission;
3. Role of schools in disease prevention;
4. Community awareness and education programs;
5. Impact of socioeconomic factors on disease prevalence;
6. Strategies for outbreak management;
7. Importance of early detection and reporting;
8. Collaboration with public health agencies;
9. Future directions in prevention research.

Successful prevention and public health are essential for the management of childhood infectious skin disease, which is extremely burdensome in most children. Information and early treatment to clean the skin are essential in reducing transmissibility. Particularly, antimicrobial stewardship programs (ASPs) in emergency departments are emerging as a good practice because they can optimize the use of antibiotics and minimize the risk of resistance in children (Mistry et al., 2017).

Furthermore, understanding the disease epidemiology of conditions such as tuberculosis among children identifies the importance of particular public health programs, for which the strategies are employed in eliminating diagnostic challenges and boosting levels of child morbidity (Seddon et al., 2014). The strategies involve collaboration between healthcare providers, families, and community organizations to offer access to resources and raise awareness. Lastly, an integrated prevention and health education plan can successfully rebut the impact of infectious skin diseases and enhance the overall well-being of children.

### 6.4.1. Importance of Vaccination in Prevention

Vaccination has a role to play in the prevention of infectious skin illnesses in children, as it not only protects the individual child but also serves to support public health programs. Vaccines such as the varicella vaccine, which protects against chickenpox, greatly reduce the incidence of diseases that present with extensive skin manifestations. In addition to avoiding current infection, vaccination creates herd immunity, a protective measure needed for those who cannot receive certain vaccines. Studies indicate that unvaccinated populations are more susceptible to outbreaks of infectious disease, providing another complexity in the management of children's health. Moreover, the etiology of diseases such as latent tuberculosis, which involves skin, underscores the need for rational vaccination strategies for minimizing overall disease burden in children (Antonina et al., 2019). With increasing knowledge of infectious diseases, it is essential to lay focus on vaccination as a cornerstone of preventive medicine in children (Seddon et al., 2014) (Figure 6.15).

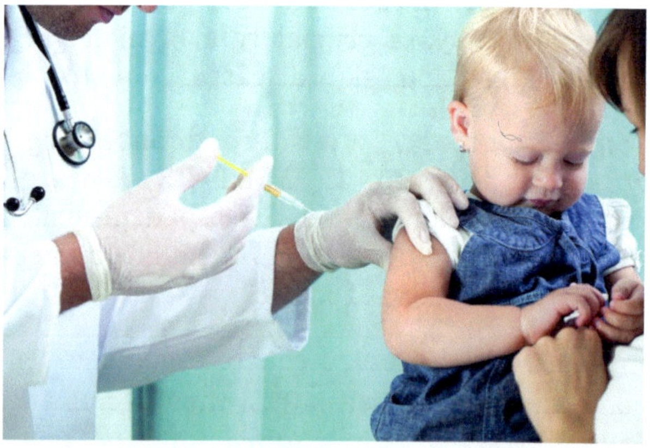

**Figure 6.15.** Vaccination plays a crucial role in the prevention of pediatric infectious skin diseases.

*Source:* https://cdn.mdedge.com/files/s3fs-public/Image/October-2017/vaccination_doc_toddler_mom_web.jpg.

### 6.4.2. Hygiene Practices to Reduce Transmission

Proper hygiene practices are key to preventing infant infectious skin infections, particularly where infants are regularly interacting with one another in places such as schools and nurseries. Frequent handwashing with soap and water is necessary because it prevents contact and fecal-oral transmission of causative agents and minimizes the risk of outbreaks. Additionally, it is crucial to instruct caregivers and children to value personal hygiene, such as the proper cleaning of skin lesions frequently and the timely treatment of infected lesions in a way that prevents the spread of contagions. Also considered should be the potential harmful impact of excessive use of antimicrobial products, resulting in skin barrier breakdown and antimicrobial resistance, making hygiene practice more difficult. Through the encouragement of a hygiene and awareness culture, communities can lower the incidence of infectious skin diseases among children and resulting in better overall health outcomes.

### 6.4.3. Role of Schools in Disease Prevention

The schools play a critical function in prevention of diseases, particularly for pediatric infectious dermatoses, as they are where health education and preventive health activities take place. They provide a structured environment where children learn about hygiene practices, such as proper hand washing and avoidance of sharing personal items, which can successfully prevent the spread of skin diseases like impetigo and scabies. Most importantly, schools can encourage early identification of infectious cutaneous diseases by means of routine health screening and timely treatment, thereby controlling the spread as well as guaranteeing individual as well as community protection. Schools also collaborate with public health authorities in establishing vaccination programs and offering valuable information concerning the prevention of cutaneous disease, particularly among ethnically diverse groups who could be at heightened risk by virtue of socioeconomic circumstance. Through the use of educational programs and community alliances, schools promote an educated student population that can assist in overall disease prevention strategies.

### 6.4.4. Community Awareness and Education Programs

Effective community education and sensitization programs are at the heart of managing childhood infectious skin diseases, particularly for vulnerable groups. The programs not only disseminate vital information about frequent infectious skin diseases, such as impetigo or fungal infections, but also enforce preventive strategies, early symptom detection, and easy access to healthcare services.

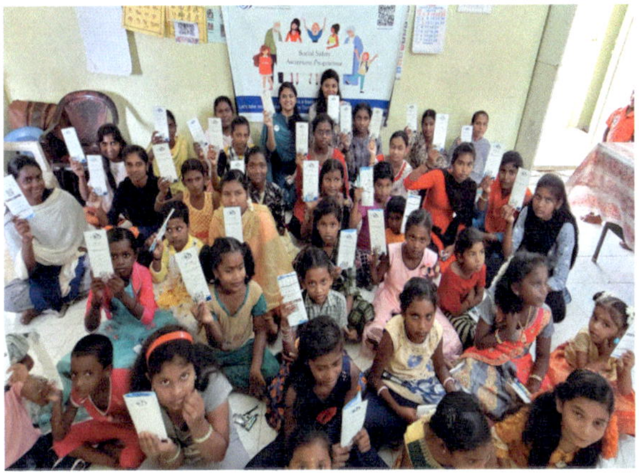

**Figure 6.16.** A large group of children and young women participates in a Social Safety Awareness Program, holding informational pamphlets aimed at promoting education on personal safety and empowerment.

*Source:* https://bewitness.world/wp-content/uploads/2022/05/16.jpg.

By working in tandem with community health agencies and schools, the programs are then in a position to reach minority populations and reinforce education on the topic of health disparities within minority communities, since the National Institute of Allergy and Infectious Diseases has highlighted the individual health concerns facing such populations. Moreover, the incorporation of culturally relevant materials can optimize the effectiveness of outreach activities to ensure that knowledge is provided and utilizable (Sandwich et al., 2016). Lastly, these combined education measures can prepare families for self-sufficiency in coping with pediatric infectious skin diseases as well as improve overall community health outcomes (Figure 6.16).

### 6.4.5. Impact of Socioeconomic Factors on Disease Prevalence

The prevalence of infectious skin diseases in children greatly relies on heterogeneous socioeconomic determinants, which influence the health outcomes of vulnerable populations. These children are likely to have increased exposure to infectious agents due to low living conditions and limited access to healthcare. For instance, the prevalence of skin diseases among Nigerian primary school students was at the level of 36.2%, with infection, particularly tinea, being highest among young individuals from lower economic status and government schools (Adah et al., 2023). These disparities indicate how economic disadvantage is associated with susceptibility to infection. Further, foreign-born children who immigrate to the United States are disproportionately burdened by tuberculosis infection, with socioeconomic status influencing access to screening and treatment (Lamb et al., 2019). As these cases illustrate, where socioeconomic status intersects with health outcomes, targeted public health interventions are necessary to diminish the infectious skin disease burden in children.

### 6.4.6. Strategies for Outbreak Management

Effective control of an outbreak is key in the management of infectious skin infections among children that can be transmitted rapidly in communal settings like schools and daycares.

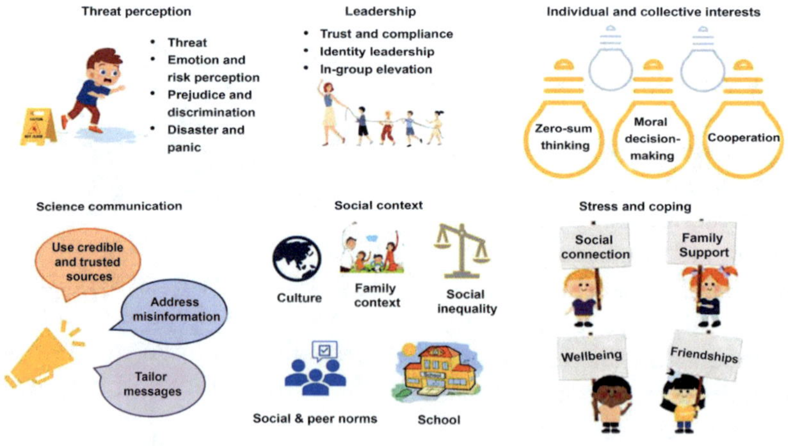


**Figure 6.17.** Effective outbreak management is crucial in controlling pediatric infectious skin diseases.

*Source:* https://covid19-sciencetable.ca/wp-content/uploads/2021/10/Figure-1-2.png.

Early identification and quarantine of infected individuals to prevent further transmission to susceptible individuals are the main measures. Implementing appropriate hygiene practices, such as disinfecting hands and washing them, is paramount in inhibiting the spread of pathogens that stem from skin infections like ringworm and impetigo. Educational programs that teach caregivers about prevention, symptoms, and the requirement for adherence to immunization schedules are also important. Targeted immunization activity against such diseases with suspected associations with cutaneous manifestations should be highlighted. There should also be surveillance and reporting systems in place to monitor the prevalence of such infections and modify public health interventions accordingly (d'Hemecourt et al., 2007). By the concerted effort of healthcare professionals, schools, and families, the impact of outbreaks can be minimized, building healthier environments for children (Figure 6.17).

### 6.4.7. Importance of Early Detection and Reporting

The necessity for early reporting and diagnosis of skin pediatric infectious diseases cannot be overstressed, given that appropriate timing in treatment is crucial to the prevention of complications and attainment of optimal health outcomes. Early diagnosis of skin infections enables health practitioners to implement effective therapeutic interventions, control infection transmission, and avert morbidity resulting from undiagnosed disease. For instance, certain infections, if left undiagnosed, can lead to serious systemic illness, thereby escalating morbidity in high-risk groups of children. Further, early reporting encourages effective surveillance, facilitating the identification of outbreaks of patterns and control action. Awareness of infectious skin disease symptoms and signs by caregivers is significant in enabling timely consultation with medical practitioners, as implicated in the association between rapid clinical assessment and successful recovery among children affected by such diseases. In this light, integration of prophylactic detection mechanisms is hence paramount in reducing the impacts of pediatric infectious skin diseases.

### 6.4.8. Collaboration with Public Health Agencies

Effective collaboration with public health agencies is crucial when it comes to managing pediatric infectious skin diseases, as they play a major role in disease surveillance, outbreak control, and educating the community. Public health agencies can implement immunization programs and provide guidelines to clinicians to enable them to implement early diagnosis and treatment of various skin infections among children using their facilities.

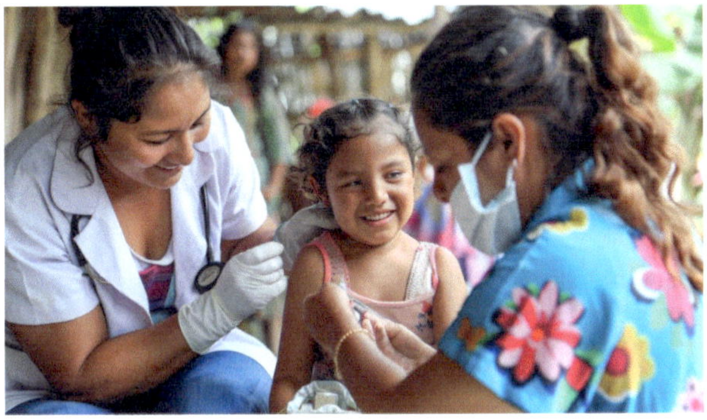

**Figure 6.18.** A young girl smiles while receiving a vaccination from a healthcare worker, with another provider offering reassurance, highlighting the role of public health outreach in community-based pediatric care.

*Source:* https://www.imagetrend.com/wp-content/uploads/2025/02/ems-public-health.jpg.

Apart from that, the cooperation can facilitate research efforts with the goal of understanding the epidemiology of such conditions so that children at the highest risk can be treated prophylactically. Efforts such as integrated surveillance and response systems, highlighted in public health emergency readiness research (Laura et al., 2004), are of crucial significance in outbreak control of infectious dermatological conditions. Moreover, the development in diagnostic technologies and availability is reflected in the importance of partnerships focusing on innovative solutions for weak populations, like children (Hesseling et al., 2011) (Figure 6.18).

### 6.4.9. Future Directions in Prevention Research

As the pediatric infectious skin illnesses evolve, the planning for the future in the area of prevention must be driven by an interdisciplinary approach, harmonizing epidemiological data with clinical insights. A case in point is new allergy trends, such as peanut allergy, where early intervention can prevent long-term health consequences compared to the previously used avoidance measures and suggests the necessity for adaptive models of preventive medicine (Kusari et al., 2018). Secondly, heightened sensitivity to such conditions as tuberculosis among kids raises the imperative of specialist research designed for specifically pediatric groups, ones that have in the past been under-represented in medical investigations (Seddon et al., 2014). Emphasizing holistic-program prevention involving schooling, early intervention, and community engagement will be instrumental in reducing infectious cutaneous diseases prevalence and severity in kids. By creating such collaborative strategies, future studies can significantly enhance healthcare outcomes for high-risk youth populations, ultimately informing public health policy and practice.

## Test Your Knowledge

1. How can proper hygiene practices help reduce the transmission of skin diseases?
2. In what ways do socioeconomic factors influence the prevalence of skin diseases, and how can collaboration with public health agencies help?

## SUMMARY

Lastly, pediatric infectious skin diseases are a significant public health challenge that must be prevented and managed using an integrated strategy. It is critical to understand the epidemiology and transmission patterns of such diseases, particularly in vulnerable populations such as refugees and children from high-prevalence areas, as highlighted in various studies, including those documenting trends in tuberculosis among immigrants (Lamb et al., 2019). Moreover, the novel evidence proposed for the role of early nutrition intervention in preventing related allergic responses, though largely confined to food allergies, puts forward the importance of adaptive actions in managing the health of children (Kusari et al., 2018). With the changing dynamics of infectious disease ecology, healthcare providers must remain vigilant and aware of newly evolving pathogens as well as changing patterns of disease prevalence. An intersectoral approach with early screening, appropriate treatment, and community education is critical in curbing the effects of these diseases on children's health and quality of life.

With pediatric infectious skin diseases, certain key aspects are noted that emphasize the complexity of diagnosis and treatment. Of interest is the range of pathogens responsible for the diseases, ranging from bacterial pathogens such as impetigo to viral infections such as molluscum contagiosum, and the importance of identification to provide optimal management. Furthermore, the consequences of pediatric antibiotic clinical trials are vast, with challenges in conducting such trials likely to lead to less-than-optimal dosage recommendations and greater risks of antibiotic resistance (Folgori et al., 2019). The accessibility of medical centers further makes disease control challenging, particularly in underprivileged communities, where delayed diagnosis aggravates the spread of diseases like scabies and eczema herpeticum (Leining et al., 2019). Therefore, enhancing the availability of health care and carers' knowledge are essential components in the prevention and control of the mentioned infectious skin diseases among children. The combined strategy might eventually improve the health status of this risk group.

## KEY TERMS FROM THIS CHAPTER

- Accurate diagnosis
- Bacteria
- Chickenpox
- Computed tomography (CT)
- Etiology
- Herpes simplex virus (HSV)
- Magnetic resonance imaging (MRI)
- Point-of-care ultrasound (POCUS)
- Antimicrobial stewardship programs (ASPs)
- Central nervous system (CNS)
- Complex landscape
- Diagnostic accuracy
- Fungi
- Infections
- Pathogens
- Potential misdiagnosis

## CRITICAL THINKING QUESTIONS

**1. The most common bacterial cause of impetigo in children is:**

a. Streptococcus pneumoniae

b. *Staphylococcus aureus*

c. Escherichia coli

d. Pseudomonas aeruginosa

**2. The characteristic lesion of impetigo is:**

a. Vesicles with black crusts

b. Erythematous papules

c. Honey-colored crusts

d. Bullae with white scales

**3. Scabies in children is caused by:**

a. Virus

b. Fungus

c. Bacteria

d. Mite

**4. The most common site for scabies lesions in infants is:**

a. Face

b. Palms and soles

c. Abdomen

d. Scalp

**5. Tinea capitis is caused by:**

a. Bacteria

b. Protozoa

c. Dermatophyte fungi

d. Virus

### *Short Answer Questions*

1. Define impetigo. What are its common causative organisms?
2. What is the difference between non-bullous and bullous impetigo?
3. Discuss the role of hygiene in preventing pediatric skin infections.
4. Describe the etiology, clinical features, diagnosis, and management of impetigo in children.
5. Explain the diagnosis and treatment of pediatric scabies. Include public health measures to prevent reinfection.
6. Discuss fungal infections of the skin in children. Include types, causative organisms, and management.

### *Answers to Critical Thinking Questions*

1. (b) 2. (c) 3. (d) 4. (b) 5. (c)

## REFERENCES


1. Ardeleanu, V., Constantin, V. D., Radaschin, D. S., Stana, P., & Tatu, A. L. (2020). *Laser Therapy in Superficial Morphea Lesions–Indications, Limitations and Therapeutic Alternatives.* ValpoScholar. https://core.ac.uk/download/304672910.pdf (accessed on 16th June 2025).
2. Bates, M., Kapata, N., Mwaba, P., O'Grady, J., & Zumla, A. (2011). *Tuberculosis in Prisons in Sub-Saharan Africa–A Potential Time Bomb.* https://core.ac.uk/download/19085580.pdf (accessed on 16th June 2025).
3. Bertram, Christie, "Evaluating Prescriber Adherence to Guideline-Based Treatment Pathways of a Newly Initiated Antimicrobial Stewardship Program at a Rehabilitation Hospital" (2017). *Undergraduate Honors Thesis Collection.* 379. https://digitalcommons.butler.edu/ugtheses/379(accessed on 16th June 2025).
4. Brador, G. M. (2019). *Long-Term Outcomes of Neonatal Herpes Simplex Virus Infection and Treatment. Information Bulletin on Variable Stars (IBVS).* https://core.ac.uk/download/287295206.pdf (accessed on 16th June 2025).
5. Burgess, J., Eisen, D., Lynch, D. P., Nordlund, J. J., Stafford, G. L., Villa, A., & Wells, M. J. (2017). *Oral Examination.* e-Publications@Marquette. https://core.ac.uk/download/213072873.pdf (accessed on 16th June 2025).
6. Mistry, R. D., Newland, J. G., Gerber, J. S., Hersh, A. L., May, L., Perman, S. M., Kuppermann, N., & Dayan, P. S. (2017). Current State of Antimicrobial Stewardship in Children's Hospital Emergency Departments. *Infection control and hospital epidemiology, 38*(4), 469–475. https://doi.org/10.1017/ice.2017.3(accessed on 16th June 2025).
7. Derinkuyu, B. E., Polat, M., Tapısız, A., & Tezer, H. (2018). *A Rare Case of Clostridium Difficile Infection-Associated Reactive Arthritis.* Bilimsel Tip Publishing House. https://core.ac.uk/download/227075472.pdf (accessed on 16th June 2025).
8. Kusari, A., Han, A., & Eichenfield, L. (2018). Recent advances in understanding and preventing peanut and tree nut hypersensitivity. *F1000Research, 7*, F1000 Faculty Rev-1716. https://doi.org/10.12688/f1000research.14450.1(accessed on 16th June 2025).
9. Folgori, L., Lutsar, I., Standing, J. F., Walker, A. S., Roilides, E., Zaoutis, T. E., Jafri, H., Giaquinto, C., Turner, M. A., & Sharland, M. (2019). Standardising neonatal and paediatric antibiotic clinical trial design and conduct: the PENTA-ID network view. *BMJ open, 9*(12), e032592. https://doi.org/10.1136/bmjopen-2019-032592 (accessed on 16th June 2025).
10. James, M. A., Manske, M. C. B., Rios Roque, J. J., & Zelaya, G. R. (2017). *Pediatric Hand Surgery Training in Nicaragua: A Sustainable Model of Surgical Education in A Resource-Poor Environment.* eScholarship, University of California. https://core.ac.uk/download/323069430.pdf (accessed on 16th June 2025).
11. Komba, E. V., & Mgonda, Y. M. (2010). The spectrum of dermatological disorders among primary school children in Dar es Salaam. *BMC public health, 10*, 765. https://doi.org/10.1186/1471-2458-10-765(accessed on 16th June 2025).
12. Larson, E. (2001). *Hygiene of the Skin: When is Clean Too Clean?* Centers for Disease Control. https://core.ac.uk/download/pdf/8251633.pdf (accessed on 16th June 2025).

13. Lau, S. K. P., Wong, S. S. Y., Yip, C. C. Y., & Yuen, K. Y. (2010). *Human Enterovirus 71 and Hand, Foot and Mouth Disease*. Cambridge University Press (CUP). https://core.ac.uk/download/37950461.pdf (accessed on 16th June 2025).

14. Markenson, D., & Redlener, I. E. (2006). *Bioterrorism*. Columbia University Libraries/Information Services. https://core.ac.uk/download/161442634.pdf (accessed on 16th June 2025).

15. Sena, T. (2019). *Managing Childhood Atopic Dermatitis: Utilizing A Written Eczema Action Plan to Improve Caregiver Self-Efficacy*. Digital USD. https://core.ac.uk/download/214384237.pdf (accessed on 16th June 2025).

16. Shehata, H., Naser, L. M., & Naser, M. (2022). *Neonatal Herpes Simplex Virus Infections: Diagnosis, Treatment, and Prevention*. Scholar AI LLC. https://core.ac.uk/download/596881966.pdf (accessed on 16th June 2025).

17. Slape, D., Thompson, R., & Westbury, S. (2021). Pediatrics: How to manage scabies. *BioExcel*. https://core.ac.uk/download/401541123.pdf (accessed on 16th June 2025).

# PEDIATRIC RESPIRATORY DISORDERS

# 7

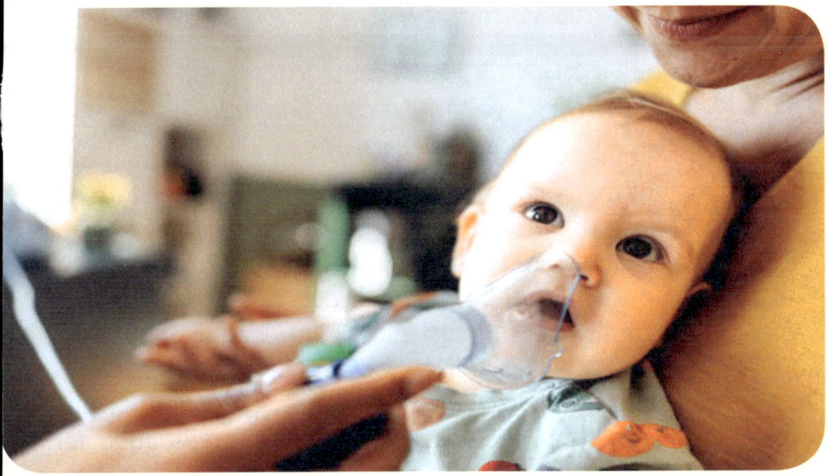

## LEARNING OBJECTIVES

**After studying this chapter, you will be able to:**

1. Discuss the anatomy and physiology of the pediatric respiratory system;
2. Explain the common pediatric respiratory disorders
3. Focus on assessment and diagnosis
4. Know nursing interventions and management;
5. Understand complications and challenges;
6. Focus on current research and advances in treatment

## Introduction

Pediatric respiratory illness is a very serious subject of concern, and therefore, the awareness of its diverse presentations and underlying pathophysiology is important. Respiratory illness encompasses asthma, bronchitis, pneumonia, and congenital anomalies of the airway. The unique anatomy and physiology of children, such as smaller airways and a more hyper-reactive immune system, account for the unique challenges posed by these illnesses. The intrinsic heterogeneity of the pediatric population mandates that healthcare providers adopt an integrative approach that attends not only to the acute clinical care but also to the broader implications on the development, growth, and quality of a child's life. Thus, an interdisciplinary team-based strategy involving nurses, physicians, and ancillary staff is essential to ensure effective management of these disorders and desirable outcomes for the patient. One of the most important aspects of pediatric respiratory disorder management is realizing the etiology and role of environmental and genetic factors responsible for their development. Research has also emphasized the increased prevalence of pediatric allergies and their relationship with respiratory disorders like asthma. It has been noted that immune-mediated hypersensitivity disorders in the pediatric population can be influenced by an array of risk factors such as genetic predisposition and environmental sensitization. It is important to understand these interconnections, as those who need to be careful in evaluating not just the respiratory symptoms that their young patients have, but also the possible underlying allergic elements that can exacerbate them.

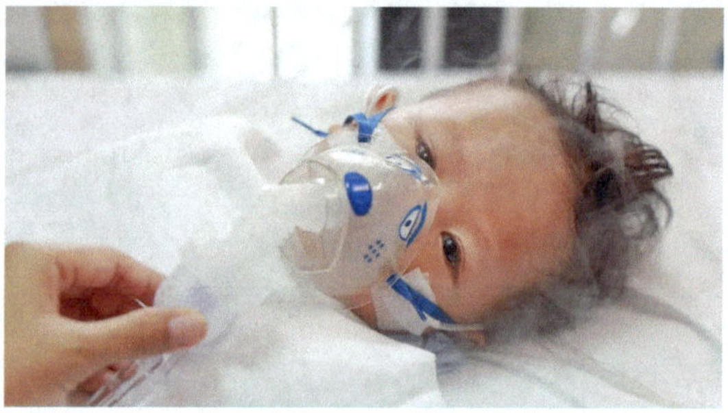

**Figure 7.1.** Pediatric respiratory disorders represent a significant area of concern.

*Source:* https://medicaldialogues.in/h-upload/2022/08/26/184318-acute-kidney-injury-in-childrenindian-academy-of-pediatric-guidelines-3.webp.

This overall vision helps the application of special interventions tackling both respiratory and allergic presentations, which ultimately helps in effective patient management. Apart from the clinical management, the application of alternative therapies has been a promising intervention in treating pediatric respiratory illnesses. Application of therapy such as pet therapy has gained recognition in the majority of pediatric hospitals, and studies have indicated positive attitudes towards their utilization among medical practitioners. This new paradigm is one of holistic care, which aims not only to treat the physical illness but also to address the emotional and psychological needs of respiratory-sick children. While early findings regarding pet therapy indicate favorable results, more research must be undertaken to determine its measures of effectiveness and inform best practice in childcare. Through incorporating such innovative methods with conventional treatments, they ultimately developed a more supportive environment for their children's patients and further improved overall health care (Figure 7.1).

## Definition and Significance of Pediatric Respiratory Disorders

Pediatric respiratory diseases are a collection of many conditions that impact the respiratory system of children and significantly impact their overall health as well as growth. Asthma, pneumonia, and bronchitis are a few of these conditions, among others, with manifestations of wheezing, coughing, and difficult breathing. They can have a multifactorial etiology, ranging from genetic predisposition to environment, such as allergens and toxins. Because the respiratory systems of children are still in development stages, even minimal respiratory abnormalities have dire implications on their physiological functioning and growth. Understanding the definition of such conditions is crucial since early detection and treatment can avoid complications and enhance patient outcomes. This understanding is the foundation on which successful nursing interventions within children's ward settings are crafted, highlighting the importance of comprehensive assessments and targeted interventions for affected children. The significance of pediatric respiratory illness extends beyond the acute aspects of illness, influencing long-term quality of life in affected individuals. Chronic respiratory illness is potentially linked to compromised physical functioning, social exclusion, and psychological morbidity in children. For instance, children with asthma not only experience physical symptoms of the illness but can also be limited in participation in sports or group activities. Besides, the prevalence of these conditions necessitates the creation of educational programs for both patients and healthcare providers aimed at fostering better management practices. By concentrating on holistic care that addresses the physical and psychosocial needs of children with respiratory illnesses, nurses can assist in defining outcomes related to health and quality of life. These practices finally reiterate the interdependence between respiratory health and overall pediatric health. Besides, pediatric respiratory disease nursing management has to consider the unique child growth and development patterns. Adult care strategies that prove effective will not necessarily translate to children due to anatomical, physiological, and psychological variations.

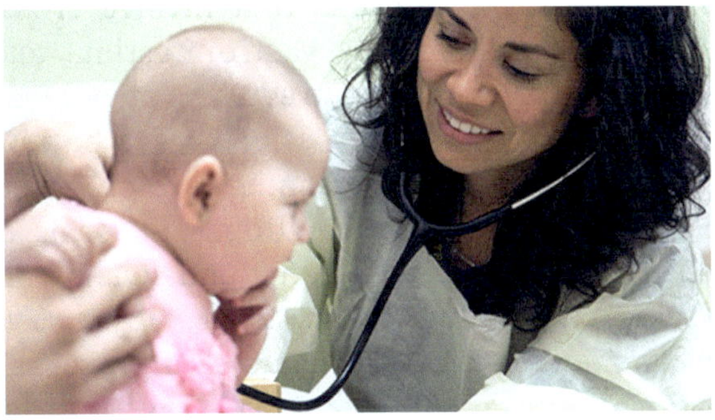

**Figure 7.2.** A pediatric healthcare provider uses a stethoscope to examine an infant during a checkup, reflecting attentive and compassionate clinical care.

*Source:* https://www.mottchildren.org/sites/default/files/styles/full_size_image/public/mottchildren%20-%20pulm%20overview%20spotlight%20graphic.png?itok=gkmr6Mt3.

As an example, interdisciplinary communication is vital in tailoring the nursing interventions to optimize pediatric patients' care. Innovations in nursing practice, including the use of age-appropriate communication and caregiver involvement in treatment regimens, are particularly successful in enhancing adherence to prescribed therapy. Research is also necessary in ongoing evaluation of pediatric respiratory disease and reframing current algorithms for selecting nursing-sensitive outcomes. Being sensitive to the complexities involved in managing such disorders, nursing professionals must be more careful and accommodating, being reminded that successful interventions can also precipitate improvements not only in the health status but also in the overall well-being of pediatric patients within medical-surgical settings (Clark et al., 2012; Doughty et al., 2014) (Figure 7.2).

## Overview of Common Respiratory Disorders in Children

Respiratory diseases in children consist of a range of conditions that can cause significant impacts on their well-being and health. Some of the most frequent disorders are asthma, bronchitis, pneumonia, and respiratory syncytial virus (RSV) infection. Asthma, with its airway inflammation and increased responsiveness, is particularly widespread among children and has a tendency to become apparent during early childhood. Environmental factors, such as air pollution and allergens, along with genetic predispositions, account for rising cases of asthma. Bronchitis, in the form of acute bronchitis, is usually a respiratory complication of viral infections characterized by cough and wheezing, while pneumonia, viral or bacterial in origin, has symptoms of fever and shortness of breath. Adequate diagnosis and early treatment are still critical because the effects of untreated respiratory illness can lead to chronic disease and frequent hospitalization in children. Because, as child health care providers, particularly, early detection of respiratory distress signs is critical to implement effective intervention processes. Breathlessness, chronic cough, and wheezing need appropriate assessment and observation to prevent potential complications. The application of equipment in diagnosis , such as chest X-rays and spirometry, allows doctors to differentiate among various respiratory conditions and develop appropriate interventions. For instance, with the exacerbation of asthma, bronchodilators and corticosteroids would be employed to alleviate symptoms, while in the management of bacterial pneumonia, antibiotics play a crucial role. Education about the management and prevention of exacerbations by families also plays an essential role in ensuring long-term health outcomes. Understanding the intricacies of each disorder informs clinical decision-making and ensures the quality of care provided to pediatric patients. Child respiratory disease management is a multidisciplinary team effort that not only treats the illness but also teaches and supports. Parents and caregivers are central to this intervention since they are typically the first to notice changes in the child's respiratory status. Teaching families to recognize symptoms and emergency procedures creates a support system for the child. Moreover, coordination with respiratory therapists can enhance the effectiveness of treatment with interventions , such as nebulizer therapy and pulmonary hygiene. Continuous education on the importance of vaccinations as a preventative treatment for respiratory infection also underscores the need for comprehensive care measures. Individually, these interventions have the effect of alleviating the impact of respiratory disease on children's daily existence, facilitating healthier futures and a diminished supply of hospitalizations among pediatric groups (Cimasi et al., 2011, 2015).

### Importance of Managing These Disorders

The is crucial in the overall care of pediatric respiratory disorders, particularly in managing complex conditions , such as congenital anomalies. Conditions , such as pectus excavatum, for instance, have direct consequences on a child's respiratory function and psychological status. Medical-surgical nurses play a crucial role not only in the preoperative evaluation and education but also in the postoperative care of these patients. They must provide empathetic care that addresses both the process of surgical recovery and the emotional challenge for children to acclimatize to their physical appearance and restriction of function. Studies reveal that nurses portraying true compassion and good communication are able to greatly optimize the patient experience and general recovery of pediatric patients who undergo corrective surgery for chest wall deformity (Donisthorpe et al., 2010). In addition, a balanced and correct knowledge of respiratory conditions in children is essential for nurses working in multidisciplinary teams for more complex aerodigestive issues. Incorporating nursing into aerodigestive programs is one way to demonstrate the benefits of multidisciplinary care, whereby conditions that involve cross-cutting issues involving gastrointestinal and respiratory systems are treated. Not only do medical-surgical nurses offer direct patient care, but also assist in planning care programs to address respiratory conditions in terms of the interplay between feeding and swallowing assessments (Acra et al., 2018). By active involvement in these systemic care processes, nurses facilitate fewer transitions across treatment phases, emphasizing the significance of their role in optimizing patient outcomes and promoting multidisciplinary intervention in managing pediatric respiratory diseases. Apart from that, the evolving nature of pediatrics and pediatric health also necessitates specialist care for pediatric respiratory disorders. As treatment mechanisms evolve and new treatment approaches become available, nurses must be responsive and keep their clinical competence current. Education and training are needed to equip nurses with the latest information on evidence-based interventions and, consequently, improve their patient care for complicated respiratory disorders. By adopting a culture of continuous learning, medical-surgical nurses are able to ensure that they are well-prepared to implement innovative care practices that effectively impact patient outcomes. Lastly, nursing's role is not just a matter of performing core care to become a critical component of the healthcare team in order to affirm that their experience is central to managing pediatric respiratory disorders effectively (Figure 7.3).

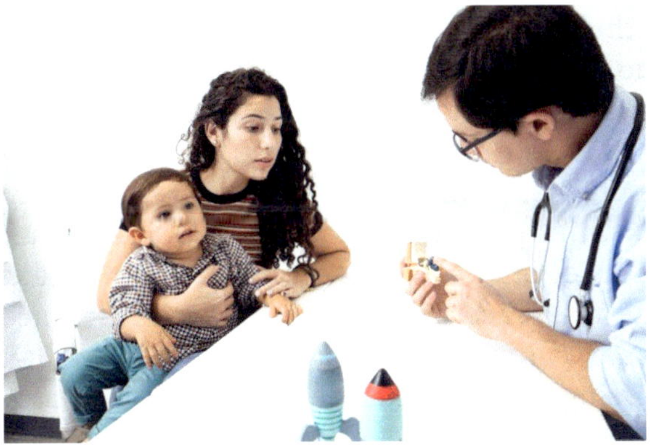

**Figure 7.3.** The role of is paramount in the comprehensive management of pediatric respiratory disorders.

*Source:* https://max-website20-images.s3.ap-south-1.amazonaws.com/Pediatric_Diseases_412272b958.jpg.

## 7.1. Anatomy and Physiology of the Pediatric Respiratory System

**Learning Outcome**

1. Differences between pediatric and adult respiratory systems;
2. Developmental changes in the respiratory system;
3. Impact of anatomy on disease presentation and management.

The anatomy and physiology of the child's respiratory system show striking differences with those of the adult, and it is important to understand these in order to appreciate respiratory disease in infants and children. The airway is of smaller diameter and shorter in infants and young children and therefore more susceptible to obstruction and trauma. The trachea is more compliant and positioned differently, contributing to airway collapse. The infants' lungs are proportionally smaller and contain fewer alveoli at birth, making them more prone to infection and secondary respiratory infection complications like asthma or bronchiolitis. These physical features necessitate specialized nursing interventions upon the treatment of pediatric respiratory diseases since the physiological reaction of the pediatric population to disease and treatment varies as the child matures and develops. An understanding of such considerations offers a foundation for competent assessment and management of respiratory illnesses within a medical-surgical practice. The physiological status of the child's respiratory system also identifies the child's nursing care complexities. Respiratory rates in neonates and infants are significantly higher than in children and adults, with infants recording 30 to 60 respirations per minute. This is accompanied by a low functional residual capacity and tidal volume, where even minor respiratory distress can lead to deoxygenation at high velocities. Furthermore, the incomplete respiratory musculature in infants under a given age limits their ability to optimize lung capacity effectively with increased respiratory effort. For this reason, pediatric nurses must be skilled at detecting early indications of respiratory distress and understanding the implications of the physiological differences of acute and chronic respiratory illness. Intervening at an extremely early period and adequate management techniques are required to avoid severe morbidity in this vulnerable group. Transition to adolescence involves major changes in the lung anatomy and physiology that affect nursing clinical care. In development, airways and lungs of children become stronger through the addition of more alveoli, thereby increasing gas exchange efficiency and the size of the lung. Endurance and strength of the respiratory muscles are also enhanced. However, this growth is not equivalent to immunity to respiratory illness because conditions , such as asthma will manifest in these stages of development. Therefore, one must take into consideration both the unique anatomy of pediatric patients and the evolving nature of their respiratory status. This in-depth knowledge is imperative for nurses to provide individualized teaching and care, preparing families adequately to address chronic conditions and encourage the general respiratory well-being of teenagers as they enter adulthood (Figure 7.4).

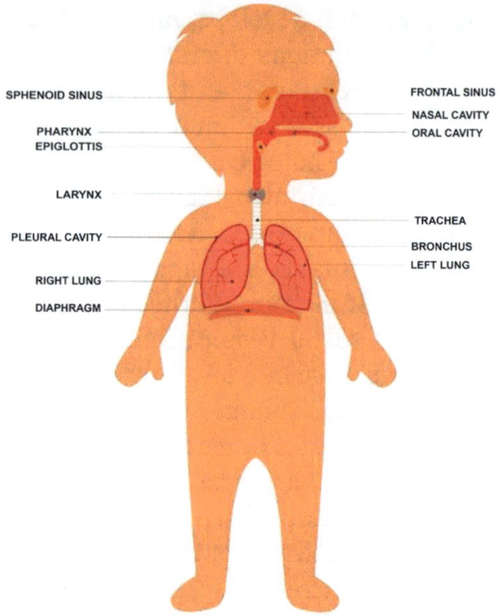


**Figure 7.4.** Anatomy and physiology of the pediatric respiratory system.

*Source:* https://external-content.duckduckgo.com/iu/?u=https%3A%2F%2Fceufast.com%2Fimgs%2Fimage-1--pediatric-respiratory-tract_800px.jpg&f=1&nofb=1&ipt=7460b22d68762332da8f04683d7fd7ea0a1e547ea7e7035705b5ef634b024e0a.

## 7.1.1. Differences Between Pediatric and Adult Respiratory Systems

The intrinsic differences between the respiratory systems of children and adults are vital in the comprehension of respiratory disease in children. Pediatric patients possess anatomically and physiologically distinct features that influence their respiratory status. For instance, children have narrower airways, implying that there is a higher potential for obstruction and higher resistance to breathing. Also, their compliance of the lungs is very different from that of adults due to the nature of the chest walls in children being less rigid and the respiratory muscles not as well developed. This situation calls for careful assessment and tailored treatments for the child patient since their response to lung disease can be quite divergent from adults. The relevance of these anatomical differences underscores the importance of special pediatric nursing training, as neglecting to consider these differences can lead to suboptimal patient outcomes and increased rates of morbidity in this vulnerable population. In the presence of respiratory disease, pediatric patients exhibit distinctive clinical presentations that may widely differ from those seen in adults. These conditions, , such as asthma, bronchiolitis, and pneumonia, have typical presentations that are anatomically and functionally specific to each of them. For instance, children with bronchiolitis have wheezing secondary to airway obstruction, compared to adults who may have a myriad of respiratory distress presentations. Diagnosis of these presentations is also further complicated by developmental variation because children cannot properly explain their symptoms; thus, precise physical examination becomes paramount. Appreciation of these distinctions in pediatric versus adult presentation nuances is essential for acute care nurses to guide treatment decision-making and monitor for unanticipated presentations that can presage rapid progression to critical status, with direct impact on clinical decision-making in pediatric nursing practice. As pediatric emergency department visits keep growing, the necessity for continued education of nursing professionals cannot be overstated. The Institute of Medicine (IOM) has also highlighted the need for improved protocols and facilities to allow health care practitioners to effectively deal with child respiratory ailments (Houten et al., 2018). Development in nursing curricula takes an essential part in equipping health care practitioners with the understanding of not just the physiological discrepancies but also the best practice guidelines for treating children. Extensive training modules could be employed to enhance knowledge of specific respiratory conditions prevalent among the pediatric age group, say, respiratory syncytial virus and croup. With a concentration on disease-specific assessments, intervention strategies, and case study evaluations in educational models, nurses are able to develop a more sensitive health environment that not only detects but competently handles the unique challenges posed by pediatric respiratory complications (Houten et al., 2018).

### 7.1.2. Developmental Changes in the Respiratory System

The alterations of the respiratory system during development in childhood are fundamental in pediatric respiratory illness. The respiratory system at birth needs significant alterations as the newborn transitions from intrauterine to extrauterine life. Neonates have a comparatively higher respiratory rate of 40–60 breaths per minute, which decreases with age. The structural maturation of the respiratory system involves alveolar development, with approximately 300 million alveoli formed by late childhood. This increase in surface area helps in efficient gas exchange, providing oxygen to meet the metabolic demands. In addition, the chest wall becomes more compliant to facilitate greater lung expansion and pulmonary mechanics. It is crucial to know these developmental milestones since variations can predispose children to respiratory illnesses and render health practitioners attuned to the fine needs of developing lung environments. Aside from the development of structures, physiological changes of the respiratory system have huge implications on child health. While growing up, children also experience changes in the volumes and capacities of the lungs, , such as increased tidal volume and functional residual capacity, to render respiration more effective. However, certain pediatric populations will have impaired respiratory function as a result of chronic medical illness. As a matter of illustration, the risk of aspiration exists in those with feeding and swallowing difficulties (FSD), and this adversely impairs their respiratory status and increases the rate of lower respiratory tract infections (LRTI).

These observations emphasize the importance of interdisciplinary collaboration in the management of children, particularly with the multifactorial etiology of respiratory diseases. Recognition of how developmental changes impact respiratory function forms the foundation for effective prevention and intervention planning to yield optimal outcomes for children (Oosthuizen, 2012). Furthermore, interactions between developmental changes and extrinsic events significantly enhance pediatric respiratory health. Environmental stimuli , such as allergens, air pollution, and infections are of particular relevance during lung developmental critical periods. For instance, kids exposed to secondhand smoke are likely to develop respiratory complications like bronchitis and asthma as their respiratory system continues to develop. The vulnerability of the pediatric group to these diseases is enhanced by the anatomical properties of narrower airways and a higher metabolic rate. For this reason, health workers must be very attentive to these risks when taking preventive measures. These systems understanding supports individualized nursing care that addresses both developmental milestones and environmental influences, ultimately promoting child respiratory health and enhancing the quality of medical-surgical care (Gleasner et al., 2019) (Figure 7.5).

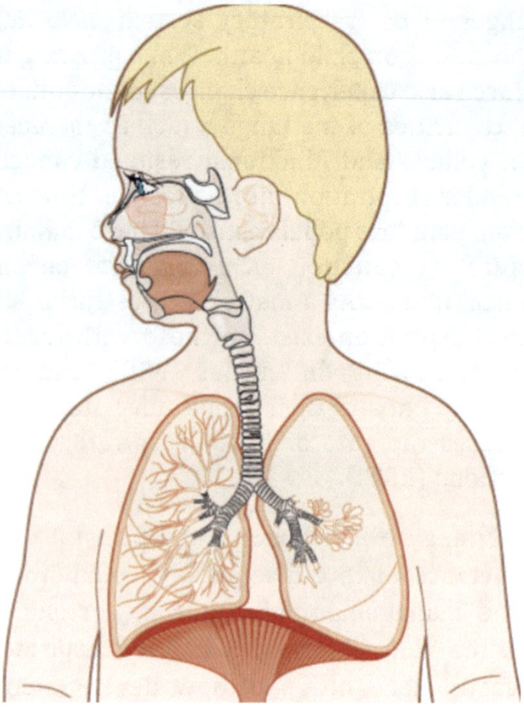

**Figure 7.5.** Developmental changes in the respiratory system.

*Source:* https://dm3omg1n1n7zx.cloudfront.net/rcni/static/journals/ncyp/aop/ncyp.2020.e1246/graphic/ncyp.2020.e1246_0001.jpg.

## 7.1.3. Impact of Anatomy on Disease Presentation and Management

Anatomical variation between children and adults has relevant implications on the presentation and treatment of respiratory disease. The pediatric airway is shorter in configuration, and the tracheobronchial tree is more compliant, making them susceptible to obstruction of the airway when there is inflammation or secretions. Anatomical structures , such as these can lead to a rapid increase in clinical deterioration, and thus early identification of signs and symptoms of respiratory distress by healthcare workers is paramount. For instance, infections like croup and bronchiolitis manifest differently from their counterparts in adults, in a way that typically makes it challenging to both diagnose and treat such infections. Therefore, the understanding of these anatomical differences is important, particularly while conducting respiratory-related examination on pediatric patients and initiating the right interventions. Treatment of respiratory disease among pediatric patients is also complicated by the developmental anatomy of the patients, which changes with growth. Younger kids also have higher metabolic and respiratory demands, hence needing more specialized therapy techniques than adults. One of the illustrations is nebulizer and inhaler administration, which is challenging as the right technique is needed, and younger children might not acquire it. Secondly, the immature pulmonary physiology of young children can lead to complications , such as respiratory distress syndrome, which needs special measures. The outcomes of these anatomical and physiological differences highlight the necessity for tailored treatment techniques that allow for effective respiratory function with the minimum risk of developing from lack of proper management in this vulnerable group. Further, the anatomical features of the pediatric breathing apparatus determine the education and training. With the ongoing development of specialized care units like neonatal/pediatric intensive care units (PICUs), nurses must acquire enhanced knowledge of the anatomical and physiological basis of disease processes in children. Advanced practice registered nurses (APRNs) starting work in such high-acuity settings often have difficulty due to their relative inexperience with critically ill children, thus affecting their respect for the anatomy in disease presentation and treatment (Callahan et al., 2019). Therefore, pediatrics curricula that provide education on the unique anatomical considerations for pediatric respiratory disease are central to developing competent practitioners. Not only does this knowledge base enhance patient care, but it also enables healthcare practitioners to be capable of responding quickly to the evolving needs of pediatric patients.

## Test Your Knowledge

1. What are two key differences between the pediatric and adult respiratory systems that impact disease presentation?
2. How do developmental changes in the pediatric respiratory system affect the management of respiratory diseases?

# 7.2. Common Pediatric Respiratory Disorders

**Learning Outcome**

1. Asthma: Prevalence and pathophysiology;
2. Bronchiolitis: Causes and clinical features;
3. Pneumonia: Types and treatment approaches.

Pediatric respiratory diseases encompass a variety of diseases that significantly affect the respiratory health of children. Among the most common diagnoses are asthma, pneumonia, and bronchitis. Asthma is a chronic inflammatory disease of the airways that often affects children and is characterized by wheezing, shortness of breath, and chest tightness. The prevalence of asthma results from environmental and hereditary risks, including allergens and air pollution. Understanding asthma pathophysiology is crucial, as it informs treatment and patient education. Treatment not only corrects symptoms but also prevents exacerbations, and hence, early identification of symptoms in pediatric patients is also very important. Pneumonia, which is another significant pediatric respiratory infection, is caused by viral, bacterial, or fungal organisms, and there is resulting inflammation of the alveoli of the lungs. This infection is an important health risk, particularly in infants and toddlers due to the immature immune system in these children. They have the triad of symptoms of cough, fever, and respiratory distress, which can quickly be followed by acute respiratory failure. Treatment of pneumonia in children requires a thorough clinical assessment and diagnostic workup with chest X-rays and laboratory investigations to determine the etiologic agent. Treatment of effective involves the use of appropriate antibiotics or antiviral medications and monitoring of response to therapy.

Furthermore, education of families regarding prevention of pneumonia, , such as immunizations and correct hand washing, is essential to morbidity reduction for this illness. Bronchitis, or wheezing bronchitis, is another frequent illness in the child population and is frequently associated with viral respiratory illness. It is characterized by inflammation of the bronchial airways, which leads to a chronic cough that can be bothersome for both the child and caregivers.

Acute bronchitis resolves within weeks, but recurrent attacks may indicate an underlying chronic illness, which requires detailed evaluation by healthcare providers. Relief of symptoms is the nursing care in this case, with fluid, humid air, and bronchodilators if wheezing is present. Besides, educating parents about how they can prevent exposure to tobacco smoke and other irritants can be an important component in preventing and controlling bronchitis. Therefore, a holistic care approach is required in managing the health problems of children with these common pediatric respiratory diseases (Figure 7.6).

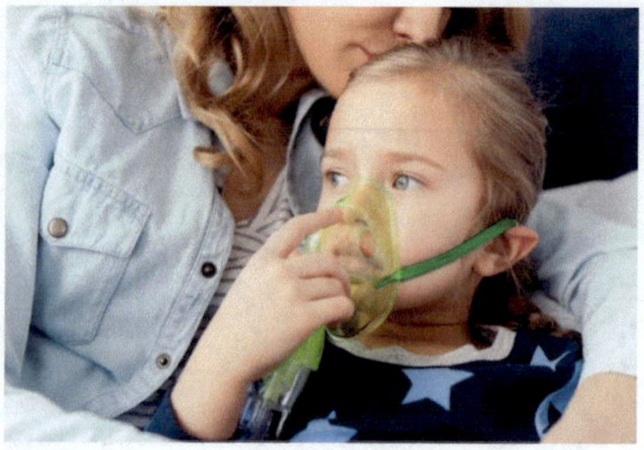

**Figure 7.6.** Common pediatric respiratory disorders.

*Source:* https://st3.depositphotos.com/13193658/35641/i/450/depositphotos_356419524-stock-photo-mother-kissing-asthmatic-daughter-respiratory.jpg.

## 7.2.1. Asthma: Prevalence and Pathophysiology

Asthma is a prevalent chronic respiratory illness, particularly in children, characterized by widespread inflammation and hyperresponsiveness of the airways. The Centers for Disease Control and Prevention estimates that asthma affects approximately 8% of children in the United States, and thus it is one of the most common chronic conditions in this population. An increase in the prevalence of asthma can be attributed to a spectrum of reasons that extend from environmental exposures to gene factors and urbanization. With increasing urbanization, children are increasingly being exposed to air pollution and allergens, which further exacerbate the condition. Socio-economic inequalities also contribute to prevalence rates in that children from lower socio-economic classes have increased rates of asthma due to increased exposure to environmental stimuli and fewer available resources with which to seek healthcare. The pathophysiology of asthma is multi-factorial and encompasses a continuum of immunologic and physiologic responses to a broad array of stimuli. The classic clinical manifestations of asthma are bronchial hyperreactivity, airway obstruction, and chronic airway inflammation that collectively cause the characteristic wheezing and dyspnea. In children, this inflammatory process is usually magnified, with a higher likelihood of airway remodeling if left untreated. The interactions between various immune cell types, including eosinophils, mast cells, and T lymphocytes, play an important role in the pathogenesis of the disease. An understanding of the mechanisms of inflammation and airway dysregulation will facilitate the development of effective targeted treatment and intervention strategies, thereby improving adequate control of the disease and patient outcomes in children. Asthma in children needs a multidisciplinary treatment strategy to include education and ongoing assessment.

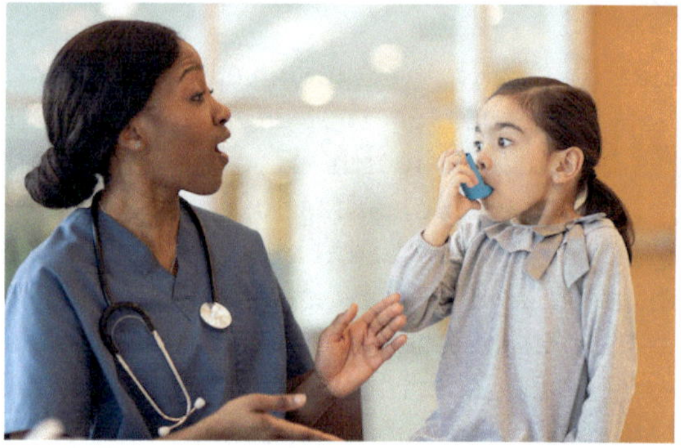

**Figure 7.7.** Pediatric asthma.

*Source:* https://s3-us-west-2.amazonaws.com/utsw-patientcare-web-production/original_images/pediatric_asthma_inhaler_600.jpg.

Pediatric practitioners and pediatric nurses play a significant role in facilitating this ongoing education by educating families about the nature of the disease, the precipitating causes, and how to manage it effectively. As acute respiratory ailments are amongst the most common complaints seen at the pediatric emergency department (Houten et al., 2018), early identification and intervention based on understanding this pathophysiology are crucial. Second, evidence-based asthma management protocols can significantly enhance clinical outcomes. This applies not only to pharmacologic measures , such as inhaled corticosteroids and bronchodilators, but also lifestyle modification and environmental control measures. The objective is to actively involve patients and caregivers in the management of asthma and therefore transform routine healthcare interactions into learning moments for education and counseling (Figure 7.7).

## 7.2.2. Bronchiolitis: Causes and Clinical Features

Bronchiolitis is a viral acute disease primarily seen in young children and infants and characterized by bronchiolar inflammation. The respiratory syncytial virus (RSV) is the key causative virus, although others , such as adenovirus and rhinovirus, contribute to its occurrence. It is most frequently observed between the ages of 2 and 6 months and mostly during winter, which usually coincides with the season of highest incidence of respiratory infections. Identification of the etiology of bronchiolitis is critical for nursing staff as early identification has extensive implications for management and treatment interventions, which are critical within a pediatric emergency environment. Immune naivety combined with the infant's narrow airway diameter makes it susceptible to the acquisition of severe respiratory distress, thereby making bronchiolitis the most predominant cause of hospitalization among children (Emergency Medical Services for Children, n.d.; Houten et al., 2018). Clinically, bronchiolitis presents with a wide range of features that are difficult to measure and intervene in from a nursing perspective. The initial clinical presentation is usually rhinorrhea, cough, and wheezing, progressively accompanied by rising respiratory effort and possible hypoxia. In the advancing disease process, clinical manifestations of tachypnea, retractions, and cyanosis may evolve and need immediate evaluation by medical personnel. The assessment process relies on intimate observation and monitoring of the vital signs, along with the utilization of such devices as pulse oximetry to assess oxygen saturation. These evaluations are critical not only for the follow-up of disease course but also for evidence-based decision-making regarding potential hospitalization or the need for interventions , such as bronchodilator therapy or supportive care interventions, underlining the importance of nursing education in the identification and management of these clinical traits effectively (Danioko, 2020).

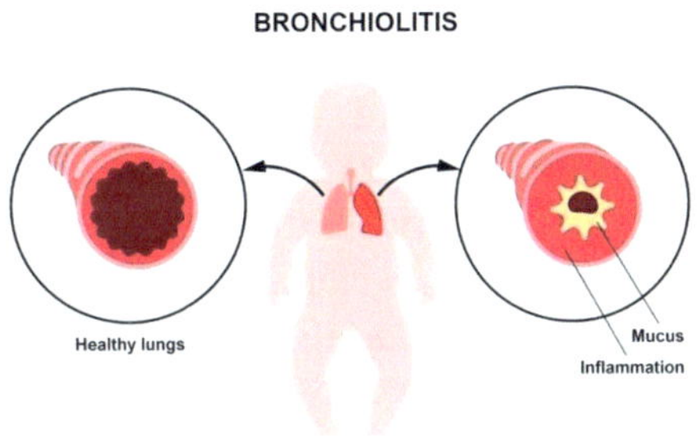


**Figure 7.8.** Pediatric bronchiolitis.

*Source:* https://stgaccinwbsdevlrs01.blob.core.windows.net/newcorporatewbsite/blogs/June2024/MlxlDGafTlifi62xRIRT.webp.

The management of bronchiolitis is supportive care primarily since there is no antiviral treatment for the etiologic viral infections. Nursing interventions play a key role in promoting optimal practices of care, , such as fluid hydration, administration of supplemental oxygen, and enhancement of airway clearance through suctioning. Monitoring of risk factors for severe bronchiolitis, , such as prematurity and underlying disease, is also helpful in designing individualized care plans for affected children. Literature highlights the significance of proper training of emergency department staff to value the nuances of respiratory conditions like bronchiolitis, which result in improved patient outcomes (Houten et al., 2018). With a general strategy that includes assessment, education, and management practices, nursing practitioners can effectively address the challenges posed by bronchiolitis in pediatric populations (Figure 7.8).

### 7.2.3. Pneumonia: Types and Treatment Approaches

Pneumonia in children is a significant concern, characterized by its variability of forms and therapeutic interventions. The most common forms of pneumonia include viral, bacterial, and aspiration pneumonia with their respective clinical dilemmas. Viral pneumonia, most commonly due to respiratory syncytial virus (RSV) or influenza, is more prevalent in young children and manifests in a wide array of symptoms from mild cough to severe respiratory compromise. Alternatively, bacterial pneumonia, commonly caused by *Streptococcus pneumoniae* or *Haemophilus influenzae*, tends to develop more abruptly and may need to be treated in-hospital for effective outcome. Pneumonia as a result of aspiration, commonly found among those with swallowing disorders, also tends to have increased risk since it can lead to further respiratory complications if treated late. Understanding the different types of pneumonia allows healthcare providers to tailor treatment modalities to the specific needs of children with respiratory disease. Effective management of pneumonia in the pediatric age group necessitates a multi-pronged approach that involves both pharmacologic and non-pharmacologic interventions. Antibiotic treatment remains the mainstay for bacterial pneumonia, and clinicians utilize guidelines to select appropriate drugs based on bacterial susceptibility patterns and patient age. With viral pneumonia, supportive care should be provided, , such as hydration, oxygen, and the use of bronchodilators if needed. The recent literature has also shown the relationship between feeding and swallowing difficulties (FSD) in children and lower respiratory tract infection, including pneumonia (Oosthuizen, 2012). Therefore, correcting the underlying FSD-related conditions may reduce incidence and patient outcomes overall. The addition of respiratory therapy, routine monitoring, and family education for preventive care further addresses the extent of nursing care in managing pneumonia within pediatric environments. Beyond the initial interventions, the long-term factors of pediatric pneumonia must also be considered, including recurrence risk and associated comorbidities. Children who repeatedly experience respiratory infections , such as pneumonia, will also have prolonged recovery time and can also experience complications , such as bronchiectasis or chronic respiratory illness. A nested mixed-effects logistic regression analysis showed that new respiratory diseases, including pneumonia itself, significantly correlated with repeated visits to the emergency departments (Danioko, 2020).

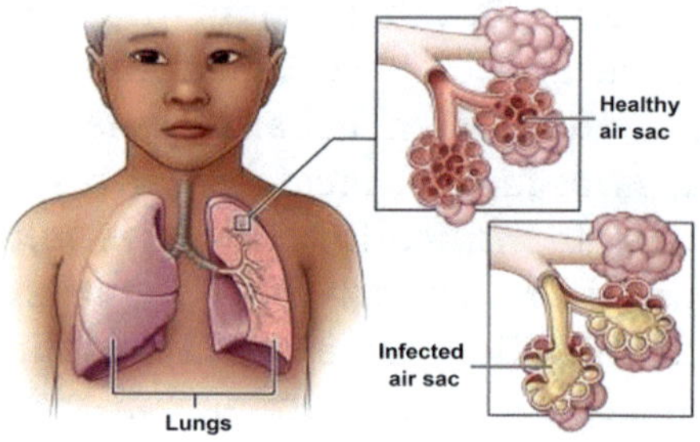


**Figure 7.9.** Pneumonia in children.

*Source:* https://content.ca.healthwise.net/resources/14.2/en-ca/media/medical/hw/acl1474_368x240.jpg.

This justifies the importance of thorough follow-up treatment and monitoring strategies. Regular assessment for underlying risk factors , such as age, nutritional status, and the presence of co-morbid medical conditions, can have a radical effect on clinical outcomes. With pediatric pneumonia management being of concern to medical providers, the emphasis on collaborative practice among interdisciplinary teams becomes key to maximizing health outcomes for affected children (Figure 7.9).

## Test Your Knowledge

1. What is the basic pathophysiology of asthma in children, and how common is it?
2. What are the typical causes and clinical features of bronchiolitis in infants, and how is pneumonia in children typically treated?

## 7.3. Assessment and Diagnosis

**Learning Outcome**

1. Clinical signs and symptoms of respiratory disorders;
2. Diagnostic tools and techniques used in pediatrics;
3. Importance of family history and environmental factors.

Diagnosis and assessment of pediatric respiratory illnesses is a critical component of the purview of. The right assessment begins with an adequate patient history where the clinicians evaluate the child's symptoms, onset, duration, and associated factors , such as environmental provocation. It is a highly critical initial step since pediatric patients will present uncharacteristic vague symptoms that can be misleading. A physical examination focusing on respiratory function, such as, , such as auscultation of lung sounds and measurement of respiratory rate, is then performed. Additionally, practitioners can utilize diagnostic tests , such as pulse oximetry and chest X-rays to assess the blood oxygen levels and determine if there is any anatomical derangement. Through a combination of these assessment techniques, practitioners are able to gain a complete idea of the patient's respiratory status and make early and effective interventions. Since pediatric respiratory diseases are multifaceted, clinical competence coupled with the incorporation of evidence-based guidelines establishes the precision of the diagnosis. As per existing literature, conventional algorithms utilized for identifying nursing-sensitive outcomes among adults cannot be used directly on children, and thus modifications should be incorporated to enhance the accuracy of the diagnosis (Clark et al., 2012). Understanding these changes is crucial as it not only improves the precision of respiratory assessment but also directs nursing intervention unique to this particular population. For instance, the pediatric age group may exhibit varying respiratory patterns or respond differently to stimuli when compared to adults and hence, prudent consideration must be taken at the time of diagnosis. Accuracy in pediatric nursing protocols, considering these factors, is hence crucial for proper patient management and optimal outcomes in respiratory care. In addition, the function of hospital records linked to each other has also become an important determinant in the improvement of diagnostic accuracy among pediatric patients. Through the use of detailed databases that cover a child's background medical history, treatment reactions, and nursing outcomes, clinicians can more effectively discriminate between disease conditions that are a direct function of care by a nurse versus those related to preceding morbidity (Danioko, 2020). This subtle perception facilitates refinement of assessment and increased nursing-sensitive outcome identification, thereby facilitating more individualized treatment regimens. Through this framework, continuous evaluation protocol assessment and redefinition during pediatric respiratory treatment are essential. This insistence serves to align interventions with the dynamic character of these disorders for higher-quality care in settings.

### 7.3.1. Clinical Signs and Symptoms of Respiratory Disorders

The presentation of pediatric patients with respiratory disease is varied and can have a significant effect on their overall health and well-being. The most frequent presentations are cough, wheeze, breathlessness, and chest retractions, which can be suggestive of the underlying existence of a condition , such as asthma, pneumonia, or bronchiolitis. Cough, for instance, is a reflex mechanism but can be suggestive of the existence of infection or inflammation of the airways. Wheezing, an expiratory high-pitched sound, is likely to be due to narrowing of the airways, a feature of disorders like asthma or infections like croup. Their explanation and significance are crucial to practitioners because they form the core of early diagnosis and management of respiratory disease, which eventually translates into improved patient outcomes and alleviation of distress (Houten et al., 2018). In addition to the more usual signs of manifestation, some of the more severe clinical symptoms in children must be treated urgently. They consist of cyanosis, as bluish coloration, typically on the lips and fingers, where there is inadequate oxygenation, and changes in mental status, which may be evidenced by irritability or somnolence in a child. The occurrence of respiratory distress can develop rapidly, and the occurrence of flaring of the nose and chest wall retractions indicate severe effort at respiration and typically require prompt action. This acute presentation is especially frequent in infants and children, who might have a lower physiological reserve than their older counterparts. Recognizing that such signs are expressions of serious health conditions is paramount for nurses who must assess and rank high-stakes care in the emergency department (Oosthuizen, 2012). Proper management of respiratory illnesses in children necessitates clear identification of signs and symptoms, leading to required intervention. The comprehensive evaluation consists of a detailed history and physical examination, augmented by pulse oximetry and auscultation to ascertain air movement in the lungs. Clinical response is often guided by standardized testing, , such as the Pediatric Respiratory Assessment Measure (PRAM), to offer an objective assessment of respiratory distress severity. A well-planned nursing curriculum with an emphasis on these assessment tools can propagate the competency of nursing staff in emergency situations, eventually resulting in improved patient care delivery. Frequent training on the insidious presentations of respiratory illnesses is essential, with the high endemic rates among pediatric patients, thus emphasizing the need for constant training and practice of evidence-based standards (Danioko, 2020) (Figure 7.10).

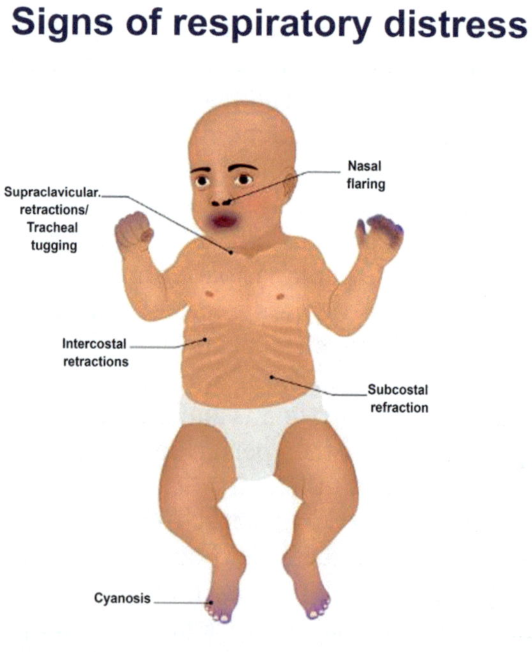


**Figure 7.10.** Clinical signs and symptoms of respiratory disorders.

*Source:* https://media.springernature.com/lw685/springer-static/image/chp%3A10.1007%2F978-3-030-63560-2_10/MediaObjects/496124_1_En_10_Fig7_HTML.png.

### 7.3.2. Diagnostic Tools and Techniques Used in Pediatrics

Pediatric respiratory disorders need the utilization of different diagnostic equipment and strategies for their management, which include careful evaluation and monitoring. Some of the most important diagnostic equipment includes the pulse oximeter, which measures the percentage of oxygen saturation in the blood without any invasive procedure. This device is most effective when used in the evaluation of children presenting with symptoms of respiratory distress and allows the healthcare provider to make a rapid determination if supplemental oxygen or intervention is necessary. Spirometry is also effective as a measure of lung function, especially where there is suspicion of chronic respiratory disease , such as asthma. Such techniques collectively enhance the clinician's ability to determine the severity of the condition and provide interventions applicable to an individual child's own needs, ultimately realizing improved health outcomes in pediatric patients with respiratory conditions. Diagnostic imaging is also crucial for the assessment of pediatric respiratory conditions. Chest X-rays are used to image thoracic cavity structures in most cases, allowing one to determine such conditions as pneumonia or congenital malformations. Where a more detailed imaging is required, computed tomography (CT) scanning provides improved visualization of lung morphology, some of which is useful in diagnosing complicated conditions like bronchiectasis or interstitial lung disease. Furthermore, ultrasound can be applied for the diagnosis of pleural effusions or guiding needle aspiration in empyema. The combination of these imaging modalities allows for the clear understanding of the associated pathologies, facilitating healthcare professionals to plan effective treatment regimens for their pediatric patients with respiratory issues. Besides physical examinations and imaging techniques, laboratory tests have a significant role in diagnostic practice in pediatric respiratory diseases. Blood tests can provide vital information on infection or inflammation, with elevated white blood cell counts indicative of possible bacterial infection or virus presence. Sputum analysis also has the capability of identifying specific pathogens responsible for respiratory disease to guide particular antimicrobial therapy. Understanding fully the child's health history, , such as previous environmental exposures and previous respiratory infections, can render such findings more understandable. The strategic use of these diagnostic techniques ensures that pediatric healthcare providers are able to diagnose and efficiently treat respiratory diseases accurately, thus attaining enhanced health outcomes among children within the context (Gleasner et al., 2019).

### 7.3.3. Importance of Family History and Environmental Factors

It is critical to appreciate the influence of family history and environment in the assessment and management of pediatric respiratory disease. Family history may yield critical information about genetic susceptibility potentially affecting respiratory diseases. For instance, familial patterns of asthma, allergic rhinitis, or cystic fibrosis can point to inherited traits that predispose a child's risk of respiratory disease. The early identification of these patterns enables the treating physician to implement preventative strategies according to the child's specific risks. Further, identification of the family history allows for more insight into the patient's history, and this is extremely relevant when creating an extensive care plan in the case of. The incorporation of family history in practice not only enhances diagnostic accuracy but also facilitates conversation between health caregivers and families about potential future health concerns. Environmental influences are just as important in causation and precipitation of respiratory conditions in children. Contact with allergens, pollutants, and other environmental stressors generally has a profound impact on respiratory well-being. As an illustration, children residing in urban communities are often exposed to increased levels of air pollution that have been correlated with increased instances of asthma and other respiratory conditions. Moreover, indoor environments, like homes with mold, cigarette smoke, or inadequate ventilation, contribute significantly toward triggering respiratory distress. Such exposures have the ability to strengthen or weaken the influence of genetic predispositions in family histories. Through the focus on both environmental and family determinants, nursing practice can adopt a more holistic approach, acknowledging modifiable risks that may mitigate the onset or severity of respiratory illnesses in children.

The addition of an ecological perspective allows for exploration of how family history and environmental concerns dynamically interact within the population of children. An understanding of these intricate interactions may inform the development of intervention strategies specific to reducing risk factors and increasing better respiratory health outcomes. By considering not only the genetic component but also the external environment, nurses are able to perform more holistic assessment and action planning that encompasses stressors that the child might have undergone during transitions in critical care, based on existing literature on medical trauma (Hanson et al., 2022). Such a multi-disciplinary practice not only facilitates clinical decision-making at the point of care but also facilitates public health efforts towards environmental interventions. Focus on family history and environmental investigations can thus be instrumental in novel approaches to the management of respiratory disease among children, ultimately contributing to improved quality of care and patient resilience across healthcare settings (Figure 7.11).

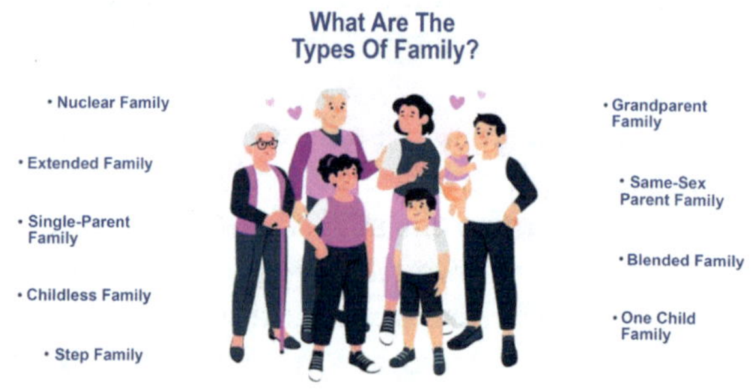


**Figure 7.11.** Importance of family history and environmental factors.

*Source:* https://ik.imagekit.io/parenting/wp-content/uploads/family-types-1024x524.jpg.

## Test Your Knowledge

1. What are common clinical signs and symptoms of respiratory disorders in children, and which diagnostic tools are commonly used?
2. Why are family history and environmental factors important in diagnosing pediatric respiratory conditions?

## 7.4. Nursing Interventions and Management

**Learning Outcome**

1. Role of nursing in acute and chronic management;
2. Medication administration and monitoring;
3. Education and support for families.

Proper intervention and management by nurses are crucial components in pediatric patients with respiratory disease. Children present unique challenges due to their anatomical and physiological differences. Monitoring of the respiratory status constantly, adequate oxygenation, and implementation of the right intervention based on the child's individual condition, whether asthma, pneumonia, or bronchiolitis, are some of the interventions. Along with this, children and their families are provided with important education for disease management. Education in the proper use of inhalers, early detection of signs of respiratory distress, and promotion of adherence to prescribed therapies are important aspects that need to be covered by clinicians. These interventions, as a nursing intervention, not only aim towards relief from acute symptoms, but also enhance long-term health care modalities that empower families for long-term care (Oosthuizen, 2012). In addition to direct patient care, management of nursing involves comprehensive assessment and interaction with the health team. Comprehensive understanding of the patient's past medical history, present symptoms, and response to prior interventions informs clinical decision making. Regular interdisciplinary conferences support this process through a coordinated treatment plan and unified homogeneity among team members. In addition, patients must have their safety advocated for by the nurses through the implementation of evidence-based practice, with strong emphasis on precise drug use and continuous monitoring for side effects (Allison et al., 2018). Standard protocols and the application of checklists can greatly reduce chances of avoidable errors and thus maintain patient safety paramount while handling complex respiratory conditions. Moreover, incorporation of an atmosphere of support, both physical and emotional, is crucial in children patients suffering from respiratory distress. The development of a soothing environment plays a significant role in a child's ability to cope with his or her condition.

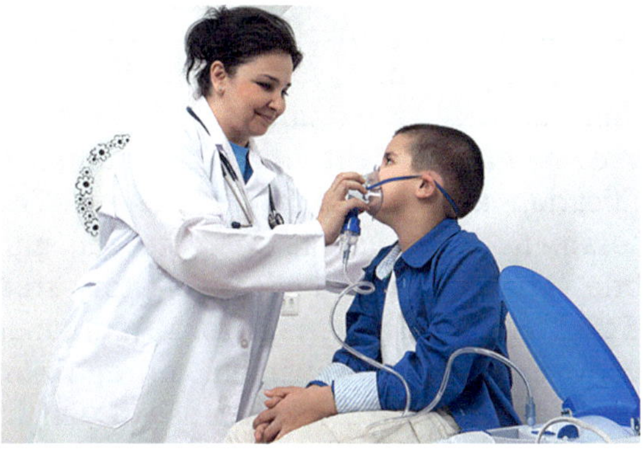

**Figure 7.12.** Nursing interventions and management.

*Source:* https://external-content.duckduckgo.com/iu/?u=http%3A%2F%2Fmy.clevelandclinic.org%2F-%2Fscassets%2Fimages%2Forg%2Fpediatrics%2Fdepartments%2Frespiratory-services.ashx&f=1&nofb=1&ipt=02b3d566c3c0932c1068d8959ebb991f41038da0832a6b09e6e9ea04aed819bf.

Providing a serene environment with required equipment and making sure parents or caregivers are involved in the care process is an illustration. Successful pain management and addressing psychological requirements are also essential factors frequently overlooked in the clinical setting. Once nurses understand the full needs of children, they can create holistic care that encompasses more than just body symptomatology to address emotional and development aspects as well. In this manner, nursing interventions not only enhance clinical outcomes but also maximize patient satisfaction, reinforcing the central role of nursing in pediatric respiratory disorders (Starre et al., 2011) (Figure 7.12).

### 7.4.1. Role of Nursing in Acute and Chronic Management

Nursing within both acute and chronic care is critical in the case of pediatric respiratory disease. Nurses act as key members of the health team, providing essential care with direct outcomes affecting the patient. Within acute care, where problems , such as life-threatening asthma attacks or pneumonia endanger life, nurses monitor patient vital signs, administer medication, and control oxygen therapy. Their assessment skills enable them to recognize subtle variations in a child's respiratory status and thus trigger early interventions. Additionally, effective communication with doctors and family members is also crucial because it ensures continuity of care and treatment regimens. This is a three-dimensional role in that not only the provision of initial care is involved but also education to empower families to understand their child's state, ultimately yielding better health pathways. In a chronic management situation, nurses extend their roles to involve long-term health instruction and family support for families with chronic respiratory illnesses, like reactive airway disease or cystic fibrosis. Nurses provide families with tools that allow them to implement effective management strategies into their daily lives. For instance, they instruct caregivers on signs of exacerbation and the importance of adhering to prescribed medication regimens. Moreover, chronic care typically requires a multidisciplinary strategy; nurses collaborate with respiratory therapists, nutritionists, and social workers in order to have appropriate comprehensive care models. This integrated model is most applicable in treating chronic respiratory conditions, where mental status and socio-economic status play an important role in influencing adherence and general health outcomes. Nurses, thus, not only supplement the medical interventions but also enable families to make them active participants in healthcare for the child. The complexities of aspiration and its intrinsic dangers, as brought out in comparable research, also add to the need for experienced nursing interventions in pediatric respiratory care. For instance, aspiration of foreign bodies is a highly dangerous risk that needs meticulous assessment and intervention tailored to the individual child's needs (Abdulwahab et al., 2017). Nurses are usually the initial specialists to assess for risk factors , such as gastroesophageal reflux or dysphagia, which can significantly jeopardize respiratory status. Through preventive care and interventions, nurses are able to significantly reduce the incidence of aspiration and the associated complications. Identification of the role of nursing in such cases is imperative, not only highlighting the clinical expertise they are providing but also the significance of their contribution to education and research in ensuring higher standards of patient care (Allison et al., 2018). Through continued professional practice development and adherence to evidence-based care, nurses are most suited to enhance pediatric respiratory management.

### 7.4.2. Medication Administration and Monitoring

Proper observation and medication management are among critical factors entered into the care of a pediatric respiratory condition in an environment. Because of the complexities entered into the pharmacologic treatment of respiratory conditions, especially among children, compliance with established standards is inescapable. For instance, utilization of sedation assessment tools like the Pasero Opioid Sedation Scale (POSS) has been found to have a significant impact on patient safety profiles. Application of standardized testing before the dispensation of opioids can lower the risk of respiratory depression due to opioids, particularly in postoperative pediatric patients who are also more vulnerable to side effects by virtue of their just completed anesthesia and drug exposure (Elliott et al., 2023). Not only does this standardized practice allow for accurate dosing, but it also facilitates intervention early if there are any issues, thereby aiding overall improved care of this vulnerable subgroup. Post-administration monitoring of results is just as important in ensuring patient safety and therapeutic efficacy in pediatric respiratory therapy. The use of integrated safety management systems, , such as the Safety-First program used in some pediatric intensive care units, is an example of how organized monitoring can both identify would-be risks and improve results. Through diligent data collection and event analysis, health workers can develop knowledge about the events and numbers of adverse events, , such as medication errors or unplanned drug interactions (Starre et al., 2011). Such an initiative underscores the importance of continuous training and education of nurses to recognize and manage drug complications promptly. Lastly, the focus on medication monitoring promotes a culture of one-on-one, effective care to each child, tailored to their own unique medical condition. Integration of technology in drug administration is another important factor in determining whether safety and effectiveness are encouraged in pediatric nursing. Auditable electronic medical record (EMR) systems can act as valuable tools for ensuring compliance with guidelines like the POSS (Elliott et al., 2023). By tracking compliance rates and medication errors in real time, healthcare professionals are able to identify areas for improvement right away. This is particularly true in the pediatric patient population, where variation in metabolic rate and body chemistry can influence medications and their margin of safety. Utilization of robust monitoring systems not only improves clinical decision making but also encourages a culture of responsibility within nursing staff. Thus, constant improvements in technology and med tech procedures for giving and monitoring medication are still essential to optimize care results for children with respiratory disease so that nurse practice is not merely safe but also effective (Figure 7.13).

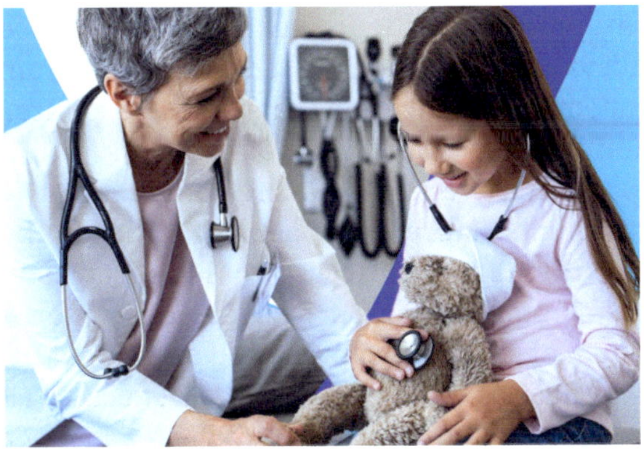

**Figure 7.13.** Medication administration and monitoring.

*Source:* https://www.performancehealthus.com/hubfs/medication%20errors%20in%20children.png.

### 7.4.3. Education and Support for Families

Education and family support are pivotal to the care of pediatric respiratory disorders in the environment. Families become the self-care providers and more often than not, the child's advocates, and an understanding of the seriousness of the child's condition can have a significant bearing on the success of the treatment. Thus, education that encompasses the nature of the disorder, the interventions offered, and their care over time is paramount. Such family members are better able to recognize signs of complications and function in healthcare systems better. Moreover, supportive interventions , such as counseling and access to resources enable the family's ability to cope with the issues of their child's illness, thereby promoting overall well-being for the child and the family as a whole. Integration of education programs into routine care for pediatric respiratory patients not only empowers families but also promotes mutual relationships between families and healthcare providers. Through the active involvement of families in treatment interventions and decision-making, clinicians have the opportunity to make interventions that are applicable to individual family processes and values. For instance, education programs that educate families on inhaler use, respiratory therapy, and lifestyle modification can be highly effective in improving compliance with treatments. Moreover, ensuring that families are provided with access to support groups and community-based services can create a system of collective support and commonalities. Consolidating the family's role as an educated ally is imperative in pediatric nursing, particularly in difficult cases that require ongoing revision of care processes, thus ensuring continuity and quality in the patients care process. Recognize the demand met by families in managing pediatric respiratory disease guides the creation of supportive interventions that directly address such needs. As health care organizations become proficient in addressing the demands of patient-centered care, the demand for customized, evidence-based educational approaches becomes increasingly evident. Health care workers must recognize families' informational and affective needs, taking approaches that are reassuring and informative amidst uncertainty. The evolving nature of pediatric care confirms the need for continuing education programs for nurses, , such as fellowship programs focused on specialized knowledge and family-centered practices. These programs can bridge theory and practice gaps to enhance a nurse's capacity to work with families in the high-acuity environment of pediatric respiratory care.

## Test Your Knowledge

1. What is the role of nursing in the acute and chronic management of pediatric respiratory disorders?
2. How do nurses ensure safe medication administration and support families in managing respiratory conditions at home?

## 7.5. Complications and Challenges

**Learning Outcome**

1. Potential complications of untreated respiratory disorders;
2. Challenges in pediatric patient compliance;
3. Socioeconomic factors affecting care and outcomes.

In pediatric respiratory disease, complications and challenges plague it to an extremely large degree, and healthcare professionals are requested to apply specialist knowledge and adapt interventions to their approach. One of the first of these complications is the accuracy of determining nursing-sensitive outcomes in pediatric patients. Research finds that algorithms for adult populations fail when applied to the younger group for the primary reason that they contain a very disparate casemix and risk profiles. Consequently, utilization of unlinked hospital records may give inaccurate estimates of rates of adverse events and consequently undermine the quality of care offered to this vulnerable patient group (Clark et al., 2012). With nurses striving to reduce the incidence of these complications, it can be seen that utilization of individualized assessment tools is imperative, reflecting the need for further research in the field of pediatric nursing practice. In addition, obesity in children has become an urgent issue associated with respiratory conditions, complicating. Obesity in children is caused by a number of comorbidities that make children susceptible to respiratory complications. For instance, obese and overweight children who undergo anesthesia most commonly are likely to experience higher risks due to airway management complication, resulting in perioperative respiratory complications. The anesthesia care team must evaluate these children thoroughly preoperatively and plan strategies for best management during and after surgery (Jacob et al., 2015). This explains the necessity of enhanced communication and teamwork among the caregivers to maximize care in the presence of the unique challenges imposed by pediatric obesity as well as respiratory disease.

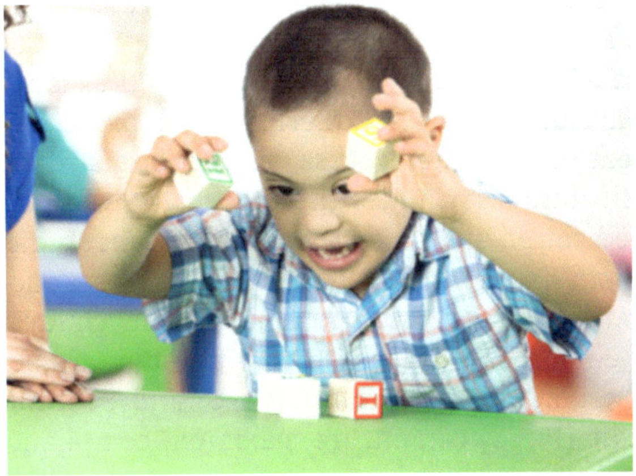

**Figure 7.14.** Supporting developmental growth through play-based learning.

*Source:* https://www.hope-amc.com/wp-content/uploads/fly-images/5337/Early-Intervention-1170x1000-c.png.

The multifactorial nature of pediatric respiratory disease also emphasizes the intensity of care required in an environment that is defined by such elements. In addition to the physiological complications, the psychological and emotional impact on the patients and their families also contributes to a heightened burden in the case of in-hospital stays. Fearful and anxious children with respiratory issues are likely to exacerbate the issue and complicate recovery. The psychological distress necessitates an integrative form of nursing care that includes counseling both the patient and the families (Clark et al., 2012). With these intricate dynamics, nurses need to be empowered not just with clinical data but also interpersonal abilities in order to maximize the therapeutic environment. Ultimately, only adherence to holistic care practices that aim to heal the body and heal the mind can tackle the intricacies and problems of pediatric respiratory diseases (Figure 7.14).

### 7.5.1. Potential Complications of Untreated Respiratory Disorders

Undiagnosed respiratory diseases in children may result in a wide range of possible complications, which could have serious effects not only on their physical well-being but also on their overall quality of life. As an example, long-term respiratory diseases like asthma or obstructive sleep apnea (OSA) might not only impair respiratory function but could also delay a child's growth and development. If not corrected, respiratory distress can cause recurrent hospital admissions, further increasing the child's anxiety and stress about medical environments. Chronic hypoxia due to undiagnosed respiratory disease is also responsible for cognitive dysfunction and developmental delay, which makes it challenging to predict long-term prognosis in these patients. Finally, it is essential that healthcare clinicians appreciate the risks of untreated respiratory conditions to intervene early and avoid potential complications and improved outcomes. In addition, untreated respiratory conditions can worsen underlying comorbidities, making the clinical presentation of a child even more complicated. Recurrent pneumonia or respiratory infection can occur, leading to prolonged courses of illness requiring complicated medical therapy, often meaning increased healthcare expenditures. Interestingly, aspects of respiratory dysfunction can affect a child's physical activity, which is integral to their total well-being and social function. Pain, as an often-overlooked symptom of respiratory distress, can have both negative physical consequences as well as cognitive consequences, i.e., anxiety and depression, in children. The use of both pharmacologic and nonpharmacologic therapy is critical in the prevention of such complications, as evidenced by current pain management and integrative treatment research (Swartzentruber, 2021). Moreover, the presence of conditions , such as unstaged obstructive sleep apnea has been linked with perioperative risks, illustrating the need for comprehensive preoperative assessments. For example, it has been noted that undiagnosed children with OSA have increased perioperative complications, highlighting the significance of the appropriate identification and management of the disorders. Involvement of organized referral programs for high-risk patients significantly enhances the prospects of accessing proper and timely interventions, as witnessed in recent studies on optimizing healthcare processes (Goforth & Roberts, 2018). By preemptively treating these respiratory ailments, healthcare practitioners not only enhance the immediate health status of juvenile patients but also remove potential long-term complications resulting from irreparable respiratory disorders. Prioritizing early treatment of respiratory ailments is thus of greatest importance, promoting an interdisciplinary approach integrating clinical and preventive care practices.

### 7.5.2. Challenges in Pediatric Patient Compliance

In pediatric nursing, patient compliance remains an enormous issue in managing respiratory disorders. Pediatric patients are unwilling or unable to adhere to medical directives as per their stage of development, and this is likely to confuse their illnesses and treatment protocols. For instance, younger children are unable even to articulate their symptoms or the need to keep their drug regimen as directed. This inadequate communication will result in under-management or inappropriate management of respiratory conditions, which will increase health issues. Also of significance is the contribution made by parents or guardians, whose beliefs, attitudes, and knowledge about medical treatment have a direct impact on a child's compliance. Interventions to educate families of the value of treatment compliance have the power to overcome the gap, creating an environment of support that allows pediatric patients to become active participants in their own care. Moreover, the physiological aspects of pediatric respiratory disease impose further complications on patient compliance. Most children with chronic respiratory diseases, , such as asthma, typically experience symptoms that are felt to be minor or transient and thus lack a sense of urgency in adhering to the prescribed treatment. In the process, parents or guardians will underestimate the necessity of daily medication and follow-up visits. Recent studies emphasize the importance of monitoring sedation and respiratory status, especially in children after surgery, where employing standardized instruments like the Pasero Opioid Sedation Scale (POSS) can ensure maximum compliance through structured assessment protocols (Elliott et al., 2023). By continuously monitoring these parameters, healthcare providers are not only in a position to monitor the efficacy of interventions but also facilitate families in recognizing signs necessitating immediate medical intervention, thereby maximizing overall compliance. Finally, pediatric patient compliance issues are also confounded by rising obesity in children, a condition that makes complications in respiratory disorders (Jacob et al., 2015). Obesity in children puts them at risk of anesthesia and other medical intervention complications, which can lead to anxiety and fear towards adhering to treatment. This fear can trigger avoidance of fully engaging in suggested therapies, hindering compliance and leading to poorer health outcomes. Pediatric clinicians must take into account the psychosocial effects of obesity when developing treatment plans. Tailored interventions incorporating lifestyle modification, education on the importance of controlling weight, and strategies to alleviate anxiety about medical interventions are required to promote compliance. Recognition of the complexity of compliance barriers allows for the formulation of more effective, individualized care plans to maximize the health benefits for children with respiratory disease (Figure 7.15).

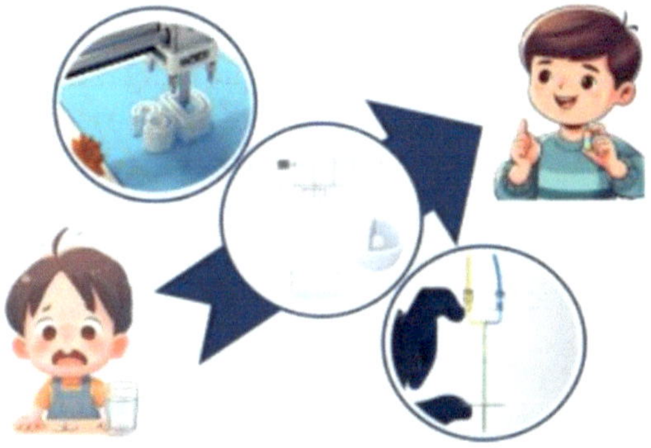

**Figure 7.15.** Challenges in pediatric patient compliance.

*Source:* https://www.pharmaexcipients.com/wp-content/uploads/2024/05/Innovative-pharmaceutical-techniques-for-Paediatric-dosage-forms-300x199.jpg.

## 7.5.3. Socioeconomic Factors Affecting Care and Outcomes

Socioeconomic conditions are a determining factor in health outcomes for pediatric patients, especially pediatric patients with respiratory diseases. Healthcare services are deeply impacted by the socioeconomic status of a family, , such as income, education levels, and housing. Underprivileged families find it difficult to afford healthcare services and medications, which results in poor management of respiratory conditions like asthma. Second, low-educational-level caregivers may be poorly educated in terms of health literacy and therefore may not be in a position to effectively manage the health system or even comply with medical instructions. Poor knowledge amplifies children's conditions by not following through on treatment regimens appropriately, highlighting the intrinsic relationship between socioeconomic determinants and pediatric respiratory outcomes. Furthermore, children's residential living conditions, where they spend the majority of their lives, influence their respiratory status. Families living in economically deprived neighborhoods are likely to be subjected to higher concentrations of air pollutants, allergens, and housing exposures that could precipitate or worsen respiratory diseases like asthma. In pediatric asthma research clinical pathways, systemic efforts need to be undertaken to address environmental determinants of health, particularly for children who are part of vulnerable populations (Oosthuizen, 2012). High rates of respiratory illness frequently occur in populations where economic disparities perpetuate poor air quality and poor access to healthcare. Thus, addressing these types of socioeconomic determinants is essential to improving the prognosis of children with respiratory disease. Lastly, policy creation and implementation that enable equal access to healthcare services and encourage healthy environments are crucial in preventing the ill effects of economic disparities. Interventions to enhance the nutrition of children and ensure safe play and exercise environments contribute significantly to their health and resistance to respiratory disease (Oosthuizen, 2012). Policymakers are able to invest in early childhood programs that provide stable relations and positive settings and, thus, create conditions that improve present and future child health outcomes. Finally, there must be an integrated response with consideration of socioeconomic factors in the scenario to enhance the care and management of respiratory disease in children.

## Test Your Knowledge

1. What are potential complications of untreated respiratory disorders in children?
2. How do socioeconomic factors affect the care and outcomes of pediatric respiratory conditions?

## 7.6. Current Research and Advances in Treatment

**Learning Outcome**

1. Innovations in pharmacological treatments;
2. Emerging therapies and technologies;
3. Importance of ongoing research in pediatric nursing.

Current advances in the management of childhood respiratory illnesses have come to increasingly emphasize the value of interdisciplinary care, as evidenced by the establishment of aerodigestive programs. These emerging models of care focus on coordinated care of complex congenital or acquired disorders involving not only respiratory function but also swallowing and nutrition development. By coordinating specialists across disciplines, these programs aim to provide multidisciplinary care that is tailored to each child's individual requirements. As a result, patient outcomes are more and more shown to be improving through organized, interdisciplinary treatment of pediatric patients with respiratory conditions, translating into improved quality of life and enhanced health milestones. Additional research seeks to examine the intricate definition and structure of aerodigestive programs, offering an emergent discussion among providers. Despite the common prevalence of these programs, there is no agreement on what constitutes an "aerodigestive patient" and what the standard components of these programs are. To alleviate this barrier, a Delphi method-based study performed with a heterogeneous group of aerodigestive providers has been employed recently. This approach yielded a broad definition and established key elements needed for effective program planning, including required constructs, functions, and indicators of research priorities in aerodigestive care, thereby laying the groundwork for subsequent clinical guidelines and standardization. To supplement structural enhancements, recent research focuses on outcome measures and funding mechanisms to secure the sustainability of aerodigestive care. Findings of multi-institutional studies indicate not only growing needs for better-defined patterns of aerodigestive care but also greater recognition of their significance for pediatric health outcomes.

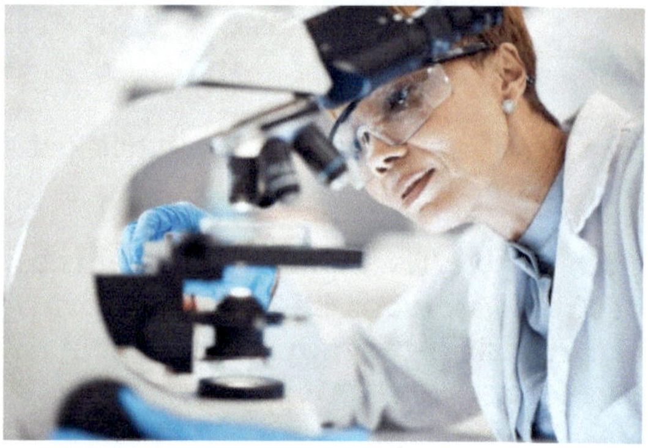

**Figure 7.16.** Current research and advances in treatment.

*Source:* https://i0.wp.com/tfscro.com/wp-content/uploads/2025/02/Next-Generation-Oncology-Research-How-CROs-Are-Accelerating-Cancer-Drug-Development_featured.jpg?fit=500%2C330&ssl=1.

Specifically, defining optimal components of care cycles between feeding and swallowing therapy is a primary use of current research on pediatric respiratory conditions. By developing strong evidence-based practice guidelines, practitioners can improve clinical interventions, fill gaps in care, and champion resources to enhance treatment opportunities. Lastly, these research directions point toward the need for continued innovation in pediatric respiratory treatment, improving overall care of the patient and enabling children to thrive in spite of the nature of their conditions (Figure 7.16).

### 7.6.1. Innovations in Pharmacological Treatments

Pharmacological innovation in the therapy of children's respiratory disease has transformed the treatment of these conditions, adapting to children's differential features with tailored therapy. Recent developments are not only intended to cure symptoms but even the causative factor itself, thereby enhancing the therapeutic result. For instance, targeted biologic drug development has revolutionized treatment modalities for asthma and cystic fibrosis with selective inhibition of particular inflammatory pathways. These drugs hold the promise to reduce the frequency and severity of exacerbations, resulting in improved lung function and quality of life. Further, the use of digital health technologies in pharmacologic management provides personalized treatment regimens and real-time monitoring of compliance with medications and symptom control in a way that ensures pediatric patients are given timely interventions that are effective and safe. Also, advancements in drug delivery systems have improved the delivery of pharmacologic treatment in pediatric patients with respiratory disease. Inhalation therapy has come to be more sophisticated, with enhanced upgrades made to ensure more deposition of medication directly within the lungs. For example, nebulizers and pediatric-ergonomic inhalers guarantee better compliance from children, who otherwise would resist therapy due to complicated delivery. On the horizon are also aerosolized medications via microparticle technology that promise more absorption and fewer side effects compared to standard preparations. These advances not only allow for increased therapeutic results but also allow pediatric patients to become active participants in the management of their disease, creating a sense of autonomy and responsibility for their health. Lastly, the integration of nonpharmacologic interventions alongside pharmacologic interventions is an integrative approach to the treatment of pediatric respiratory disease. Research highlights incorporating drug treatment with supporting therapies , such as breathing techniques and cognitive behavior techniques, to maximize patient outcomes. The methods are designed to address what is known by doctors as the reality that pain and distress resulting from respiratory diseases can drastically change a child's lifestyle. As stated, while pharmacologic methods manage the immediate symptoms, the use of adjunct therapies maximizes treatment efficacy in reducing long-term effects on physical and mental well-being (Swartzentruber, 2021). Most importantly, management of pain among pediatric populations must be done; otherwise, chronic pain conditions prevail into adulthood, finally impacting health throughout the lifespan (Oosthuizen, 2012). Through a multi-dimensional treatment strategy, health professionals can provide comprehensive care that not only ends symptoms but also maximizes the overall health of children.

### 7.6.2. Emerging Therapies and Technologies

Within the pediatric respiratory disease context, new therapies and technologies play a crucial role in improving patient outcomes and quality of care nursing. Advances in respiratory medical equipment and supplies (RMES) , such as advanced ventilation systems and continuous positive airway pressure (CPAP) machines, are examples of the power of technology to address the needs of children with complex chronic illness. As they become more sophisticated, they not only provide vital assistance to patients but also yield significant information that can be employed in clinical decision-making. Sophisticated monitoring devices, for instance, enable clinicians to monitor respiratory function in real time, so appropriate interventions can be undertaken that can prevent the occurrence of an acute respiratory crisis. These innovations demonstrate the imperative intersection of technology and patient care, which ultimately leads to better treatment of pediatric respiratory disease. Additionally, research demonstrates the impact of RMES on healthcare utilization and related expenses for children with respiratory disease. For instance, research indicated that children who utilized RMES experienced significantly higher health costs per year compared to children who were not receiving RMES, since they exhibited higher medical needs in this category. Kids on equipment like ventilators and tracheostomy care not only represent a special class of children's patients but also the multilateral challenges that face in caring for complex cases. The emergent treatments not only facilitate respiratory function but also dictate the necessity for an entire level of comprehension from nursing practitioners regarding the implications for patient care, including the necessary protocols for equipment use and upkeep. These findings underscore the need for an interdisciplinary approach to optimize delivery of care for this at-risk population (Gaur et al., 2017). Finally, pediatric respiratory care with telehealth further demonstrates novel technologies designed to improve outcomes. This modality has potential for real-time monitoring of patients and real-time consultation, reducing in-person visits to the hospital. Telehealth not only enhances specialist care access for children in underserved or remote areas but also facilitates chronic respiratory disease management by readily available healthcare resources. Through these technologies, healthcare clinicians are able to create personalized treatment plans, which are more responsive to the individual patient's needs. As new areas of pediatric respiratory care emerge, the use of novel strategies like telehealth is a representation of the ongoing desire to improve nursing competencies so that children afflicted with respiratory diseases can be offered comprehensive, individualized, and effective treatments (Barra et al., 2023) (Figure 7.17).

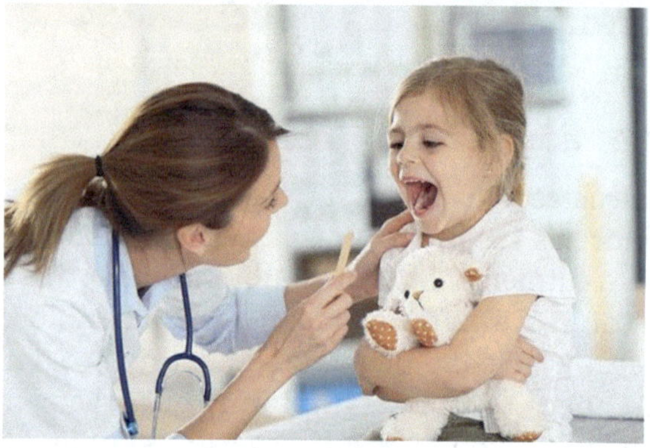

**Figure 7.17.** Emerging therapies and technologies.

*Source:* https://neonest.in/wp-content/uploads/2024/01/a6bd8b7bb8cc92d4f3501fe87df11e01.jpg.

### 7.6.3. Importance of Ongoing Research in Pediatric Nursing

The role of research in pediatric nursing can never be overemphasized, particularly in pediatric respiratory disorders. Research continues to refine treatment modalities and develop new care patterns in response to the unique needs of children. Pediatric patients, unlike their adult counterparts, have varying physiological and developmental characteristics that demand a predefined method. The increased prevalence of chronic respiratory diseases among children underscores the necessity for research. Further research can lead to enhanced understanding of such disorders, essential to the development of effective interventions and the enhancement of nursing practice. Nursing practitioners, while involved in research, reinforce evidence-based practice, which ultimately leads to improved patient outcomes and more efficient delivery of care in medical-surgical practice among children. Research informs clinical interventions in pediatric respiratory nursing that assist in treating long-term conditions requiring prolonged management. The evolving care context, driven by emerging technological advances in medicine and in respiratory assistance, demands ongoing investigation of best practice in at-risk children. As an example, literature emerging in the area of home mechanical ventilation (HMV) highlights the need for expert guidelines covering the particularities of pediatric care. There is a great disparity in comprehensive guidelines on children with respiratory disorders who require long-term ventilation, as noted by Adderley et al. (2017). By conducting research among these patients, clinicians can create evidence-based guidelines that maximize care, improve the quality of life of patients, and maximize overall efficiency in health. This, thus, brings to the fore the urgent necessity for systemic learning and understanding of pediatric respiratory problems in the nursing industry. In addition to this, the interprofessional nature of pediatric care underscores the importance of nursing scholarship. Interprofessional collaboration between various healthcare professionals, doctors, respiratory therapists, and nurses, is central in managing complex pediatric respiratory cases. Ongoing research facilitates seamless interdisciplinary communication so that the whole team can have a current consensus about best practice from recent evidence. For instance, the findings of ongoing research into the ethics of children's long-term ventilation, and particularly into issues of informed consent and quality of life, can significantly shape practice and policy. With the application of a research-based practice, pediatric nursing not only enhances its quality of care but also fosters a culture of shared knowledge and collaboration. This collaboration ultimately supports in enhancing treatment outcomes, providing holistic and understanding care to pediatric patients with respiratory illnesses.

## Test Your Knowledge

1. What are some recent innovations in pharmacological treatments and emerging therapies for pediatric respiratory disorders?
2. Why is ongoing research important in the field of pediatric nursing, especially for respiratory care?

## SUMMARY

The studies on pediatric respiratory illness in the context illustrate the crucial requirement for peak assessment and intervention strategies. The employment of standardized assessment instruments, for instance, the Pasero Opioid Sedation Scale (POSS), has proven effective in the avoidance of adverse effects like opioid-induced respiratory depression in pediatric patients undergoing surgery. Given that such patients are generally more susceptible due to other causations like anesthetic effects and opioid use, the requirement to enhance practice monitoring becomes indispensable. The results wherein greater than 99.9% adherence to documented sedation assessments indicate the potential of such guidelines not merely to guarantee patient safety but to improve the quality of care in pediatric wards, eliminating problems concerning unintended sedation and respiratory complications (Elliott et al., 2023). Additionally, ongoing education and familiarization with detailed curricula specifically tailored for addressing pediatric respiratory care requirements are required for emergency and medical-surgical nurses. As noted in the emergency department nurse curriculum plan for the Kaiser Permanente Central Valley Area, structured training modules on respiratory assessment, pathophysiology, and interventions can significantly contribute to nurses' knowledge base and competencies. The curriculum provision of case studies and simulation ensures nursing professionals are better equipped to deal with frequent respiratory conditions in pediatric patients, , such as asthma and bronchiolitis. The positive participant evaluation outcomes further solidify the necessity for educational interventions highlighting pediatric respiratory complaints to improve the clinical outcome in this vulnerable age group (Houten et al., 2018). As a whole, pediatric respiratory disorder practice needs to be improved through a multi-faceted strategy of embracing stringent assessment instruments, education, and the development of evidence-based guidelines. With growing pediatric health requirements, the need for better nursing skills becomes ever more compelling. By addressing the educational needs of nurses along with embracing effective assessment methods, health care organizations can reduce the risks associated with respiratory disorders to a great extent. Enhancements in education and compliance with protocol not only enhance patient safety but also foster the unified comprehension of pediatric respiratory needs, ultimately leading to improved health outcomes among this vulnerable patient population. The inclusion of quality improvement initiatives is a key enhancement to the development of nursing practice for pediatric care.

In the field of child respiratory illnesses, a significant focus is placed on the occurrence and implications of obstructive sleep apnea syndrome (OSAS) in children. OSAS is seen in approximately 0.7% to 3% of children, with a peak prevalence during preschool age. The condition is caused by recurrent episodes of upper airway obstruction during sleep, leading to unwanted consequences , such as hypoxia and sleep disruption. Children may exhibit certain signs, , such as nighttime snoring, pauses in breathing, and mouth breathing, which have a negative impact on their daytime functioning and development. The causes of OSAS, , such as anatomical and functional abnormality, need to be examined for correct diagnosis and treatment. The most recognized etiology is adenotonsillar hypertrophy, underscoring the importance of early treatment and appropriate referral settings modalities so that this common disorder is addressed sufficiently (José et al., 2025). The other major aspect of pediatric respiratory disorders is the challenge rural hospitals face. Rural hospitals play a vital role in providing health services to underprivileged populations, , such as rural patients. However, the financial viability of the facilities has been under constant threat, and this has led to their shutdowns, significantly impacting the delivery of required medical services, including treatment of respiratory diseases in children. Evidence indicates that patients prefer to stay away from rural hospitals to access urban centers with more advanced services and technologies. Such evasion creates critical gaps in the delivery of care, as rural residents come to depend on regional hospitals for timely medical treatment. All these variations must be addressed through planning strategies to enhance hospital care, and this might indeed improve pediatric patient outcomes in such regions (José et al., 2025). Also, management of pediatric respiratory ailments cuts across various treatment methodologies, including surgical and clinical care. Surgical interventions, , such as adenotonsillectomy or craniofacial deformity correction, are often necessary in children suffering from OSAS to reliably reestablish airway patency. In addition, clinical interventions like continuous positive airway pressure (CPAP) therapy and sleep hygiene practices are also crucial as part of well-rounded treatment plans. All of these approaches together are needed to ensure evidence-based treatment that intervenes for acute symptoms as well as long-term health status. The nurses play a significant role in observation and counseling families about the complexities involved in pediatric respiratory disease management, to give them thorough care encompassing medical as well as emotional aspects at all phases of treatment (Balbani et al., 2005).

## KEY TERMS FROM THIS CHAPTER

- Asthma
- Deoxygenation
- Genetic factors
- Physiology
- Respiratory disorders
- Respiratory syncytial virus (RSV)
- Vulnerable population
- Bronchitis
- Feeding and swallowing difficulties (FSD)
- Lower respiratory tract infections (LRTI)
- Pneumonia
- Respiratory illnesses
- Respiratory tract

## CRITICAL THINKING QUESTIONS

1. **The most common cause of bronchiolitis in infants is:**
   a. Influenza virus
   b. Respiratory Syncytial Virus (RSV)
   c. Streptococcus pneumoniae
   d. Adenovirus
2. **A classical "barking cough" in a child suggests:**
   a. Bronchial asthma
   b. Bronchiolitis
   c. Croup
   d. Pneumonia
3. **Which of the following is a typical sign of pneumonia in children?**
   a. Bradycardia
   b. Chest in-drawing
   c. Polyuria
   d. Abdominal distention
4. **Wheezing is most commonly associated with:**
   a. Asthma
   b. Tuberculosis
   c. Croup
   d. Epiglottitis
5. **What is the most common bacterial cause of community-acquired pneumonia in children?**
   a. Escherichia coli
   b. Streptococcus pneumoniae
   c. Klebsiella pneumoniae
   d. *Staphylococcus aureus*

### Short Answer Questions

1. Define bronchiolitis. What is the most common causative virus?
2. What are the clinical features of pneumonia in a child?
3. Differentiate between viral and bacterial pneumonia.
4. Describe the clinical features, diagnosis, and management of bronchiolitis in infants.
5. Explain upper vs. lower respiratory tract infections in children with examples.
6. Discuss the role of immunization in preventing respiratory infections in children (e.g., pertussis, measles, influenza).

### *Answers to Critical Thinking Questions*

1. (b); 2. (c); 3. (b); 4. (a); 5. (b)

# REFERENCES


1. Acra, S., Balakrishnan, K., Benscoter, D. T., Boesch, A., et al. (2018). Structure and functions of pediatric aerodigestive programs: A consensus statement. https://core.ac.uk/download/161627653.pdf (accessed on 16th June 2025).
2. Allison, M., Beloat, A., Daugherty, S., Hanson-Abromeit, D., et al. (2018). Reporting quality of music intervention research in healthcare: A systematic review. https://core.ac.uk/download/227054380.pdf (accessed on 16th June 2025).
3. Balbani, A. P., Weber, S. A., & Montovani, J. C. (2005). Update in obstructive sleep apnea syndrome in children. *Brazilian journal of otorhinolaryngology*, *71*(1), 74–80. https://doi.org/10.1016/s1808-8694(15)31288-x(accessed on 16th June 2025).
4. Barra, M. E., Zink, E. K., Bleck, T. P., Cáceres, E., Farrokh, S., Foreman, B., Cediel, E. G., Hemphill, J. C., Nagayama, M., Olson, D. M., Suarez, J. I., & Curing Coma Campaign, its contributing members (2023). Common Data Elements for Disorders of Consciousness: Recommendations from the Working Group on Hospital Course, Confounders, and Medications. *Neurocritical care*, *39*(3), 586–592. https://doi.org/10.1007/s12028-023-01803-4 (accessed on 16th June 2025).
5. Burns, H. (2019). The development of hypersensitivity reactions in the pediatric population: A review. https://core.ac.uk/download/213464303.pdf (accessed on 16th June 2025).
6. Cabana, M. D., Cattamanchi, A., Gupta, N., Jennings, T., et al. (2021). Implementing pediatric inpatient asthma pathways. https://core.ac.uk/download/323082497.pdf (accessed on 16th June 2025).
7. Cimasi, R. J., & Zigrang, T. A. (2015). *Adviser's Guide to Health Care, Volume 2: Consulting Services*. https://core.ac.uk/download/551513559.pdf (accessed on 16th June 2025)
8. Clark, A., Sedman, A., Beal, A. C., Tourangeau, A. E., Lawthers, A. G., Agency for Healthcare Research and Quality (US), Bremner, A. P., et al. (2012). Identifying pediatric nursing-sensitive outcomes in linked administrative health data. https://core.ac.uk/download/195649158.pdf (accessed on 16th June 2025).
9. Copeland, L. I. B. T., James, D., Duinkerken, M. S. I., Gordon, K., et al. (2019). Jefferson Digital Commons quarterly report: October–December 2019. https://core.ac.uk/download/286097805.pdf (accessed on 16th June 2025).
10. Danioko, S. (2020). A novel correction for the adjusted box–Pierce test–New risk factors for emergency department return visits within 72 hours for children with respiratory conditions–General pediatric model for understanding and predicting prolonged length of stay. https://core.ac.uk/download/345021292.pdf (accessed on 16th June 2025).
11. Doughty, M. W. (2014). Determining the health problems of Alaska Military Youth Academy participants. https://core.ac.uk/download/162576817.pdf (accessed on 16th June 2025).
12. Gaur, D. (2017). Characteristics of children enrolled in Medicaid using respiratory equipment and supplies. https://open.bu.edu/bitstream/2144/23777/6/Gaur_bu_0017N_12674.pdf (accessed on 16th June 2025).
13. Goforth, Martha Kate and Roberts, Price, "Referral Policy for Moderate to High-Risk Obstructive Sleep Apnea Patients Identified by the STOP-Bang Questionnaire: A Quality Improvement

Project" (2018). Doctoral Projects. 93. https://aquila.usm.edu/dnp_capstone/93 (accessed on 16th June 2025).

14. Hassan, M., & Mousa, H. (2017). Gastroesophageal reflux disease. https://core.ac.uk/download/324162916.pdf (accessed on 16th June 2025).
15. Oosthuizen, N. (2012). A profile of a pediatric population with feeding and swallowing difficulties at a tertiary hospital in the Western Cape. https://core.ac.uk/download/185445474.pdf (accessed on 16th June 2025).
16. Potter, K. (2004). Pet therapy uses in pediatric hospitals: An internet-based pilot study. https://core.ac.uk/download/223074365.pdf (accessed on 16th June 2025).
17. Swartzentruber, Miriam, "The Importance of Providing Multimodal Analgesia: A Literature Review of Nonpharmacologic Pain Treatments" (2021). *Senior Honors Theses*. 1092. https://digitalcommons.liberty.edu/honors/1092(accessed on 16th June 2025).

# PEDIATRIC GASTROENTEROLOGY

# 8

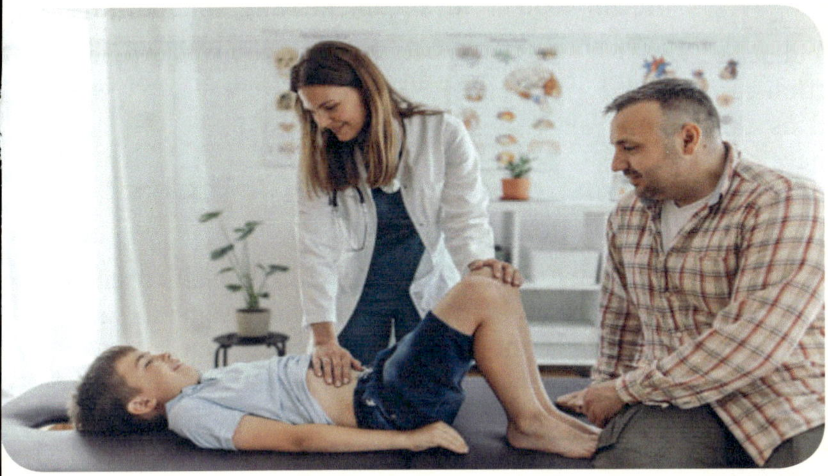

## LEARNING OBJECTIVES

**After studying this chapter, you will be able to:**

1. Explain the anatomy and physiology of the pediatric gastrointestinal system;
2. Discuss the common gastrointestinal disorders in children;
3. Explain the diagnostic approaches in pediatric gastroenterology;
4. Learn about treatment modalities in pediatric gastroenterology;
5. Know the impact of gastrointestinal disorders on child development;
6. Focus on advances in pediatric gastroenterology

## Introduction

Pediatric gastroenterology is a medical subspecialty concerned with the diagnosis and care of gastrointestinal illness in infants, children, and adolescents. The specialty spans a very broad range of disorders, a few examples of which include but are not limited to inflammatory bowel disease, celiac disease, and functional gastrointestinal disorders. One of the features of an innovative challenge in this specialty is handling the unique physiological and psychological requirements of pediatric patients. On account of the realization that children's bodies and immune systems are still developing, treatment regimens in most cases will require conservative adjustments in contrast to what will be applied to adults. Additionally, pediatric gastroenterologists must also contend with families by providing education and reassurance as parents grasp the intricacies of diagnosing and treating their children's gastrointestinal issues. Thus, building rapport and trust becomes necessary in the entire process of treatment. One of the salient aspects of pediatric gastroenterology is the central position of nutrition in managing gastrointestinal disease. Most of the conditions have malabsorption or dietary restriction as a consequence, and a sound understanding of nutritional requirements based on children's growth and development is warranted. The use of restrictive diets, for example, , such as low-FODMAP dieting, has been popularized for managing gastrointestinal symptoms. However, while this method appears promising, data on its safety and efficacy in children remain sparse (Thomassen et al., 2022). In fact, studies are purported to indicate that nutrient inadequacies resulting from untimely dietary restriction can impact the nutritional status as well as the psychosocial well-being of children. Therefore, pediatric gastroenterologists ought to be endowed with the skills to appropriately counsel families such that nutritional management is both safe and beneficial.

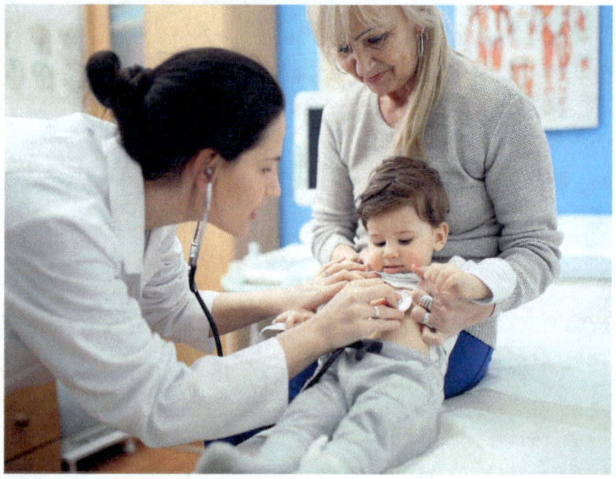

**Figure 8.1.** Pediatric gastroenterology is a specialized branch of medicine focusing.

*Source:* https://dam.northwell.edu/m/49be39825998ef50/Drupal-Web_GettyImages-514835994.jpg.

New methods and technologies are reshaping the landscape of pediatric gastroenterology, enhancing diagnostic and treatment modalities. New advancements in machine learning and data science, for instance, are capable of refining the standard of pediatric care with better data structuring, analysis, and modeling (Maier et al., 2021). These innovations bring opportunities to enhance existing clinical practices with more effective and tailored treatment regimens. Additionally, the addition of multidisciplinary teams, including nutritionists and mental health specialists, will further improve the model of holistic care most important to children with gastrointestinal challenges. Thus, as pediatric gastroenterology advances, staying abreast of technological advancements and collaborative approaches will become paramount to optimizing patient outcomes in this essential area of care (Figure 8.1).

## Definition and Scope of Pediatric Gastroenterology

Pediatric gastroenterology is a specialty branch of medicine involved in the diagnosis and management of gastrointestinal conditions in children, encompassing a wide range of diseases from infancy through early adulthood. The specialty addresses various complications, , such as but not restricted to chronic abdominal pain, inflammatory bowel disease, celiac disease, malnutrition, and liver ailments. Pediatric gastroenterologists learn about the unique physiological variations between kids and adults, understanding that children's gastrointestinal systems can manifest diseases differently. Since children's bodies are in the process of development, the treatment may be considerably different, requiring a collection of skills that integrate child-centered care methods with modern medical practices. As the prevalence of gastrointestinal disease is increasing, the significance of pediatric gastroenterology has increased immensely in providing children with quality and timely care. Pediatric gastroenterology is not limited to disease treatment alone. It encompasses preventative health care measures, dietetics, and family education concerning gastrointestinal health. Pediatric gastroenterologists usually work together with experts, dietitians, and general physicians to promote an integrative treatment methodology. Multidimensionality plays a significant role in addressing ongoing concerns and attending to overall development and well-being in children. Moreover, the development of new diagnostic tools , such as endoscopy and imaging enhances professionals' capabilities in assessing and tracking gastrointestinal well-being accurately. With ongoing research and development, pediatric gastroenterology is always striving to optimize care procedures, not only the health of children in medical terms but also their psychological and social well-being.

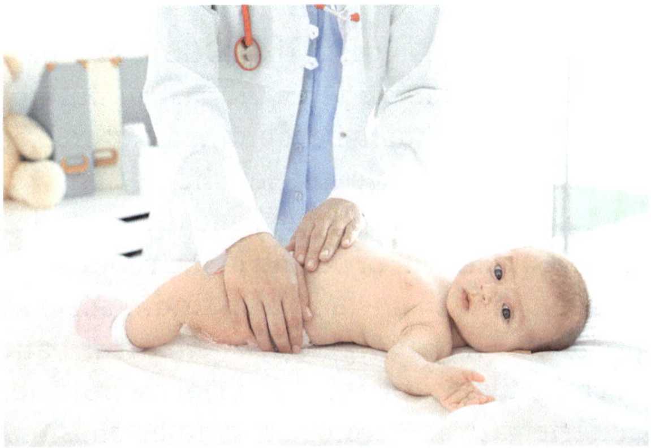

**Figure 8.2.** The scope of pediatric gastroenterology.

*Source:* https://www.drrupalijain.com/img/services/pediatric-gastroenterology.jpg.

Besides, pediatric gastroenterology is increasingly embracing the precepts of precision medicine, which target tailored care based on genetic, environmental, and lifestyle factors. This new paradigm offers even more individualized treatment options that more effectively enhance patient outcomes and minimize side effects. Research activities in this regard have found the influence of social determinants of health on gastrointestinal illnesses in children that can also involve aspects related to weight stigma and its implication in the healthcare setting (Rubino et al., 2020). Interaction between physiological and societal determinants needs to be understood in order to provide equal healthcare. As the specialty evolves, integrating multidisciplinary methodologies will be at the forefront of dealing with growing pediatric gastrointestinal complexity and delivering children with comprehensive care that is attuned to their unique needs and circumstances (Figure 8.2).

## Importance of Specialized Care for Children

In pediatric gastroenterology, the necessity of children needing specialist treatment cannot be overplayed. Physiological and growth phases in children necessitate a unique method of diagnosis and treatment, particularly concerning gastrointestinal disorders. Specialist treatment guarantees that pediatric patients receive interventions tailored to their unique needs, considering variations in their metabolic rate, growth curve, and overall well-being. For instance, illnesses , such as obesity, now epidemic in teenagers, require thorough acquaintance with child-specific factors that contribute to weight gain. There is no solitary approach to management; hence a personalized strategy for dietary interventions and exercise advice plays a critical role towards improving patient results as well as facilitating long-term well-being. Additionally, the psychological and social conditions of childhood obesity need to be treated with special care to avoid complications of associated comorbidities. According to recent studies, obese children have increased risks of Type 2 Diabetes Mellitus and hypertension. Obesity stigma may also complicate treatment with a tendency to avoid health services. Expert pediatric care therefore becomes absolutely essential not only in the treatment of the physical aspects of concomitant disorders but also in facilitating an unhospitable environment. Pediatric gastroenterology-trained healthcare providers are capable of employing empathetic communication skills and realizing the psychological implications, reducing a feeling of isolation in such children and fostering positive self-concept and health behaviors.

Finally, the evolving treatment landscape for pediatric obesity, , such as drug therapy, reiterates the necessity for specialized treatment. New drugs that have been proven to be beneficial in the weight reduction process, , such as GLP-1 agonists, need to be rigorously tested for efficacy and safety in pediatric populations—a step that requires pediatric expertise. As nearly 6% of adolescents are technically severely obese, higher-level treatment is dependent on well-educated decision-making. Multidisciplinary treatment with gastroenterologists but also with mental health professionals might be the best overall treatment plan, addressing both clinical and psychosocial issues. Indeed, pediatric gastroenterology subspecialty care not only prepares health professionals to deal with bodily wellness but also allows for a holistic intervention strategy to child health, fostering on-the-spot as well as long-term health outcomes.

## *Overview of Common Gastrointestinal Disorders in Children*

A complete understanding of pediatric gastrointestinal conditions involves exploration of the most common complaints seen in this population. Of these, functional gastrointestinal disorders (FGIDs) are most frequent, with a significant number of cases having no underlying organic illness. In one important discovery, it is found that children with FGIDs are disproportionately affected by chronic abdominal pain and its attendant increased frequency of school absence. In fact, research has established that these children miss more than three days of school per month due to their symptoms, highlighting the extent to which FGIDs can influence their everyday lives and school participation (Seth et al., 2024). This case highlights the need for healthcare providers not just to diagnose but to take charge of the psychosocial aspects of FGIDs in children. In addition, gut-brain interaction disorders (DGBIs) are a critical group in the context of pediatric gastrointestinal diseases. They are characterized by dysfunction in gut-brain communication and are highly prevalent among children, particularly in Latin America. A cross-sectional investigation showed that approximately 34.5% of the tested children had a DGBI and that the highest prevalence diagnosis was functional constipation at 23.4% across all ages (Velasco-Benítez et al., 2024).

This trend suggests that DGBIs can be a major determinant of pediatric gastrointestinal symptoms and should be identified and treated in order to improve the quality of life for children with these disorders and their families. Effective treatment of pediatric gastrointestinal disorders has to include a multidimensional approach involving both medical and educational treatments. A priority role for pediatric gastroenterologists is to establish an open setting in which these affected children can receive definitive care. This includes open discussion with families about the features of the disorder and how it affects daily living, particularly school attendance and psychosocial well-being.

Additionally, comorbid conditions, , such as anxiety associated with functional gastrointestinal disorders, need to be managed in order to achieve optimal overall health (Seth et al., 2024). By integrating medical treatment with psychological treatment and school facilities, medical professionals can curb the effects of gastrointestinal illnesses in children, paving the way for improved outcomes in their health and performance at school (Figure 8.3).

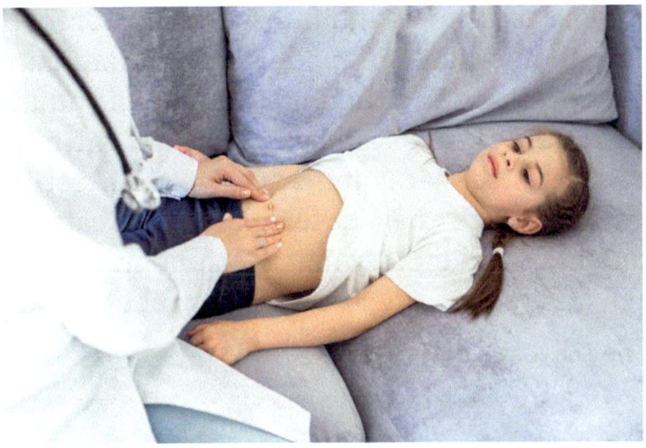

**Figure 8.3.** Overview of common gastrointestinal disorders in children.

*Source:* https://www.ankurahospitals.com/wp-content/uploads/2024/09/pediatric-gastrointestinal-infections.jpeg.

## 8.1. Anatomy and Physiology of the Pediatric Gastrointestinal System

**Learning Outcome**

1. Differences between pediatric and adult gastrointestinal anatomy;
2. Developmental changes in the gastrointestinal system;
3. Common physiological functions and their significance.

The pediatric gastrointestinal system is characterized by anatomical and physiological distinctions that are quite different from those of adults. The GI tract is significantly shorter in neonates and toddlers, which has implications for their digestion and absorption of nutrients. The esophagus is narrower, and the stomach is small and more alkaline, which leads to variations in gastric acid secretion and digestive enzyme activity. This unformed anatomy plays a critical role in pediatric nutrition because babies are primarily sustained on fluid diets, which demands modification in the mode of feeding. The presence of immature liver enzyme activity also impacts metabolic processes, which is of other concern in disease control , such as in metabolic disorders and imbalance of bilirubin, common in neonates. Identification of such anatomical nuances is important in pediatric GI conditions, which may not occur exactly like their adult equivalent, emphasizing the need for specialized knowledge in pediatric gastroenterology (Alvina et al., 2021). The physiological functions of the pediatric GI tract shift enormously as the child grows. Initially, infants use breast milk or formula to build gut microbiota for digestion. As the child transitions towards solid foods, the GI system needs to accommodate a variety of nutrients, which will necessitate further digestive enzyme maturation and systemic response. Of particular significance, the surface area for absorption in intestines, which expands during the progression, contributes to nutrient uptake and intestinal health. Additionally, infants undergo more frequent gastrointestinal motility compared to adults, which affects feeding and digestive patterns. Such physiological changes illustrate the dynamic interaction of growth and gastrointestinal function, where pediatric-specific assessments become mandatory to validate optimal nutritional results and counteract possible complications , such as feeding intolerance and malabsorption, which are prevalent in numerous pediatric illnesses (Alvina et al., 2021). Pediatric gastroenterology must also consider the impact of congenital anomalies and acquired disease on the GI tract anatomy and physiology. Esophageal atresia and congenital malformations of the gastrointestinal tract may disrupt development and function and need to be diagnosed early and treated. Additional specific management strategies are also required for conditions , such as celiac disease and inflammatory bowel disease. The pathophysiologic responses to illness can be vastly dissimilar due to the dissimilar metabolic rate and individual immunological pictures of the children. Such specificity underscores the necessity for extensive knowledge of both the normal anatomy and of the range of pathophysiological possibilities. As such, pediatric gastroenterologists will need to have a sharp sense of understanding how all these factors interact, especially when taking into account treatment regimes based on initial involvement and ongoing monitoring of the child's adjustability to dietary regimen and medical treatments (Alan et al., 2012).

## 8.1.1. Differences Between Pediatric and Adult Gastrointestinal Anatomy

Knowledge of pediatric rather than adult anatomy differences in the gastrointestinal system is key to pediatric gastroenterology. The gastrointestinal tract in young children and infants is smaller in proportion to the adult, not just impacting digestion but even the amount and type of food that can be efficiently processed. For instance, the intestines, stomach, and esophagus differ in size and length considerably. The pediatric GI tract is less elongated. This anatomical consideration is a very important factor when it comes to diagnosing food intolerance. And disorders. Of. Nutrient. Absorption. Since pediatric patients will generally have symptoms that need. To. Know. Their. Specific. Anatomical. Structure. Accurately. Furthermore, irregular anatomical development or growth patterns, i.e., congenital gastrointestinal malformations, pose additional challenges, hence emphasizing the necessity for a specialized method of addressing children's gastrointestinal health (Pennazio et al., 2022). Another fundamental difference lies in the histological structure and function of the gastrointestinal tract in children versus adults. In children, the mucosal lining is immature, and this can affect nutrient absorption and susceptibility to gastrointestinal disease. For example, undifferentiated digestive enzymes can hinder optimal food digestion and nutrient uptake, leading to gastrointestinal pathology less commonly seen in adults. This aspect of development is imperative to health care providers because it highlights the need for age-related assessment and intervention. Moreover, the gut microbiota responsible for immunity and digestion varies among children and adults. These differences necessitate an intimate acquaintance with pediatric gastrointestinal anatomy since they determine the treatment modalities and dietary management practices in the vulnerable population (Barker et al., 2020).

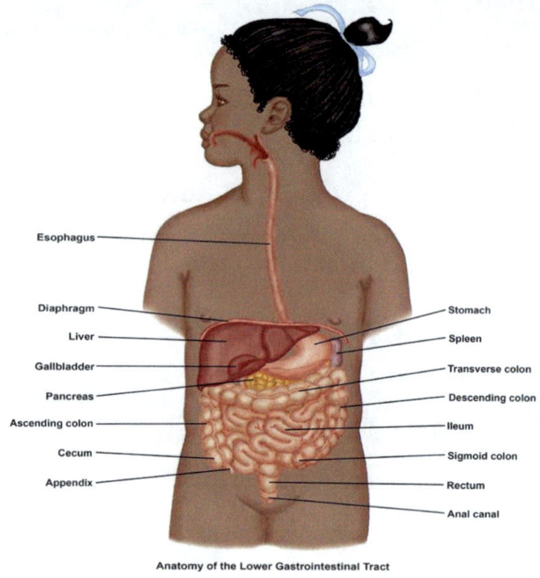


**Figure 8.4.** The differences in gastrointestinal anatomy between pediatrics and adults are crucial for pediatric gastroenterology.

*Source:* https://nursekey.com/wp-content/uploads/2016/10/F000435u43-02-9781437727753.jpg.

Pediatric gastroenterologists must also consider the functional differences in gastrointestinal anatomy while managing children. Differences in motility, including esophageal peristalsis and intestinal transit time, are more pronounced in children than in adults. For example, infants may develop gastroesophageal reflux secondary to diminished tone of the lower esophageal sphincter, which in most adults is less of a problem. In addition, the GI tract of children is more permeable to pathogens, becoming infected and inflamed with a presentation unlike that of adults. Awareness of these functional differences enables more accurate diagnosis and effective treatment plans based on children's unique physiological response. Since gastrointestinal anatomy varies with age, it is important that healthcare providers are aware of the difference to achieve the maximum potential of pediatric patients' health and growth (Pennazio et al., 2022) (Figure 8.4).

## 8.1.2. Developmental Changes in the Gastrointestinal System

The gastrointestinal system also undergoes intense development changes from childhood through to adolescence, accounting for both physiological maturation and response to modified dietary needs. During early infancy, the gastrointestinal tract is immature in large part, and this can manifest as challenges , such as gastroesophageal reflux and feeding. As the child grows, the structure and function of the intestine experience a transformation that facilitates improved digestion and absorption of nutrients. One of the essential points of consideration at this point is how nutrition impacts the development of the gut. For instance, breast milk provides the appropriate nutrition and promotes healthy gut flora, which is central in digestive functionality. Contrarily, premature introduction to inappropriate solid foods may lead to gastrointestinal distress, shedding light on the need for proper nutrition advice during critical developmental stages in pediatrics. Another significant aspect of gastrointestinal development is the role played by the gut microbiome, which increases in diversity throughout early life. Exposure to a diverse range of foods provokes microbial community changes, which can affect metabolic health and immune system maturation. Administration of antibiotics and delivery type (cesarean versus vaginal) can affect composition of the gut microbiome and can predispose children to gastrointestinal illness. Current advances in pediatrics gastroenterology emphasize the importance of promoting a healthy microbiome to prevent adult diseases , such as allergies, obesity, and inflammatory bowel disease. It is, therefore, critical to know the alterations in the gastrointestinal tract during development and their impact on the microbiome to guide pediatricians in using preventive interventions against gastrointestinal disease. Furthermore, gastrointestinal illnesses in children tend to originate from congenital abnormalities or systemic illness that impede normal development.

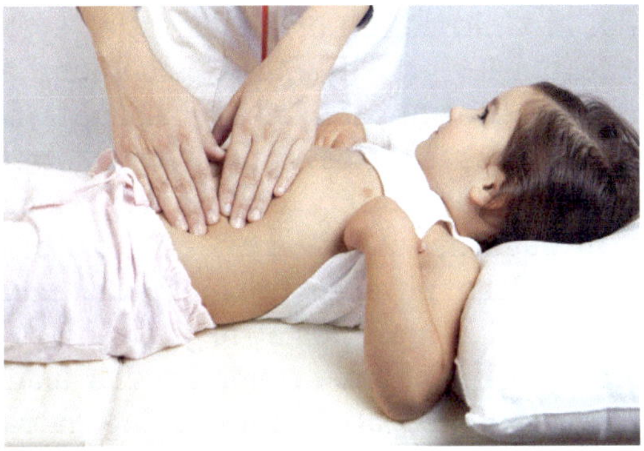

**Figure 8.5.** A healthcare provider performs an abdominal examination on a young child, demonstrating pediatric assessment in the context of gastrointestinal care.

*Source:* https://www.sitarambhartia.org/wp-content/uploads/2018/10/Pediatric-Gastroenterology-1024x683@2x.jpg.

Hirschsprung disease and congenital gastrointestinal anomalies are the best examples where early diagnosis and treatment are crucial. Such conditions can yield severe complications, not just to digestion but to overall health and development as well. Improvements in imaging technologies, , such as gastric emptying scintigraphy and intestinal transit scintigraphy, have improved the capability of pediatric gastroenterologists to detect and treat such illness effectively. Identification of developmental adjustments in the gastrointestinal tract helps in building effective treatment strategies and offering a comprehensive management of pediatric cases (Garganese et al., 2024; Khafizova et al., 2024) (Figure 8.5).

### 8.1.3. Common Physiological Functions and Their Significance

In pediatric gastroenterology, understanding of the normal physiological processes is essential in the diagnosis and treatment of gastrointestinal illnesses. The process of digestion performs important roles , such as the breakdown of food, nutrient absorption, and elimination of waste. In children, a normal digestive system is essential for growth and development, and therefore identification of any disruption in these processes is essential. For instance, gastrointestinal motility, or the movement of food through the digestive tract, is one of the more significant physiological functions that can be expressed in most pediatric gastrointestinal disorders. Disruptions in motility can lead to diarrhea or constipation, threatening nutrient acquisition and thus affecting the overall health of the child. Research on the gastrointestinal tract reveals the crossroads of pediatric patients in the context of inflammation and immune status. In particular, interaction between the host immune system and the gut microbiota is a key determinant of homeostasis and prevention of inflammation. For example, studies of diseases , such as colitis highlight the utility of pharmacological interventions aimed at specific receptors to promote mucosal healing and enhance physiological function. For example, current research on the 5-HT4 receptor activation indicates the protection of colitis experimental models, and it proposes that therapy based on these receptors can achieve notable advantages for children suffering from inflammatory bowel diseases (Mylie et al., 2018). It becomes important to understand these dynamics in order to develop target therapies that can benefit pediatric patients' quality of life. Along with motility and inflammation, advances in imaging techniques have also significantly advanced pediatric gastrointestinal physiology. The use of gastrointestinal ultrasound (GIUS) has been widely popularized in recent years and provides the clinician with a non-invasive means by which to observe and evaluate the anatomical and physiologic characteristics of the gastrointestinal tract of the child. Such an approach is particularly precious with its ability to conduct early diagnosis of many conditions without exposing the patient to radiation (Nylund et al., 2016). With enhanced proficiency in interpreting normal sonoanatomical information, clinicians can be more sensitive to identifying abnormalities that may indicate underlying pathologies. Consequently, the synergy of high-tech imaging equipment with knowledge of physiological processes not only enhances the diagnostic accuracy but also facilitates early and required treatment in pediatric gastroenterology.

## Test Your Knowledge

1. How does the anatomy of the pediatric gastrointestinal system differ from that of adults?
2. What are key developmental changes in the pediatric GI system, and why are physiological functions like digestion and absorption significant?

## 8.2. Common Gastrointestinal Disorders in Children

**Learning Outcome**

1. Gastroesophageal reflux disease (GERD)
2. Inflammatory bowel disease (IBD)
3. Celiac disease and gluten sensitivity

In pediatric gastroenterology, a good knowledge of prevalent gastrointestinal disorders is important for proper diagnosis and treatment. Of the several disorders that children could be suffering from, gastroesophageal reflux disease (GERD) proves to be one of the most common conditions in children. Defined by the regurgitation of contents from the stomach, GERD can cause considerable distress, irritability, and feeding difficulties among infants and toddlers. With the growing incidence of obesity in the pediatric population, it has also been noted that there exists a strong correlation between child obesity and GERD because obesity itself can exacerbate the condition by increasing intra-abdominal pressure. Treating GERD in an obese child thus means formulating an integrative treatment regimen with weight management forming the central part of it. Understanding of these relationships is essential for planning targeted interventions and maximizing outcomes for these children. Constipation is another common gastrointestinal disorder that poses challenges to children and parents. Constipation is often characterized by infrequent passage of bowel movements, straining, and hard stools that result in both physical and emotional distress. Food habits and fluid status in children often play a key role in the development of constipation. The relationship between obesity and constipation is increasingly well understood, as obese children often have altered dietary patterns which make them susceptible to gastrointestinal impairment. Therapy for constipation in this population must adopt an evidence-based strategy with dietary alterations, augmented physical activity, and potentially the use of medication. By prioritizing prevention and education regarding good bowel habits, healthcare providers can enhance the quality of life in affected kids significantly as well as cut short long-term consequences of chronic constipation to their health. Functional abdominal pain is a common complaint in the pediatric population that can significantly affect a child's everyday living and overall health. This is a condition of periodic abdominal pain or discomfort without any organic basis, eventually leading to anxiety and school avoidance. Obesity has come under suspicion as one of the likely causes in the genesis of functional abdominal pain in recent studies, thus complicating the management of this condition.

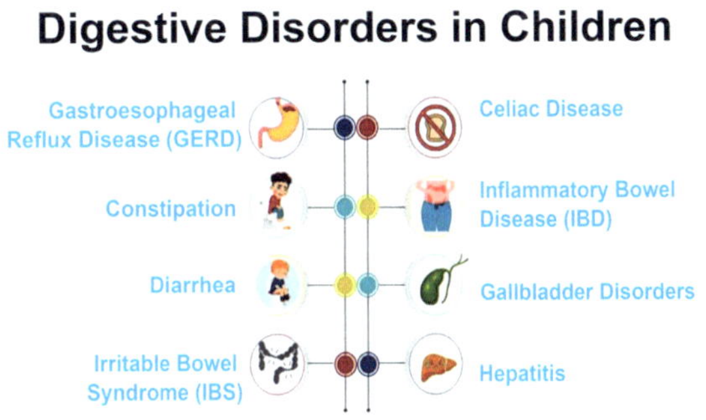


**Figure 8.6.** Common gastrointestinal disorders in children.

*Source:* https://drmagnusjayaraj.b-cdn.net/wp-content/uploads/2023/10/Digestive-Disorders-in-Children-1024x671.webp.

Obese children tend to be stressed more and have their lifestyle curtailed, additionally exacerbating their gastrointestinal symptoms. With these findings, physicians are advised to consider weight control as an integral part of treatment for functional abdominal pain. As obesity in children gains more prevalence, diagnosing and resolving these gastrointestinal complaints become all the more crucial to provide patients of a younger age group with physical and psychological comfort in clinical practice (Sen et al., 2024). Additionally, the impact of the COVID-19 pandemic on gastrointestinal illness has brought additional nuance to this setting that needs ongoing research and renovation of treatments (Röckert et al., 2023) (Figure 8.6).

### 8.2.1. Gastroesophageal Reflux Disease (GERD)

Understanding Gastroesophageal Reflux Disease (GERD) in children is necessary as it may present quite differently than in adults. Although it is easy for adults to equate regurgitation and heartburn, their children might present in unusual uncharacteristic symptoms like failure to thrive, wheezing, and chronic cough. These atypical presentations must be carefully assessed clinically by clinicians so that they do not miss the diagnosis and apply appropriate treatment. In addition, communication issues resulting from children's stages of development can complicate diagnosis. Clinicians therefore have to employ a combination of patient history, physical exam, and tests to establish GERD accurately, employing imaging modality , such as pH monitoring and upper gastrointestinal endoscopy in eliminating the occurrence of reflux and complication thereof (Raza et al., 2025). The management of pediatric GERD is a three-way approach consisting of lifestyle modification, pharmacotherapy, and, in serious cases, surgery. Non-invasive treatment can first start with feeding regimen changes, counseling positional therapy, and proper weight maintenance. In the event that symptoms persist after instituting these practices, pharmacotherapy can be started with emphases on proton pump inhibitors (PPIs) and histamine-2 receptor antagonists to reduce gastric acid secretion. Treatment approaches need to be adjusted for medical professionals based on the age, symptom severity, and complications of the individual child. Surgical procedures, like fundoplication, are also selected in cases of refractoriness when normal medical management does not result in benefit (Ivashkin et al., 2024). Personalized care guarantees better patient outcomes and addresses the unique needs of the child patient. Complications that arise from untreated or inappropriately treated GERD have significant long-term implications for children. Esophagitis, stricture, Barrett's esophagus, and indeed adenocarcinoma of the esophagus are some of the complications involved, particularly when the GERD is chronic and left untreated. The consequences of these complications go to underline the importance of early diagnosis coupled with continuous treatment in avoiding complications. Also, pediatric patients with extraesophageal symptoms of GERD , such as respiratory complaints without conventional symptoms must be closely monitored, often requiring advanced diagnostic studies like 24-hour pH-impedance monitoring. By tackling all of these factors in an all-encompassing manner, clinicians are able to significantly enhance the quality of treatment and achieve better long-term outcomes for children suffering from GERD, thereby reducing the possibility of serious complications (Ivashkin et al., 2024; Raza et al., 2025) (Figure 8.7).

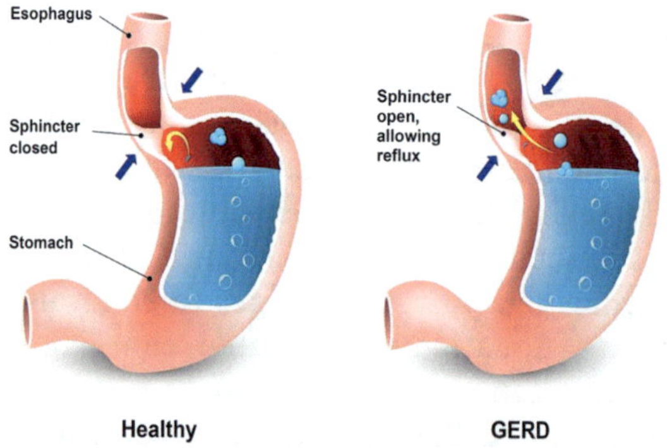


**Figure 8.7.** Understanding gastroesophageal reflux disease (GERD).

*Source:* https://gastrohealth.com/-/media/news/patient-care-photos/gastroesophageal-reflux-disease-1024x676.ashx.

## 8.2.2. Inflammatory Bowel Disease (IBD)

Inflammatory bowel disease (IBD), including both ulcerative colitis and Crohn's disease, is a significant challenge to pediatric gastroenterology due to its multifactorial etiology and clinical heterogeneity. The illness is characterized by chronic inflammation of the intestinal tract and in many instances can be accompanied by debilitating manifestations , such as abdominal pain, diarrhea, and malnutrition. Early identification in children is important since IBD can have a profound impact on growth and development during this formative stage. Furthermore, the increasing prevalence of IBD in pediatric populations means it is imperative to have an in-depth understanding of its pathophysiology, clinical diagnostic criteria, and the potential problems associated with treatment approaches tailored to young patients. Management of IBD must be multidisciplinary in children, with dietary interventions, pharmacologic intervention, and, in some cases, surgical interventions. Current recommendations, for instance, those of the European Crohn's and Colitis Organization (ECCO), are centered on personalized treatment. For instance, nutritional supplementation and enteral nutrition can reverse malnourishment while pharmacotherapy with immunosuppressants , such as corticosteroids and biologics suppresses inflammation and lessens the severity of symptoms. Yet, adherence to these recommendations varies at times among providers. A survey of adult and pediatric gastroenterologists' practices finds that adherence to ECCO guidelines can be extremely variable, implying greater training and resources within specialties to achieve the optimal management approaches for the patient group (Elimeleh et al., 2023). An emerging area of interest in the effective management of IBD in childhood is the use of non-invasive diagnostic techniques, one being intestinal ultrasound (IUS). The technique represents an accurate and radiation-free tool to assess disease activity, quantify bowel wall thickening, and diagnose complications like abscess formation. Current studies emphasize the rising incorporation of IUS into standard evaluation in pediatric patients with IBD, ensuring timely intervention without risking young patients through exposure to more destructive methods. Adoption remains feasible but is sporadic and dependent on physician training and institutional resources. Findings from a national survey of Türkiye's gastroenterologists show that there is immense disparity between the potential of the tool as commonly endorsed and its usage, calling for educational efforts to increase the application of IUS in pediatric clinics (Bilican et al., 2025) (Figure 8.8).

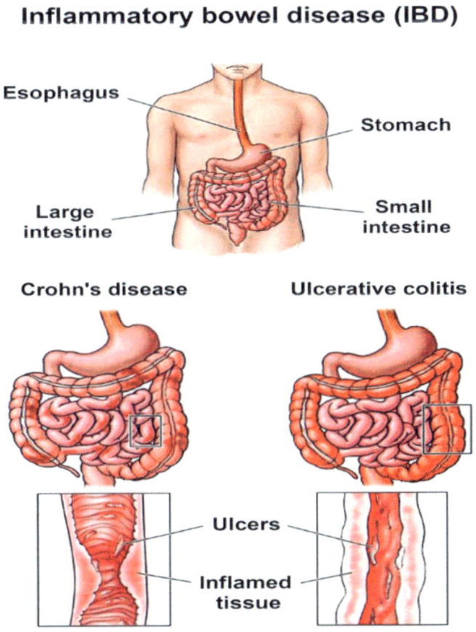


**Figure 8.8.** Inflammatory bowel disease (IBD).

*Source:* https://my.clevelandclinic.org/-/scassets/images/org/health/articles/15587-inflammatory-bowel-disease-ibd.jpg.

## 8.2.3. Celiac Disease and Gluten Sensitivity

Celiac disease (CeD) is an autoimmune, multifactorial disorder of the small intestine in most instances, elicited by the ingestion of gluten foods by individuals with a genetic predisposition. Presentation of CeD in children can be very dissimilar, whereby gastrointestinal manifestations may be dominated by diarrhea, abdominal distension, and pain, while non-gastrointestinal manifestations are characterized by growth retardation and behavioral disturbances. Increased recognition of celiac disease has led to the development of diagnostic algorithms including serological screening and biopsy analysis. Notably, the European Society for Pediatric Gastroenterology Hepatology and Nutrition (ESPGHAN) has provision made for a no-biopsy diagnostic approach under specific conditions, though it is shown that this will result in poorer long-term outcomes than in the case of traditional biopsy-confirmed diagnoses, so emphasizing the implication of overall management strategies in the cases concerned (Enache et al., 2025). Gluten sensitivity, though distinct from celiac disease, presents similar clinical challenges in pediatric gastroenterology. This disorder is characterized by extraintestinal and gastrointestinal manifestations that occur after gluten consumption but do not lead to intestinal mucosal injury characteristic of celiac disease. There is a need to differentiate gluten sensitivity from celiac disease, as misdiagnosis will lead to inappropriate dietary restriction or inadequate treatment. Recent evidence has suggested that gluten sensitivity may be linked to alterations in gut microbiota and immune response, indicative of an intricate interaction between diet, environment, and genes. Accurate identification and management of gluten sensitivity are hence crucial to avoid adverse effects of unnecessary gluten avoidance in children, which can impact development and growth. New therapeutic options and innovative approaches are revolutionizing the management of both gluten intolerance and celiac disease in children. Promising new treatments, , such as zonulin inhibitors and gluten-hydrolyzing enzymes, are at various stages of clinical trial, ushering in a new era of personalized gastroenterology. There is growing interest in utilizing immunotherapy and microbiota manipulation as adjunct therapies to conventional gluten-free diets. These advances suggest that the future of celiac disease management may extend beyond diet regimes to include pharmacologic therapies that have the potential to reduce symptoms and heal. However, more research is needed to validate the safety and effectiveness of such new treatments in the pediatric population, reflecting on the developing arena of treatment and the need for continuous advances in the management of pediatric gastroenterology (Dipasquale et al., 2020).

## Test Your Knowledge

1. What are the typical symptoms and causes of GERD and celiac disease in children?
2. How does inflammatory bowel disease (IBD) present in children, and how is it different from gluten sensitivity?

## 8.3. Diagnostic Approaches in Pediatric Gastroenterology

**Learning Outcome**

1. Clinical evaluation and history taking;
2. Imaging techniques and their applications;
3. Endoscopic procedures and their relevance.

The etiologic diagnosis of disease in the pediatric gastrointestinal system is a complex and multifaceted process that demands an appreciation for many diagnostic modalities. Endoscopic evaluation of the gastrointestinal system is one of the fundamental tools employed in pediatric gastroenterology. Endoscopy allows direct visualization of the mucosal surface and can identify abnormalities in the form of ulceration, inflammation, or neoplasia. The utility of the diagnostic tool is demonstrated by its ability to enable biopsies to be performed for histological assessment, thereby enabling accurate diagnoses for such conditions as celiac disease and infections like Helicobacter pylori. Stressing the role of endoscopic therapy, the guidelines instituted by the Japanese Society for Pediatric Gastroenterology place particular emphasis on not only active infection diagnosis but antimicrobial susceptibility testing for the best possible treatment strategy for *H. pylori*, an area of particular concern in pediatric gastrointestinal clinical practice and research (Kato et al., 2020). Apart from endoscopy, a combination of sophisticated imaging modalities plays an important role in diagnosing gastrointestinal illnesses in children. Techniques , such as ultrasound, computed tomography (CT), and magnetic resonance imaging (MRI) are particularly useful in evaluating pancreatitis, inflammatory bowel disease, and anatomical defects. These techniques provide accurate anatomical information and functional data, allowing clinicians to develop appropriate treatment plans. Their use must also take into account special anatomical and physiological differences that occur in children compared to adults. Pediatric patients, for instance, may develop atypical symptoms that must be interpreted sensitively through imaging findings. As part of an aim to enhance diagnostic accuracy, present research within the specialty is aimed at designing homogeneous guidelines to direct appropriate imaging in an effort to prevent unnecessary radiation exposure and obtain effective disease control. With the emphasis on specific disorders, that of achalasia in children illustrates the necessity for the utilization of a multidisciplinary approach, involving different diagnostic modalities. According to existing evidence, medical history and physical examination are vital in arriving at an initial diagnosis, backed by manometry and contrast swallow studies.

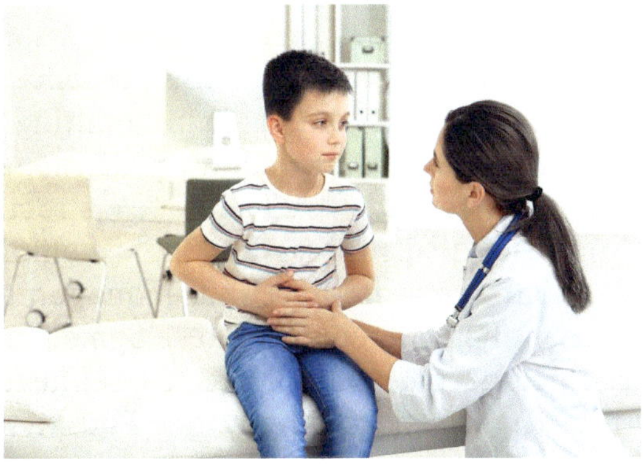

**Figure 8.9.** A healthcare provider evaluates a young boy experiencing abdominal discomfort, illustrating a clinical consultation in pediatric gastroenterology.

*Source:* https://productimages.withfloats.com/serviceimages/tile/6503ea7a6c38a85a3eec7042paediatric-gastroenterology-1024x705.

A survey highlighted that the majority of centers adopt a multidisciplinary strategy for treatment, with pediatric gastroenterologists and surgeons in the majority of instances, to provide optimal care (Marinde et al., 2018). This practice heterogeneity underscores the necessity of concordant guidelines that can harmonize diagnostic approaches from center to center, particularly because achalasia is a rare but sinister disease requiring prompt treatment. Through its encouragement of collaboration among specialists and use of various diagnostic tools, pediatric gastroenterology aspires to maximize outcomes for patients with gastrointestinal illness (Figure 8.9).

### 8.3.1. Clinical Evaluation and History Taking

In pediatric gastroenterology, effective clinical evaluation and detailed history-taking are fundamental to accurate diagnosis. Because children often lack the capacity to clearly articulate their symptoms, clinicians must rely heavily on caregivers to provide comprehensive information. This includes a thorough account of the child's feeding history, bowel habits, developmental progress, and the presence of symptoms such as abdominal pain, vomiting, or diarrhea.. A good history allows practitioners to identify trends related to specific gastrointestinal disorders and hence inform subsequent examination and management plans. Identifying the stages of development and special perspectives of children, as delineated by the American Academy of Pediatrics, emphasizes the importance of including the family within the evaluation process, in the end enriching the accuracy and effectiveness of the clinical assessment (Laura et al., 2022). While taking a history, clinicians must utilize standardized questionnaires and symptom checklists for pediatric patients to be able to take a more structured approach to gathering pertinent information. Utilization of such tools is useful in identifying patterns of symptoms that may indicate underlying gastrointestinal pathology, e.g., inflammatory bowel disease or malabsorption syndromes. Inclusion of psychosocial factors is also imperative since the gastrointestinal symptoms in children can easily superimpose upon emotional distress or functional disorder. Furthermore, an understanding of the impact of family and cultural influences on eating will enable the clinician to put the child's symptoms into the broader context of their life. The medical history and previous medical conditions or operations should also be taken into account in an attempt to have a comprehensive picture of the child's condition, as these might be determinative of the way the gastrointestinal complaints present (Lauren et al., 2020). In pediatric gastroenterology, ongoing assessment and follow-up are crucial in the management of complex cases with the evolving symptomatology and extrinsic influences, , such as the COVID-19 pandemic. With many children with postacute sequelae of SARS-CoV-2 infection, careful clinical evaluation can reveal new or worsening gastrointestinal symptoms, which require monitoring and management in watchfulness. Pediatric clinicians need to be cognizant of such comorbidities since they ensure that they treat any psychiatric problems that may arise during the pandemic. Intensive collaboration with interdisciplinarity teams, including mental health specialists, nutritionists, and pediatric subspecialists, enhances the care process and ensures that the child is presented with an integrative service. The ultimate outcome is a holistic evaluation and individual treatment based on a thorough understanding of medical as well as psychosocial factors involved in pediatric gastroenterological health (Dipasquale et al., 2020).

### 8.3.2. Imaging Techniques and Their Applications

In pediatric gastroenterology, imaging techniques have a valuable role in diagnosis, monitoring, and treatment planning. High-resolution ultrasonography, for instance, is ideally positioned for pediatric patients in being painless and not involving the use of ionizing radiation. The technique is better than others in imaging abdominal organs , such as the liver, spleen, and pancreas, and is helpful in diagnosing conditions , such as hepatomegaly and biliary atresia. Furthermore, the applicability of ultrasound technology enables point-of-care applications, and it is a key initial imaging evaluation in children presenting with acute abdominal pain. The ability to provide feedback in real time enhances pediatric gastroenterologists' decision-making and, in turn, significantly affects patient outcomes. Magnetic resonance imaging (MRI) is also a key modality in pediatric gastroenterology's diagnostic toolset for evaluating complex gastrointestinal disease. MRI, with newer modalities , such as MR enterography, plays an important role in the diagnosis of subtle small intestinal pathologies and the assessment of diseases , such as Crohn's disease. Its excellent soft tissue contrast allows the precise imaging of inflammation, strictures, and transmural complications that are challenging to detect with routine imaging methods. Furthermore, MRI is also a radiation-free option, a consideration of paramount importance when dealing with the pediatric age group, where ionizing radiation exposure is to be kept at a bare minimum. The imaging modality is not only diagnostic but also facilitates long-term management through the provision of critical information for monitoring of disease and assessment of response to treatment. Computed tomography (CT) imaging likewise has important applications in pediatric gastroenterology, specifically for rapid assessment of acute situations that demand prompt diagnosis. While use of CT in children is alarming with regards to radiation exposure, more advanced methods like iterative reconstruction and dose-saving approaches have yet to make it more feasible. CT is extremely useful for defining intricate intra-abdominal pathology , such as appendicitis, abscesses, and tumors. Studies indicate that wise use of CT supplemented with clinical assessment can lead to a process-oriented diagnosis without causing unwarranted surgery. Further, the use of multiphasic imaging techniques in combination produces maximal diagnostic benefit by providing global impressions of organ and vascular architecture that are necessary in the management of complex pediatric cases (Prad et al., 2020; Jaffer et al., 2022) (Figure 8.10).

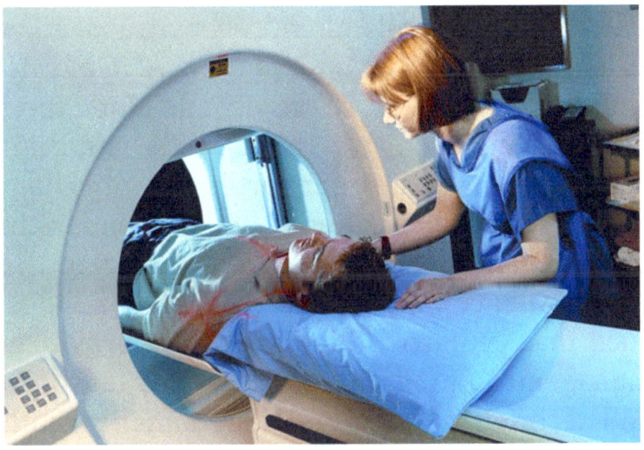

**Figure 8.10.** Imaging techniques and their applications.

*Source:* https://cdn.expresshealthcare.in/wp-content/uploads/2017/05/27123918/201705ehm39.gif.

## 8.3.3. Endoscopic Procedures and Their Relevance

Endoscopic procedures occupy a pivotal place in pediatric gastroenterology, offering a least-invasive method of diagnosis and treatment of many pediatric gastrointestinal illnesses. Procedures , such as esophagogastroduodenoscopy (EGD) and colonoscopy enable gastroenterologists to see the mucosal lining of the gastrointestinal tract and take biopsies and intervene accordingly. For instance, endoscopic techniques allow for the diagnosis of inflammatory bowel diseases (IBD) like Crohn's disease and ulcerative colitis. Direct visualization of lesions, retrieval of histological data, and interventions, i.e., stricture dilation or polyp removal, considerably ease the treatment of these difficult cases in a pediatric age group. Endoscopy's ability to diagnose exceeds mere visualization, as evidenced by a study of Crohn's disease of the esophagus that demonstrated a high percentage of patients with endoscopy-induced clinical remission and mucosal healing after directed therapy. Endoscopic findings can have treatment implications, causing caregivers to modify standard therapeutic regimens in hopes of better outcomes. Particularly, the capacity to detect strictures or fistulas in the gastrointestinal tract makes intervention possible with a direct impact on symptom resolution and quality of life in pediatric chronic gastrointestinal disease. In this respect, the role of endoscopy transcends the aspect of diagnostic capability and becomes an essential therapeutic intervention. Also of relevance is the value of endoscopic procedures in their ability to assess disease activity and guide therapeutic interventions in inflammatory bowel disease. In a study involving ulcerative colitis, clinical indexes were found to correlate well with endoscopic activity and therefore supported the importance of endoscopic assessment of treatment plans. The data revealed that patients who had undergone endoscopic mucosal healing were at substantially improved risk of recurrence, highlighting the active role of endoscopy in disease management. Such evidence validates the inclusion of endoscopic examination in standard monitoring programs such that pediatric IBD patients are provided with timely and appropriate modifications in their management program. Last but not least, the continuous refinement of endoscopic techniques and technology can potentially enhance both diagnostic and therapeutic outcomes in pediatric gastroenterology, underscoring its irreplaceable significance in this field of medicine (Figure 8.11).

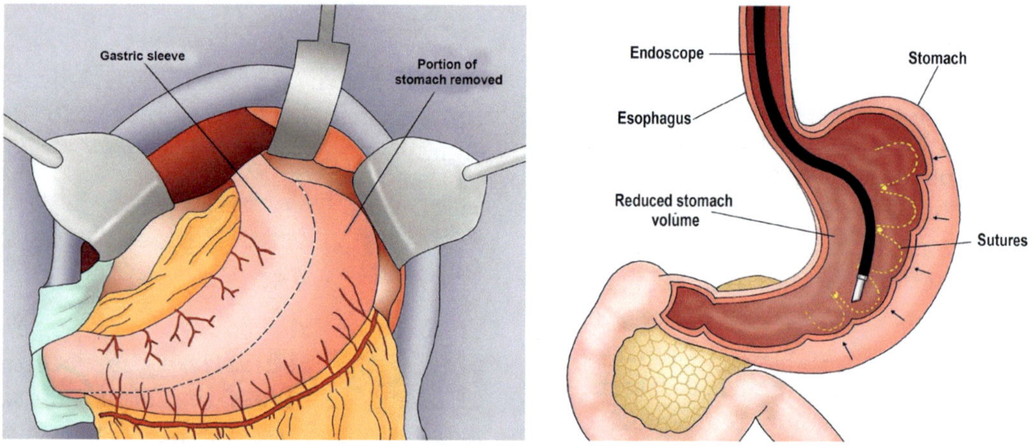


**Figure 8.11.** Endoscopic procedures play a pivotal role in the field of pediatric gastroenterology.

*Source:* https://www.ghadvances.org/cms/10.1016/j.gastha.2023.10.013/asset/fac67638-6749-4539-84e6-e37a8f2cd5c1/main.assets/gr3_lrg.jpg.

## Test Your Knowledge

1. Why are clinical evaluation and history taking important in diagnosing pediatric gastrointestinal disorders?
2. What roles do imaging and endoscopic procedures play in pediatric GI diagnosis?

## 8.4. Treatment Modalities in Pediatric Gastroenterology

**Learning Outcome**

1. Pharmacological treatments and their indications;
2. Nutritional management and dietary interventions;
3. Surgical options for severe gastrointestinal conditions.

Therapeutic strategies in pediatric gastroenterology are evolving rapidly, reflecting advances in medicine and expanding knowledge on pediatric gastrointestinal disease. For instance, management of gastrostomy granulomas, a frequent presenting complication in children with gastrostomy tubes, has classically included painful interventions like silver nitrate. Current data suggest that other interventions, , such as table salt, may bring dramatic benefits. A study at San Antonio Children's Hospital showed that the reduction in median granuloma size was greater using table salt compared to silver nitrate with increased parental satisfaction and fewer side effects. This points to a potential of less invasive, lower-cost treatment options, which are crucial in pediatric practice where patient comfort and family influence considerations are paramount. Therefore, exploring diverse treatment options is essential in the improvement of outcomes in pediatric gastroenterology (Jack et al., 2025). Apart from local complications like gastrostomy granulomas, pediatric gastroenterology also addresses functional gastrointestinal disorders like functional constipation (FC), which is a prevalent disorder in children. Traditional management has targeted lifestyle change and osmotic laxative treatment, yet approximately 30% of affected children are still symptomatic even with these interventions. The development of novel pharmacologic treatments has introduced new weapons against FC, including the FDA-approved drug linaclotide in children aged 6–17 years. Evaluation of these novel treatments emphasizes the need for ongoing research into their effectiveness and safety, since FC pathophysiology is different in the child compared to the adult population. This requirement as a basis for personalized therapeutic approaches marks a new tendency toward more tailored therapy in pediatric gastroenterology to enhance therapeutic outcomes in children (Wolfson et al., 2024). Incorporation of new therapeutic modalities requires complete understanding of their consequences in the pediatric group. Although the development of pharmacological as well as non-pharmacological modalities seems encouraging, the uniqueness of pediatric patients requires careful consideration for safety and side effect profiles. In addition to innovative treatment, standardization of methodologies and outcomes is required for effective treatment of gastrointestinal disorders in children in order to make comparisons between therapies. As evidenced by recent studies, there is a consensus emerging for the necessity to create individualized treatment plans that are a mirror of personal clinical requirements of every child. An innovative strategy based on current and future therapeutic modalities will ultimately lead to improved management strategies in pediatric gastroenterology such that the young patient will be given the best and most humane available care (Wolfson et al., 2024).

### 8.4.1. Pharmacological Treatments and Their Indications

Pharmacological therapy plays a key role in the treatment of most gastrointestinal diseases in pediatric gastroenterology due to the multifactorial and complex nature of most diseases. Pain syndrome is one such disease, which is common among children admitted to hospitals. Despite the availability of numerous analgesics , such as paracetamol, non-steroidal anti-inflammatory drugs (NSAIDs), and opioids, pain is often underdiagnosed and remains incompletely treated. The literature indicates that an understanding of the indication for each of the analgesics can be crucial, as well as their respective dosing and routes of administration. Opioids like morphine and fentanyl, for instance, are key drugs in managing severe pain but are potential candidates for serious side effects. By increasing the clinician's awareness of these medicines, quality of care in pediatric pain syndrome can improve dramatically, both acute and chronic pain needs being adequately addressed (Bykov et al., 2025). Of gastroenterological diseases in general, Cyclic Vomiting Syndrome (CVS) stands out due to its cyclical nature and massive impact on a patient's quality of life. Management of pediatric CVS often involves pharmacological interventions, which have evolved from expert opinion to evidence-based practice guidelines. Abortive and prophylactic treatments are highlighted in the guidelines. Anti-migraine medications are one of the pharmacological interventions, which are recommended in patients with a family or personal history of migraine. Drugs , such as 5-hydroxytryptamine 3 (5-HT3) and neurokinin 1 (NK-1) receptor antagonists are useful for abortive treatment. Further, beta-blockers and tricyclic antidepressants are suggested for prophylaxis, but caution regarding their side effects is advised. This multi-treatment approach emphasizes the efficacy of customized pharmacological therapy in the treatment of CVS in pediatric gastroenterology (Karrento et al., 2025). Additionally, not only does the application of pharmacological treatments offer relief from mere symptoms, but they also make a substantial contribution to the management of the disease and the prognosis of patients. The addition of nonpharmacologic therapies, along with pharmacologic therapy, is essential in the overall regimen of treatment for gastrointestinal pediatric illnesses. Interventions , such as trigger avoidance and behavioral changes complement the pharmacologic treatments, enhancing overall efficacy. Pharmacologic drugs should, however, be carefully selected and monitored for potential side effects, particularly in children. The intersection of customized pharmacologic therapy and a combined understanding of pediatric patient needs can lead to optimized outcomes and fewer complications. Ultimately, an advanced style of medication management is integral to the practice of pediatric gastroenterology, indicative of the multiple needs of pediatric patients (Karrento et al., 2025) (Figure 8.12).

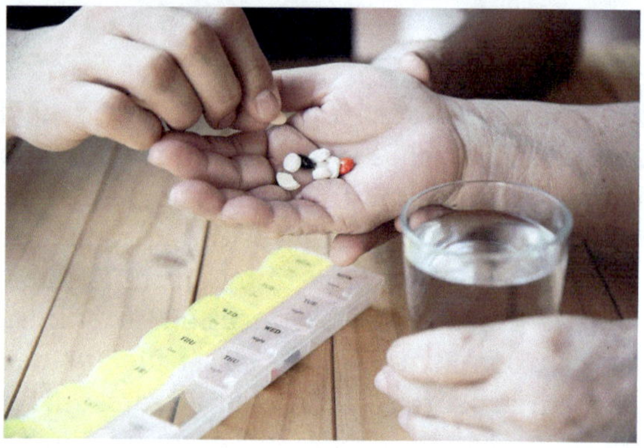

**Figure 8.12.** Pharmacological treatments and their indications.

*Source:* https://nirvanhospital.com/wp-content/uploads/2023/12/Integrating-Medication-Management.png.

### 8.4.2. Nutritional Management and Dietary Interventions

Nutritional care and dietary management are central to the practice of pediatric gastroenterology, and especially in the management of conditions like Crohn's disease. Specialized formulas have become an essential treatment in caring for this population, as identified in systematic reviews of the literature pointing towards their effectiveness. For instance, one research summarized 23 individual studies in over 1,000 children and concluded that the patients receiving specialized formulas had significantly higher rates of mucosal healing and remission compared to those receiving standard formulas. Specifically, the evidence indicated that mucosal healing rates between 63% and 89% were achieved following eight weeks of treatment, which indicated the potential of directed dietary interventions in bringing about healing. By means of individualization of nutritional supply according to pediatric patients' needs, medical professionals are able to maximize the impact of treatment and promote long-term management of health in pediatric gastroenterology, substantiating the need for such interventions as a fundamental part of clinical practice (Richard et al., 2025). Food Insecurity, Increasing across the United States, is a different type of challenge in pediatric gastroenterology as it impacts the nutritional status of these children. Providers are most often best positioned to advise families who are food insecure due to their specialized training in nutrition support. Recent studies indicate that the majority of caregivers report not being properly screened for food insecurity within health centers; only 10–15% of caregivers reported ever being asked about their level of food security during consultations. Furthermore, while over half of the healthcare providers reported feeling comfortable to administer screenings, few of them did so on a regular basis. This discrepancy highlights a significant barrier that can interfere with successful nutritional care. Closing these gaps with disciplined screening routines and empowering families with adequate resources can lead to improved nutritional condition and general well-being in children with gastrointestinal illnesses (Morrow et al., 2024). Effective diet management also calls for careful attention to the individual needs and preferences of pediatric patients while fostering an environment that invites open discussion between caregivers and families. Individualized diet regimens will enhance compliance and therapeutic outcomes, as diets that are viewed by patients as acceptable and achievable will be adhered to. Additionally, disseminating education on the importance of nutrition for gastrointestinal health will enable families to make informed food choices. Gastroenterology clinicians, as a result, play a significant role in educating families about the contribution of diet to disease management, including its value for the addition of varied and nutrient-dense food to children's diets. Through the provision of dietary interventions compatible with family belief systems and patient preference, health providers can improve dietary adherence and promote the long-term health and well-being of pediatric patients (Richard et al., 2025).

### 8.4.3. Surgical Options for Severe Gastrointestinal Conditions

Severe gastrointestinal disease in the pediatric patient can be treated surgically when conservative measures are not mitigating the illness or when the condition is severely jeopardizing the health of the patient. Malrotation or atresia, inflammatory bowel disease, and perforated diverticulitis are classic surgical indications. Pediatric gastrointestinal surgery has evolved significantly over the past few decades with the progress in minimally invasive surgery introducing a number of benefits associated with it compared to open surgery. These surgeries reduce postoperative discomfort and recovery time and have lower complication rates, which makes them extremely useful in younger patients who can have comorbidities to be dealt with accordingly. In addition, pediatric surgeons possess specialized training designed to equip them to deal with the unique anatomical and physiological parameters of children, allowing for individualized surgical techniques optimizing outcomes. Surgical intervention for severe gastrointestinal disorders encompasses a variety of procedures ranging from repair operations in anatomical deformities to resection of diseased segments of intestine. In inflammatory bowel disease, bowel resection or strictureplasty can be performed by surgeons to prevent severe injury or obstruction. In congenital conditions , such as gastroschisis, early surgery is necessary so that normal feeding and development are possible.

Postoperative care is crucial in the pediatric patient since complications may be induced by growth issues and ongoing patient growth. Ongoing interdisciplinary communication among surgeons, gastroenterologists, and nutritionists is important in an effort to offer maximal care that addresses immediate surgical requirements as well as sustained gastrointestinal function. The integration of the use of technological capabilities, , such as imaging and endoscopy, also optimizes preoperative planning and postoperative care in an effort to enable surgical results to be maximized. The scope of the surgical role is not only acute resolution of serious gastrointestinal illness but also long-term care of resultant complications and overall quality-of-life improvement for the patient. Children postoperation can have numerous problems, including nutritional deprivation, which require a multidisciplinary team to assure a healthy growth and development. Individualized dietetic support is necessary, particularly in the case where resection of the bowel may hamper absorptive capacity. Psychological counseling and education of patients and family members become vital components of postoperative care, addressing any anxiety or fear towards surgery. As pediatric gastroenterology continues to grow, ongoing research and clinical trials are required to enhance surgical techniques and patient care so that children with complex gastrointestinal disease receive effective and safe treatment. The emphasis must remain on an individualized, patient-centered model that involves the medical, surgical, and psychosocial elements of care and ultimately improves the overall well-being of this vulnerable population (Andrew et al., 2022; Laura et al., 2022) (Figure 8.13).

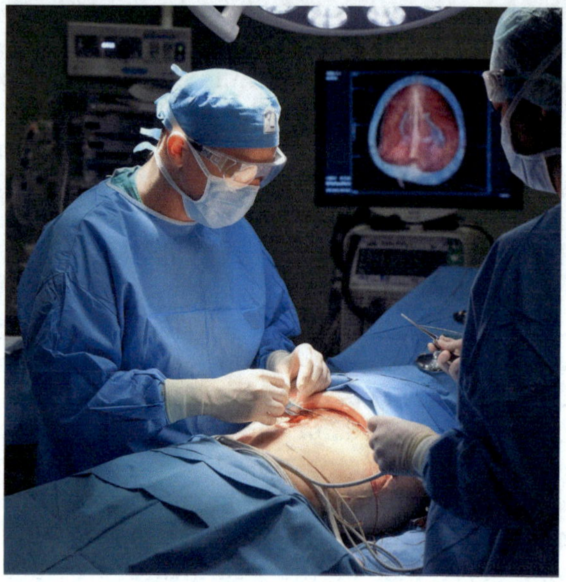

**Figure 8.13.** Surgical options for severe gastrointestinal conditions.

*Source:* https://drtejasdharia.com/wp-content/uploads/2025/04/image3-10.webp.

## Test Your Knowledge

1. What are common pharmacological treatments used in pediatric gastrointestinal disorders, and what are their indications?
2. How do dietary interventions and surgical options contribute to managing severe gastrointestinal conditions in children?

## 8.5. Impact of Gastrointestinal Disorders on Child Development

**Learning Outcome**

1. Physical growth and nutritional status;
2. Psychological effects and emotional well-being;
3. Social implications and quality of life.

Gastrointestinal disease in children is closely linked to developmental problems, possibly inhibiting physical and intellectual growth. Malnutrition caused by illnesses , such as celiac disease or persistent diarrhea may lead to disrupted nutrient absorption, thus disrupting a child's growth pattern and health. For example, a child's potential to thrive is greatly dependent on proper nutrition of essential nutrients, which facilitate such fundamental processes as brain growth and immune function. In severe cases, undiagnosed conditions can manifest themselves as failure to thrive, wherein there is impaired height and weight growth, coupled with retardation in social and mental development.

These children can also experience academic functioning disturbance due to fatigue and discomfort, ultimately affecting social and emotional development too. Thus, early diagnosis and intervention are needed in order to avoid the negative impacts of poor gastrointestinal function and to enable optimal developmental outcome in children. The global spread of the COVID-19 pandemic has added more issues for children suffering from gastrointestinal disease, as diagnosis and management have become more complex. As observed in many clinical cases, early medical treatment has been compromised, leading to delayed diagnosis and treatment. A nice example is a situation where gastrointestinal symptoms of celiac disease spiraled into life-threatening features due to lockdown. During the pandemic, the majority of healthcare professionals were reallocated to address COVID-19, shortening their availability for routine pediatric evaluation and care of chronic conditions. The psychological effect associated with these intermissions, including heightened fear and tension regarding health conditions, may even impact the child's overall development. This intersection, therefore, of gastrointestinal disease and pandemic restriction has ominous implications for the physical, as well as the mental, welfare of affected children, imposing a requirement of increased sensitivity and expert healthcare concern.

The interplay between gastrointestinal disease and child development is multifaceted, particularly with consideration of the psychosocial nature of children's lives. Dysfunctional gastrointestinal performance can generate significant emotional disruption through such effects as anxiety, depression, and social withdrawal. Researchers have noted that kids with chronic gastrointestinal issues often exhibit behavioral changes that affect their social interactions with peers, which further contributes to isolating them during key development stages. For example, it was reported in one study that behavioral and mental illness phenomena occur on a regular basis in kids with conditions , such as functional gastrointestinal disorders, in which presenting symptoms may resemble those of depression or anxiety. Thus, treatment of the psychosocial facets of gastrointestinal disease is central to maximizing care. Pediatric gastroenterologists must adopt an interdisciplinarity team approach, integrating mental health care into treatment plans in order to maximize overall developmental outcomes for children with such life-long gastrointestinal challenges (Figure 8.14).

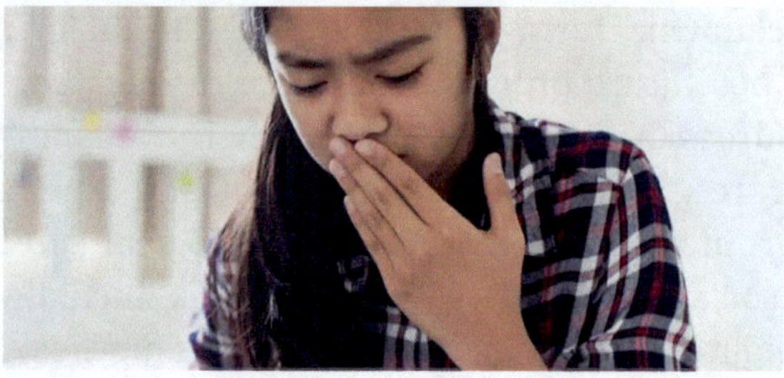

**Figure 8.14.** A young girl covers her mouth, appearing nauseous, which may indicate symptoms of an underlying gastrointestinal issue.

*Source:* https://cdhf.ca/wp-content/uploads/2022/08/holdingmouth.jpg.

## 8.5.1. Physical Growth and Nutritional Status

In pediatric gastroenterology, monitoring the growth of children as well as their nutrition is of primary importance, particularly in those with risk factors , such as preterm birth or long-standing gastrointestinal disease. Regular monitoring by weight, length, and head circumference has particular relevance in the detection of potential growth faltering or undernutrition, most significantly in discharged neonatal infants. The need for tailored nutritional treatment is best understood when growth measures indicate significant variation, , such as loss of over −2 standard deviations of weight or length. Aggressive early intervention through staged nutrition can trigger recovery and return infants to normal growth trajectories, underlining the importance of continued follow-up with healthcare providers to optimize outcomes (Haiden et al., 2025). Infant nutrition care necessitates a comprehensive understanding of changing nutrition needs with every developmental milestone. For instance, infants transitioning from breast milk to solids need to be observed by their brain development rather than age per se. The precise strategy not only promotes healthy growth patterns but also prevents complications created by early feeding regimens. For supplements, in the case of supplementation needs, addition of human milk fortifiers in breast-fed children or adequate protein-to-energy ratio in formula-fed children is crucial in catch-up growth. Nutritional intervention, so optimally tailored to particular needs, underscores the close interplay between habits in diet and development of the body, and demonstrates the value of timely and well-differentiated dietary adjustment in prevention of peril associated with growth retardation (Haiden et al., 2025). Particularly for inflammatory bowel diseases like Crohn's disease, the role of nutrition is not only confined to caloric but also includes the significant role of nutritional parameters and their implications on physical growth. Based on research, exclusive enteral nutrition (EEN), especially short-peptide preparations, has been extremely effective in inducing remission in children with active Crohn's disease.

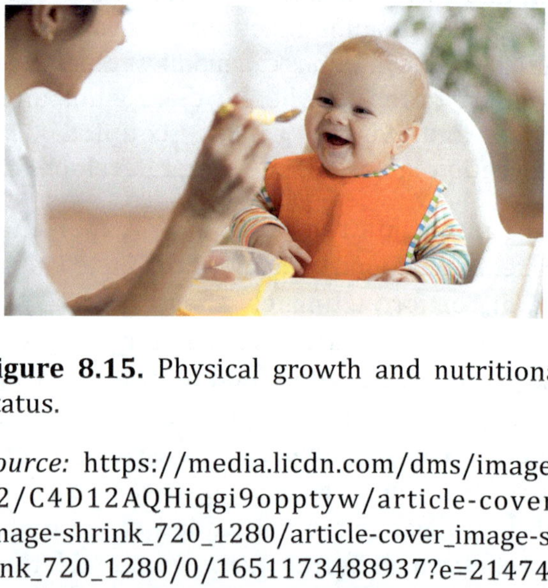

**Figure 8.15.** Physical growth and nutritional status.

*Source:* https://media.licdn.com/dms/image/v2/C4D12AQHiqgi9opptyw/article-cover_image-shrink_720_1280/article-cover_image-shrink_720_1280/0/1651173488937?e=2147483647&v=beta&t=pB4hMlkI49VVA2hY8rD2O6Kif_IFG1Rbl8-dgZqf-To.

The positive results that are associated with EEN, including improved Z-scores for weight-for-age and body mass index, indicate significant changes in both indices of growth and overall nutritional status. These data corroborate the necessity for gastroenterology practitioners to implement evidence-based nutrition therapies that are particularly aimed at healing gastrointestinal inflammation as well as at maximizing growth, thereby further supporting the overall health and development of children in pediatric clinics (Figure 8.15).

### 8.5.2. Psychological Effects and Emotional Well-Being

In pediatric gastroenterology, the emotional well-being and psychological effects on adolescents with inflammatory bowel disease (IBD) are of utmost concern. Studies have indicated a heightened risk for social impairment, emotional symptoms, and anxiety in this group of patients. Specifically, adolescents with IBD may experience more psychosocial difficulties and sleep disturbances that adversely affect their quality of life. The evidence of association of IBD symptom severity with psychosocial issues highlights the requirement of proper assessment during clinic consultations. The evidence highlights that although adolescents may describe comparable levels of psychosocial symptoms to those described by comparable peers, parental report tends to be indicative of increased frequencies of emotional distress and social problems, reflecting differential perception that can render treatment planning difficult (Pirinen, 2012). In addition, psychological morbidity spillovers into physical symptoms that can potentially exacerbate the challenges faced by young patients. Empirical research accentuates how depression and anxiety may lead to non-compliance with treatment guidelines, thereby complicating IBD management. Literature points out risk factors , such as increased severity of disease and decreased socioeconomic status that are responsible for a large share of psychological burden for such patients. Furthermore, young and adolescent patients also experience physical symptoms , such as abdominal pain and sleep disturbances directly related to their emotional state. These associated factors need to be addressed by healthcare providers because psychologically based interventions can contribute significantly to the improvement in patient outcomes through the facilitation of medication compliance and overall quality of life for adolescents and children with IBD (Benchimol et al., 2016). In conclusion, the association of psychological health with physical IBD symptoms demands treatment using a multi-dimensional framework. Doctors must incorporate psychosocial evaluation as part of their routine medical assessment on a regular basis to ensure integrative treatment. Adolescents with IBD difficulties typically require special psychological treatment specifically tailored to their unique emotional and social needs. By involving adolescents, parents, and medical providers in partnership, one can create a culture that encourages open dialogue regarding mental health. Not only does this collaborative approach allow for the identification of psychosocial issues but it also enables patients and families to manage the complexity of chronic illness and ultimately foster resilience and optimize long-term outcomes in pediatric gastroenterology (Pirinen, 2012).

### 8.5.3. Social Implications and Quality of Life

Social consequences of pediatric gastroenterology suggest a range of challenges faced by caregivers and families in the case of diagnosis with gastrointestinal diseases in a child. The diseases not only impact the physical health of the child but also put emotional and psychological burdens on family dynamics. Parents are typically fighting to navigate a healthcare system, attempting to receive adequate treatment and support while they work with their child's illness. The need for frequent medical appointments, diet changes, and potential hospitalizations will disrupt everyday life, affect the family's routine and instill a sense of instability. Although the caregivers have the burden, their own mental health is also compromised, creating tension and anxiety, further complicating the entire family situation and quality of life for the child and siblings as well. As older children grow up with gastrointestinal disease, their social lives are affected, which affects their quality of life. Symptoms , such as food restrictions, frequent bathroom trips, and unpredictability of symptoms lead to social withdrawal or anxiety in school and peer situations. Social withdrawal can precipitate feelings of inadequacy or embarrassment, which negatively affects the child's self-esteem as well as his or her mental well-being. In addition, the necessity for medical accommodations while at school may expose children to stigmatization or misinterpretation by teachers as well as peers, hindering social development. It is essential that schools implement support measures that promote inclusion so that children with gastrointestinal disorders can excel both academically and socially and have a more balanced perception of their health. Additionally, children's chronic gastrointestinal disorder prognosis is also very much dependent on proper management and access to healthcare. For instance, active interventions , such as specialized nutritional care, mental health services, and palliative care options will greatly enhance a child's quality of life. The growing recognition of the benefit of a multidisciplinary approach to treatment in pediatric gastroenterology allows for individualized therapy addressing both the physical and psychological features of these conditions. As noted in clinical guidelines, including those for metastatic gastric cancer, the role of genetic risk assessment is forward-facing in early management and eventual long-term outcome in susceptible populations. By targeting these more complex aspects, health professionals can enhance their approach to enhancing the social consequences and living conditions of pediatric patients (Figure 8.16).

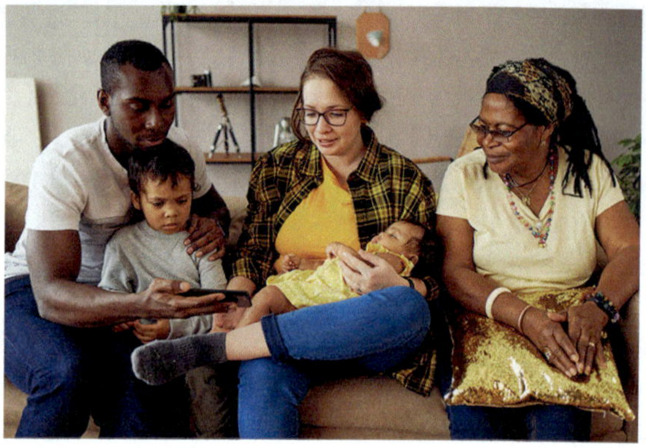

**Figure 8.16.** Social implications and quality of life.

*Source:* https://www.eurofound.europa.eu/sites/default/files/2025-01/image_activity_living_conditions_quality_life.png.

## Test Your Knowledge

1. How do gastrointestinal disorders affect a child's physical growth and nutritional status?
2. What are the psychological and social impacts of chronic GI disorders on children?

## 8.6. Advances in Pediatric Gastroenterology

**Learning Outcome**

1. Emerging research and clinical trials;
2. Innovations in diagnostic technologies;
3. Future directions in treatment and management.

Recent innovations in pediatric gastroenterology have greatly improved the diagnosis and treatment of numerous gastrointestinal diseases in children. Among the most significant advances is the incorporation of sophisticated imaging methods, including high-resolution endoscopy and magnetic resonance imaging (MRI), which allow for more detailed and enhanced visualizations of the gastrointestinal tract. These methods allow for less invasive treatment and increased accuracy in the detection of abnormalities, thus making it easier to intervene and treat at an early stage. In particular, the ability to test mucosal health at the microscopic level has revolutionized the treatment of inflammatory bowel disease (IBD) and celiac disease. As medical technology continues to evolve, ongoing investigation into new imaging modalities will continue to improve diagnostic accuracy in pediatric gastroenterology, eventually resulting in improved patient outcomes and reduced demand for more invasive surgical procedures. The use of biomarker testing has become increasingly prevalent in pediatric gastroenterology, particularly in the diagnosis and management of complex gastrointestinal diseases. Recent studies indicate the potential of biomarkers that are useful in identifying genetic predisposition towards certain disorders, , such as familial adenomatous polyposis and hereditary non-polyposis colorectal cancer. Furthermore, non-invasive biomarkers for conditions like lactose intolerance have been found to be efficient, changing the overall trend from application of outdated invasive diagnostic methods to more patient-oriented processes. These developments underscore the necessity of a multimodal approach that combines genetics, clinical evaluation, and biopsy results for formulating individualized treatment regimens, as in the case of chronic liver disease and the related complications. As these advancements continue to progress, they will enable maximization of modality management and enhanced quality of care in the pediatric population. In addition to diagnostic advancements, advancements in therapy in pediatric gastroenterology have also transformed management strategies for liver disease and gastroenterological illness.

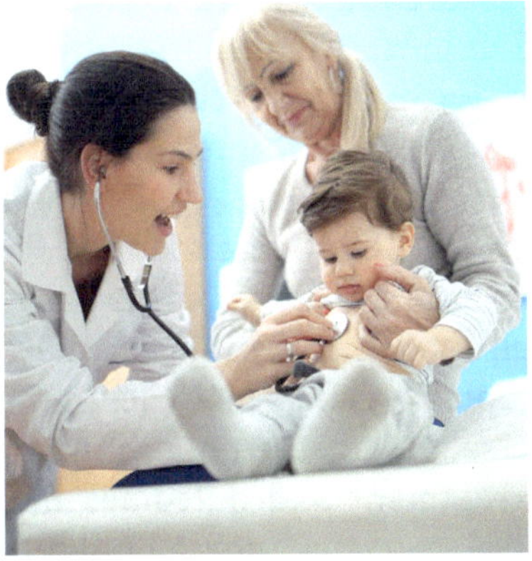

**Figure 8.17.** Advances in pediatric gastroenterology.

*Source:* https://tursium.com/wp-content/uploads/2022/04/Pediatric-Gastroenterology-i1-1008x1024.jpg.

The European Society for Pediatric Gastroenterology, Hepatology and Nutrition (ESPGHAN) has made a very significant step forward in disseminating information regarding acute liver failure (ALF), with recent conferences revolving around its intricacies and its treatment options. With improved understanding of the etiology and treatment of ALF, treatment strategies have now evolved to include both acute care modalities as well as long-term follow-up regimens. Featured developments are intensive care therapies, novel imaging modalities, and even personalized treatment paradigms designed specifically for the pediatric patient. Early diagnosis and curative therapies reflect the commitment to enhancing the quality of life for infected children, as they emphasize the significance of continuous research advancements and clinical practice in this rapidly evolving discipline (Jaffer et al., 2022; Zellos et al., 2021) (Figure 8.17).

### 8.6.1. Emerging Research and Clinical Trials

With emerging pediatric gastroenterology, evolving research and clinical trials are assuming increased importance in shaping the treatment protocols for some of the gastrointestinal conditions. Of especial interest are conditions , such as celiac disease (CeD), eosinophilic esophagitis (EoE), inflammatory bowel disease (IBD), and autoimmune hepatitis (AIH) that are at the forefront of these advancements. Emerging drug therapies , such as biologics and precision medicine treatments are under investigation to simplify treatment and outcomes in pediatric patients. For instance, novel gluten-degrading enzymes and zonulin blockers are some of the promising drugs for changing CeD's course. By tailoring interventions according to proteomics breakthroughs, doctors can better treat the unique characteristics of these conditions among children, ultimately providing improved care (Dipasquale et al., 2020). Clinical trials are essential to establish a therapy's safety and efficacy in newly introduced treatments among pediatric patient populations. With scientists looking to the therapeutic horizon for EoE, they are testing biologics that act on specific immune pathways, thereby offering a more tailored strategy compared to current therapies. Drugs , such as dupilumab and other IL-13 antagonists form the focus of such studies, and there is evidence of disparate efficacy between various patient groups. This emphasizes the requirement for additional pediatric-specific data in order to completely support these decisions. Likewise, in IBD, studies revolve around biologics like vedolizumab and small molecules like tofacitinib, which show promise in treating refractory disease. These clinical assessments are crucial since novel therapies require careful examination to determine their safety and effectiveness in pediatric populations (Dipasquale et al., 2020). Yet another essential element of ongoing research involves the investigation of the efficacy of nonconventional therapies, including cannabinoid-based ones, which have been found to be effective in treating resistant conditions.

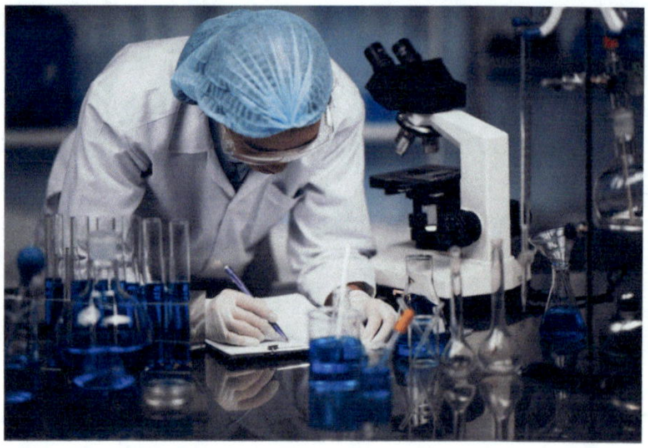

**Figure 8.18.** A scientist records observations in a laboratory surrounded by microscopes and glassware containing blue solutions, representing active research and experimentation in a clinical or biomedical setting.

*Source:* https://attraxcdnprod1-freshed3dgayb7c3.z01.azurefd.net/1481126/e40ce6f4-d08e-41da-9b68-65e34e789e42/2025.4.23.14553/img/10977109-1a28-4022-fdef-08db669d4adc.

New findings suggest that Cannabidiol (CBD) may be useful for children experiencing diseases , such as Dravet syndrome, a life-threatening epilepsy condition that may also present in conjunction with gastrointestinal conditions. Systematic reviews of various clinical trials indicate that CBD can reduce seizure frequency substantially, representing a worthwhile adjunct therapy. Inasmuch as findings of this type are not particularly relevant to gastroenterology, they do point towards the interrelatedness of much pediatric disease and the need for multidisciplinary treatment strategies. As these discoveries continue to develop, the pediatric gastroenterology profession needs to stay alert and prepared to incorporate effective new treatments into practice, providing holistic care for affected children (Figure 8.18).

## 8.6.2. Innovations in Diagnostic Technologies

Improved diagnostic technologies over the past few years have significantly advanced pediatric gastroenterology with increased detection and management of gastrointestinal disease in children. Some of the significant advances include the use of high-definition endoscopy, where there is far more vibrant visualization of the gastrointestinal tract. This has become imperative for identifying very subtle mucosal changes, and thus it is a very valuable tool for the early diagnosis of gastric and intestinal cancer. Moreover, the innovation of technologies , such as narrow-band imaging has enabled more precise discrimination among various tissues, hence enhancing efficiency in diagnosis. Such technologies, along with empowering healthcare professionals to provide early intervention, also reduce the need for more invasive interventions, eventually leading to better patient outcomes. The integration of artificial intelligence into imaging interpretation is another frontier, making pattern recognition and diagnostic capabilities better, thus making practice in pediatric gastroenterology revolutionized. Aside from endoscopic technology, advancements, new methods in biomarker discovery have revolutionized pediatric gastroenterology diagnostic practices. More recognition of the role of biomarkers in gastrointestinal disease has led to developing non-invasive tests capable of complementing traditional imaging modalities. For instance, fecal calprotectin and serum inflammatory markers provide such vital information in inflammatory bowel disease (IBD) that earlier diagnosis and better disease activity monitoring are possible in children. All this makes for more personalized treatment approaches, with physicians being able to administer focused interventions according to biomarker profiles. Also, continuous research and development of new biomarkers are constantly enriching the armory of gastroenterologists with diagnostic tools. This trend is also an indicator of the need for interdisciplinarity in pediatric medicine, as advances in the laboratory are transferred into clinical expertise with even more patient management results overall. Lastly, the monumental leaps in imaging devices, , such as magnetic resonance enterography (MRE) and computed tomography (CT) enterography, are welcome additions to pediatric gastroenterology's diagnostic toolkit. MRE is a non-radiation technique, particularly valuable in monitoring conditions like Crohn's disease in children, as it minimizes the associated risks from ionizing radiation that is common with CT scans. These newer imaging technologies allow for complete studies of the small intestine and surrounding structures, which are crucial for accurate diagnosis and evaluation of complications. Furthermore, advances in technology , such as three-dimensional imaging have improved visualization and understanding of anatomical variations and pathology. All these advances highlight further concern for continued improvement in diagnostic accuracy and safety in pediatric gastroenterology, resulting in effective management plans for gastrointestinal disorders in young patients.

## 8.6.3. Future Directions in Treatment and Management

The future of treatment and management in pediatric gastroenterology is bound to transform profoundly with the advent of more sensitive forms of treatment aimed at specific disorders.

Recognition of illnesses , such as Cyclic Vomiting Syndrome (CVS) makes it distinguishable as an illness requiring customized therapy with specific consideration given to the patient's unique symptoms and triggers. With recent scientific advances revealing multifactorial etiologies of CVS, including abnormal brain-gut mechanisms and gastrointestinal motility disorders, clinicians can now better design specific treatment approaches. Symptomatic and supportive care still remain the foundation in the midst of acute attacks, but prophylactic abortive attack stopping with early therapy can now attempt to abort attacks. Thus, strategic individualizations of management can decidedly enhance the quality of life of a child to such an extent that post-management protocols get increasingly sophisticated and attuned to patient experiences (Raucci et al., 2020). As functional gastrointestinal disorders (FGIDs) continue to become widespread in pediatric practice, the future of gastroenterological management has to be centered around maximizing diagnostic and therapeutic protocols. Recent criticisms of the classification schemes offer an incentive to underscore the multifactorial etiology of the FGIDs and their convergence with other categories, complicating treatment. However, through the use of standardized diagnostic criteria, improved understanding of these diseases can be achieved, and epidemiologic studies can inform new directions in research. Through the analysis of subgroups by symptom patterns, subsequent studies may reveal critical information concerning the pathophysiologic processes involved, leading to more optimal modes of treatment. Detailed research is essential in developing targeted interventions that depart from empirical therapies, so treatment is evidence-based and patient-specific to the specific nature of pediatric patients (Taminiau et al., 2005). Also essential is the multidisciplinary team collaboration in breaking open the future progress in pediatric gastroenterology between researchers, geneticists, and practitioners. Genetic susceptibility and environmental factors influencing gastrointestinal health will be investigated to yield more information on common as well as on unusual illnesses. Analysis of single gene mutations and phenotypic expression can indicate pathways toward individualized medicine so that clinicians can anticipate and tailor treatment based on genetics. Furthermore, enhanced education and training of healthcare providers will be required in order to integrate these advances into daily practice. By being at the forefront of current research and fostering collaboration, the specialty can optimize management strategies, which in turn benefits outcomes for children suffering from gastrointestinal disease (Raucci et al., 2020; Taminiau et al., 2005) (Figure 8.19).

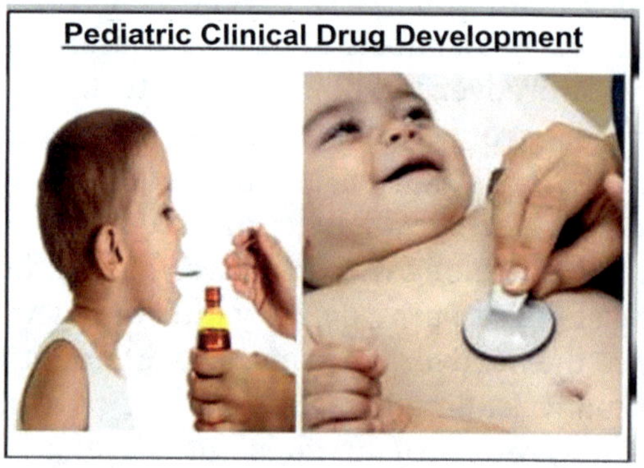


**Figure 8.19.** The future of treatment and management in pediatric gastroenterology.

*Source:* https://s3.amazonaws.com/images.powershow.com/7087717.pr.jpg.

## Test Your Knowledge

1. What are some recent innovations in diagnostic technologies for pediatric gastrointestinal disorders?
2. What are the future directions in the treatment and management of pediatric GI disorders?

## SUMMARY

The pediatric gastroenterology is a vital section of specialty intended to fulfill the unique gastrointestinal needs of children. As highlighted in our analysis, the image of pediatric gastroenterology is defined by multiple determinants, including disease prevalence like inflammatory bowel disease as well as the impact of infectious diseases. Also, identification of these complexities is not only crucial for effective diagnosis and treatment, but also for constructing preventive strategies that can significantly reduce the prevalence of these disorders. Continued research is imperative to advance our understanding of pediatric gastrointestinal disorders and improve clinical outcomes in affected children. Beyond that, there is a need to overcome the challenges faced in pediatric gastroenterology, particularly in low- and middle-income countries, to increase healthcare accessibility and quality. The unavailability of specialized health care facilities leads to delayed diagnosis and inadequate treatment, exacerbating the morbidity of gastrointestinal diseases. Strengthening healthcare infrastructure and training of health professionals are important measures. As it has been researched in the literature, long-term support and investment in health care facilities can supplement efforts in global health to provide improved health services to vulnerable populations, ultimately leading to better pediatric health outcomes (Rao et al., 2025). Finally, the treatable nature of most pediatric gastrointestinal diseases underscores the need for integration of care that combines both medical and socio-economic considerations. Pediatric gastroenterology's nuances require a multi-disciplinary approach that incorporates clinical expertise as well as appreciation of the various socio-cultural determinants of child health. Instituting preventive measures, , such as nutritional and hygiene education, along with the best available treatment modalities, can significantly minimize risks and provide better health in children. The overlap of findings from diverse research indicates the need for a systemic and collaborative approach to pediatric gastroenterology, as evidenced by findings pointing to the positive outcomes of coordinated care and interventions, particularly in disorders with significant inflammatory components, , such as pustular psoriasis (Tang et al., 2025).

One area of concern in the field of pediatric gastroenterology is the management of eosinophilic esophagitis (EoE), a condition that must be treated throughout childhood and into adulthood. Transferring patients from pediatric gastroenterology (pGI) to adult gastroenterology (aGI) presents critical issues of continuity of care. Key findings: An alarming majority were lost to follow-up, with results indicating that 16% of patients did not begin care with aGI specialists following the transition. In addition, the median time from the last pGI visit to the first aGI visit was surprisingly long, averaging approximately 299 days for clinic visits and 730 days for endoscopy evaluations. This lag complicates patient management and accentuates the need for clear protocols to facilitate seamless transitions among care in pediatrics and adults, pointing to an imperative gap that needs to be urgently filled in the expanding arena of pediatric gastroenterology (Webber et al., 2025). In examining the effect of this transition period on patient outcomes, it is important to consider the role of drug non-adherence as well as symptom worsening. The study pointed out a disparity in medication adherence rates, where the latter rose from 7% in pGI care to 26% in aGI care, pointing to an alarming pattern where the patients get a higher frequency of symptoms like heartburn on transfer. The fact that endoscopic and histologic severity remained consistently unaltered despite these clinical alterations suggests that the changeover in care does not favorably augment the care of the patients. The importance of such results is significant; they highlight the requirement of interventions that not just reduce the transition process but also facilitate continuity of care in EoE patients. Hence, developing comprehensive protocols for this group is important as it goes a long way in averting potential deterioration in health outcome with pGI to aGI transition (Webber et al., 2025). Moreover, the broader implications of effective pediatric gastroenterology extend beyond treatment of specific conditions like EoE; they address an institution-wide need for innovation in the delivery of patient care mechanisms across all pediatric arenas. Emphasizing the development of combined models of care will provide young patients with receipt of both necessary clinical evaluations as well as psychosocial interventions as they move forward. This multi-faceted approach addresses the intricacies of the needs of pediatric patients and encompasses elements of education, dietary management, and ongoing monitoring in clinical practice. These approaches are crucial in ensuring that not only are the patients provided with clinical care, but also that they have an understanding of their health conditions, thereby leading to greater participation in their treatment plans. As pediatric gastroenterology evolves, multidisciplinary practice and patient-centered practice should remain the central focus of practice, enhancing overall outcomes across a lifetime.

## KEY TERMS FROM THIS CHAPTER

- Celiac disease (CeD)
- Disorders of gut-brain interaction (DGBIs)
- Gastric acid production
- Gastroesophageal reflux disease (GERD)
- Magnetic resonance imaging (MRI)
- Microbial populations
- Collaboration
- Functional gastrointestinal disorders
- Gastroenterology
- Inflammatory bowel disease (IBD)
- Mental health

## CRITICAL THINKING QUESTIONS

1. **The most common cause of acute diarrhea in children worldwide is:**
   a. *Salmonella*
   b. Rotavirus
   c. *E. coli*
   d. *Giardia*
2. **A child with persistent vomiting, visible peristalsis, and a palpable olive-shaped mass likely has:**
   a. Gastroesophageal reflux
   b. Pyloric stenosis
   c. Intussusception
   d. Appendicitis
3. **Which condition presents with currant jelly stools and a sausage-shaped abdominal mass?**
   a. Meckel's diverticulum
   b. Intussusception
   c. Hirschsprung's disease
   d. Pyloric stenosis
4. **Celiac disease in children is caused by sensitivity to:**
   a. Casein
   b. Lactose
   c. Gluten
   d. Fructose
5. **The most common cause of lower gastrointestinal bleeding in infants is:**
   a. Intussusception
   b. Meckel's diverticulum
   c. Anal fissure
   d. Hirschsprung's disease

## Short Answer Questions

1. Define celiac disease. Name the offending dietary protein.
2. What is the function of Oral Rehydration Solution (ORS)?
3. Describe the etiology, clinical features, diagnosis, and management of acute diarrhea in children.
4. Discuss gastroesophageal reflux disease (GERD) in infants, presentation, diagnosis, and treatment.
5. Explain the pathophysiology, clinical presentation, and treatment of Hirschsprung's disease.

## Answers to Critical Thinking Questions

1. (b); 2. (b); 3. (b); 4. (c); 5. (c)

## REFERENCES


1. Abusuliman, M., Jamali, T., & Zuchelli, T. E. (2025). Advances in gastrointestinal endoscopy: A comprehensive review of innovations in cancer diagnosis and management. *World Journal of Gastrointestinal Endoscopy*. https://www.semanticscholar.org/paper/22cce6368c3fee9d868e7855f466e99c866b6bb7 (accessed on 16th June 2025).
2. Aderinto, N., Olatunji, G., Kokori, E., Ajayi, Y. I., Akinmoju, O., Ayedun, A. S., Ayoola, O. I., et al. (2024). The efficacy and safety of cannabidiol (CBD) in pediatric patients with Dravet syndrome: A narrative review of clinical trials. *European Journal of Medical Research, 29*. https://www.semanticscholar.org/paper/175ac81b2555be7bb3d56e64b05c0215a45ce4e6 (accessed on 16th June 2025).
3. Beaton, D., Chaparro, M., Ellul, P., Katsanos, K., et al. (2019). Diagnosis and outcome of esophageal Crohn's disease. https://core.ac.uk/download/288156918.pdf (accessed on 16th June 2025).
4. Bilican, G., Karakan, T., Eğritaş Gürkan, Ö., Sabhan, H., Hedin, C., Forss, A., Petrousis, G., et al. (2025). P0376 advancing intestinal ultrasound for IBD in Turkey: Results of a national survey. *Journal of Crohn's and Colitis*. https://www.semanticscholar.org/paper/30611e47cd0b36def50c23f1da2c6676be6ab456 (accessed on 16th June 2025).
5. Nylund, K., Maconi, G., Hollerweger, A., Ripolles, T., Pallotta, N., Higginson, A., Serra, C., Dietrich, C. F., Sporea, I., Saftoiu, A., Dirks, K., Hausken, T., Calabrese, E., Romanini, L., Maaser, C., Nuernberg, D., & Gilja, O. H. (2017). EFSUMB Recommendations and Guidelines for Gastrointestinal Ultrasound. EFSUMB-Empfehlungen und Leitlinien des Gastrointestinalen Ultraschalls - Teil 1: Untersuchungstechniken und Normalbefund (Langversion). *Ultraschall in der Medizin (Stuttgart, Germany : 1980), 38*(3), e1–e15. https://doi.org/10.1055/s-0042-115853(accessed on 16th June 2025).
6. Catassi, G., Vallorani, M., Cerioni, F., Lionetti, E., & Catassi, C. (2020). A negative fallout of COVID-19 lockdown in Italy: Life-threatening delay in the diagnosis of celiac disease. *Digestive and Liver Disease, 52*, 1092–1093. https://doi.org/10.1016/j.dld.2020.05.016 (accessed on 16th June 2025).
7. Corleto, V. D., D'Ambra, G., Delle Fave, G., Delle Fave, F., et al. (2015). Application of clinical indexes in ulcerative colitis patients in regular follow-up visit: Correlation with endoscopic 'mucosal healing' and implication for management. https://core.ac.uk/download/54524888.pdf (accessed on 16th June 2025).
8. Daly, M. B., Pal, T., Berry, M. P., Buys, S. S., Dickson, P., Domchek, S. M., Elkhanany, A., et al. (2021). Genetic/familial high-risk assessment: Breast, ovarian, and pancreatic, Version 2.2021, NCCN Clinical Practice Guidelines in Oncology. *Journal of the National Comprehensive Cancer Network, 19*, 77–102. https://doi.org/10.6004/jnccn.2021.0001 (accessed on 16th June 2025).'
9. Dipasquale, V., Serra, G., Corsello, G., & Romano, C. (2020). Standard and Specialized Infant Formulas in Europe: Making, Marketing, and Health Outcomes. *Nutrition in clinical practice : official publication of the American Society for Parenteral and Enteral Nutrition, 35*(2), 273–281. https://doi.org/10.1002/ncp.10261
10. Horne, A. W., & Missmer, S. A. (2022). Pathophysiology, diagnosis, and management of endometriosis. *BMJ*. https://doi.org/10.1136/bmj-2022-070750 (accessed on 16th June 2025).

11. Kansra, A. R., Lakkunarajah, S., & Jay, M. S. (2021). Childhood and adolescent obesity: A review. *Frontiers in Pediatrics, 8*. https://doi.org/10.3389/fped.2020.581461 (accessed on 16th June 2025).

12. Kyryk, V. (2024). *'Cell and Organ Transplantology*. https://www.semanticscholar.org/paper/6a1b536f3691ad0d162e4187a4a2e2ffd1507b5f (accessed on 16th June 2025).

13. Maier-Hein, L., Eisenmann, M., Sarıkaya, D., März, K., Collins, T., Malpani, A., Fallert, J., et al. (2021). Surgical data science – From concepts toward clinical translation. *Medical Image Analysis, 76*, 102306–102306. https://doi.org/10.1016/j.media.2021.102306 (accessed on 16th June 2025).

14. Morrow, R., Stahl, M. G., Liu, E., Shull, M., Germone, M. M., Nagle, S., Griffith, I., et al. (2024). Food insecurity screening practices in a pediatric gastroenterology population. *JPGN Reports, 5*, 135–139. https://www.semanticscholar.org/paper/5a9f109218c7d871230054a4570afe8b87074bdd (accessed on 16th June 2025).

15. Mylie, Q. (2018). The effects of 5-HT4 receptor agonists on interleukin-10 knockout mice. https://core.ac.uk/download/215153814.pdf (accessed on 16th June 2025).

16. Pirinen, T. (2012). Psychosocial symptoms and sleep in adolescents with pediatric inflammatory bowel disease. https://helda.helsinki.fi/items/697437b4-0d5b-4735-9de4-fdcd8de389d0(accessed on 16th June 2025).

17. Röckert Tjernberg, P., Malmborg, K., & Mårild, K. (2023). Coronavirus disease 2019 and gastrointestinal disorders in children. *Therapeutic Advances in Gastroenterology, 16*. https://www.semanticscholar.org/paper/7930e68859f5ac19ff1c60f299c8ab63daaee564 (accessed on 16th June 2025).

18. Rubino, F., Puhl, R. M., Cummings, D. E., Eckel, R. H., Ryan, D. H., Mechanick, J. I., Nadglowski, J., et al. (2020). Joint international consensus statement for ending stigma of obesity. *Nature Medicine, 26*, 485–497. https://doi.org/10.1038/s41591-020-0803-x (accessed on 16th June 2025).

19. Sen, S., & Misra, S. (2024). Pediatric obesity and non-hepatobiliary gastrointestinal disorders: A comprehensive review. *Gastroenterology, Hepatology & Digestive Disorders*. https://www.semanticscholar.org/paper/3e7e2fa8b72252f2c00d2e25e62b187db3c0f367 (accessed on 16th June 2025).

20. Tang, J., Hou, Z., Liao, W., Wang, Y., Zhang, G., Luo, Y., Gao, X., et al. (2025). Pediatric pustular psoriasis in Southern China: A 12-year retrospective analysis of 41 cases focusing on clinical characteristics and treatment outcomes. *Psoriasis: Targets and Therapy, 15*, 185–195. https://www.semanticscholar.org/paper/b53dbb77adad19704ec9ff1db5487f19cc0de5c1 (accessed on 16th June 2025).

21. Thomassen, R. A., Luque, V., Assa, A., Borrelli, O., Broekaert, I., Dolinsek, J., Martin-De-Carpi, J., et al. (2022). An ESPGHAN position paper on the use of low-FODMAP diet in pediatric gastroenterology. *Journal of Pediatric Gastroenterology and Nutrition, 75*, 356–368. https://doi.org/10.1097/mpg.0000000000003526 (accessed on 16th June 2025).

22. van Lennep, M., van Wijk, M. P., Omari, T., Salvatore, S., Benninga, M. A., & Singendonk, M. (2018). Clinical management of pediatric achalasia. *Journal of Pediatric Gastroenterology and Nutrition, 68*, 521–526. https://doi.org/10.1097/mpg.0000000000002221 (accessed on 16th June 2025).

# PEDIATRIC HEMATOLOGY AND ONCOLOGY

# 9

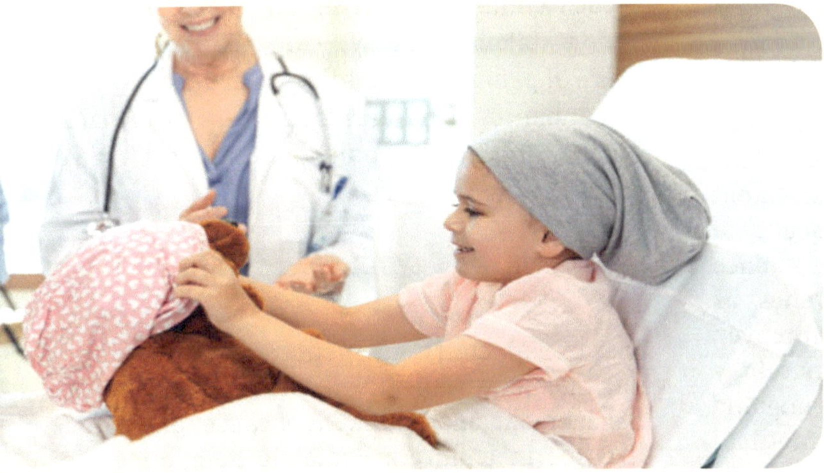

## LEARNING OBJECTIVES

**After studying this chapter, you will be able to:**

1. Give an overview of hematological disorders in children;
2. Understand the oncological disorders in children;
3. Discuss the role of pediatric hematologists and oncologists;
4. Focus on advances in research and treatment;
5. Explain psychological and social impacts on patients and families;
6. Know ethical considerations in pediatric hematology and oncology.

## Introduction

Pediatric hematology and oncology is a wide spectrum of conditions in children, which in the majority of instances calls for specialized medical intervention to realize optimal care and management. Underpinning this field is knowledge of hematologic disorders , such as anemia, hemophilia, and malignancies, including leukemia and tumors. As these conditions present issues that are different from each other, the treatment setting encompasses not just traditional chemotherapy and radiation but also innovative treatments , such as targeted therapy and immunotherapy. Multidisciplinary management is required, encompassing not just medical therapies but supportive care for addressing the psychological and emotional demands of the young patient as well as his family. The inclusion of hospitalists to manage care, especially in complex cases, has proved effective in improving education outcomes for medical professionals as well as streamlining care processes, thus increasing the overall patient satisfaction levels among caregivers and physicians (An et al., 2023). One characteristic of pediatric oncology is the increasing emphasis on minimizing long-term therapy complications. As an example, radiation therapy, while often necessary in the treatment of tumors, is full of risks, particularly to younger patients whose bodies are still developing and are more susceptible to damage. It is here that innovations like proton beam therapy (PBT) have become more popular, lower in toxicity compared to the older photon therapies. One of the benefits of PBT is reducing collateral damage to the surrounding healthy tissues from the target, hence a viable alternative in the treatment of tumors in the central nervous system in children (Smirnova et al., 2023). This adjustment is not only a scientific advancement but also an ethical need to improve the quality of life of cancer survivors in children since science still encourages the focus on the effectiveness as well as safety of treatment modalities. Moreover, the dynamic course of pediatric hematology and oncology underscores the worth in ongoing research and interaction among medical caregivers.

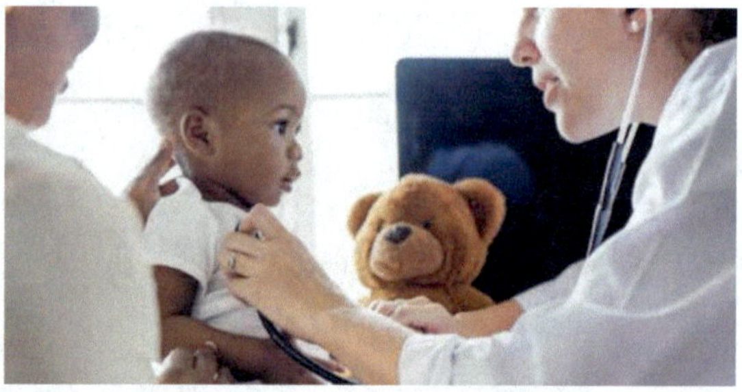

**Figure 9.1.** The field of pediatric hematology and oncology encompasses a wide range of conditions affecting children.

*Source:* https://external-content.duckduckgo.com/iu/?u=https%3A%2F%2Fwww.apolloinformationcentre.com%2Fwp-content%2Fuploads%2F2023%2F02%2FPediatric-Hematology-Oncology.jpg&f=1&nofb=1&ipt=a350ef74bef3182dc3daa3b062a5c674896d103ef0efbc67c2c8e42326add83f.

With every new treatment comes hope of improved outcomes for patients with dismal prognoses. Clinical trials represent a critical vehicle for increasing knowledge and opportunities for treatment, affording pediatric patients' exposure to novel interventions not otherwise available. Moreover, it requires active involvement of caregivers and parents in the care process as they assist in creating personalized care plans that are tailored to the unique needs of each child. By fostering an open discourse among stakeholders, we can ensure that the future of pediatric hematology and oncology not only enhances survival rates but also prioritizes the overall health of young patients first (An et al., 2023) (Figure 9.1).

## Definition of Pediatric Hematology and Oncology

The subspecialty of pediatric hematology and oncology is involved with the diagnosis, management, and treatment of cancer and blood diseases in children. Pediatric hematology is involved with a wide range of blood disorders , such as anemia, hemophilia, and sickle cell disease with emphasis on the uniqueness of blood diseases in a developing pediatric population. Pediatric oncology, however, is involved with various malignant disorders of the child , such as leukemia, lymphomas, and solid malignancies. The inherent physiological and developmental characteristics of children require special methods, since response to disease and treatment modalities might differ significantly from adults. The interplay of these two specialties highlights the essential role of interdisciplinary cooperation in providing optimal care and improving outcomes in children with hematological and oncologic disorders. One of the basic problems of pediatric hematology and oncology is the problem of risk of toxicity due to treatment regimens. Although better survival for certain diseases , such as acute lymphoblastic leukemia has been obtained, treatment-induced toxicity remains a cause of concern for both families and healthcare providers. Recent studies have underscored the need for uniform definitions of acute toxic effects since differences in reporting render it difficult to properly judge treatment outcomes by various protocols. Studies have identified fourteen specific acute toxic effects from hypersensitivity reactions to severe neurological complications that necessitate close monitoring. The consensus reached due to the convergence of global specialists assists in deciding standardized reporting indicators for enhancing comparison capacity of treatment modalities and designing more effective side effects management strategies (Attarbaschi et al., 2016).

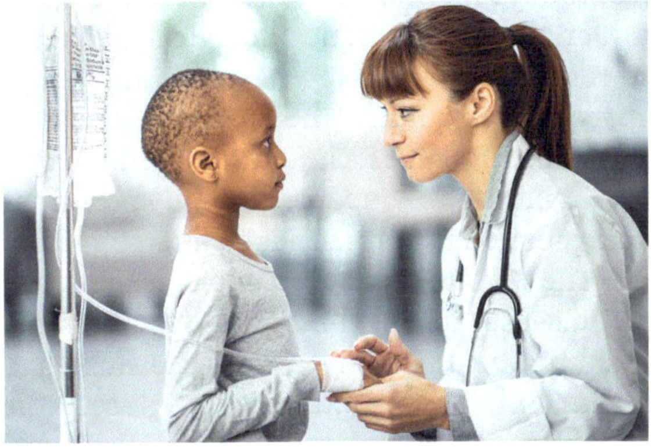

**Figure 9.2.** The specialized field of pediatric hematology and oncology focuses on diagnosis.

*Source:* https://pediatrics.med.jax.ufl.edu/images/flip-flop-pediatric-hematology-and-oncology-fellowship.jpg.

Another component that is similarly paramount to pediatric hematology and oncology is the accuracy of pathological diagnoses, particularly of central nervous system tumors, which can present certain special diagnostic challenges. With over a hundred types of tumors falling in this category, intra-heterogeneity in histopathological diagnoses can complicate treatment. New approaches , such as DNA methylation-based classification provide a potential answer, significantly improving diagnostic accuracy compared to conventional methods. Not only does this aid in understanding tumor biology better, but it also makes targeted therapy possible that can match the specific nature of the malignancy. By utilizing free online classifier tools designed for accessibility, health professionals can enhance pediatric cancer diagnostic practice to enhance patient outcomes as well as adjust treatment protocols accordingly (Aronica et al., 2018) (Figure 9.2).

## Importance of Specialized Care for Children

The requirement of specialized treatment in pediatric hematology and oncology cannot be stressed enough, given the special developmental problems involved in the treatment of children. A child with cancer or a blood disorder does not only impact the patient but the family as well. Because children may not be able to grasp the complexity of their condition, specialized education and counseling are required. As children's cognitive and affective capacities are far removed from those of adults,' family-centered education approaches must be highlighted by specialist care teams. Evidence verifies that open communication and tailored educational strategies are critical for attaining preferred patient outcomes, particularly in dealing with the overwhelming process of receiving a cancer diagnosis, which can compromise the information processing capacity and decisional involvement of a family (Ahern et al., 2016). By addressing these specific needs, specialized pediatric treatment is able to establish an environment conducive to both comprehension and adjustment. Furthermore, the intricacies of managing such illnesses as sickle cell disease (SCD) demonstrate the need for specialized methods of treating pediatric patients. Teenagers with SCD are generally at risk of increased mortality due to improper transition of care from pediatric to adult care, emphasizing the necessity for special care addressing their specific needs during this phase. Evidence indicates that psychological and social aspects play a great role in these patients' health care transitions, and therefore a multi-faceted approach should be adopted for proper management (Clayton-Jones et al., 2021). Caregivers must not only administer medical care but also goal-setting discussions and support networks that address feelings of isolation and stigma. Through cooperative partnerships and cultural familiarity with the environments in which each patient resides, physicians and other healthcare providers can enhance their assistance with transition, ultimately achieving enhanced health outcomes.

Furthermore, the incorporation of interdisciplinary collaboration into pediatric hematology and oncology care is essential to achieving maximum treatment outcomes and patient satisfaction. Total care is not left to oncologists and hematologists alone but also encompasses nurses, social workers, psychologists, and child life specialists who work together to form an integrated treatment plan. Blending of these disciplines enhances patient-family education, empowering families to be involved participants in their child's treatment. Thus, they are better able to cope with the complexities of healthcare, which are more likely to overwhelm them. Evidence is available that upholds a unifying framework of education, with emphasis placed on guaranteeing consistent communication between care teams and families (Landier et al., 2016). Implementing these interprofessional practices not only ensures patients are given timely and thorough care but also empowers families to stand effectively on behalf of their children's needs, thereby promoting the quality of care in pediatric hematology and oncology.

## 9.1. Overview of Hematological Disorders in Children

**Learning Outcome**

1. Common hematological disorders;
2. Symptoms and diagnosis;
3. Treatment options and management.

The range of hematological disorders in children encompasses an array of diseases that profoundly influence their well-being and quality of life. They are both malignant and non-malignant diseases, with the malignancies covering leukemia and lymphoma and the non-malignancies covering anemia and thrombocytopenia. Childhood cancers are characterized by unique biological behaviors and responses to therapy, necessitating unique approaches. Pediatric hematology therefore focuses on the research and understanding of these conditions, encouraging advancements in diagnostic tests, treatments, and supportive care. The emotional and psychological effect of these diseases on the children and their families should not be downplayed since the challenges of adapting to chronic disease necessitate multilevel approaches to care that go beyond the mere alleviation of physical distress. The evolving hematology care environment for pediatric hematologic diseases is nothing short of astounding, incorporating emerging therapies and multimodal interventions. Improved developments in immunotherapy and targeted therapy have also illuminated the outlooks for children diagnosed with advanced hematologic malignancies. The research on integrative modalities of medicine (IMMs) has also grown, as physicians seek to reconcile the multimodal needs of care for children. Research indicates that the majority of pediatric hematology-oncology (PHO) practitioners exhibit a desire to become more informed about IMMs, reflecting an eagerness to integrate complementary modalities , such as massage and mindfulness into patient care (Holly et al., 2025). These findings highlight the necessity of embracing an integrative model of treatment that combines evidence-based medical treatments with supportive interventions to best treat the patient. Moreover, the role of patient preferences and cultural traditions towards hematological disorder care has emerged as a significant factor.

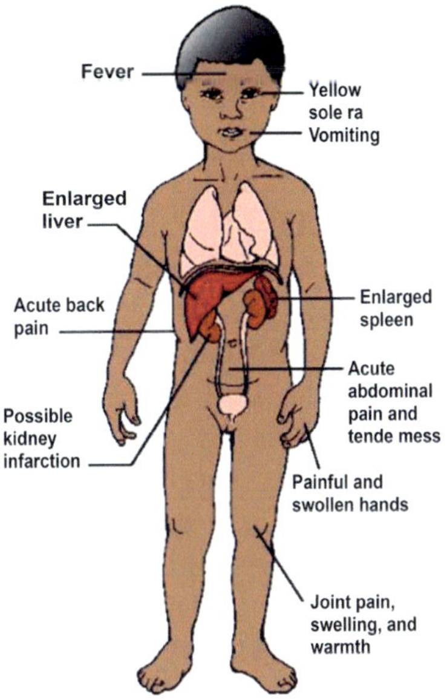


**Figure 9.3.** Overview of hematological disorders in children.

*Source:* https://nursekey.com/wp-content/uploads/2016/07/C52-FF1.gif.

For instance, a recent study highlighted that a considerable number of hospitalized children expressed a preference for inclusion of Kampo, Japanese traditional herbal medicine, as part of their treatment protocol (Kawashima, 2023). This indicates increased interest among patients and providers in adopting complementary therapies alongside conventional care. Knowledge of the disparate attitudes regarding treatment modalities and perceived effectiveness can assist healthcare professionals in individualizing care plans to improve compliance with patient needs. As pediatric hematology remains challenged by these issues, it is essential to involve families in the decision-making process in an environment that values their preferences and beliefs but also pursues optimal health outcomes (Figure 9.3).

### 9.1.1. Common Hematological Disorders

Pediatric hematological conditions embrace a wide range of diseases that bear significantly on the health and overall well-being of children afflicted by them. The most prevalent conditions are anemia, leukemia, and bleeding diseases , such as hemophilia and thrombocytopenia. Anemia, a deficiency in red blood cells or hemoglobin, can result from nutritional deficiencies, chronic disease, or genetic illness. It is thus essential to determine the causative agent so that effective treatment protocols can be undertaken. Similarly, leukemias in children, particularly acute lymphoblastic leukemia (ALL), are a significant challenge in pediatric oncology. These malignancies disrupt the normal hematopoiesis and produce diversified clinical manifestations which require extensive management protocols that blend pharmacological intervention, supportive therapy, and psychological support for both families and patients. The psychosocial impacts of the hematological disease on child patients cannot be overstated. Research has evidenced that children with such diseases are found to exhibit higher levels of psychological distress which can affect their quality of life and development. A family assessment of children with hematological and oncological illness revealed that while high adaptive functioning families fared better than maladaptive families, the latter displayed a significant amount of emotional load despite treatment. Furthermore, the pivotal role of family environment in creating resilience in children with the disease attests to the interdependent nature of medical and psychological intervention. Through improving supportive family interactions, healthcare providers can create healing and supportive environments for families to cope with the issues presented by pediatric hematological disorders (Sumrall et al., 2023). Besides psychological problems, thromboembolic complications present a huge issue in treating hematological malignancies. Venous Thromboembolism (VTE) has a high prevalence among patients, complicating treatment outcomes. Pediatric patients with blood malignancies typically present with thrombocytopenia, making anticoagulation treatment challenging in general. Thus, treatment is based on guidelines established for adult patients and modified for pediatric application. The delicate balance between preventing thrombosis and minimizing hemorrhagic complications reflects the complexity of treatment protocols for children with such conditions. Current literature emphasizes the need for evidence-based guidelines specifically directed towards such issues in the pediatric setting, culminating in safe and effective practice in pediatric hematology and oncology (Annibali et al., 2018) (Figure 9.4).

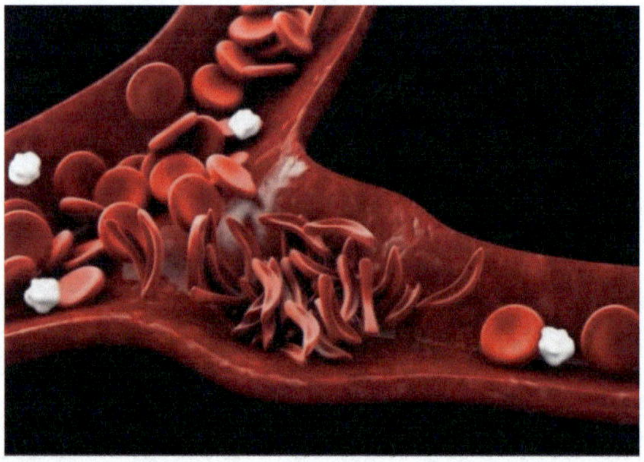

**Figure 9.4.** Common hematological disorders.

*Source:* https://www.matrixdiagnostics.net/wp-content/uploads/2024/11/What-Are-the-Most-Common-Hematological-Disorders-and-Their-Symptoms.webp.

## 9.1.2. Symptoms and Diagnosis

The recognition of symptoms in pediatric oncology and hematology is determinant for early diagnosis and appropriate treatment. Symptoms of inexplicable weakness, pallor, or bruising are commonly attributed to benign conditions and can retard essential treatment. Pallor and jaundice children, with obvious symptoms, were found to be consulted by a doctor sooner, with the visibility of the symptoms having an inverse correlation with the need for diagnosis (Al-Nassan et al., 2024). Also, some studies indicate that the presence of some symptoms is a determinant of the diagnostic schedule. For instance, central nervous system tumors were found to be accurate predictors of diagnostic delay, and patients with them had significantly longer time lags to therapy (Al-Nassan et al., 2024). Therefore, awareness of the clinical presentation of various hematological disorders is of utmost significance to pediatricians to facilitate early referral and reduce time delays to commence treatment. Diagnosis of childhood cancers encompasses various diagnostic mechanisms and devices. First, thorough medical history, as well as complete physical examination, is critical in assessing potential hematological disorders. This is then typically followed by the application of laboratory investigations, imaging, and, if necessary, biopsies to arrive at a proper diagnosis. One cannot overemphasize the application of imaging modalities, particularly for tumor visualization or infiltrative processes, as early detection of abnormal growth certainly impacts on therapeutic planning. In addition, the interpretation of lab tests, , such as bone marrow biopsies and complete blood counts, adds further complexity to the diagnostic process, which forces the clinician to interpret results against age-related reference values. Generally, these diagnostic approaches place emphasis on the need for a multidisciplinary approach in enhancing accuracy and speed of diagnosis of childhood hematology and oncology. In studying the relationship between symptom severity and diagnosis in pediatric cancer, symptomatology and age enter into the frame as determinants of outcomes. Research suggests that increasing age is associated with longer diagnostic delays and hence there is a need for increased sensitivity among healthcare providers towards symptom presentation at different ages (Al-Nassan et al., 2024). Moreover, the occurrence of B symptoms, unintentional weight loss, night sweats, and fever, has been correlated with poor prognosis and higher rates of relapse in numerous cancers, including Hodgkin lymphoma, showing their significance at diagnosis. As physicians attempt to prolong diagnostic periods and treatment courses, the integration of education schemes directed towards care providers and caregivers as well can reinforce symptom recognition and reduce referral times. Therefore, an integrated understanding of symptoms and how they impact treatment will remain central to improving patient outcomes in pediatric oncology and hematology.

### 9.1.3. Treatment Options and Management

Effective management of pediatric hematologic malignancies is multidisciplinary, particularly when considering therapeutic approaches to high-risk disease , such as neuroblastoma. New data indicate that the treatment situation is heterogeneous and often personalized to address the unique character of each patient's disease. In a report available on relapse/progressive and refractory high-risk neuroblastoma, chemotherapy was employed in 97% of patients, reflecting its pivotal role in upfront therapy. Moreover, immunotherapy was applied in nearly half the patients, with a tendency toward the addition of new biological agents to enhance the efficacy of conventional methods. Importantly, enrollment in clinical trials was noted in 34% of the cases, indicating the requirement for continuous research and development in clinical practice to achieve the best outcomes in this high-risk population (Mart et al., 2025). Chronic myeloid leukemia (CML) in children possesses a distinct clinical presentation compared with its adult counterpart and necessitates treatment protocols that are distinct. Imatinib, a first-generation tyrosine kinase inhibitor (TKI), remains the pillar of therapy with a satisfactory initial response but with lagged molecular response in children. Second-generation TKIs may be considered in patients with imatinib resistance or intolerance, indicating that dynamic treatment planning is needed due to evolving therapeutic needs. Long-term follow-up should also be considered due to potential side effects , such as growth retardation and endocrine abnormalities, particularly in children, who are still developing. This vigilance in management not only attempts to achieve remission but also offers extensive observation for treatment sequelae (Rafi et al., 2025).

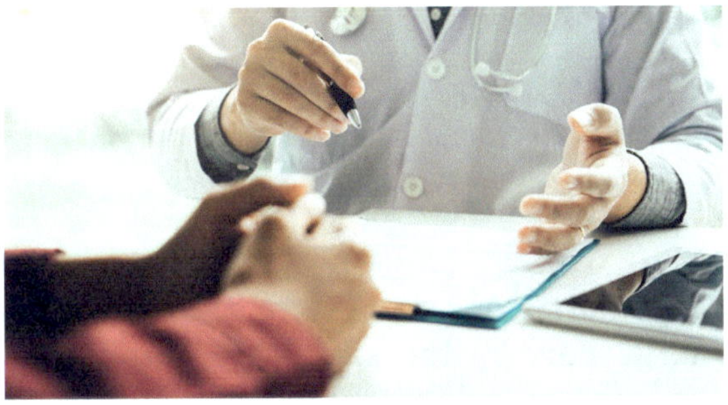

**Figure 9.5.** A healthcare provider discusses medical information with a patient, emphasizing shared decision-making and informed consent in a clinical consultation.

*Source:* https://cdn.cancercenter.com/-/media/ctca/images/others/blogs/2021/03-march/blog-advanced-cancer-l.jpg.

Generally, the treatment strategies and care measures in pediatric oncology and hematology are characterized by a penchant for individualized treatment and ongoing monitoring of therapeutic effectiveness. The blend of two or more modalities , such as chemotherapy, immunotherapy, and targeted therapy brings a multidimensional approach to address the multidimensionality of pediatric malignancies. Moreover, participation in clinical trials not only gives access to new treatments but is also valuable to gain information that can be used to make current protocols better. As the specialty evolves further, the emphasis on individualized therapies, meticulous follow-up, and a multidisciplinary team will continue to be instrumental in optimizing outcomes in children with these fatal disorders (Figure 9.5).

## Test Your Knowledge

1. What are some common hematological disorders in children, and how are they typically diagnosed?
2. What are the main treatment options for pediatric hematological disorders?

## 9.2. Overview of Oncological Disorders in Children

**Learning Outcome**

1. Types of pediatric cancers;
2. Early signs and diagnostic procedures;
3. Treatment modalities and their implications.

The pediatric oncology setting is dominated in large part by the specificity and relative prevalence of childhood cancers. Children are different from adults with neuroblastoma, Wilms tumor, and acute lymphoblastic leukemia, to name a few cancers, with their own discrete biologic characteristics and sites of growth. They are not only pathophysiologically heterogeneous, but also in prognosis and with respect to treatment response. Even though not very frequent in comparison to adult cancers, childhood cancers disproportionately account for deaths from disease among children. Early detection and treatment are therefore the chief determinants of outcome, necessitating the provision of specialist pediatric hematology and oncology services. Improved understanding of such conditions facilitates individualized intervention that can optimize diminution of the physical and psychological impact on children and their families. A multidisciplinary symptom management program has emerged as a top priority within the pediatric hematology and oncology community, as kids with cancer have physical as well as psychological symptoms. The incorporation of complementary therapies, or integrative medicine modalities (IMMs), has gained popularity to effectively manage symptoms. While a majority of pediatric hematology-oncology (PHO) providers are interested in applying IMMs, major concerns remain regarding their safety and efficacy. Research indicates that nearly 78% of such practitioners are uncertain about communicating with families about IMMs. Although fears related to some modalities persist, the overall opinion among health practitioners is the potential usefulness of methods , such as massage and mindfulness. Responses signal a need for ongoing education and structured integration of accepted IMMs into patient care pathways to improve quality of life in families and patients (Holly et al., 2025). A more complex examination of the referral processes in pediatric hematology and oncology clinics provides valuable information on treating oncologic disorders. A recent study of outpatient specialty clinic inpatients explained the overutilization of these services by pediatricians who have poor initial workups. The 4,210 patient charts reviewed retrospectively indicated that a mere 0.95% of them had life-threatening diagnoses, showing questionable appropriateness of these referrals. Such data emphasizes the necessity for higher-level diagnostic procedures at primary care settings prior to referral, while only such patients as require specialist oncology treatment are referred to the latter clinics. This approach not only alleviates oncology services but also enhances the efficacy and efficiency of patient care across the continuum of care (Özlem, 2024).

### 9.2.1. Types of Pediatric Cancers

Childhood cancer topography is diversified, and cancers of various types are in categories based on where they happen and their histology. The hematologic cancers are a significant category, and the prominent ones are the leukemias and the lymphomas. Among these, the acute lymphoblastic leukemia (ALL) is prevalent in children. ALL is derived from immature lymphocytes and is an aggressive tumor to manage since it is extremely aggressive. Research has established that a history of a prior malignancy has a significant influence on the risk of developing ALL, particularly secondary ALL (s-ALL) after prior cancers. Patients with a prior malignancy were at increased risk of ALL as per a population-based analysis, highlighting close monitoring in survivors of cancer in childhood (Rosenberg et al., 2017). This grouping calls for an awareness of not just the types but the interdependent nature of pediatric cancers and their prognostic meaning. In addition to leukemias, pediatric solid tumors form another critical group in the spectrum of child neoplasms. These tumors can occur in a range of tissues, including the brain, kidney, and soft tissue. Neuroblastoma, for instance, is an extremely common solid tumor of early childhood and most frequently occurs in the adrenal glands. Neuroblastoma pathophysiology involves the disorganized development of the neural crest cells, which results in various tumors and consequences. Meanwhile, Wilms tumor is another common pediatric solid tumor. The management of these tumors involves complex diagnostic procedures, like imaging and histopathological examination, to guide management plans. Furthermore, new approaches , such as liquid biopsies using cell-free DNA profiling, are being implemented in pediatric oncology with the promise of earlier detection and monitoring of these solid tumors (Astrahantseff et al., 2020). These developments represent a giant leap towards precision medicine and improved prognostic assessments for younger patients. The heterogeneity of childhood cancers presents not only the challenges of new diagnostic and treatment modalities but also the need for continuous research in biomarkers and novel therapies. Continuous research on the genetic underpinnings of various cancers, including leukemias and solid tumors, reveals important information that may influence treatment and enhance patient survival. For the case, understanding the exact genetic alterations that characterize a variety of childhood cancers can assist in investigating targeted therapy protocols that maximize responses. Simultaneously, prevent unwanted side effects. Additionally, the integration of technologies like liquid biopsies into clinical practices enables the optimization of monitoring approaches and the identification of relapse, eventually leading to more effective treatment control. As pediatric hematology and oncology continue to advance, such advancements should be used to optimize care for those children afflicted with these complex diseases (Figure 9.6).

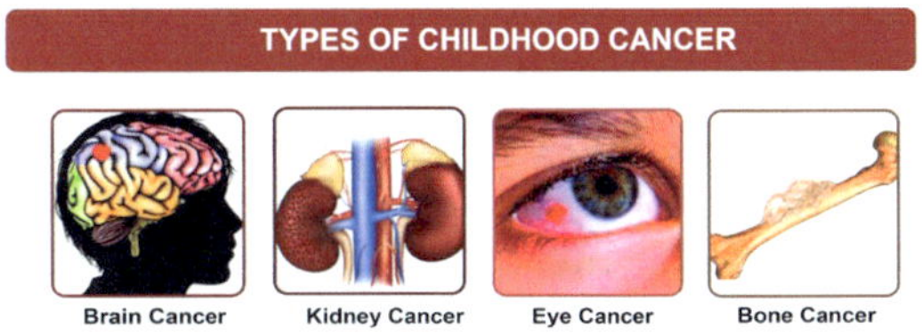


**Figure 9.6.** Types of pediatric cancers.

*Source:* https://external-content.duckduckgo.com/iu/?u=http%3A%2F%2Fwww.medindia.net%2Fimages%2Fcommon%2Fpatientinfo%2F950_400%2Ftypes-of-childhood-cancer.jpg&f=1&nofb=1&ipt=46b5b49d06a680d61bac941b9af72583e4787fc21291bc7bcf38896c5e39dd3d.

### 9.2.2. Early Signs and Diagnostic Procedures

Early recognition of symptoms pertaining to pediatric hematology and oncology diseases is essential in improving patient outcomes. These symptoms that are typically observable at an early time comprise bruising without any visible cause, persistent fatigue, and recurrent infections, which may reveal underlying issues , such as leukemia or other hematological disorders. Detection of these symptoms typically leads to an extensive assessment that typically begins with a detailed clinical history and physical exam. Physicians must be careful since children will not always describe their symptoms accurately, needing very sensitive detection of subtle signs that might signify malignancy. Caution can enable timely treatment, enhancing outcomes through positive treatment responses and survival rates along with it. Pediatrics' hematology and oncology diagnostics keep advancing, technology advancements that enhance accuracy and performance. Blood tests usually form the basis on initial diagnosis, with full blood counts to assess hematocrit and hemoglobin levels, together with white blood cell count assessment for abnormality. Bone marrow biopsies and imaging studies, including MRIs and CT scans, also assist in diagnosing cancers. These diagnostic tests not only determine the presence of a disease but also provide useful information about its staging, which is crucial in formulating an appropriate treatment plan. With the development of new diagnostic modalities, an interdisciplinary team with the cooperation of pathologists, radiologists, and pediatric oncologists becomes essential to deliver comprehensive care to children. At the same time, the inclusion of updated definitions for invasive fungal diseases (IFDs) in diagnostic criteria enhances the capacity to manage co-morbid conditions commonly present in immunocompromised pediatric oncology patients. Clinical practice based on broad definitions and rigorous classifications of "proven," "probable," and "possible" IFDs, as defined by the Infectious Diseases Group, becomes highly useful in practice. These definitions guide healthcare professionals how to risk-stratify and choose the most appropriate diagnostic tests, particularly among high-risk patients. Due to the increased morbidity among IFDs in these patient groups, the employment of higher-tech imaging and laboratory diagnostic methods is called for. Thus, constructing a cooperation model with stress on early identification of symptoms and the use of robust diagnostic procedures can immensely improve outcomes in children with hematological malignancies (Akan et al., 2019; Abdelhafeez et al., 2021).

### 9.2.3. Treatment Modalities and Their Implications

Treatment modalities in pediatric hematology and oncology do indeed play a deciding role in determining the clinical outcomes of patients with malignancies. Choice of therapy is often based on the type and stage of cancer, patients' overall condition, and their personal biological characteristics. As a general rule, the core treatment pillars are chemotherapy, radiation therapy, and surgery. The strategic application of these modalities is to eliminate malignancies and improve survival rates with minimum side effects. For instance, in osteosarcoma, surgical excision of pulmonary metastasis is a common consideration that may encompass significant heterogeneity between medical practitioners in terms of timing and technique, reflective of an unstandardized practice in the profession (Bhattasali et al., 2015). These disparities point to the critical necessity of guidelines that can facilitate therapeutic uniformity and optimize patient outcomes. In addition, infection control is a central challenge in pediatric oncology, particularly in aggressively treated patients like chemotherapy and hematopoietic stem cell transplant recipients. These patients have an increased risk of acquiring bacterial, fungal, and viral infections due to immunosuppression.

Conventionally, fungal and bacterial infections used to be the top priority in fever and neutropenia attacks; however, recent studies have revealed an alarming frequency of viral infections being etiologies of morbidity and mortality among this vulnerable population (Fisher et al., 2012). Development of successful pre-exposure and post-exposure prophylaxis strategies, as well as stringent infection control practices, is important. This multi-dimensional approach not only helps to manage acquired infections but also to prevent their establishment, ultimately influencing the overall treatment trajectory and quality of life in children with hematological malignancies. Treatment modalities have implications that extend beyond immediate clinical treatment; they also encompass long-term survivorship and quality-of-life concerns. Pediatric cancer survivors tend to develop severe sequelae that can be caused by aggressive treatment, including cardiovascular toxicities, secondary malignancies, and psychosocial disturbances. Thus, a global treatment plan needs to include long-term follow-up and survivorship care, with respect to physical and psychological needs of patients. Besides this, familiarity with potential late effects associated with various treatment approaches is required for the individualization of ongoing management plans. Thus, clinicians must be cautious not only in selecting treatment modalities but also in the care of survivors overall so that the benefits of aggressive treatment do not come at an unacceptable cost in patients' future well-being (Figure 9.7).

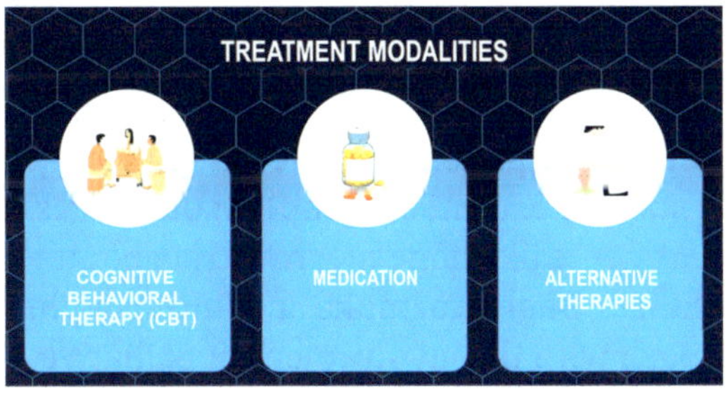


**Figure 9.7.** Treatment modalities and their implications.

*Source:* https://external-content.duckduckgo.com/iu/?u=https%3A%2F%2Furpbehavioralhealth.com%2Fwp-content%2Fuploads%2F2023%2F10%2Ftreatment-modalities.jpg&f=1&nofb=1&ipt=7f1bb2ee8bc4818e6d62b828db192c424cf4d3b5abd570a391af439bb40c80ec.

## Test Your Knowledge

1. What are the most common types of pediatric cancers, and how are they typically diagnosed?
2. What are the main treatment modalities for pediatric cancers, and what are some of their implications?

## 9.3. The Role of Pediatric Hematologists and Oncologists

**Learning Outcome**

1. Education and training requirements;
2. Responsibilities in patient care;
3. Collaboration with multidisciplinary teams.

Pediatric hematologists and oncologists have a vital role to play in the management of children's diseases, particularly those related to cancers and blood disorders. These experts are trained in diagnosing, managing, and treating entire patients suffering from conditions , such as leukemia, lymphoma, and other blood disorders. Their function not only involves chemotherapy administration and utilization of newer modalities like bone marrow transplantation, but also dealing with the complex psychosocial problems of their patients and families.

Successful treatment of these childhood diseases frequently requires treating the emotional and psychological problems that arise in the course of treatment. This interdisciplinary framework is essential, as it is vital in the overall recovery and health of adolescent patients and their families, showing the vital role pediatric oncology and hematology care continues to have in current medicine. The incorporation of palliative care interventions into pediatric oncology and hematology has become an essential component of overall patient care. With such an enormous symptom burden as that of treatments like bone marrow transplantation, specialists ought to make a multidisciplinary approach with the involvement of palliative care services a priority. Such incorporation allows better communication with relatives, well-informed decision-making, and resolution of challenging prognostic discussions. Studies have established that palliative care can enhance the quality of life in cancer patients undergoing aggressive treatment regimens, increasing symptom management and emotional support through family involvement (Johnson et al., 2024). Despite this, hospitals have recorded low levels of palliative care integration, and there is an urgent need for pediatric oncologists to promote protocols that put such high-priority care activities at the forefront of their treatment regimens. The COVID-19 pandemic has also posed unprecedented challenges for pediatric hematology and oncology clinics, with global impacts on the delivery of services. New information shows there is substantial disruption of cancer care, including the disruption of treatments and lower new diagnoses, particularly in low-income and middle-income countries (Agulnik et al., 2021). The pandemic necessitated rapid modifications in care provision, and healthcare professionals were forced to develop new procedures to ensure continuity of care, remain in contact with families of patients, and manage deficiencies in resources. Pediatric hematology and oncology professionals react to this new environment while their focus on quality and safety of care remains the overweening one. The hardship faced during this period refers to the resilience of these professionals and to the compelling need for integrated support systems, where even during moments of crisis, children with cancer receive timely and efficient interventions to get the best possible outcomes.

### 9.3.1. Education and Training Requirements

Pediatric hematology and oncology education and training requirements are critical components of preparing healthcare professionals for addressing the challenges of patient care in the specialty. Potential practitioners must undergo an intensive education process beginning with a medical degree, followed by a pediatrics residency. Such fundamental training provides them with the required abilities in common child medical care before advancing into a pediatric hematology-oncology fellowship. These fellowships are typically three years in duration and involve training in specialty which comprises diagnosis and treatment of hematologic malignancies and cancers of childhood and training in more advanced therapeutic techniques. Also important is the fact that inclusion of training in communication skills in these fellowship programs is crucial so that fellows can manage difficult conversations with families in a better way (Kerri et al., 2024). Since the practice of medicine is growing, there is also an imperative to incorporate health equity and the influence of systemic factors on patient care into their education. Certain new businesses have taken the initiative in perceiving the value of teaching structural and interpersonal racism as part of medical education. In pediatric oncology and hematology, teaching this is valuable in overcoming disparity in treatment, especially concerning pain management and timing of intervention for vulnerable groups. Programs like the Health Equity Conference Series at UCSF reflect an engaged response, attempting to equip healthcare professionals with tools and knowledge to combat bias and improve outcomes in vulnerable populations (Jain, 2024). This awareness and ability to recognize health disparities are an important aspect of educating future pediatric hemato-oncologists. Aside from clinical training, professional upkeep and life-long education are most essential in pediatric hematology and oncology. Practitioners must update themselves with the recent research, treatment, and innovations in patient care in order to successfully treat complicated cases. Ongoing learning through workshops, conferences, and learning networks not only increases practitioners' level of knowledge but also fosters a culture of shared learning among the multidisciplinary teams that define this specialty. Besides, participation in simulation educational programs will improve communication skills and clinical judgment to a significant level, making practitioners competent to deliver empathic and effective care to patients and families. Lastly, the whole training program should comprise both clinical competency and the element of social justice in healthcare in order to make pediatric hematologists and oncologists competent to cater to the diverse needs of their patient populations (Figure 9.8).

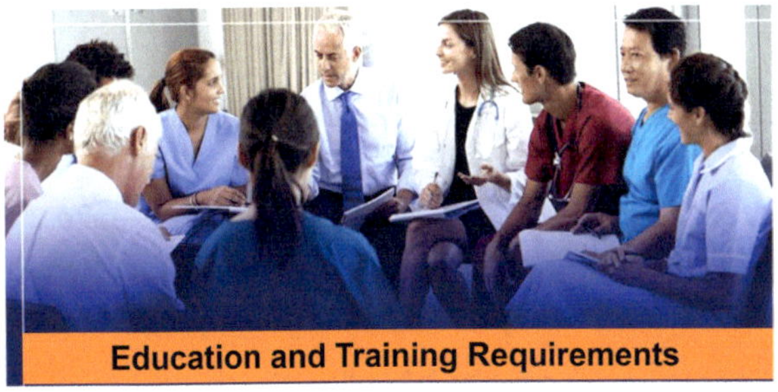


**Figure 9.8.** Education and training requirements for pediatric hematology and oncology.

*Source:* https://ams.londondms.com/backend/images/blog/upload/AMS-00W088b16Z-education-and-training-requirements-in-health-social-care-png.png.

## 9.3.2. Responsibilities in Patient Care

The patient care responsibilities within the field of pediatric hematology and oncology include a range of significant factors that attempt to optimize patient outcomes and provide equitable care. Broadly concentrating this effort is the identification of the unique needs of children with hematologic and oncologic disease. Healthcare professionals must navigate the nuances of creating treatment plans that are medicinally sound as well as sensitive to the developmental stages and emotional contexts of their pediatric patients. Through the implementation of intervention approaches that foster effective communication and engagement with both patient and family, professionals can maximize understanding and adherence to treatment protocols. Emphasis on collaboration among multidisciplinary teams is essential in this respect, ensuring that all aspects of care from diagnosis to palliative therapies are in the best interest of the patient and his/her family. Equally as important inpatient care duties are determining social determinants of health, most particularly in pediatric patients and their families. These determinants have strong influences on health outcomes and can complicate the delivery of care. Socioeconomic status, access, and language are also obstacles to effective communication and the influence of care. In pediatric hematology-oncology, where treatment regimes are also complex, clinicians must be knowledgeable about such barriers and make an effort to implement culturally and linguistically concordant interventions. Research on language-discordant interactions highlights the risk of decreased quality of care and complications when proper communication does not exist; therefore, developing a multilingual, welcoming healthcare environment is essential to ensure equal accessibility and outcomes for all patients (Ruiz et al., 2025). Besides, acute condition management , such as respiratory failure in pediatric hematology and oncology patients, emphasizes specific duties that medical professionals need to carry out. The use of high-flow nasal cannula (HFNC) therapy has been shown to be a crucial intervention in the management of acute respiratory failure in vulnerable patients. Yet, HFNC treatment's reported failure rate, up to 27% in certain research, is proof of the necessity for continuous monitoring and responsive care protocols within the ICU setting (Alayed et al., 2025). Professionals must determine predictors of failure with HFNC, , such as initial pH and complicating factors like cardiac failure or sepsis, so that they can change treatment procedures immediately and effectively. Such commitment not only depicts the complexity involved in childcare but also sustains the keen emphasis on safeguarding patient welfare during the course of treatment.

### 9.3.3. Collaboration with Multidisciplinary Teams

Effective collaboration between multidisciplinary teams is essential in the practice of pediatric oncology and hematology, whereby these multidisciplinary teams apply diverse specialties to meet the multilateral care of the child with cancer or blood disorder. Through a collaborative care approach, medical caregivers can access different specialties, from hematology and oncology to surgery and palliative care, to fashion integrative treatment plans for dealing with the multilateral needs of a child. The group discussion in multidisciplinary team (MDT) meetings brings about balanced consensus in terms of the treatment modalities, thereby bringing about a climate wherein patient-centered care becomes crucial. The involvement of the patients in such decisions might also enhance treatment adherence and satisfaction overall, as a sign of the significance of shared decision-making in current medical practice (Naeem et al., 2025). Patient preference and inter-professional communication coordination is also better proven through special training courses, , such as the ones conducted in the St. Jude Global Academy Neuro-Oncology Training Seminar. This seminar has succeeded in developing teamwork among various groups of physicians, , such as oncologists, neurosurgeons, and pathologists, coming from resource-limited settings (Daniel et al., 2024). By fostering a spirit of teamwork, these training programs have had transformative effects on clinical practice, like the implementation of multidisciplinary tumor boards (MDTB), otherwise absent in these involved institutions.

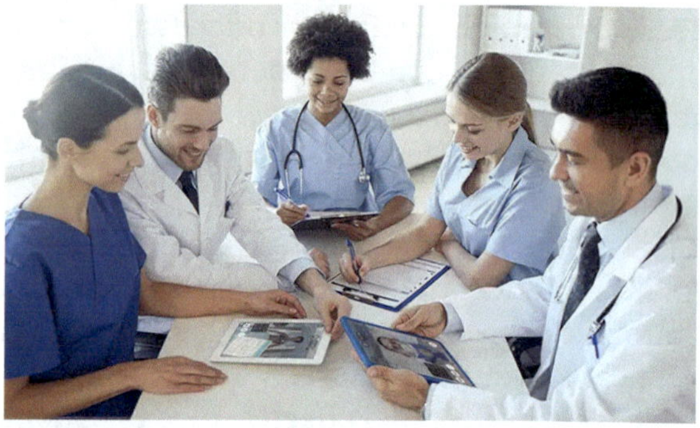

**Figure 9.9.** Collaboration with multidisciplinary teams.

*Source:* https://bodyinteract.com/wp-content/uploads/2024/07/multidisciplinary-teams-healthcare-1.webp.

The impact of such collaboration, as evidenced through participants' feedback, demonstrates how strengthening communication and cooperation within these MDTBs has direct impacts upon the results of patient care, hence forging a vital link between educational interventions and the provision of healthcare. Resolving the issues of multidisciplinary teams remains a priority in pediatric oncology and hematology. Common hurdles are pragmatic issues of time constraints and inconsistent attendance by key team players, which may interfere with teamwork. The efficacy of MDTs is, to a large extent, reliant on the commitment of all the specialists to attend sessions and contribute during discussions. Furthermore, the lack of clinical knowledge and awareness of the vision of each discipline can negatively impact decision-making processes. With maturing practices, there will be ongoing need to examine these working frameworks and integrate patient insight to counteract systemic pressures to ultimately enhance the provided care for pediatric patients with hematologic and oncologic disorders (Naeem et al., 2025) (Figure 9.9).

## Test Your Knowledge

1. What education and training are required to become a pediatric hematologist/oncologist, and what are their primary responsibilities in patient care?
2. How do pediatric hematologists and oncologists collaborate with multidisciplinary teams in caring for children?

## 9.4. Advances in Research and Treatment

**Learning Outcome**

1. Recent breakthroughs in pediatric hematology;
2. The impact of clinical trials on patient outcomes;
3. Innovations in cancer treatment for children.

There have been significant advances in pediatric hematology and oncology research that have resulted in improved survival and quality of life for children diagnosed with cancer. Over the past two decades, improvements in new modalities of treatment, , such as targeted therapy and immunotherapy, have transformed treatment paradigms. As an example, newer research has commented that pooled cumulative weighted mortality in children with cancer admitted into pediatric intensive care units (PICUs) is approximately 27.8%, and this necessitates further studies into practices of care and interventions that could play a beneficial role in these statistics. Methods for enhancing treatment intervention accuracy are being aggressively researched, and this now allows caregivers to tailor interventions to the patient's own profile and cancer-specific features. This is a historic step forward in personalized medicine with the potential to provide more effective interventions and better outcomes for this high-risk subgroup. In addition to pharmacological advances, innovative supportive care modalities are in the process of being developed to improve symptom management in children with cancer undergoing treatment. One such example is the use of acupressure as an adjunctive treatment to alleviate symptoms of treatment in the form of nausea and pain. A randomized controlled trial, Acupressure for Children in Treatment for a Childhood Cancer (ACT-CC), attempts to assess the efficacy and practicality of acupressure interventions among children receiving chemotherapy or hematopoietic stem cell transplantation. This study has value not only as a potential clinical contribution but also in its focus on the global nature of care and the recognition that management of aversive symptoms is central to optimizing overall quality of life through treatment. Through the integration of non-pharmacologic modalities into standard care, healthcare providers can be a part of a more comprehensive treatment model. The incorporation of newer study results and treatment regimens in pediatric hematology and oncology mirrors a broader transformation in the area, with an emphasis both on efficacy and safety in treatment regimens. While survival rates have enormously improved for children with cancer with time, morbidity from intense treatments remains a concern. The identification of causative factors for elevated PICU mortality in cancer-stricken children is most significant, as this information will be in a position to guide the creation of more successful care interventions. More precisely, ascertaining the risks posed by mechanical ventilation and other supportive care can lead to improved management techniques within the PICU. Together, these advances in research and treatment not only aim to enhance survival rates but also aim to encourage improved quality care for those children and families, so that physical and emotional needs are met along the way during the process of treatment.

## 9.4.1. Recent Breakthroughs in Pediatric Hematology

Advances in pediatric hematology in recent times have significantly influenced the treatment and diagnosis of blood disease in children. The development of new therapies that utilize gene editing technologies, , such as CRISPR-Cas9, is one of the new developments aimed at treating inherited genetic hemoglobinopathies like sickle cell disease and beta-thalassemia. Not only does this enable precision treatment approaches, but it also points to the importance of precision medicine for children. Continuing clinical trials are also proving very promising, with the potential for curative treatments that can greatly improve patient outcomes. By shifting treatment paradigms, these advances are of hopeful prospect for children suffering from formerly untreatable blood diseases, thereby improving their quality of life along with survival rates. Another great advancement in pediatric hematology is the improved understanding of lymphoblastic leukemia, particularly acute lymphoblastic leukemia (ALL). Current research has focused on applying sophisticated genomic profiling and biomarker-based therapy, allowing more individualized treatment avenues. For instance, scientists have made decisions regarding certain gene alterations that dictate therapy, such that oncologists are able to tailor therapy in accordance with patient profiles. Evidence demonstrates that the all-encompassing strategy not only makes treatment regimens work better but also decreases the toxic effects of treatment. These advancements speak to the necessity of continued research in pediatric hematology to further streamline treatment regimens and combat the complexity present in pediatric patients so that treatment modalities are as effective and as non-toxic as possible. The rate at which immunotherapy has also evolved has also made significant contributions to pediatric hematology, namely in combating malignancies , such as juvenile myelomonocytic leukemia (JMML).

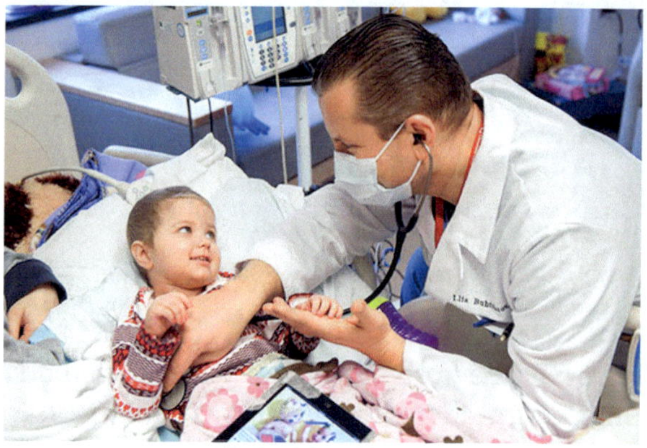

**Figure 9.10.** Recent breakthroughs in pediatric hematology.

*Source:* https://www.petalschildrenhospital.in/assets/Specialities/Pediatric_Hematology_1.jpg.

Next-generation treatments, including monoclonal antibodies and CAR T-cell therapy, have been making waves in the press because they have the ability to leverage the body's own immune system to target cancer cells directly. Researchers now are exploring the efficacy of such treatments in kids, and along with that, the earliest indication of success in enhancing treatment outcomes and minimizing rates of relapse. These developments not only mark a turning point in strategy but also reflect a growing sense of the need for individuated treatment regimens sensitive to a child's unique underlying biology. Such developments highlight the value in integrating multidisciplinary strategies in the practice of pediatric hematology and oncology and provide renewed hope for children with complex hematologic diseases (Figure 9.10).

### 9.4.2. Innovations in Cancer Treatment for Children

Current advancements in the treatment of childhood cancer have tremendously transformed pediatric hematology and oncology, improving survival and quality of life among children. One of the most astonishing advancements is the emergence of precision medicine, which aligns treatments with the genetic profile of tumors in patients. This approach offers more focused therapies that reduce damage to normal cells and enhance the effectiveness of therapy. Specifically, therapies that inhibit single pathways critical to cancer cell survival are being developed for most pediatric cancers, offering hope to cancers that have had no decent treatment. As scientists continue to illuminate the specific genetic mutations in childhood cancers, possibilities for individualized treatment plans remain promising, paving the way for improved outcomes in this precious population. Additionally, breakthroughs in radiation therapy represent a further milestone in the treatment of childhood cancers. Techniques , such as proton therapy, in which the high doses of radiation are delivered directly to the tumors and bypass healthy tissues surrounding them, have proven to be valuable for the oncologist's arsenal. Proton therapy differs from conventional photon treatments since it offers accuracy and is particularly beneficial in treating tumors that are close to critical organs, sparing potential late effects that might affect children in adulthood. With approximately half of all cancer patients requiring radiation therapy, the study of these treatments, as well as their rates of success over previous treatments, reflects why more research in this field is necessary. The persistence of refining and developing radiation-based treatments ensures that pediatric patients are given the most current treatment available while minimizing risks associated with their treatments (Collins et al., 2017). Chemotherapy is also still at the base of children's cancer treatment, changing with advances in new agents, delivery methods, and safety protocols. Though chemotherapy has significantly enhanced survival rates of numerous pediatric cancers to nearly 90% in the last sixty years, their delivery comes with risks associated with each. Extensive levels of administration errors are a significant problem, with errors ranging from 4% to 18% in various environments (Bertram et al., 2015). In a bid to mitigate these problems, programs , such as the Pediatric Chemotherapy and Biotherapy Provider Program have been established to educate healthcare providers on safe administration practices, hence reducing the likelihood of errors. These training programs reflect a greater commitment across pediatric hematology and oncology to enhance the safety and efficacy of chemotherapy in children to ensure that their care is innovative and responsible.

### 9.4.3. The Impact of Clinical Trials on Patient Outcomes

The performance of clinical trials in pediatric hematology and oncology has a massive impact on patient outcomes by introducing evidence-based therapy that improves the quality of care. Clinical trials are systematic procedures under which novel treatments are evaluated, with the guarantee that the drugs given to children with hematologic cancers are not only safe but also effective. For instance, progress in the genetics of blood diseases has led to more targeted therapies that can decrease side effects severity of traditional treatments. As indicated in most experiments, such breakthroughs directly influence enhanced survival rates and the quality of patients' lives. The evolution of patient-reported outcomes (PRO) measures, indicated by ongoing calls for credible instruments in clinical trials for hematological diseases like pyruvate kinase deficiency, demonstrates the necessity of attending to patient perceptions in treatment evaluations (Salek et al., 2018). Clinical trial trends further indicate the imperative need for pediatric-oriented research in order to address the unique issues of children with hematological diseases. As treatment approaches become more complicated, for example, with new immunotherapy and bone marrow transplant techniques, clinical trials give researchers the opportunity to assess not only efficacy but also the long-term impact of these therapies on children's health. For example, research studies performed on graft-versus-host disease (GVHD) in child patients have illustrated that heterogeneous approaches to transplantation may produce different outcomes in terms of relapse and quality of life. The multivariate analysis of new research indicates significant differences in graft-versus-host rate by donor type, which is key information for the refinement of transplantation protocols (Mehta et al., 2019). Thus, continued study of clinical trials must be done to further clarify pediatric-specific responses to hematologic treatment. Lastly, the ethical implications surrounding clinical trials highlight their influence on future practice in pediatric hematology and oncology. Offering informed consent by the patients and families, coupled with their safety and well-being during clinical trials, is proof of the ethical responsibility of the medical community. With novel treatments emerging from such trials, including those for orphan diseases like pyruvate kinase deficiency, it becomes imperative that researchers come up with valid frameworks that determine and offer the connected benefits and risks. Also, with the pediatric group generally being vulnerable, trials must take into account not only clinical efficacy but also psychosocial factors that influence children being subjected to prolonged therapy. Overall, clinical trials not only take forward the frontiers of the treatment available in pediatric oncology and hematology but also provide an integrated approach consisting of patient safety, ethical concerns, and the likelihood of improved outcomes (Figure 9.11).

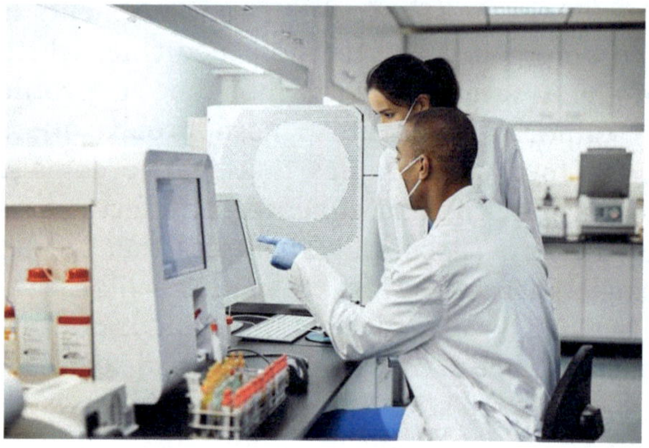

**Figure 9.11.** The impact of clinical trials on patient outcomes.

*Source:* https://imageio.forbes.com/specials-images/imageserve/65ba93ac6615590d62359701//960x0.jpg?height=474&width=711&fit=bounds.

## Test Your Knowledge

1. What are some recent breakthroughs in pediatric hematology and how have clinical trials improved patient outcomes?
2. What innovations in cancer treatment are transforming care for children with oncological disorders?

# 9.5. Psychological and Social Impacts on Patients and Families

**Learning Outcome**

1. Emotional challenges faced by children;
2. Support systems for families;
3. Long-term effects of treatment on quality of life.

The psychological suffering of children with hematological and oncological conditions is overwhelming and multifaceted. These children can battle fear, anxiety, and ambiguity around their health, and this can give rise to extreme emotional disturbance. The suffering of diagnosis and long-term medical treatment can hinder their sense of normalcy and have a damaging effect on their development and socialization. Besides, chronic disease also tends to keep them away from daily activities , such as play and school, resulting in isolation and lower self-esteem. Literature on pediatric patients' health-related quality of life also brought forth the need to take into account such psychological considerations and that supportive therapy would enhance coping mechanisms and overall well-being, thereby enhancing the ability of these children to deal with the physical as well as the emotional load of their diseases (Salek et al., 2018). Family adaptation is crucial in determining how children with blood diseases and cancer would psychologically react. Family functioning has a direct impact on a child's emotional well-being because the strain of taking care of an ill child can test family relationships and stability. Studies have determined different patterns of family functioning among the caregivers, from adaptive to maladaptive styles. For instance, a study on families with children suffering from chronic diseases categorized families based on their adaptability and identified that maladaptive families can face problems in the areas of child psychological distress and compromised quality of life (Sumrall et al., 2023). In contrast, highly adaptive families facilitate resilience by providing a health-promoting environment that can overcome stress associated with illness. This poses the demand for family-based interventions to create better coping strategies and emotional support within the family. The social impact of pediatric hematology and oncology diseases extends beyond the patient to the siblings, parents, and ultimately the community as a whole. Siblings are made to feel neglected or develop emotional disturbances as a result of all the attention accorded to the ill child, leading them to feel jealous or abandoned. Apart from that, parents typically experience a lot of stress, balancing care demands with their own emotional needs and commitments. Stigma about chronic illness can also isolate families from their networks of support, leaving them with less social support and increasing perceptions of loneliness. An understanding of these dynamics is critical for healthcare professionals, as helping to establish a supportive network and facilitating relationship building with other families experiencing similar circumstances can foster resilience and enhance results for all members of the family unit.

## 9.5.1. Emotional Challenges Faced by Children

Emotional problems faced by pediatric patients with hematologic or cancerous diseases are usually profound and sophisticated. Such children become more apprehensive and fearful regarding their outcomes and treatment protocols. Uncertainty of their disease can manifest in helplessness and isolation because they are unable to comprehend their situation in the framework of their young lives. In addition, the stress of frequent hospitalization, painful procedures, and missing school may exacerbate withdrawal and sadness. Children are not very good at verbalizing their feelings, so it might result in behavior issues complicating treatment and social interactions too. It is thus essential that healthcare practitioners, , such as nurses, adopt an integrated model when treating not just the physical but also the psychological needs of such patients, with psychological care being part of the clinical care they provide. A very important aspect of effective support for children with such emotional problems is creating open and interprofessional communication among healthcare practitioners, patients, and families. It is revealed that by incorporating nurses in the prognosis-related communication (PRC) process, they can provide important emotional support and counseling to enhance the care experience of the child and family. This integration is the foundation for eradicating feelings of loneliness and uncertainty, as the children are comforted by a better understanding of their condition. However, current processes tend to exclude nurses from such important considerations, possibly limiting the effectiveness of the provided emotional support. There must be a paradigm shift that aims to prioritize the active engagement of nurses in PRC, leading to improved outcomes not only for patients but also for families struggling with the complexities of pediatric hematology and oncology diseases (Sisk et al., 2019). As children advance to adolescent and young adult (AYA) stages, their emotional struggles may shift, presenting new challenges, particularly as they enter adulthood health care systems. The study of the factors that impact health care transition is such that emotional and psychological support remains paramount during this period. Youths with disorders like sickle cell disease report stigma and isolation perceptions, highlighting their ongoing need for accessible emotional resources and support systems. These determinants have the potential to exert a significant influence on their self-management and utilization of health care, validating the need for culturally congruent interventions that address their unique needs. By doing so, health care providers are better positioned to assist children and AYAs with tailored educational and psychosocial interventions, in the end, improving their quality of life and outcomes within the pediatric hematology and oncology clinic (Clayton-Jones et al., 2021) (Figure 9.12).

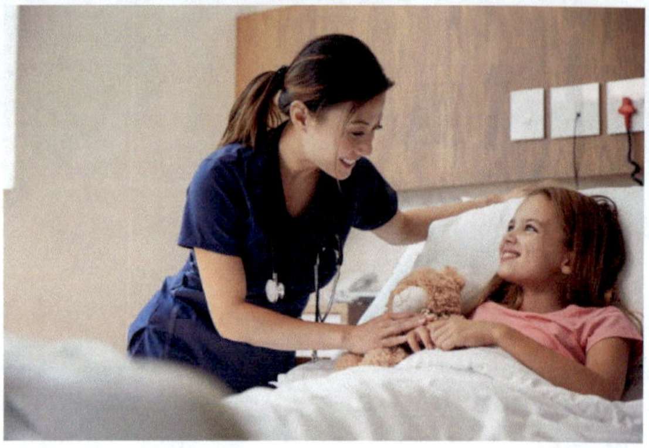

**Figure 9.12.** Emotional challenges faced by children diagnosed with hematological or oncological conditions.

*Source:* https://external-content.duckduckgo.com/iu/?u=https%3A%2F%2Fprismcareerinstitute.edu%2Fwp-content%2Fuploads%2F2020%2F01%2Fprism-medical-assistant-children-challenges.jpg&f=1&nofb=1&ipt=393b7ab180f55f8caad5f0a43259b834f0e678f17e02cba08b9aceb766e38401.

## 9.5.2. Support Systems for Families

The experience of navigating pediatric hematology and oncology is riddled with affective and pragmatic obstacles for families. The most critical aspect of support systems is the utilization of extensive education programs specifically designed to meet the diverse needs of families with a childhood cancer diagnosis. According to a consensus developed by an expert panel for the Children's Oncology Group, effective patient and family education is intrinsically family centered. Understanding the significant implications of such a diagnosis, it is essential that families are given ample time to cope with the news and create strategies for coping with ongoing life needs. These programs not only impart necessary information about the disease and therapy but also assist in readiness of families to face the psychosocial impacts of cancer diagnosis, especially the need for institutional and community support along the treatment process (Landier et al., 2016). Any supportive system in pediatric hematology and oncology is based on communication. Families in particular are particularly assisted by healthcare professionals skilled in prognosis-related communication (PRC). Such a difficult task in delivering prognostic information necessitates collaboration between the healthcare team, with nurses playing a key role. The work in one study demonstrated the importance of nurses being involved in this process because patients and families place greater reliance on what they observe and empathetic care. Sadly, the current model tends to leave nurses out of such critical decision-making, thereby undermining their ability to effectively support families. It is important that educational programs include training for physicians and nurses in a way that nurses are prepared as active decision-makers in PRC, thereby enhancing family comprehension and coping strategies (Sisk et al., 2019). Moreover, developing support networks among families goes beyond hospital walls. Both informal and formal social support groups provide essential networks for families dealing with the strain of pediatric hematology and oncology. Social support groups create a space of experience, advice, and emotional support sharing that builds strength among families dealing with the intricacies of a cancer process. Hospitals and treatment centers can strengthen family support by assisting in connecting family with such resources, providing a more comprehensive form of care. The use of family-based education in conjunction with supportive community networks is priceless in lightening the pediatric cancer burden and promoting the general health and well-being of patients and their families. Through continued advocacy for effective support systems, stakeholders can alleviate some of the emotional challenges that come with the treatment of child cancer (Landier et al., 2016).

### 9.5.3. Long-Term Effects of Treatment on Quality of Life

Pediatric cancer treatment has long-term effects on the quality of life as survivors grow up. Children with cancer are at high risk of developing neurocognitive late effects, which can have a negative impact on their educational attainment, vocational achievement, and overall satisfaction with life. Research has verified that formal educational support can be essential to their success, but it will heavily rely on parents' sensitivity and ability to obtain resources needed. It is important to have provision for identifying perceived support that parents receive in the process of retranscription back to school so that such households are able to navigate the educational readjustment process without any difficulties and gain access to appropriate intervention. This assistance not only aids academic achievement but also promotes the creation of some form of normalcy in the existence of such child survivors, thereby their overall well-being in spite of the adversity they face (Parrillo et al., 2023). Aside from academic challenge, physical and psychological impacts of cancer therapy on children are profound and widespread. The treatment protocols employed, particularly in the case of acute leukemia, can have long-term influences on several organ systems, including the respiratory, cardiovascular, and endocrine systems. Perhaps most intriguingly, survivors frequently experience cognitive function and emotional abnormalities, which can have a profound impact on their quality of life. Experts have highlighted the need to differentiate between survival and a lack of toxicity-related impairment of quality of life. As survival rates from childhood cancer improve, there is an increasing demand for a comprehensive understanding of these late effects. Ongoing research persists across the globe to evaluate quality of life and identify means of avoiding and controlling treatment-associated side effects, thus improving the outcome for survivors of childhood cancer (Orlova et al., 2023). The evolving landscape of pediatric oncology and hematology necessitates a multidisciplinary approach to understanding and improving the quality of life in survivors of childhood cancer. With increasing survival rates, there must be a focus not just on prolonging life but also on enhancing the quality of lived life in such individuals. This is a call that necessitates a concerted effort from medical professionals, educators, and families to create robust support systems that cater to the unique needs of this population. In addition, continued research into the long-term outcomes of treatment for childhood cancer will allow for the establishment of effective follow-up treatment and therapeutic regimes. By addressing the physical, cognitive, and psychological impacts of treatment, stakeholders can establish an environment that supports resilience and flourishing among survivors. Lastly, the objective is not only to help survive these children but also thrive in all aspects of their lives (Orlova et al., 2023; Parrillo et al., 2023) (Figure 9.13).

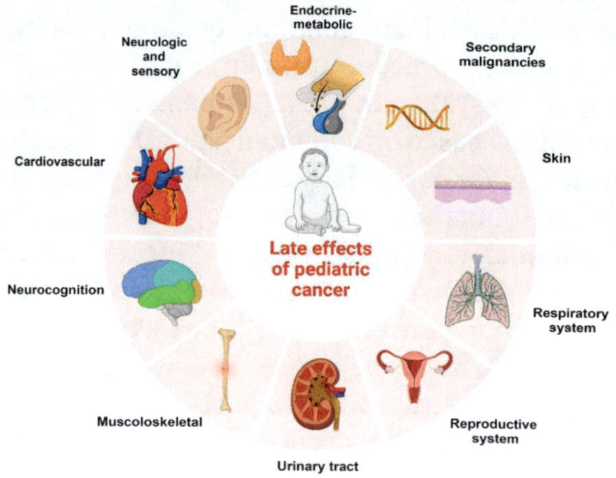


**Figure 9.13.** The long-term effects of treatment for pediatric cancers significantly impact the quality of life as survivors grow into adulthood.

*Source:* Pancaldi, A., Pugliese, M., Migliozzi, C., Blom, J., Cellini, M., & Iughetti, L. (2023). Neuropsychological Outcomes of Children Treated for Brain Tumors. Children, 10(3), 472. https://doi.org/10.3390/children10030472

## Test Your Knowledge

1. What emotional challenges do children with serious hematological or oncological conditions commonly face, and what support systems can help families cope?
2. How can long-term treatments for pediatric blood disorders and cancers affect a child's quality of life over time?

# 9.6. Ethical Considerations in Pediatric Hematology and Oncology

**Learning Outcome**

1. Informed consent and decision-making;
2. Balancing treatment benefits and risks;
3. The role of palliative care.

Ethics in pediatric hematology and oncology is particularly complex due to the vulnerable status of the patient group in question. Since children, given their age and phase of development, can typically be expected not to have the capacity to fully understand the implications of medical procedures , such as hematopoietic stem cell transplantation (HSCT), the procedure, while potentially lifesaving, raises significant ethical issues with regard to informed consent, particularly when the donor is also. Patients need to be appropriately informed about the risks, likelihood of adverse events, and total cost of both the donation and transplant process. As noted, there are ethical obligations to provide assurance that the potential advantages of any treatment must outweigh the inherent risk to the donor, highlighting the importance of careful deliberations among healthcare providers, patients, and families to make such delicate decisions (Russa et al., 2017). Furthermore, the problem of conflict of interest surfaces most visibly in pediatric hematology and oncology whenever a single physician is charged with both the duty of choosing donors and taking care of patients. Such a situation could present difficulties in giving full attention to the best interests of both donor and recipient. The non-maleficence ethical rule requiring health professionals not to cause harm is particularly strained in such circumstances. Doctors are compelled to walk that thin rope of objectivity while still providing appropriate protection and care to all concerned parties, donors, recipients, and their families, respectively. Donor and recipient coverage by insurance raises the level of complexity, as the provision of such can be a treatment determiner. It is therefore essential to formulate strict regulatory frameworks to govern such transactions, and ethical practice has to be maintained at every level of patient management (Russa et al., 2017). The advent of liquid biopsy techniques in pediatric oncology is a giant leap towards non-invasive cancer diagnosis, but it also creates new ethical challenges. The hope of cell-free DNA profiling as a tool to enhance therapeutic decision and monitoring of treatment response also complicates issues on standardization of these techniques in clinical practice. While early work promises to connect liquid biopsies to tumor markers, gaps remain in the type of tumor tested and detection methods. Ethical issues are around equitable access to these emerging technologies, especially considering the disparities that pervade the healthcare system. While such methodologies become a part of pediatric treatment protocol, stakeholders must examine their implications on patient confidentiality, consent, and the overall scenario of customized medicine. The deployment of established liquid biopsy-based technologies must be done with caution so that technological superiority is balanced with ethical integrity.

## 9.6.1. Informed Consent and Decision-Making

In pediatric hematology and oncology, informed consent is crucial, particularly where complex therapies , such as allogeneic hematopoietic stem cell transplantation (allo-HSCT) are under consideration. From the outset, the medical team must ensure that families are aware of the complexity of the procedure and both the potential benefits and risks involved. The ethical duty of providing comprehensive information requires that parents or guardians be given clear data to enable them to make informed decisions in the best interest of their children. Basic principles include clarification of possible bad occurrences, the weight of health complications with possible occurrences, and balancing such risks against possible benefits of the transplant. In addition, a sound ethical consent process would have to consider conflicts of interest, particularly where the same physician is involved in donor selection and recipient care, to provide a firm adherence to the ethical principles guiding the making of treatment choices (Russa et al., 2017). Decision-making in pediatric oncology is also complicated by the need for effective communication of prognostic information. Nurses occupy the middle of this scenario, usually the interface between the medical team and the family. However, the existing practice has the tendency to leave nurses out of the process of prognosis-related communication (PRC), and therefore they are not able to fully inform and counsel families. This exclusion creates loopholes in the decision-making framework, as caregivers may not entirely understand the patients' prognosis, treatment options, and outcomes. As can be observed from existing studies, it is feasible to augment the provision of prognostic information and involve families more actively in children's care choices through the facilitation of teamwork between healthcare providers, particularly nurses (Sisk et al., 2019). Furthermore, a cultural shift within pediatric oncology must also take place so that nurses are key players in the PRC process. Training is critical for doctors and nurses in terms of the importance of engaging nursing staff in having empathetic conversations with patients about prognosis and treatment. Empowering them can lead to more positive outcomes for both patients and families and enhance the cohesiveness of healthcare teams. With regard to collaboration and the facilitation of communication strategies, healthcare professionals can facilitate informed consent that reflects the general opinion of all involved. These advances will not only enhance informed consent but also enhance decision-making overall, resulting in better experience and outcomes for children with hematology and oncology problems (Sisk et al., 2019) (Figure 9.14).

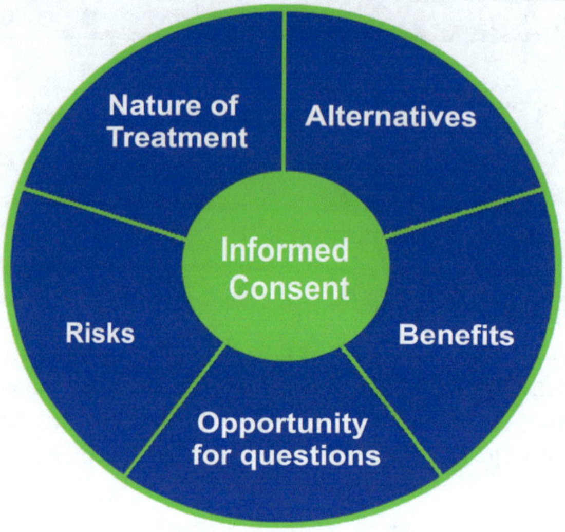


**Figure 9.14.** Informed consent and decision-making.

*Source:* https://external-content.duckduckgo.com/iu/?u=https%3A%2F%2Funderstandingmyositis.org%2Fwp-content%2Fuploads%2F2016%2F09%2Finformed-consent-1.jpg&f=1&nofb=1&ipt=c0fb8f5f49854f67fb4f2a8e480ebbc3fc09ffdd3402b814bc25fb1f6f0b8650.

## 9.6.2. Balancing Treatment Benefits and Risks

Within pediatric oncology and hematology, balance is everything as far as treatment benefits and risks, especially for patients , such as children who have vulnerabilities. Combined with variation in treatment modalities like chemotherapy, radiation, and stem cell transplantation, the therapy then has to be that much more complex in the way that it needs to be chosen. Every therapy carries with it its own set of pros and cons, and the patient's present health status and prognosis has to be carefully weighed. For instance, because chemotherapy is so potent at killing cancer cells, it also has the potential for causing great short-

and long-term toxicity hazards. Practitioners are therefore compelled to weigh projected outcomes against dangers of potential ill effect in designing the most beneficial treatment regimen for their children. In planning therapy regimens , such as allogeneic hematopoietic stem cell transplantation (allo-HSCT), the balance between benefit and risk takes on an increased importance. Allo-HSCT has transformed the treatment of various hematological disorders but is also beset with inherent dangers like graft-versus-host disease, organ toxicity, and potentially fatal infection. Ethical concerns over donor safety, especially in the case of children, further complicate the decision process.

As stated, donor selection standards and recipient care must guarantee the safety of all individuals and require that donors assume no greater risk than the potential gain by recipients (Russa et al., 2017). This comprehensive approach guarantees ethical integrity in addition to maximum patient benefit. The outcomes for single conditions show this exquisite balancing act, particularly in relapse conditions like Wilms tumor. Research indicates that high-dose chemotherapy coupled with autologous hematopoietic cell transplant performs mediocrely, with approximately 45% overall survival being reported in relapsed patients (Mehta et al., 2019). The promising figures, however, hide the critical underlying risks, including treatment-related morbidity and mortality long after therapy has been stopped. As clinicians move toward further optimization of treatment protocols, the focus now shifts to optimizing therapeutic modalities with improved patient event-free survival without excessively compromising quality of life. Finally, ongoing research endeavors must work to define therapies that control disease recurrence effectively with decreased long-term risk, validating the role of balanced treatment paradigm in pediatric cancer (Figure 9.15).

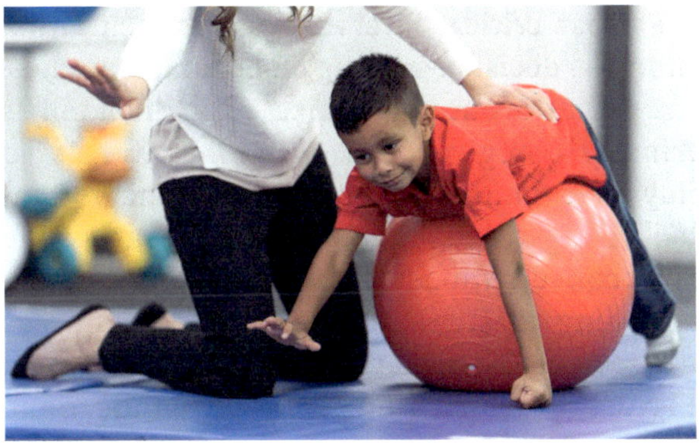

**Figure 9.15.** Balancing treatment benefits and risks.

*Source:* https://candokidspediatrics.com/wp-content/uploads/2024/03/Benefits-of-Pediatric-PT.webp.

## 9.6.3. The Role of Palliative Care

Palliative care plays a critical role in the management of children with hematological conditions and their families, particularly as they battle through diagnosis, treatment, and decisions regarding end-of-life care. Palliative care is not only focused on alleviating physical symptoms like pain, nausea, and fatigue, but it is also meant to treat the psychological, emotional, and spiritual issues of pediatric patients and their families. Through their interaction with an interdisciplinary group of personnel that often includes doctors, nurses, social workers, and psychologists, families are treated to an integrated process that seeks to optimize quality of life. Effective communication between healthcare providers, patients, and families lies at the core of palliative care, a setting in which fears over symptoms, choice of treatment, and emotional issues can be expressed freely. These are important considerations, especially for children with severe prognoses about hematologic malignancies, in which the integration of palliative care can improve ultimate outcomes and family satisfaction (Sisk et al., 2019). Also, provision of prognostic information within the context of palliative care is a most critical intervention for facilitating informed decision-making on behalf of families. The pediatric oncology nurse, often the family's primary caregiver, has a significant role to play in communicating prognosis news and facilitating treatment options and end-of-life care conversations. Too frequently, though, according to studies of recent years, nurses are seen to be excluded from the process of disclosure, which can potentially undermine their care for both patients and families (Sisk et al., 2019). This exclusion requires a paradigm shift, catalyzing nurses to engage actively within these required conversations. Improved education and communication among caregivers can close the gap, allowing families to be given holistic advice during challenging moments. Palliative care is therefore integrated into the entire treatment regime in pediatric hematology and oncology settings. In addition to symptom management and communication, palliative care also has a high value on the emotional and psychosocial support of the patient and his or her family. The psychological effect of chronic illness, especially in children, can be staggering, reaching to siblings, parents, and the family as a whole. Psychological support and counseling as well as support groups are covered in palliative care to allow families to cope with the emotional burden of life-threatening illness. Furthermore, the social resources and dynamics are also critical to be addressed in the home care context while managing care. Proofs have shown that this is able to more effectively alleviate anxieties and increase care service satisfaction through involving families in care planning and decision-making. Through the integration of these components within pediatric hematology and oncology treatment, palliative care not only maximizes patient experience but also strengthens the family's ability to cope with the brutal realities of serious illness (Sisk et al., 2019). Through whole-person care, palliative care is ultimately a progression toward creating more authentic and compassionate healthcare experiences.

## Test Your Knowledge

1. What ethical challenges are involved in informed consent and decision-making in pediatric hematology and oncology?
2. How do healthcare teams ethically balance treatment benefits and risks, and what role does palliative care play in this context?

## SUMMARY

In pediatric hematology and oncology, the importance of complicated treatment regimens in patient outcomes cannot be downplayed. The incidence of acute lymphoblastic leukemia (ALL) and its associated consequences, , such as hospitalization duration, underscore the necessity for integrated care strategies. Results indicate that children with high-risk and very high-risk ALL tend to experience adverse consequences, , such as extended hospitalization, and intense healthcare resource consumption. Therefore, implementation of strict discharge planning and follow-up care is crucial to the prevention of complications from inpatient care (Althouse et al., 2018). Proactive interventions also contribute significantly to reducing hospital readmission and enhancing the overall quality of life in young patients, which underscores the holistic nature of effective treatment outcomes. Additionally, the control of complications , such as fever and neutropenia (FN) is essential to enhance the comfort of patients. Proper intervention techniques that empower healthcare workers, especially nurses, are essential to maximize the quality of care delivered to this high-risk group. Educational programs designed to advance the competency of nurses in the detection and management of FN can significantly shift the pattern of patient care. By equipping medical professionals with the information and tools they require, patients and families can benefit from timely intervention and home care management, leading to reduced hospitalization and improved quality of life (Makarovich, 2024). These results underscore the imperative relationship between training, competency, and outcomes in pediatric oncology. Finally, the complexities of pediatric hematology and oncology require a multidisciplinary and collaborative approach. The stakeholders must meet up, among healthcare providers, families, and care support agencies, to craft an environment conducive to integrative care for patients. As research and practice advance, integration of findings from studies , such as those on longer inpatient stays and FN care can facilitate further knowledge of patient needs. Continuing evaluation of treatment protocols and outcomes will foster an adaptive healthcare system, one that respects the physical and emotional aspects of healing. Such commitment to forward-thinking care practices remains paramount in addressing the unique challenges faced by pediatric patients with hematologic and oncologic diseases, ultimately striving to build a world in which treatment effectiveness and quality of life are no longer incompatible.

In pediatric hematology and oncology, management of acute lymphoblastic leukemia (ALL) has become highly sophisticated and has led to very high rates of survival among children afflicted with the disease. However, along with this progress lies the awareness that therapy can cause an entire spectrum of toxicities. A recent Ponte di Legno working group consensus has listed 14 significant acute toxicities of ALL treatment protocols. Such toxicities are varied in incidence and severity, posing problems in instilling complete management within different treatment modalities. International collaboration has been enhanced by the Delphi technique, which allowed for consensus of standardized definitions of the toxicities. This has enhanced the accuracy of comparison of outcomes of treatments. Treatment of such toxic effects is essential to optimize treatment modalities and develop guidelines that minimize risks while maximizing chances of survival in children with ALL (Attarbaschi et al., 2016). The other critical area within the realm of pediatric hematology is the management of immune thrombocytopenia (ITP) and its unpredictable behavior in the affected patients. Though most young patients with ITP recover spontaneously, a few can still go on developing symptoms for which second-line therapy becomes necessary. Decision-making in the initiation of such a therapy was determined by the Pediatric ITP Consortium of North America in one of their studies. Factors that influence treatment choices include parental and patient preferences, side effect profiles of the treatments themselves, and perceived efficacy of the alternatives. Especially significant is the likelihood of long-term remission and underscores the value of personalized care strategies. Such regard for patient preference helps ensure an open environment among families, patients, and providers when making treatment plans (Grace et al., 2018). Moreover, the relationship between treatment response and quality of life in pediatric oncology and hematology underscores the requirement for continued investigation to further develop current protocols. Evolution of definitions and meanings of treatment-related toxicities not only maximizes care outcome but also informs future clinical practices and research fields. As testified by the experience of ITP treatment, shared decision-making must remain at the heart of therapeutic approaches to ensure that treatments remain aligned with the values and preferences of patients and families. These observations emphasize the importance of well-conducted comparative effectiveness research that can guide treatment recommendations and improve patient experience in the rapidly changing domains of pediatric hematology and oncology (Attarbaschi et al., 2016; Grace et al., 2018).

## KEY TERMS FROM THIS CHAPTER

- Acute lymphoblastic leukemia (ALL)
- Chronic myeloid leukemia (CML)
- Hemophilia
- Leukemia
- Malignancy
- Patients
- Sickle cell disease (SCD)
- Toxicity
- Chemotherapy
- Hematology
- Integrative medicine modalities (IMMs)
- Lymphomas
- Oncology
- Pediatric hematology-oncology (PHO)
- Thrombocytopenia
- Tyrosine kinase inhibitor (TKI)

## CRITICAL THINKING QUESTIONS

1. **The most common type of childhood leukemia is:**
   a. Chronic myeloid leukemia (CML)
   b. Acute lymphoblastic leukemia (ALL)
   c. Acute myeloid leukemia (AML)
   d. Hairy cell leukemia
2. **Iron deficiency anemia is most commonly caused by:**
   a. Genetic mutation
   b. Iron loss or inadequate intake
   c. Vitamin B12 deficiency
   d. Hemolysis
3. **Thalassemia major is primarily treated with:**
   a. Vitamin C
   b. Bone marrow transplant
   c. Regular blood transfusions and iron chelation
   d. Antibiotics
4. **Sickle cell anemia is caused by a mutation in the gene coding for:**
   a. White blood cells
   b. Platelets
   c. Hemoglobin
   d. Iron
5. **Which of the following is a common symptom of leukemia in children?**
   a. Hyperactivity
   b. Enlarged lymph nodes and fatigue
   c. Constipation
   d. Frequent urination

### Short Answer Questions

1. Discuss iron deficiency anemia in children: causes, clinical features, diagnosis, and treatment.
2. Describe thalassemia major: clinical features, diagnosis, and management.
3. Explain the pathophysiology, diagnosis, and management of sickle cell disease.
4. Write a detailed note on acute lymphoblastic leukemia (ALL) in children.
5. Discuss the nursing care of a child undergoing chemotherapy.
6. What are the psychosocial challenges faced by children with cancer and their families?

### *Answers to Critical Thinking Questions*

1. (b); 2. (b); 3. (c); 4. (c); 5. (b)

## REFERENCES


1. Mehta, R. S., Holtan, S. G., Wang, T., Hemmer, M. T., Spellman, S. R., Arora, M., Couriel, D. R., Alousi, A. M., Pidala, J., Abdel-Azim, H., Ahmed, I., Aljurf, M., Askar, M., Auletta, J. J., Bhatt, V., Bredeson, C., Chhabra, S., Gadalla, S., Gajewski, J., Gale, R. P., ... Weisdorf, D. J. (2019). GRFS and CRFS in alternative donor hematopoietic cell transplantation for pediatric patients with acute leukemia. *Blood advances*, *3*(9), 1441–1449. https://doi.org/10.1182/bloodadvances.2018030171 (accessed on 16th June 2025).
2. Adcock, R., Banerjee, A., Dvorak, C. C., Golden, T., et al. (2019). Acupressure to reduce treatment-related symptoms for children with cancer and recipients of hematopoietic stem cell transplant: Protocol for a randomized controlled trial. https://core.ac.uk/download/323079284.pdf (accessed on 16th June 2025).
3. Agulnik, A., Bhakta, N., Chantada, G., Chen, Y., et al. (2021). Global effect of the COVID-19 pandemic on pediatric cancer care: A cross-sectional study. https://core.ac.uk/download/394997177.pdf (accessed on 16th June 2025).
4. Akan, H., Alexander, B. D., Andes, D., Azoulay, E., et al. (2019). Revision and update of the consensus definitions of invasive fungal disease from the European Organization for Research and Treatment of Cancer and the Mycoses Study Group Education and Research Consortium. https://core.ac.uk/download/287649722.pdf (accessed on 16th June 2025).
5. Fisher, B. T., Alexander, S., Dvorak, C. C., Zaoutis, T. E., Zerr, D. M., & Sung, L. (2012). Epidemiology and potential preventative measures for viral infections in children with malignancy and those undergoing hematopoietic cell transplantation. *Pediatric blood & cancer*, *59*(1), 11–15. https://doi.org/10.1002/pbc.23417(accessed on 16th June 2025).
6. Althouse, S. K., Batra, S., Rahrig, A., Rupenthal, B., et al. (2018). Factors associated with a prolonged hospital stay during induction chemotherapy in newly diagnosed high-risk pediatric acute lymphoblastic leukemia. https://core.ac.uk/download/160755266.pdf (accessed on 16th June 2025).
7. Angaard Nielsen, J. S., Brierley, J., Dohna-Schwake, C., Krause, J., et al. (2019). PICU mortality of children with cancer admitted to pediatric intensive care unit: A systematic review and meta-analysis. https://core.ac.uk/download/227040533.pdf (accessed on 16th June 2025).
8. Annibali, O., Napolitano, M., Avvisati, G., & Siragusa, S. (2018). Incidence of venous thromboembolism and use of anticoagulation in hematological malignancies: Critical review of the literature. *Critical reviews in oncology/hematology*, *124*, 41–50. https://doi.org/10.1016/j.critrevonc.2018.02.003(accessed on 16th June 2025).
9. Aronica, E., Becker, A., Benner, A., Beschorner, R., et al. (2018). DNA methylation-based classification of central nervous system tumors. https://core.ac.uk/download/323063278.pdf (accessed on 16th June 2025).
10. Attarbaschi, A., Barzilai, S., Escherich, G., Frandsen, T. L., et al. (2016). Consensus definitions of 14 severe acute toxic effects for childhood lymphoblastic leukemia treatment: A Delphi consensus. https://core.ac.uk/download/42370388.pdf (accessed on 16th June 2025).
11. Grace, R. F., Despotovic, J. M., Bennett, C. M., Bussel, J. B., Neier, M., Neunert, C., Crary, S. E., Pastore, Y. D., Klaassen, R. J., Rothman, J. A., Hege, K., Breakey, V. R., Rose, M. J., Shimano, K. A., Buchanan, G. R., Geddis, A., Haley, K. M., Lorenzana, A., Thompson, A., Jeng, M., ... Lambert,

M. P. (2018). Physician decision making in selection of second-line treatments in immune thrombocytopenia in children. *American journal of hematology, 93*(7), 882–888. https://doi.org/10.1002/ajh.25110(accessed on 16th June 2025).

12. Bertram, L. A. (2015). *Pediatric Oncology Nurses' Knowledge of Safe Administration of Chemotherapy/Biotherapy.* https://core.ac.uk/download/232575633.pdf (accessed on 16th June 2025).
13. Bhattasali, O., Geller, D., Gill, J., Gorlick, R., et al. (2015). Variability in the reported management of pulmonary metastases in osteosarcoma. https://core.ac.uk/download/323068150.pdf (accessed on 16th June 2025).
14. Rosenberg, A. S., Brunson, A., Paulus, J. K., Tuscano, J., Wun, T., Keegan, T. H. M., & Jonas, B. A. (2017). Secondary acute lymphoblastic leukemia is a distinct clinical entity with prognostic significance. *Blood cancer journal, 7*(9), e605. https://doi.org/10.1038/bcj.2017.81(accessed on 16th June 2025).
15. Clayton-Jones, D., Matthie, N., Treadwell, M., Field, J. J., Mager, A., Sawdy, R., George Dalmida, S., Leonard, C., Koch, K. L., & Haglund, K. (2021). Social and Psychological Factors Associated With Health Care Transition for Young Adults Living With Sickle Cell Disease. *Journal of transcultural nursing : official journal of the Transcultural Nursing Society, 32*(1), 21–29. https://doi.org/10.1177/1043659619896837(accessed on 16th June 2025).
16. Collins, C. (2017). *Radiation Therapy Medical Physics Review–Delivery, Interactions, Safety, Feasibility, and Head-to-Head Comparisons of The Leading Radiation Therapy Techniques.* https://core.ac.uk/download/215516487.pdf (accessed on 16th June 2025).
17. Sisk, B. A., Schulz, G. L., Mack, J. W., Yaeger, L., & DuBois, J. (2019). Communication interventions in adult and pediatric oncology: A scoping review and analysis of behavioral targets. *PloS one, 14*(8), e0221536. https://doi.org/10.1371/journal.pone.0221536(accessed on 16th June 2025).
18. Salek, M. S., Ionova, T., Johns, J. R., & Oliva, E. N. (2019). Appraisal of patient-reported outcome measures in analogous diseases and recommendations for use in phase II and III clinical trials of pyruvate kinase deficiency. *Quality of life research : an international journal of quality of life aspects of treatment, care and rehabilitation, 28*(2), 399–410. https://doi.org/10.1007/s11136-018-2025-y(accessed on 16th June 2025).
19. Landier, W., Ahern, J., Barakat, L. P., Bhatia, S., Bingen, K. M., Bondurant, P. G., Cohn, S. L., Dobrozsi, S. K., Haugen, M., Herring, R. A., Hooke, M. C., Martin, M., Murphy, K., Newman, A. R., Rodgers, C. C., Ruccione, K. S., Sullivan, J., Weiss, M., Withycombe, J., Yasui, L., ... Hockenberry, M. (2016). Patient/Family Education for Newly Diagnosed Pediatric Oncology Patients. *Journal of pediatric oncology nursing : official journal of the Association of Pediatric Oncology Nurses, 33*(6), 422–431. https://doi.org/10.1177/1043454216655983
20. Makarovich, S. (2024). *Inservice Education: Management of Fever and Neutropenia Among the Pediatric Oncology Population.* https://core.ac.uk/download/619706193.pdf (accessed on 16th June 2025).
21. Spraker-Perlman, H. R., Heidelberg, R. E., Wright, R. P., Ly, A. G., Meyer, M., Vukadinovich, C., Baker, J. N., et al. (2025). Pediatric hematology-oncology provider attitudes and beliefs about the use of integrative modalities for their patients: A cross-sectional survey. *Journal of Integrative and Complementary Medicine.* https://www.semanticscholar.org/paper/01036899964d0253db0eefe6515f84e6c8b046c4 (accessed on 16th June 2025).

# PEDIATRIC ENDOCRINOLOGY

# 10

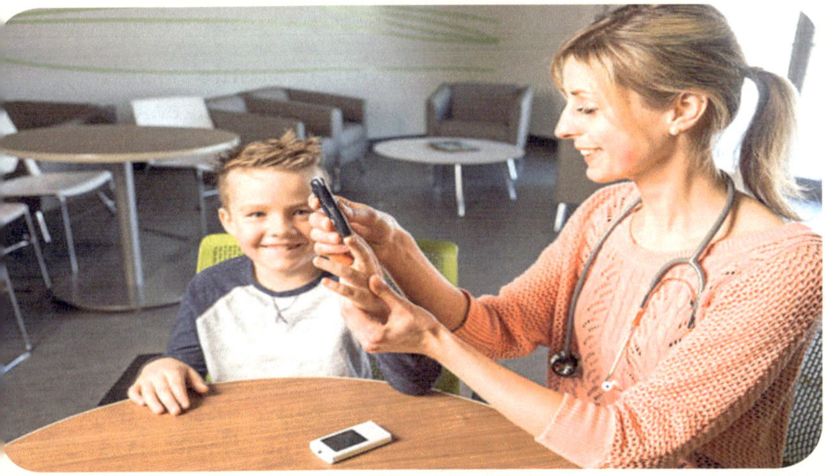

## LEARNING OBJECTIVES

**After studying this chapter, you will be able to:**

1. Discuss the hormonal development in children;
2. Explain the common endocrine disorders;
3. Focus on the diagnosis of endocrine disorders;
4. Know treatment options in pediatric endocrinology;
5. Understand psychological and social implications;
6. Evaluate advances in pediatric endocrinology.

## Introduction

Pediatric endocrinology refers to the medical study and treatment of endocrine disorders in children, a specialty crucial in offering optimal growth and development in the initial years of life. During the various stages of growth of a child, the endocrine system has an active role to regulate the metabolism, reproduction, and physical and mental health. The specialty manages a wide range of diseases , such as diabetes, obesity, thyroid diseases, and sexual differentiation disorders. The complexity of diagnosing and treating these disorders makes the clinician's deep understanding of normal and abnormal endocrine function critical. Exposure to pediatric endocrinology is the background upon which to understand these complicated interactions and the powerful influence they have on the course and quality of the child's development. In explaining specific conditions that are treated under this specialty, type 1 diabetes mellitus is an outstanding example, indicating the necessity of successful management and transfer from pediatric to adult care. Adolescents with this long-term condition are likely to face enormous challenges, particularly in transferring to adult health care services. Research indicates that without suitable guidance, substantial deteriorations in glycemic control are experienced during this period, highlighting the need for well-designed models of transition based on education and patient as well as family support. A knowledge of these facilitators and barriers is necessary for healthcare workers so they can institute an uninterrupted process of transition that maintains the health and wellbeing of the patient. The nuances of managing diabetes in adolescents mirror the general issues of pediatric endocrinology, where multidisciplinary management and family involvement are paramount for maximum success. Family support systems and dynamics serve a role that cannot be overstated in being able to control endocrine conditions.

Family involvement in pediatric endocrinology becomes part of the treatment team, as it influences adherence to treatment and health outcome. For instance, empirical studies employing measures like the family interaction macro-coding system (FIMS) have established that parenting behavior and family cohesion, acceptance and behavioral control, say, are determinants of treatment outcomes for conditions like type 1 diabetes and spina bifida. These findings illuminate some degree of interdependence of physical and family functioning and suggest that an interdisciplinary treatment plan that emphasizes addressing familial roles can be more effective. Thus, the exploration of the convergences of pediatric endocrine disease and family functioning provides an overall impression of the challenges and strategies required to navigate through these complex health landscapes, thus promoting improved patient outcomes in pediatric endocrinology (Figure 10.1).

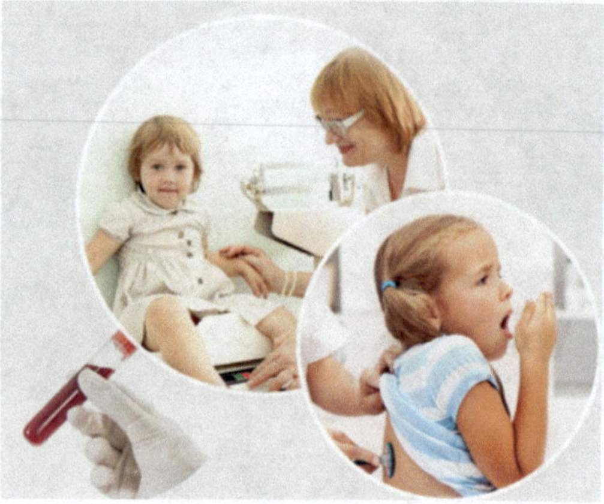

**Figure 10.1.** Pediatric endocrinology encompasses the study and management of hormonal disorders in children.

*Source:* https://cradlehospital.com/wp-content/uploads/2018/07/lab-testing.png.

## Definition and Scope of Pediatric Endocrinology

Pediatric endocrinology is a subspecialty of medicine that focuses on the diagnosis and management of endocrine and metabolic disorders in children. Pediatric endocrinology is an intersection of evidence from various fields of endocrinology and pediatrics to treat unique physiological differences between pediatric and adult populations. Pediatric endocrinologists assess growth-related conditions, sexual maturation, metabolic syndrome, and diabetes, among others. Furthermore, the scope of practice encompasses evaluation of congenital disorders that affect endocrine function, , such as sexual differentiation disorder or adrenal gland disorder. In providing targeted interventions for the latter, pediatric endocrinology encourages not just physical but also psychological and developmental management of affected children, accentuating the integrated character of practice within this specialty. The definition of pediatric endocrinology is also enriched by the reality that it is an interdisciplinary medicine, which often coordinates with other medical specialties in order to optimize patient care. For instance, pediatric endocrinologists may collaborate with nutritionists, geneticists, and psychologists to develop comprehensive treatment plans based on each patient's distinct needs. This collaborative nature is particularly evident in treating obesity and diabetes, where lifestyle modification, medication, and counseling are necessary to deliver proper treatment. Moreover, the pace of genetic research has also advanced the understanding of disorders, enabling earlier diagnosis and intervention. These collaborative and dynamic processes continue to advance the field of pediatric endocrinology as an essential component of healthcare in adolescents. Apart from clinical responsibilities, pediatric endocrinologists also play significant roles in education and research. They contribute towards training prospective healthcare professionals through mentorship and academic programs in a bid to advance information on endocrine disorders in childhood. Research in pediatric endocrinology enhances treatment guidelines and discovers novel therapeutic options, further expanding the field's contribution to children's health. Pediatric endocrinology, in the real sense of the term, transcends the treatment of disease; it encompasses efforts to improve the welfare of endocrine diseased children. As health care evolves further, the relevance of this subspecialty is all the clearer and underscores the absolute need for continuous research and development in pediatric endocrinology (Cox et al., 2013).

## Importance of Endocrine Health in Children

The significance of endocrine well-being in children is underlined by the intricate interaction between hormone control and growth and development. Endocrine diseases may lead to profound disruption of physical, emotional, and intellectual development during periods of optimum growth. Disorders , such as Turner syndrome, caused by chromosomal defects, exemplify the intricate interaction between genetics and endocrine activity. One large-scale study of karyotype-confirmed Turner syndrome cases revealed that short stature and delayed puberty were among the most common presentation problems, with a high prevalence of patients who had cardiac and urinary pathologies, as well as psychosocial pathology. These findings explain the necessity of continuous monitoring and intervention to treat these multifaceted problems in pediatric patients presenting with endocrine disorders (Yeşilkaya et al., 2015). Early identification and comprehensive management are essential, both in order to optimize physical health as well as overall well-being and development. Pediatric endocrinology is more than hormonal imbalance and entails an integrative model of the child's health. Disorders of sex development (DSD), for instance, reflect the complexity of endocrine disorders, in that they often co-exist with numerous other conditions. International DSD Registry reports indicate that 26% of the cases presented with other health conditions, , such as cardiac malformations and central nervous system abnormalities. Such correlations necessitate a multi-disciplinary team, as treatment for such complexity would require coordination among various specialist doctors to provide integrative care particular to each child's needs. By using a holistic perspective, pediatric endocrinology can mitigate the impact of endocrine disease on the life of children in not only physical but also psychosocial and emotional development (Cox et al., 2013). In light of these understanding, the importance of endocrine well-being in children becomes apparent in maintaining long-term health outcomes. Early diagnosis and effective control of endocrine disorders can significantly improve the health of such children and allow them to reach their full potential. Preventive care , such as regular checkup and parents' education on growth patterns and endocrine changes is extremely useful in such situations. With advancements in pediatric endocrinology, ongoing research and development are necessary in streamlining diagnostic equipment and treatment modes to enable children with the best possible care for optimal endocrine function. With all these considered, medical professionals can better serve children and their families, which eventually results in healthier generations gifted with optimal physical, emotional, and social thriving (Figure 10.2).

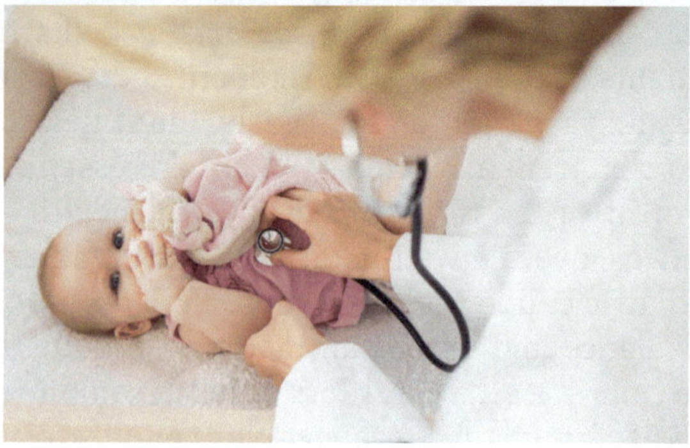

**Figure 10.2.** The significance of endocrine health in children.

*Source:* https://www.providence.co.in/wp-content/uploads/2020/03/PEDIATRIC-ENDOCRINOLOGY-sub-banner.png.

## Overview of Common Endocrine Disorders in Pediatrics

In pediatric endocrinology, the most pressing of problems is sexual development disorders, like hypospadias. Such a birth defect, characterized by a boy's abnormal urethral opening, can occur with varying degrees of severity. There is evidence of an intriguing genetic etiology; severe forms in some boys are caused by mutations in the steroidogenic factor 1 (SF-1, NR5A1) gene. Analysis has revealed that certain mutations are linked with significant clinical presentations, including decreased testosterone secretion and undescended testes. The results highlight the utility of genetic testing in assessing severe cases of hypospadias, as SF-1 mutations may have not only physical implications but also long-term implications for the health of individuals involved. This new information underpins a more refined approach to diagnosis and treatment, particularly in complex cases in children (Achermann et al., 2009). Obesity is yet another pervasive endocrine disorder prevalent among children and adolescents, and with increasing alarm levels globally. The Centers for Disease Control and Prevention recognizes that around 17% of American children and adolescents are obese, and of these, severe obesity has alarming percentages. This increase is linked to many comorbidities, , such as cardiovascular disease and type 2 diabetes, which carry long-term health implications.

The multi-factorial basis of obesity as a chronic illness with both genetic and environmental influences necessitates a multi-modal treatment regimen to be effective. Treatment in most instances involves behavioral therapy, diet, and exercise, but the majority of treatments are unsuccessful, especially in those with severe obesity. Evidence-based and patient-tailored treatments addressing pediatric obesity-specific physiology remain critical to effective intervention (Ameer et al., 2018). Besides hypospadias and obesity, disorders of growth and metabolism rank highest in pediatric endocrinology. Growth hormone deficiency (GHD) is one such instance of complexity in the diagnosis as well as management of endocrine illnesses in children. GHD can be produced by various causes , such as pituitary or genetic mutations and is associated with delayed onset of puberty and growth retardation. Very much better outcomes can be obtained following early treatment with synthetic growth hormone, which emphasizes the importance of early treatment. Other conditions , such as congenital adrenal hyperplasia (CAH) also present with disturbances in metabolism, which add to the clinical presentation. CAH particularly underlines the necessity of robust screening and management guidelines, as it may lead to adrenal insufficiency and undervirilization or genitalia virilization, which has a significant impact on a child's physical and psychological well-being. Treatment of these intricate conditions requires a highly coordinated effort from clinicians, parents, and specialists (Achermann et al., 2009).

## 10.1. Hormonal Development in Children

**Learning Outcome**

1. Stages of hormonal development from infancy to adolescence;
2. Role of hormones in growth and development;
3. Impact of hormonal imbalances during developmental stages.

Hormonal growth in childhood is a complex process and is influenced by an endless array of genetic, environmental, and nutritional factors. The endocrine system is a vital player in growth and development control through hormones , such as growth hormone, thyroid hormones, and sex steroids. These hormones each contribute to physical growth, the development of the brain, and the sexual maturation of the reproductive organs. Misregulation or deficiency of any one of these hormones can lead to severe health issues, , such as stunted growth or precocious puberty. For instance, the impact of congenital illnesses on hormone function or activity can be manifested early in life, necessitating careful metabolic monitoring and management strategies. Understanding these hormonal alterations is significant for pediatric endocrinologists when it comes to addressing the issues of disorders of growth and development and long-term impact on health outcomes. Hormonal growth in children is typically evaluated from birth, where variations can be very difficult to address clinically. Disorders of sex development (DSD) are one instance of the complexity of hormonal expression and function. DSD diagnosis is through extensive assessment by means of hormonal testing, imaging, and genetic studies, accompanied by multidisciplinary treatment to help affected families. Today's information has explained the biological underpinning of the disorders, emphasizing the importance of individualized treatments tailored to be gender variance-sensitive in accordance with societal attitudes. Since they are pediatric endocrinologists, there is a responsibility not only to heal hormonal disorders but also to guide and counsel families about sensitive social expectations in terms of development and identity. Thus, a greater understanding of hormonal intricacies becomes essential in promoting physical and emotional well-being in such children (Ahmid et al., 2016).

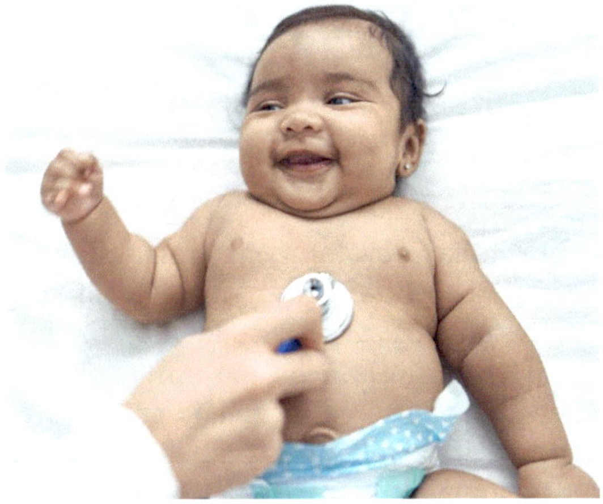

**Figure 10.3.** A smiling infant undergoes a routine checkup as a healthcare provider listens to the chest with a stethoscope, highlighting the importance of regular pediatric assessments.

*Source:* https://www.geetanjalihospital.co.in/img/media/cache/blogs/02/1200x630/1010/2%20(5).jpg.

Linear growth is a significant indicator of the metabolic health of children, particularly in the context of some hormonal disorders , such as congenital adrenal hyperplasia (CAH). New studies indicate that early diagnosis and intervention through the use of newborn screening will help alleviate the impact of growth generally seen in children with CAH. Treatment involves the administration of low doses of hydrocortisone, which, based on current research, has been found to stabilize growth measures against population norms. In tracking development, height standard deviations (H-SDS) offer a quantifiable indicator to evaluate treatment outcome over time. Notably, while initial measurements of height can be above the mean at birth, children can develop to their genetic size potential as they mature through directed interventions. This fine understanding of growth patterns is critical to pediatric endocrinologists since it allows them to design treatment regimens optimally to optimize health outcomes (Bonfig et al., 2011) (Figure 10.3).

### 10.1.1. Stages of Hormonal Development from Infancy to Adolescence

The hormonal development from infancy to puberty is characterized by a series of stages of intricate biological activity. Infancy, the initial stage, is characterized by the influence of the mother's hormones, estrogen and progesterone, which are involved in sexual differentiation and development of various body systems. As infants grow into early childhood, the levels of these hormones decline, and there follows a comparatively inactive sexual development stage. This hormonal suppression state is needed, allowing children to grow steadily before puberty sets in. It is also at this period that the hypothalamus-pituitary-gonadal (HPG) axis is suppressed, setting the stage for ensuing development milestones that occur in adolescence and require a timely activation of hormone signals. When children reach the stage of prepuberty, a cascade of endocrine changes begins to manifest, culminating with the triggering of the HPG axis. This is often termed adrenarche, typically at age 6 to 8, characterized by increased secretion of adrenal androgens , such as dehydroepiandrosterone (DHEA). These androgens are responsible for triggering the early development of secondary sex characteristics , such as pubic hair and changes in body odor. Furthermore, the pubertal development is regulated by various factors, , such as psychosocial and environmental signals, which can influence the timing of hormone fluctuation. Indeed, according to more recent studies, the modulation between genetic predispositions and extrinsic stimuli can notably affect the process of the puberty onset, illustrating the concept of adaptive plasticity in this formative phase of development (Templeton et al., 2013). The onset of actual puberty is signaled by the activation of the HPG axis, which triggers significant hormonal imbalances leading to bodily growth. This process typically starts at about ages 9 to 14 in females and 10 to 15 in males, during which the hypothalamus enhances the release of gonadotropin-releasing hormone (GnRH).

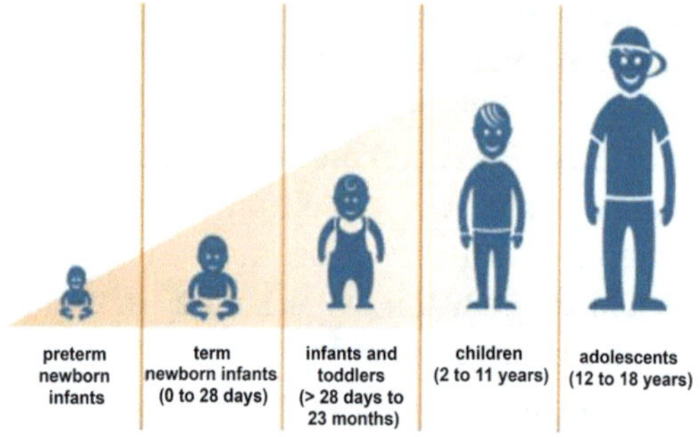


**Figure 10.4.** Stages of hormonal development from infancy to adolescence.

*Source:* https://www.rnpedia.com/wp-content/uploads/2014/12/Human-Growth-and-Development.gif.

This, in turn, causes the anterior pituitary gland to secrete luteinizing hormone (LH) and follicle-stimulating hormone (FSH), activating gonadal function and the secretion of sex steroids. In males, this results in testosterone levels increasing, while females undergo an increase in estrogen and progesterone secretion. Interestingly, Klinefelter syndrome, among others, may complicate these hormonal developments, as evidenced by studies tracking testicular dysfunction in such males. It is crucial that pediatric endocrinologists comprehend these hormone stages since identification and regulation of abnormalities at this phase can establish good health outcomes in children who have developmental issues (Carlomagno et al., 2023) (Figure 10.4).

### 10.1.2. Role of Hormones in Growth and Development

Hormones also play an essential role in the growth and development of children, regulating physiological changes from pre-natal stages to adolescence. The endocrine system, which secretes hormones into the bloodstream, regulates numerous disparate biological processes, including metabolism, growth, and sexual development. As an example, growth hormone (GH) plays a fundamental role in regulating the growth of height and skeletal development in children and adolescents. Also, sex hormones, , such as testosterone and estrogen, are responsible for secondary sexual characteristics and help to develop the reproductive apparatus. Any deficiency or excess of any of them can lead to severe developmental disorders, which may induce the development of dwarfism or precocious puberty. In this sense, understanding the intricate balance of hormones is essential for pediatricians in the process of diagnosing growth disorders and defining the correct interventions. In addition to growth hormone, thyroid hormones also have a function in metabolic regulation and overall growth. Thyroid hormones affect the development of the central nervous system and contribute significantly to mental capacity and physical growth. Those with hypothyroidism, for example, may exhibit delayed growth and developmental delays; early diagnosis and treatment must be done to avoid such outcomes. The mechanisms for hormone regulation by feedback challenge the complexity of pediatric endocrinology, where not only hormones but also the environment and overall condition control growth. Moreover, hormones like insulin exert a considerable impact on controlling the metabolism of energy and growth, hence influencing children's development, both physically and mentally.

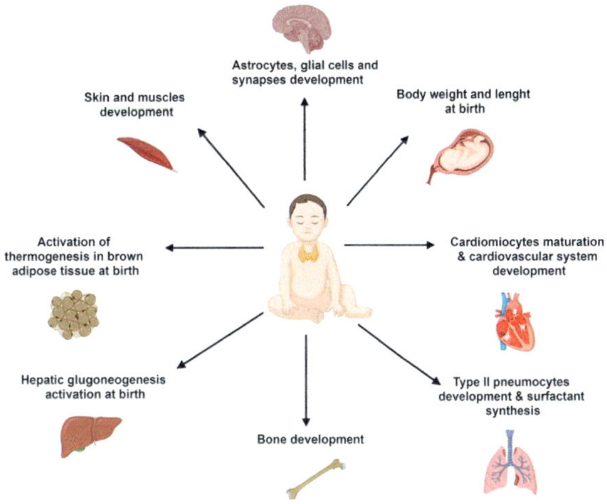


**Figure 10.5.** Hormones play a pivotal role in the growth and development of children.

*Source:* https://www.researchgate.net/publication/359341035/figure/fig2/AS:11431281258649712@1720126059841/The-role-of-thyroid-hormones-in-fetal-and-infant-development-Thyroid-hormones-are.tif.

Thus, detailed examination of hormone mechanisms explains the complexities and conundrums in the management of pediatric growth disorders. Recent developments have illuminated the function of including gender differences, as mediated by sex hormones, in understanding growth and development. For instance, the differential effects of estrogen and testosterone can lead to differences in growth patterns and metabolic processes in male and female children. Not only do gender determine physiological states, but also are enmeshed with social expectations, the latter of which can affect pathways to health. Psychosocial and hormonal influences are complex; environmental stressors in a child may accelerate development, as according to some theory, psychosocial family stress can enhance adaptations to a reduced life history strategy, perhaps towards earlier maturation (Templeton et al., 2013). These reflections underscore the necessity to merge biological and environmental factors into pediatric endocrinology, emphasizing the intricate interaction between hormones, growth, and development in children (Appetecchia et al., 2018) (Figure 10.5).

### 10.1.3. Impact of Hormonal Imbalances During Developmental Stages

The impact of hormonal imbalance at critical times of development is paramount in shaping most physiological and psychological outcomes in children. Such imbalance could be the consequence of an endless array of possible causes, including genetic predispositions, environmental influences, and dietary deficiencies. As illustration, derangement in the secretion or regulation of hormones , such as testosterone, estrogen, and insulin could yield adverse effects on development, metabolism, and overall well-being. The implications are most striking under the conditions of rapid expansion, , such as puberty, when the body radically changes to prepare for adulthood. The full appreciation of how hormonal fluctuation impacts developmental trajectories is essential for medical practitioners as it lays the ground for the design of early intervention techniques to avert long-term morbidity. In pediatric endocrinology, it is essential to consider the interaction between hormonal imbalance and conditions that develop during developmental stages. Conditions like Klinefelter syndrome, with an extra X chromosome in males, show how hormonal malfunction will manifest physically and emotionally. Individuals with such a syndrome can enjoy high rates of anxiety, depression, and poor social performance, particularly if growing up and developing during their childhood and adolescence. It has been argued that developmental results can significantly be improved through interventions during the early stages, hence repeating the importance of early treatment and diagnosis in order to intervene effectively into hormonal disturbances. How genetic susceptibility interacts with environmental stressors in influencing neuroendocrine reaction is a lot to say about the challenge of these conditions in children (Panvino et al., 2024). Hormonal disturbances would also have serious effects on reproductive health as well as quality of life in young people. For example, male infertility could be closely linked with hormonal disturbances that include major hormones , such as testosterone and follicle-stimulating hormone. The disturbances in these hormones could affect normal spermatogenesis and lead to fertility problems later in life. Hormonal disturbances typically require a multidisciplinary management that includes pharmacological treatments , such as replacement of hormones and lifestyle modifications that are tailored to the patient. Understanding the character of these treatment regimens is important for clinicians to formulate effective management strategies that address both the physiological and psychological demands associated with hormonal imbalance. Adopting a holistic strategy that combines the developmental model and individual variation is critical in order to enhance health outcomes within pediatric endocrinology (AlAsmi, 2025).

## Test Your Knowledge

1. What are the key stages of hormonal development from infancy to adolescence, and what roles do hormones play in growth and development?
2. How can hormonal imbalances during childhood and adolescence affect development?

## 10.2. Common Endocrine Disorders

**Learning Outcome**

1. Diabetes mellitus in children;
2. Growth hormone deficiency;
3. Thyroid disorders in pediatric patients.

The study of endocrine disorders common in children encompasses a range of conditions with broad impacts on child growth, development, and health. One is congenital adrenal hyperplasia (CAH), a condition present at birth caused by an inherited disorder affecting the adrenal glands' synthesis of steroids and leading to excessive production of androgens. It is especially critical because it can result in ambiguous genitalia in newborns, which must be carefully assessed by clinicians and addressed accordingly. Early diagnosis is paramount, as early interventions avert long-term complications, including those affecting sexual development and adjustment to psychosocial issues. Recent research indicates the complexity of managing these cases, necessitating a multidisciplinary intervention to ensure complete care and support to families overcoming such issues (Ahmid et al., 2016). Another serious endocrine disorder includes juvenile diabetes, also referred to as Type 1 diabetes mellitus. This autoimmune disease typically manifests in childhood or adolescence and results in the destruction of insulin-secreting beta cells within the pancreas. The ensuing lack of insulin necessitates lifetime management by insulin therapy and monitoring of blood sugar. The outcome of poorly controlled diabetes in children can be severe, with complications , such as growth inhibition, reduced academic achievement, and early onset of cardiovascular disease in adulthood. Literature indicates that effective management practices that emphasize education and self-management skills can significantly improve health outcomes in pediatric patients (Ernst et al., 2010). Lastly, thyroid disease, , such as hypothyroidism and hyperthyroidism, is increasingly being seen as common endocrine conditions in pediatric practice. Hypothyroidism, or the generation of insufficient thyroid hormone, can cause delayed growth, reduced intellect, and weight gain, while hyperthyroidism, or overproduction of the hormone, can result in symptoms like hyperactivity and weight loss. Early diagnosis and correct management of the disorders are crucial in the preservation of sound development and growth. Of particular note, children with endocrine disorders have also been described as having more psychiatric symptoms, even necessitating a critical assessment of mental health alongside endocrine assessment (Ernst et al., 2010). This information highlights the necessity of an integrated model for treatment of the multi-dimensional aspects of endocrine disorders in children (Figure 10.6).

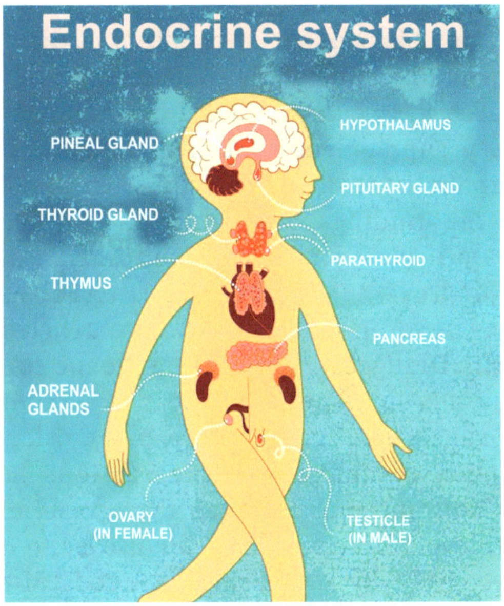


**Figure 10.6.** The study of common endocrine disorders.

*Source:* https://www.momjunction.com/wp-content/uploads/2020/10/Endocrine-System-Diagram-Parts-And-Functions-For-Kids1-1.jpg.webp.

### 10.2.1. Diabetes Mellitus in Children

Diabetes Mellitus, particularly Type 1 Diabetes (T1D), is a critical issue in the pediatric population, with direct effects on their physical health and mental well-being. T1D children are not only burdened with the inconvenience of daily insulin therapy but are also at risk for long-term complications , such as retinopathy and nephropathy. These complications have a poor potential to severely impair their quality of life and need close follow-up throughout their development and growth. The American Diabetes Association (ADA) established screening guidelines to facilitate early diagnosis of such disorders with emphasis on ongoing follow-up as well as adherence to prescribed care protocols. Through the adoption of universal screening procedures, medical practitioners can identify potential complications at an early stage, thus improving health outcomes for children suffering from T1D (Bartz et al., 2019). Nutritional control is also crucial in overall diabetes management in children, particularly in sustaining optimal glycemic control. Of late, research has been conducted on the effects of dietary supplements , such as vitamin D on metabolic control in children with diabetes, and the findings are promising. Research revealed that vitamin D supplementation may improve hemoglobin A1c (HbA1C) levels among children with T1D who are deficient in vitamin D, suggesting that the glycemic control is causally linked to the status of vitamin D. This suggestion presents the potential for the inclusion of nutritional interventions along with conventional diabetes therapy, offering multi-level management of the disease to treat it effectively. By addressing the needs of both diet and medicine, healthcare professionals can also support an improved holistic treatment of diabetes in children (Fatahi et al., 2015). Additionally, technology in diabetes care has revolutionized the children's care environment for patients with this chronic illness. Continuous glucose monitoring and insulin pump regimens provide real-time feedback, allowing for precise dosing of insulin and enhanced glycemic control. Such technological advances enable children and their parents to make rational decisions about their health, preventing the occurrence of hypoglycemic attacks and other diabetes complications. As the health care system continues to develop, the use of best practice alerts in computerized medical records can also improve adherence to proven clinical guidelines for diabetes care. This synergy of evidence-based and technological practice underscores the imperative requirement of ongoing education and assistance to families who provide care for pediatric diabetes (Bartz et al., 2019).

### 10.2.2. Growth Hormone Deficiency

Growth hormone deficiency (GHD) among children is a significant problem among health practitioners in the field of pediatric endocrinology. Patients with GHD are known to exhibit less linear growth, raising concern about reaching normal height as an adult. Undiagnosed and untreated GHD impinges not only on the height but also on psychosocial aspects of a child's life, , such as self-esteem and social interaction. Child endocrinologists utilize a series of diagnostic methods to determine GHD, including assessment of growth, hormone stimulation tests, and bone age evaluation. Early diagnosis is important since appropriate treatment can significantly enhance growth outcomes, and thus the quality of life of the afflicted children. But the complexity of the condition demands a multidisciplinary management that involves not only endocrinologists but also nutritionists and psychologists, who can deal with the overall developmental care of these patients. The management of GHD is most commonly in the form of recombinant human growth hormone (rhGH) therapy, which has proved beneficial for growth stimulation in these children. Yet the therapy of GHD raises some issues regarding long-term compliance with treatment schedules. According to studies, non-compliance with growth hormone (GH) treatment can result in suboptimal clinical outcomes, specifically on linear growth and quality of life (Carlo et al., 2017). Healthcare providers should understand the determinants of therapy compliance, including the efficacy of various injection devices and support systems in patients. Advanced technologies that facilitate administration and monitoring, , such as electronic devices for automated monitoring, have promise in promoting adherence rates. However, the acceptance and practicability of new solutions depend heavily on rigorous research to ensure the patient's ongoing compliance throughout treatment. While rhGH use has been historically focused on height normalization, recent evidence suggests it has crucial functions to play in sustaining bone health and cardiovascular status as well, expanding its therapeutic scope. Studies have established that deficiencies of these aspects in adults who have developed GHD in childhood highlight the need for a more adaptive approach to therapy at adulthood onset (Ahmid et al., 2016).

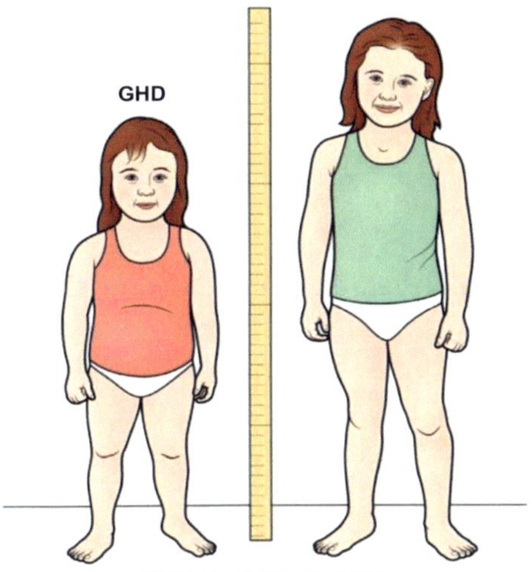


**Figure 10.7.** Growth hormone deficiency (GHD) in pediatric patients poses significant challenges for healthcare professionals in the field of pediatric endocrinology.

*Source:* https://images.saymedia-content.com/.image/t_share/MTc2NDU4NjQ0OTIwMjE0NzQx/is-your-child-growing-okay.jpg.

The long-term benefits of prolonged rhGH treatment during this critical period are not sufficiently studied and are, therefore, the subject of further research. As the specialty of pediatric endocrinology continues to evolve, practitioners are faced with the challenge of reconciling the cost and clinical benefit of rhGH therapy across the lifetime of their patients. An in-depth understanding of the impact of GHD on overall well-being is crucial in order to develop effective treatment interventions that not only address growth but also cater to the overall well-being of the affected persons and therefore ongoing research is an essential requirement (Figure 10.7).

### 10.2.3. Thyroid Disorders in Pediatric Patients

Pediatric thyroids diseases are a major area of interest in the field of pediatric endocrinology and have implications for growth, metabolism, and health. Hypothyroidism and hyperthyroidism are the two most frequent conditions encountered in children and are both etiologies of severe developmental complications if left untreated early. One of the more ominous characteristics of these conditions is their association with autoimmune disorders. For example, Hashimoto's thyroiditis, an autoimmune etiology of hypothyroidism, has been documented in various studies, and their findings indicated that up to 11.1% of patients with Turner syndrome can develop thyroid dysfunction and this complicates their clinical management and treatment planning (Abací et al., 2015). The severity of these diseases warrants aggressive screening and monitoring protocols; hence early detection is critical in avoiding long-term consequences like cognitive impairment and failure to grow. Apart from the physiological consequences, thyroid disease in children has significant psychological and social consequences. The conditions make the children emotionally challenged due to their own physical symptoms, hence presenting with looming social stigmatization and isolation. A study has indicated that pediatric patients with Turner syndrome also exhibit learning and psychosocial issues, occurring in 39.1% of screened patients (Yeşilkaya et al., 2015). Primary care physicians should thus consider both psychological and medical support when developing integrated care plans for such patients. Coordination of care and communication are essential since families are important stakeholders in the therapy and psychosocial care of the child. Moreover, early intervention measures can minimize some psychological impacts of these disorders, enhancing the well-being of children with these disorders. Routine screening practices should be implemented for improved detection and treatment of thyroid disorders in children. Formal guidelines suggested by the American Diabetes Association (ADA) include the identification of comorbidities in diabetes among children with thyroid disorders, and routine screening is recommended. Utilizing electronic medical record systems to prompt reminders for physicians has the potential to enhance adherence to such standards, ultimately increasing the quality of care for pediatric patients. Studies have demonstrated that interventions like this have the potential to achieve dramatic increases in screening rates, so that significant issues are detected prior to becoming additional severe complications. With advancing pediatric endocrinology, attention to evidence-based practice and care integration strategies will remain of utmost relevance in addressing the multifaceted challenges posed by thyroid diseases and their comorbidity.

## Test Your Knowledge

1. What are the key symptoms and management strategies for diabetes mellitus and growth hormone deficiency in children?
2. What are common thyroid disorders in pediatric patients, and how do they affect development?

## 10.3. Diagnosis of Endocrine Disorders

**Learning Outcome**

1. Clinical evaluation and patient history;
2. Laboratory tests and imaging studies;
3. Importance of early diagnosis for treatment outcomes.

Accurate diagnosis of endocrine disease in children depends on an empathetic understanding of the several clinical and biological parameters. History and physical examination are normally conducted in a comprehensive manner and suitable to the age and level of development of the child. Care should be taken by the health professionals to consider the unique presentation of endocrine disease in children, rather than in adults. Diseases , such as Growth Hormone Deficiency (GHD) or Congenital Hypothyroidism may have insidious symptoms that must be diligently watched in order to detect at an early stage. High-technology diagnostic methods, like biochemical investigations of the levels of hormones, are included in the confirmatory process after the generation of suspicion based on clinical evaluation. Furthermore, imaging studies can be employed when structural endocrine gland abnormalities are suspected. Through bringing together clinical understanding with modern diagnostic technology, experts can accurately diagnose endocrine disorders, providing access to early and effective intervention. Genetic and molecular tests are increasingly being used in diagnosing endocrine disorders. Some conditions, , such as Disorders of Sex Development (DSD), often have complex genetic histories that routine diagnosis will overlook. The international DSD Registry reflects the observation that associated conditions tend to occur together with instances of DSD, and thus a multi-angled diagnostic process is required. For instance, the information provides varying karyotypes and incidence rates of associated anomalies, , such as cardiac and skeletal issues among individuals with this condition. The applicability of such findings extends beyond mere diagnosis; it also underscores the requirement for clinicians to adopt a more integrated approach while guiding treatment and management strategies. By integrating genetic data into the diagnostic process, doctors are able to tailor interventions according to each child's unique profile, thereby facilitating better patient care and outcomes overall (Cox et al., 2013).

Further, the diagnosis of endocrine disturbances is not only based on physical examinations and genetic analysis but also needs an interdisciplinary model. There needs to be coordination between pediatric endocrinologists, primary care physicians, geneticists, and allied healthcare professionals in order to address the multifactorial cause of these conditions in an appropriate way. Such conferences as the one held in Novosibirsk on the state of progress in endocrinology are typical of this interdisciplinary dialogue through the sharing of information on new diagnostic procedure and treatment modalities for endocrine diseases (Cox et al., 2013). Through cooperative contributions, the discipline has made advances in disease mechanisms, accuracy in diagnosis, and in the management of patients. These efforts finally result in more individualized and comprehensive care for endocrine disease children, thereby improving the quality of their health and life (Figure 10.8).

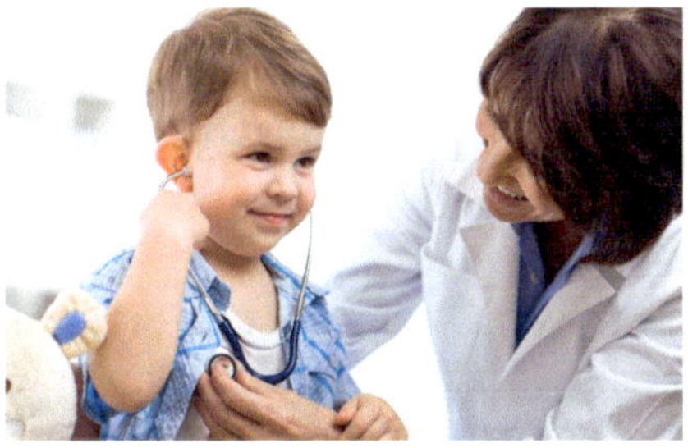

**Figure 10.8.** Fostering a positive and engaging experience in pediatric care.

*Source:* https://medika.bg/img/pediatric-endocrinology-nurse.jpg.

## 10.3.1. Clinical Evaluation and Patient History

In pediatric endocrinology, proper diagnosis and treatment of endocrine disorders are determined by comprehensive clinical evaluation and extensive patient history. History taking, being the first step, is often comprised of gathering in-depth information regarding growth patterns, developmental milestones, and family histories. This information enables clinicians to distinguish between normal physiological development and pathological changes. For instance, short children may require extensive growth chart evaluations and endocrine hormone levels in order to assess for such factors as Turner syndrome or other growth hormone deficiency. In such instances, early identification of clinical markers can significantly influence treatment response and options. A thorough patient history is thus the foundation upon which target investigations and interventions are derived, determining a child's trajectory of health care. Addition of findings from karyotype analysis further firm the clinical diagnostic process. It has been proven that girls with Turner syndrome may present with characteristic features, including delayed puberty and heart disease, besides abnormal karyotypes , such as 45,X. Systematic analysis of clinical data in such individuals has proved to reveal a high incidence of congenital abnormalities that are not necessarily evident during the initial assessments. Because of the nature of Turner syndrome, detailed patient history with an emphasis on such risk factors becomes important. This enables clinicians to implement stringent monitoring regimens for such conditions as Hashimoto's thyroiditis and osteoporosis with individualized therapy. Hence, merging genetic information with conventional clinical evaluation leads to improved patient care. Moreover, awareness of genetic predisposition in pediatric endocrinology adds scope to the clinical assessment presented with diseases like pituitary adenomas. Identification of germline mutations like those in the MEN1 and AIP genes is linked with early presentation of aggressive tumors in children. Diligent family history has the potential to detect patterns of these genetic disorders suggestive and provoke earlier and better interventions. Screening criteria based on genetic risk factors can also guide clinical evaluation in the tertiary setting such that high-risk patients are given proper attention. By appreciating the interface between patient history and genetic susceptibility, clinicians not only maximize diagnostic specificity but also modify treatment protocols addressing both acute concerns and long-term health effects, thereby optimizing pediatric endocrinologic outcomes.

## 10.3.2. Laboratory Tests and Imaging Studies

Laboratory and imaging procedures are key to the diagnosis and management of endocrine conditions in children. Laboratory and imaging procedures play a crucial role in the diagnosis of conditions , such as growth abnormalities, pubertal disease, and metabolic disorders. Significantly, hormonal tests that measure levels of some hormones in blood or urine are significant in establishing the presence of conditions , such as Turner syndrome or sexual development disorder. The ability to precisely measure hormone concentrations enables clinicians to distinguish among different disorders and therefore direct appropriate treatment modalities and monitoring regimens. Furthermore, imaging tests , such as ultrasound or MRI provide valuable information regarding anatomical abnormalities that invariably follow endocrine disorders, for instance, congenital adrenal hyperplasia or pituitary gland malformation. In conditions like Turner syndrome, when diagnosis early in life dictates long-term prognosis, such laboratory tests as karyotyping assume a very important function. In a study using a pediatric Turkish population, the prevalence of the karyotype 45,X in Turner syndrome patients was reported with an emphasis placed on the function of laboratory diagnostics to uncover genetic abnormalities with concomitant clinical features , such as short stature and delayed puberty (Yeşilkaya et al., 2015). In the severity of such conditions, the coincidence between laboratory findings and clinical presentation allows for detailed interpretation of each patient's individual case. Regular follow-up by way of these diagnostic channels then becomes important in optimizing individual treatment regimens, ranging from hormone replacement therapies to monitoring for growth. With emerging medical technologies, harmonization of laboratory assessments between regions has also come into prominence. For instance, the EU COST Action BM 1303 guidelines emphasize standard application of advanced techniques , such as mass spectrometry in the analysis of steroid hormones across different developmental disorders. The uniformity is not only important for correct diagnosis but also for comparing results from different healthcare units. By coordinating lab activities, medical professionals will be in a position to ensure that therapeutic interventions guided by diagnostic results are not only effective, but also timely. The facilitation of an operational partnership in laboratory medicine, therefore, will not only enhance diagnostic accuracy but also enhance improved delivery of care to children with endocrine disorders (Figure 10.9).

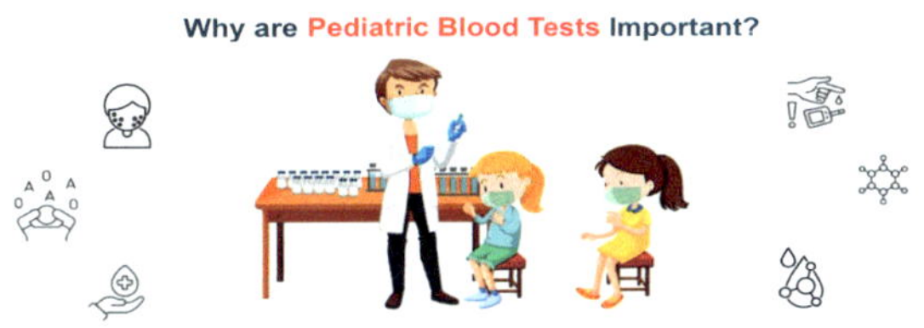


**Figure 10.9.** Laboratory tests and imaging studies.

*Source:* https://www.ganeshdiagnostic.com/admin/assets/images/product-section/Why%20are%20Pediatric%20Blood%20Tests%20Important_1705055819.jpg.

### 10.3.3. Importance of Early Diagnosis for Treatment Outcomes

Pediatric endocrinology early detection is essential to optimize treatment and prevent long-term complications of endocrine disorders. Early detection of disorders , such as growth hormone deficiency, congenital adrenal hyperplasia, and disorders of sex development may result in successful treatment plans. Intervention in children with growth disorders, for instance, not only guarantees normal growth but also affects psychosocial development positively. As attested in existing literature, proactive and well-informed management practices with individualized interventions can optimally reduce secondary complication risk and enhance overall quality of life in affected children. The significance of early diagnosis cannot be overestimated as it directly influences downstream treatment pathways and long-term well-being. Furthermore, differences in disease severity can be influenced by demographics too, emphasizing the need for timely diagnosis. For example, studies indicate that racial and socioeconomic disparities are responsible for variability in presentation and severity of conditions , such as Cushing disease in children. According to research, Hispanic/Latino and African–American children developed more severe symptoms and greater long-term risks compared to non-Hispanic Whites. These variations underscore the need for vigilant observation and open-minded approach to diagnosis and treatment across populations. Existence of awareness about the impact of such factors enables healthcare professionals to implement effective screening methods that enable early diagnosis, thereby allowing timely interventions and tailored treatment regimens in response to each child's unique condition. Introduction of a multidisciplinary approach further enhances the initial diagnosis and subsequent management of endocrine disorders in children. Medical professionals like endocrinologists, pediatricians, and mental health professionals collaborate in creating comprehensive management strategies that account for both the physiological as well as psychosocial aspects of endocrine conditions. Coordination is particularly critical for disorders with unusual presentation, , such as disorders of sex development. As emphasized by recent reports, the inclusion of clinical expertise in a multidisciplinary setup not only streamlines patient management but also provides an ideal environment for caring for families with challenging diagnoses. Therefore, early diagnosis development through collaboration can significantly improve treatment outcomes and ensure an integrated care approach in pediatric endocrinology encompassing both the medical and emotional well-being of patients and their families.

## Test Your Knowledge

1. How do clinical evaluation and patient history contribute to diagnosing endocrine disorders in children?
2. What diagnostic tools are used for endocrine disorders, and why is early diagnosis important?

## 10.4. Treatment Options in Pediatric Endocrinology

**Learning Outcome**

1. Hormone replacement therapies;
2. Lifestyle modifications and dietary interventions;
3. Surgical options for endocrine disorders.

Pediatric endocrinology care is broad and uniquely tailored to address the specific needs of children with endocrine conditions. Early intervention plays a crucial role in the treatment of conditions , such as growth hormone deficiency, congenital adrenal hyperplasia, and sex development disorders. Pediatric endocrinologists provide global care by employing an array of healthcare professionals in collaboration with other care providers. For instance, in unusual genitalia, a thorough understanding of the etiology and the complications that have ensued is crucial to organize an individualized treatment plan. Co-management with experts enables the medical team to manage the psychosocial effects of the conditions, thus counseling both the patient and the family through often difficult decision-making. As per the recent advances, there is increasing recognition of the need for careful strategies that consider changing societal perception of diversity and inclusion in the management of such conditions (Ahmid et al., 2016). The treatment with growth hormone remains one of the best-established treatment methods in pediatric endocrinology, particularly in children with growth hormone deficiency. The timing and adherence to this treatment are critical for best success, since non-adherence has been associated with adverse outcomes of growth and decreased quality of life in involved individuals. Current controversy in the practice of endocrinology emphasizes the value of identifying factors influencing adherence, including not only the suitability of the delivery mode but also the ongoing support to families and patients. Modern injectable devices that incorporate electronic technology have been designed to enhance compliance by enabling monitoring and recording of the injection regimen. These technologies aim at providing consistency of treatment, hence increasing the potential for favorable growth responses and overall health outcomes (Carlo et al., 2017). Furthermore, the treatment protocol for endocrine diseases in childhood is continuously evolving with technology and clinical practice innovation reshaping the management of chronic conditions. New therapeutic options and precision medicine approaches allow more refined interventions according to the individual patient profile, particularly for such multifactorial diseases as metabolic disorders and sexual development disorders.

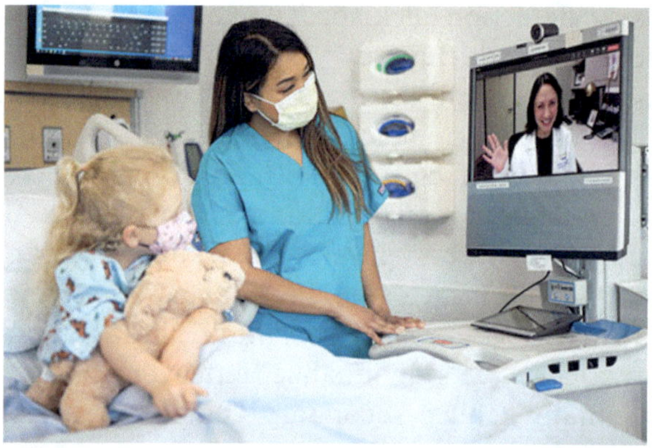

**Figure 10.10.** The treatment options in pediatric endocrinology.

*Source:* https://health.ucdavis.edu/media-resources/children/images/Promo/pediatric-telehealth-program.jpg.

Combined with genetic screening, diagnostic accuracy has increased, allowing clinicians to diagnose accurate anomalies and tailor interventions even further. Furthermore, the development of standardized registries and protocols allows for information to be gathered about rare conditions so that future therapeutic interventions are evidence-based and guided by wide clinical experience. With ongoing evolution of the practice, there continues to be a need for clinicians to create treatment strategies to address the needs of children and ensure that both their emotional and physical well-being are considered in the management of endocrine disorders (Figure 10.10).

### 10.4.1. Hormone Replacement Therapies

The application of hormone replacement therapies (HRT) in pediatric endocrinology is increasingly becoming significant in the treatment of various endocrine disorders. Accurate therapeutic interventions are needed to correct conditions , such as hypogonadism, deficiency of growth hormone, and congenital hyperplasia of the adrenal gland so that children can develop into physical and secondary sexual features needed for their age group. HRT offers a potential remedy in substituting the deficient hormones, hence guaranteeing normal growth patterns and development of secondary sexual features. However, the initiation of HRT in children must be carried out with a critical perspective since the long-term outcomes of the treatments remain under investigation. Furthermore, collaboration between pediatricians, endocrinologists, and families must be conducted to develop treatment plans in view of each child's unique physiological and psychological requirements, in addition to societal attitudes regarding gender identity and growth. In recent years, advances in knowledge of gender and sex differences have made a more differentiated approach to HRT in children necessary. The fact that sex hormones can influence not only physical but also psychological development has markedly widened the area of treatment. With the distinct functions of estrogen and testosterone, for instance, clinicians must be attuned to how these hormones affect behavior and expectation during times of development. As has been observed in the evolving dialogue on gender identity and expression, a multidisciplinary approach that considers these observations is vital. This awareness will not only make therapeutic intervention medically appropriate but also socially appropriate, hence fulfilling the comprehensive needs of HRT children and facilitating inclusiveness and acceptance among children's care (Appetecchia et al., 2018). Furthermore, the use of rule-governed and standardized procedures in HRT for children is critical to maintaining the quality and safety of care. Compilation of clinical data on hormone treatments is necessary for the development of useful guidelines and protocols that will further improve the outcome of patients. As stated in relation to disorders of sex development (DSD), treatment decisions should be guided by individualized needs and wants, particularly in difficult cases, where there is the need to thoroughly evaluate biological and psychosocial considerations. By documenting and publishing clinical experience in a collective registry, clinicians can build a robust evidence base supporting best practice. These ventures are not only designed to improve individual treatment pathways but also improve the knowledge of pediatric endocrine disorders as a general entity, ultimately shaping an overall approach to management (Ahmid et al., 2016).

### 10.4.2. Lifestyle Modifications and Dietary Interventions

The rising prevalence of obesity and related metabolic diseases among children underscores the importance of lifestyle modification and diet interventions as key components of pediatric endocrinology. Child obesity, with its close link to prediabetes and Type 2 Diabetes (T2D) onset, merits special interventions to improve the health status of such children. Applications that contain meal tracking software, , such as Nourishly©, have been promising to decrease Glycosylated Hemoglobin A1c (HbA1c) and Body Mass Index (BMI) through guided dietary feedback and education. Despite statistically significant reductions in such measures being problematic, technology use in the form of dietary interventions is a growing approach, and the need for more research and optimization to enhance its impact in clinical settings is paramount, particularly in overweight or obese adolescents (Torhorst et al., 2024). Aside from technology application, dietetic interventions must be tailored to meet the special physiological and psychological needs of children and young people. The success of lifestyle modification is more than a modification of food consumption; it is the promotion of good eating habits and physical exercise on a continual basis. Multi-faceted education programs incorporating children and their families have been found to be of utmost significance for the instillation of sustainable behavior changes. By providing not only nutritional information but also hands-on teaching in meal planning and portion control, pediatric endocrinologists can empower families to self-manage their health. This multifaceted process not only addresses critical concerns of weight and diabetes management but also transferring lifetime habits that create a holistic state of wellness and prevention of other comorbid conditions (Bartz et al., 2019). In addition, adherence to screening guidelines and early detection of diabetes complications, , such as those highlighted by the American Diabetes Association (ADA), also highlights the importance of integrating lifestyle modification into treatment strategies. Employing best practice alerts within electronic medical records for guiding compliance with such guidelines is an example of how health care technology can optimize health outcomes. Engaging youth with Type 1 Diabetes (T1D) in ongoing monitoring and education about probable comorbidities empowers youth and their families to optimize their conditions. Not only does this holistic method optimize patient care, but it can also have an effect on community health overall by reducing the long-term cost of diabetes and its complications. Therefore, combining lifestyle change with evidence-based interventions is critical in the establishment of effective pediatric endocrinology interventions (Bartz et al., 2019) (Figure 10.11).

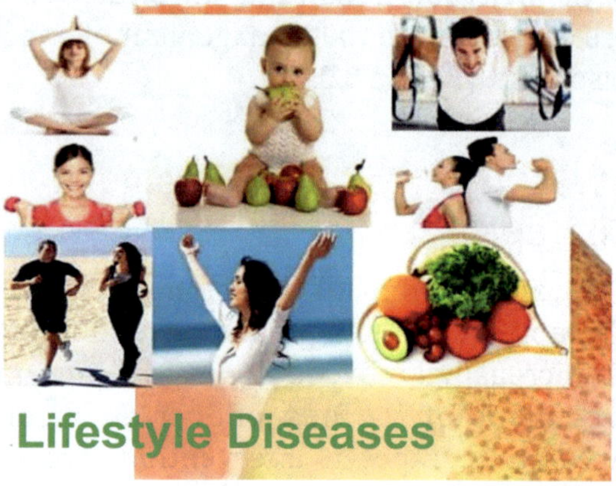


**Figure 10.11.** Lifestyle modifications and dietary interventions.

*Source:* https://cdn.slidesharecdn.com/ss_thumbnails/lifestylediseasesppt-180203174909-converted-200902072215-thumbnail.jpg?width=560&fit=bounds.

## 10.4.3. Surgical Options for Endocrine Disorders

Surgery is a central part of the management of most endocrine disorders in children when conservative therapy fails. Imbalance of hormones or anatomical defects in conditions , such as congenital adrenal hyperplasia (CAH) and disorders of sex development (DSD) are typically managed with surgery. Adrenalectomy is a consideration in CAH if medical management is unable to contain the hormone levels, particularly with severe cases of the condition or if adrenal tumors develop as a result of excessive long-term stimulation. Such interventions through surgery in this instance aim not only at alleviating hormonal excess but also at preventing potential complications in the form of adrenal crises and infertility at a later point in life, hence enhancing overall welfare of such affected children. The scope of surgery for endocrine disorders also covers instances of patients diagnosed with endocrine gland tumors, , such as thyroid and parathyroid tissues. In children with thyroid nodules or malignancies, resection is still the treatment of choice to avoid both disease progression and complications. Preoperative and postoperative assessment is also necessary, in view of the fact that the surgery may directly influence the level of thyroid hormones and thus necessitate life-long monitoring and potential hormone replacement therapy. Laparoscopic techniques in thyroid surgeries have become popular due to reduced recovery times and less scarring, making them particularly appealing when treating endocrine issues in children who are extremely sensitive to surgical stress and cosmetic issues. Finally, the advancements that have taken place in minimally invasive surgical techniques have transformed the management of endocrine disorders in children with many benefits over traditional surgery. Laparoscopy and robotic-assisted operations provide accuracy without producing trauma to surrounding structures, leading to quick recovery and reduced postoperative morbidity. For instance, laparoscopic adrenalectomy for Cushing's syndrome allows for definitive treatment of the disease along with preservation of adrenal function when needed. Moreover, in the case of DSD patients, operations like gonadal surgery can correct ambiguous genitalia or hormone secretion issues. The emphasis on careful evaluation and multidisciplinary model ensures the surgical decision is made based on children's endocrine condition, promoting constructive outcomes in their long-term health and development (Nasir, 2024).

## Test Your Knowledge

1. What are common hormone replacement therapies and lifestyle interventions used in treating pediatric endocrine disorders?
2. When are surgical options considered in pediatric endocrine disorders, and what are some examples?

## 10.5. Psychological and Social Implications

**Learning Outcome**

1. Impact of endocrine disorders on mental health;
2. Social challenges faced by affected children;
3. Importance of family support and counseling.

The psychological effect of endocrine disorders among children extends beyond disease symptoms, deeply influencing emotional states and self-worth. Kids who grapple with diseases , such as obesity, typically resulting from endocrine imbalance, tend to experience heightened anxiety and depression. Obesity has been established by studies to have a profoundly negative effect on various psychological and social factors among children, exhibiting significant differences in depressive mood and quality of life when compared to their non-obese peers. As noted, emotional symptoms were more pronounced in girls, while conduct problems were more prevalent in boys, illustrating the muted psychological picture dictated by pediatric endocrine disorders (Behdani et al., 2018). It underlines the necessity to incorporate mental health as a natural component of treatment plans, given that children's self-esteem can be irreparably damaged by their physical health conditions. Social implications also occupy a very important position in children suffering from endocrine diseases. Children who are faced with issues , such as obesity tend to become victims of social stigma and, thus, face exclusion and isolation from society and peer groups and participation in group activities. This tends to perpetuate a trend of low self-esteem as well as other mental illness , such as depression and anxiety. Social reactions to such children tend to reflect society's attitudes towards health and bodily image. Thus, endocrine diseases and social acceptance need to be acknowledged by teachers, health professionals, and parents. Supportive intervention promoting social interaction and healthy self-image is crucial as it can significantly enhance the quality of life for such children (Behdani et al., 2018). Increasing community awareness can also reduce stigma and facilitate an integrative setting. Finally, the integration of psychological support into pediatric endocrinology is of the highest priority to cope with both psychological and social consequences.

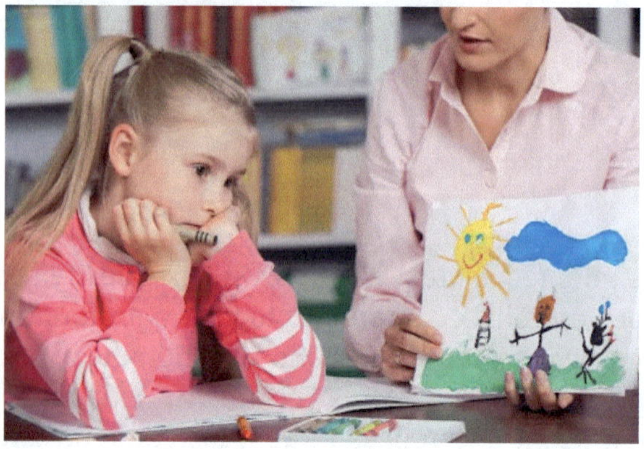

**Figure 10.12.** Psychological and social implications.

*Source:* https://njpediatricneurosurgery.com/wp-content/uploads/2023/10/important-of-child-psychology.webp.

Multidisciplinary interventions by psychologists, social workers, and endocrinologists can give more unified care able to cope with these children in its multidimensionality. Education programs alerting families about the psychological consequence of chronic diseases can strengthen parents to cope with their children better through the emotional dimension of endocrine disorders. Through facilitative models of collaborative care, health clinicians are empowered to build resilience in children and improve coping relative to their health and social life. It is achievable through establishing environments for emotional and physical well-being and highlighting interdependence of these critical factors in pediatric endocrinology (Figure 10.12).

### 10.5.1. Impact of Endocrine Disorders on Mental Health

The intricate endocrine interdependence of disturbance and mental status necessitates careful examination, particularly in children. Endocrine disturbances , such as Turner Syndrome (TS) illustrate that hormonal imbalance leads not only to physical but also to very evident psychological impairment. Studies refer that approximately 39.1% of TS children have learning problems and psychosocial disturbances, highlighting a crucial confluence of endocrinology and mental health. The intricate interplay between growth hormone levels and psychosocial adaptation makes clinical presentation even more challenging; children with chronic endocrine diseases are also at higher risks of anxiety, depression, and social withdrawal secondary to stigma concerning their diseases. It is hence essential that the psychological implications of endocrine disease are recognized when designing treatment programs for meeting the twin physiological and psychological demands. In addition to Turner Syndrome, disorders of sex development (DSD) provide a second vantage point from which to consider the impact of endocrine disorders on mental health within the pediatric population. The international Registry for DSD reported a variety of associated conditions, where 26% of them had another disorder, which helps in increasing mental health concerns. For instance, there are different karyotypes, including 45,X and 46,XY, that come with a range of psychological conditions, i.e., anxiety and identity issues. These complexities call for coordinated care to ensure that psychological resources supplement medical care. Given that the endocrine system is deeply intertwined with emotional regulation, the intricate aspects of DSD necessitate an interprofessional collaboration among healthcare professionals to foster children not only physically, but also psychologically. Furthermore, the high prevalence of comorbidities in endocrine disorders , such as cardiac abnormalities and central nervous system abnormalities increases the psychological concerns that confront the afflicted children. For instance, cardiac anomalies are found in 20% of patients with 46,XY DSD, which can impose several levels of stress and anxiety related to health management. The combined effect of such endocrine illnesses can result in increased vulnerability for mental illness disorders, , such as depression and self-esteem problems, which can continue into adolescence and adulthood. Therefore, addressing the psychological aspects of endocrine illnesses is critical in pediatric endocrinology. Integration of mental health testing and interventions into standard treatment regimens will offer comprehensive care that addresses and acknowledges the emotional wellbeing of affected children throughout their course of development.

### 10.5.2. Social Challenges Faced by Affected Children

Individuals with disorders of sex development (DSD) suffer severe social challenges that impair their psychological adjustment and undermine their capacity to adjust to alternative environments. Their condition's nature leads to the development of an incoherent gender identity and self-concept, which impacts their interactions with others in the long term. It is essential to recognize these challenges as they might appear in the forms of bullying and exclusion, which might cause already fragile self-esteem. Moreover, research indicates that exposure to stigmatizing environments is likely to have long-term mental and emotional health outcomes, rendering affected children at greater risk for anxiety and depression. Managing the social aspects of DSD entails a lot of peer and community education to engender an environment of inclusiveness and tolerance that accommodates difference rather than advancing stigma. Parent experiences have a significant influence on the social reality of DSD children. In a process that tends to be complicated and involving intricate decision-making, parents have to go through the intricacies of gender assignment, surgery, and disclosing information about their child's condition. Parents' decisions not only impact the child's current social interactions but also determine how they will be viewed and accepted in the long term. Parents typically feel anxious and confused regarding the child's diagnosis and the treatment options available, thereby indirectly validating the child's feelings of inadequacy. Moreover, parents experience the conflict of desiring secrecy about the condition versus requiring social support, thus further burdening the family system. Thus, the psychological burden placed on the parents can have a negative impact on the social adjustment of their children, hence the need for an effective communication process between families and healthcare providers aimed at suitably supporting the impaired children (Carr et al., 2011). As more information and awareness about pediatric endocrinology become available, addressing the broader social issues faced by the impaired children remains crucial. Some of these factors are the exposure to polluted environments that can aggregate health issues into developmental challenges impacting the social life of a child. For instance, children who are exposed to toxic chemicals may experience learning disabilities and behavioral disorders that also make it harder for them to connect with other children on different levels. The role of policy reforms should also be emphasized as the capability to make environments secure can significantly lower such risks and enhance the quality of life for such children. By integrating strategies that encompass both the medical and social domains, medical professionals can develop more holistic care that encompasses not only physiological well-being but also children's social development, who often live with such endocrine disorders (Madsen & Hitchcock, 2011) (Figure 10.13).

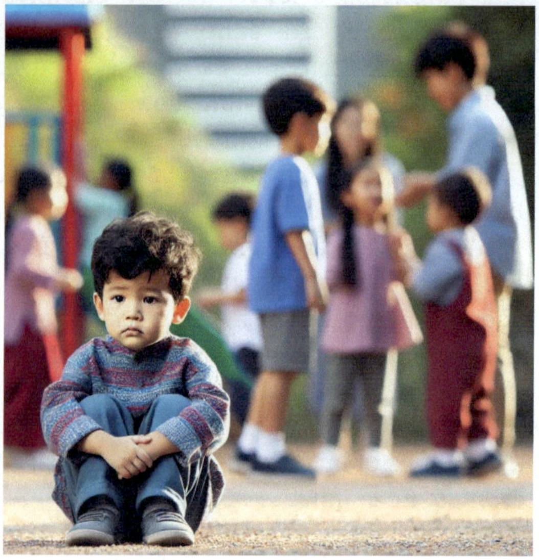

**Figure 10.13.** Social challenges faced by affected children.

*Source:* https://www.mywellnesshub.in/blog/wp-content/uploads/2025/03/social-challenges-1.webp.

## 10.5.3. Importance of Family Support and Counseling

In pediatric endocrinology, family support is a fundamental element in the care of endocrine disorders in children. Families are the primary support figure, providing psychological, emotional, and practical support throughout the diagnosis and treatment of a child. For instance, when kids are facing challenges pertaining to conditions , such as diabetes or growth disorders, it will mostly be the family that assists with daily management tasks , such as monitoring blood sugar or medication. Having assistance from members of family will greatly reduce anxiety and loneliness among children, resulting in a sense of security that is essential for healthy adaptation. Furthermore, support from their families makes treatment compliance better because children also stick to doctor's orders when they are loved and supported by all the people who surround them. Counseling also plays a revolutionary part in the support system of children with pediatric endocrine disorders. A targeted counseling approach may provide families with key coping skills and assistance to enhance overall well-being for both the child and the adult caregivers. Education-based integrative treatment that incorporates information on some endocrine diseases can empower families to make informed decisions regarding the well-being of their child. For example, information regarding disease like polycystic ovary syndrome (PCOS), a complex endocrine disorder, may prove immensely useful.

The counselors can offer specialized intervention appropriate for the particular challenges offered by such disorders and therefore enhance the capacity of the family to adapt to the simultaneous physical and psychological impacts. The active involvement of counseling not only enhances awareness but also the strengthening of family bonds, enhancing the resilience of children living with chronic conditions even more (Annagur et al., 2018). Moreover, family support and counseling are significant in developing an active climate where children are comfortable talking about their experience and fears related to their illnesses. Open communication within the family allows children to express their feelings regarding treatment, fears, and expectations. This is important because it develops a culture of trust and confirmation and eradicates psychological burdens that often accompany chronic illnesses. Moreover, counseling offers a place where families can be taught effective communication skills to enable them to collaborate in the attainment of treatment goals. Through collaboration, counseling promotes healthy family cohesiveness and health literacy, ultimately leading to better health outcomes. Thus, integrating professional counseling with family support not only aids in the child's management plan but also enables wholistic development and growth in the family system during coping with the complexity of pediatric endocrine disorders (Hanna et al., 2019).

## Test Your Knowledge

1. How can endocrine disorders affect a child's mental health and social life?
2. Why are family support and counseling important in managing pediatric endocrine disorders?

## 10.6. Advances in Pediatric Endocrinology

**Learning Outcome**

1. Recent research and clinical trials;
2. Technological advancements in treatment;
3. Future directions in pediatric endocrine care.

Advances in pediatric endocrinology over recent years have tremendously improved our care and understanding of disorders of sex development (DSD)-related conditions. When clinicians meet newborns with unusual genitalia, the development of multidisciplinary practice becomes vital. The merging of specialized knowledge enables a holistic practice that treats not only the biological cause but also addresses the psychosocial and family implications. Through the creation of personalized management plans, medical professionals can maneuver complex sex assignment decisions when ambiguity prevails. This delicate coordination enhances the quality of care given, creating a supportive framework for families as the social climate of DSD keeps changing. The need for standardized collection and dissemination of clinical information highlights the critical need for strong evidence in guiding subsequent medical practice. Therefore, the advances signify a paradigm shift towards more sympathetic and holistic care model of pediatric endocrinology (Ahmid et al., 2016). In addition, examination of racial and socioeconomic disparities in pediatric endocrinology has come to signify a necessary area of inquiry. Particularly in the setting of Cushing disease (CD), it has been demonstrated that minority groups, , such as Hispanic/Latino and African-American children, experience greater severity and poorer outcomes compared to their non-Hispanic White counterparts. The literature also provides support that the extent of the degree of hypercortisolemia levels and tumor characteristics have important roles in these outcomes. The effects extend beyond the simple clinical presentation and demonstrate that socio-economic status and access to care have significant effects on health outcomes. While clinicians and researchers work to correct such disparities, the evidence is evidence that underlines the necessity for evidence-based, inclusive healthcare interventions and policies. Such awareness provides an environment within which disparities can be addressed systematically and all children are provided with equitable and effective pediatric endocrinology care (Gkourogianni et al., 2017). Furthermore, the ongoing progress in molecular genetics has transformed diagnostics and treatment approaches in pediatric endocrinology. Genetic predispositions also play a central role in the majority of endocrine diseases, dictating the pattern and expression of the disease. Improvements in genomic medicine now enable clinicians to pinpoint certain mutations associated with various diseases, including adrenal insufficiency and growth disorders. Such precision facilitates early treatment and tailored management regimens, thereby markedly improving patient results. In addition, the ability to screen for at-risk patients before they become symptomatic also has the promise of reducing the incidence of serious complications. Pediatric endocrinologists, with technology improving with the integration of genetic data, will be better positioned to tailor therapy, and this will have breakthroughs that not only improve physical well-being but also overall health in affected children (Figure 10.14).

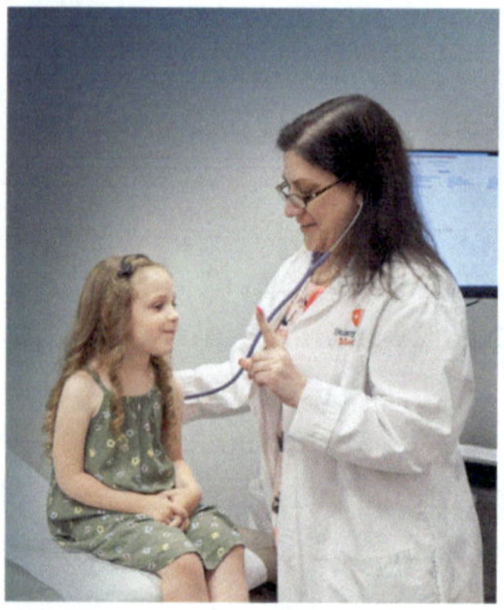

**Figure 10.14.** Demonstration of compassionate care in a clinical setting.

*Source:* https://www.stonybrookmedicine.edu/sites/default/files/cckimages/page/Pediatric-Endocrinology-Hero-MOBILE_1080X1240.jpg.

## 10.6.1. Recent Research and Clinical Trials

Recent research in pediatric endocrinology has emphasized the importance of sex and gender differences in the diagnosis and treatment of endocrine disorders. Research into the influences of sex hormones on human physiology has increased our understanding of numerous conditions, and individualized treatment in medicine has followed. Different endocrine milieus, dictated by sex hormones , such as estrogens and testosterone, could lead to male and female differences in physiological and pathophysiological responses. While the traditional approach in medicine has ignored such differences, there is mounting evidence to support including gender-associated factors in practice. As there is a growing emphasis on gender in medicine, information regarding its impact on disease course and treatment response is an area of significance that requires more research eventually, optimizing therapeutic strategies in pediatric endocrinology (Appetecchia et al., 2018). For type 1 diabetes (T1D), there are ongoing clinical trials suggesting the value of evidence-based screening to avoid long-term complications of this illness. One of the more intriguing interventions at Texas Children's Hospital employed best practice alerts (BPA) within electronic medical records to increase adherence to the American Diabetes Association's (ADA) screening guidelines. There was a notable increase in screening rates of important areas like urine microalbumin-to-creatinine ratio and lipid panel. This quality improvement project not only targeted early diagnosis of comorbidities but was also able to maintain greater than 90% compliance in screening behavior for many years. Moving to EMR-based decision support is an incredible step toward maximizing patient outcomes in pediatric endocrinology, validating that structured approaches can enhance implementation of established standards of care (Bartz et al., 2019). Furthermore, ongoing clinical research continues to explore new treatments for the improved management of endocrine disease in children. Clinical trials evaluating the efficacy of new pharmacologic agents and new monitoring techniques are necessary to maximize outcomes in this vulnerable population. New evidence suggests that tailored treatment regimens, with allowance for individual variation, whether genetic, hormonal, or indeed environmental, can lead to better outcomes compared with the traditional one-size-fits-all regimen. Besides, incorporation of growing awareness of the psychosocial implications of such disorders ensures formation of more comprehensive models of care addressing not only the physical health of pediatric patients but also their social and emotional health. With the progress of pediatric endocrinology with such information from recent research and clinical tests, it seeks to form more advanced and supportive paradigms of care for affected youth (Appetecchia et al., 2018).

## 10.6.2. Technological Advancements in Treatment

The continuous technology innovation has largely changed the face of pediatric endocrinology, particularly endocrine disease treatment. New modes of treatment , such as continuous glucose monitoring systems and insulin pump devices, have significantly transformed diabetes care in children. These technologies allow for dynamic, real-time monitoring of blood glucose levels, which allows patients and their caregivers to be capable of responding dynamically to fluctuations and optimizing blood sugar control. Furthermore, mobile health app integration means that both healthcare workers and patients are able to communicate effectively, and from afar, modify treatment regimens. In such a manner, endocrine disorders may be handled in cooperation. Clinical outcomes are maximized via continuous development of these apps, while the quality of life for patients is enhanced by the provision of a reduction in diabetes complications. Along with managing diabetes, genetic engineering and molecular therapy advances are on the verge of playing a fundamental part in the management of pediatric endocrine disorders. Genes for conditions like growth hormone deficiency and congenital adrenal hyperplasia can be corrected by targeted gene therapy, which has the aim of repairing underlying genetic defects. Advances in CRISPR technology have resulted in unprecedented levels of precision when it comes to editing genes, hence offering potential curative interventions for infrequently seen endocrine disorders. In addition, long-acting hormone preparations , such as growth hormone have improved compliance in children with more uniform therapeutic effects. These advances show the transition toward individualized medicine with the offering of tailored treatment approaches based on a specific child's individualized genetic and phenotypic characteristics, leading ultimately to better healthcare outcomes.

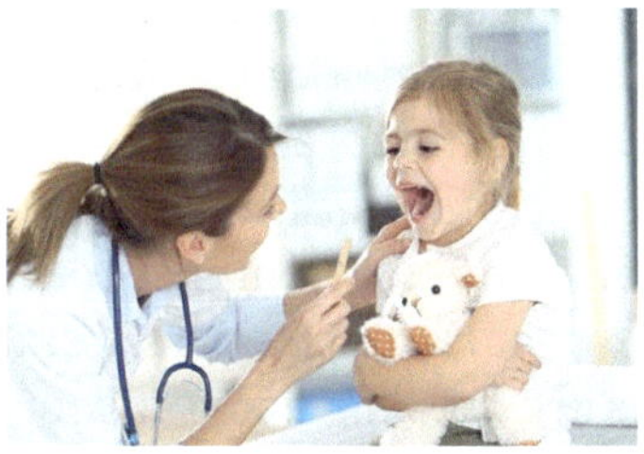

**Figure 10.15.** Technological advancements in treatment.

*Source:* https://neonest.in/wp-content/uploads/2024/01/a6bd8b7bb8cc92d4f3501fe87df11e01.jpg.

In the future, the integration of artificial intelligence (AI) in pediatric endocrinology is an enormous promise for the enrichment of treatment procedures. AI programs are capable of learning through large amounts of clinical data and recognizing patterns in them that may be used to create predictive models for disease progression and for response to therapy. Moreover, machine learning applications are being investigated for their potential in tailoring hormone replacement therapies, thus maximizing efficacy while minimizing side effects. This technological revolution is also extended to telemedicine, which is now more pivotal as far as managing chronic endocrine disorders are concerned, particularly in the wake of the COVID-19 pandemic. Through telehealth platforms, specialists can treat patients from remote or disadvantaged regions, thereby ensuring equal access to quality endocrinological care. These innovations emphasize not just pediatric endocrinology's plasticity in response to evolving healthcare settings but also its commitment to applying new technologies to the betterment of patient outcomes (Figure 10.15).

### 10.6.3. Future Directions in Pediatric Endocrine Care

The pediatric endocrine care of the future is set to change fundamentally, primarily with the help of developments in digital technologies and artificial intelligence. Recent expert debate has pinpointed exciting changes being made in electronic monitoring systems and novel algorithms that improve the referral process for conditions like short stature. Such innovations are opening doors to more sensitive and precise detection of children who require intervention. Furthermore, the introduction of sophisticated imaging techniques provides safer diagnostic options with preserved sensitivity and effectiveness. Utilizing these technologies, pediatric endocrinologists will not only be able to attain better clinical results but also enhance their practices on a general efficacy basis. The emphasis on introducing such technologies into routine care shows commitment to creating a more data-driven approach to working in the assessment and management of endocrine disorders in children so that care can be tailored to individual patient needs and situations (Guazzarotti et al., 2021). In addition, the transfer from pediatric to adult health is also another big challenge and opportunity in pediatric endocrinology, especially in adolescents with obesity. Attention to this age group is critical because they are transitioning and are susceptible to health-related difficulties if managed improperly. Currently, the lack of standards for this transition means that there is a gap in care that is desperately required. Incorporating formal transition processes will not only provide better adolescent outcomes but also engage them more with care systems. Acquiring specialized training for medical professionals will be paramount to equip them with the knowledge and skills required to treat such patients effectively. Fostering discussions on disparities and care obstacles will be paramount in creating comprehensive healthcare services for adolescents, thus all patients will receive necessary care during this sensitive transitioning period (Barazzoni et al., 2024). In addition to technological advancements and improved transition practice, concern for standardizing the process of testing will be the key advance in pediatric endocrine practice. With newer technology evolving, being able to quantify accurately key markers like insulin-like growth factor-1 (IGF-1) levels becomes crucial in assessing the outcome of growth hormone therapy. The use of computer-learning models can greatly increase the validity of , such assessments, enabling more precise predictions to suit unique patients. This holistic strategy not only prioritizes patient-centered care but also improves clinical decision-making by being based on standardized information in a variety of patient populations. With pediatric endocrinology becoming more open to these advancements, the paradigm will shift towards a more efficient and streamlined healthcare system that will ultimately benefit the younger patients as they establish their unique endocrine disabilities (Guazzarotti et al., 2021).

## Test Your Knowledge

1. What are some recent research developments and technological advancements in the treatment of pediatric endocrine disorders?
2. What are the future directions in pediatric endocrine care, and how might they improve outcomes?

## SUMMARY

Pediatric endocrinology is a specialty of medicine that comes a great distance in addressing the polyphyletic issue posed by various hormonal disturbances in children. In its further advancement, there is increasing awareness regarding the necessity for an approach that is patient-centered. This includes not just awareness of the endocrine dysfunction itself but also of the circumstances that usually arise with it. Over a quarter of cases noted in the global DSD Registry report concomitant medical conditions, which supports the use of a multimodal treatment strategy. According to Cox et al. (2013), the detection of these associations is able to illuminate potential for genetic etiology and emphasize the importance of comprehensive management, enabling affected individuals to receive thorough evaluation and interventions tailored to their complex presentation. This multidimensional model of care is essential in optimizing outcomes and improving quality of life in children with endocrine disorders. Furthermore, progress in therapeutic and diagnostic approaches is ushering in new treatments in pediatric endocrinology. The introduction of new technologies, , such as salivary bioscience, represents a paradigm shift for evaluating endocrine function in the child. This non-invasive method gives scientists the potential to analyze several biological markers in a single oral fluid sample, obtaining an understanding of complex biological systems, including the endocrine and immune systems. As described by Granger et al. (2014), such advances will enable the investigation of gonadal steroid exposure through windows of critical development, yielding essential information that can be used to guide preventive intervention and therapeutic treatment. The transition towards such advanced diagnostic equipment heralds the prospect of high-impact applications, finally comprehending endocrine disorders and how they affect children's development and growth. In summary, the integrated and interdisciplinary approach towards pediatric endocrinology is the solution to addressing the needs of the affected children effectively. As more evidence confirms the relationship between endocrine disorders and comorbid conditions, clinicians are forced to battle for the care practices that incorporate. This is not just the building block for the improvement of clinical results, but also essential in assisting families with the support they require throughout the course of their healthcare. Through the application of research developments and embracing holistic practices, pediatric endocrinologists are able to strive for more personalized and effective care. With ongoing investigation, the mysteries of hormonal disorders will continue to be illuminated, and this will ultimately result in enhanced comprehension and creative practice that benefits the pediatric patient in the future.

The subject of pediatric endocrinology entails a number of important topics, with a focus on endocrine disease affecting the growth and development of children. An important topic of discussion is congenital adrenal hyperplasia (CAH), especially its non-life-threatening forms, which can go unnoticed via newborn screening. Inadequacy in detection will deprive the child of early diagnosis and management, leading to complications , such as excessive growth and premature bone aging among affected children. Besides the short-term physiological effects, the forfeited potential of earlier treatment highlights the importance of ongoing vigilance on the part of pediatric healthcare professionals, so that symptomatology of CAH is recognized and addressed as quickly as possible. Ongoing focus on targeting the genetic causes of endocrine disease in children, the activity of specific genes like CABLES1 has also become of interest. Mutations in CABLES1 have been discovered through research that may predispose children to corticotropinomas, pituitary tumors. Notably, mutations were identified in Cushing's disease-affected children, indicating there may be a genetic basis for presentation of the disease. Understanding the mechanisms behind such mutations contributes to the overall pool of information about how genetic factors influence pediatric endocrine disease. This forms the basis for subsequent studies to clarify the relationship between genetic abnormalities and the etiology of some of the disorders the endocrine system of children is prone to, advocating for certain therapies and preventive measures. In addition, the study of the growth pattern in untreated boys with classic CAH informs us about the endocrine influence on child health. One study discovered that although early height velocity in affected infants is not appreciably raised, marked growth rate increases are noted after the first six months of life, in correspondence to elevated androgen levels. Thus, detection of the nuances of growth pattern can enhance care in such children, particularly for glucocorticoid treatment. This means that reducing hydrocortisone doses in the first few months would be more beneficial, thereby decreasing potential side effects while continuing to control symptomatically for CAH. Such evidence reaffirms the merit of integrative approaches in pediatric endocrinology by considering both therapeutic and physiological factors in the treatment of conditions related to hormones in children.

## KEY TERMS FROM THIS CHAPTER

- Abnormal endocrine function
- Cardiac anomalies
- Central nervous system disorders
- Complex health landscapes
- Congenital adrenal hyperplasia (CAH)
- Diabetes
- Disorders of sex development (DSD)
- Endocrinology
- Family interaction macro-coding system (FIMS)
- Follicle-stimulating hormone (FSH)
- Growth hormone deficiency (GHD)
- Hypothalamus-pituitary-gonadal (HPG)
- Luteinizing hormone (LH)
- Metabolism
- Psychological health
- Reproduction

## CRITICAL THINKING QUESTIONS

1. **The most common cause of congenital hypothyroidism is:**
   a. Iodine deficiency
   b. Thyroid agenesis or dysgenesis
   c. Maternal diabetes
   d. Pituitary tumor
2. **A child with short stature, delayed bone age, and obesity is likely to have:**
   a. Type 1 diabetes
   b. Growth hormone deficiency
   c. Hyperthyroidism
   d. Addison's disease
3. **The most common type of diabetes in children is:**
   a. Type 2 diabetes mellitus
   b. Type 1 diabetes mellitus
   c. MODY (Maturity-Onset Diabetes of the Young)
   d. Secondary diabetes
4. **Which of the following is NOT a typical symptom of Type 1 Diabetes Mellitus in children?**
   a. Polyuria
   b. Polydipsia
   c. Weight gain
   d. Fatigue
5. **The hormone responsible for lowering blood glucose is:**
   a. Glucagon
   b. Cortisol
   c. Insulin
   d. Adrenaline

### Short Answer Questions

1. Define congenital hypothyroidism. Mention two early signs in infants.
2. Describe the causes, clinical presentation, diagnosis, and management of congenital hypothyroidism.
3. Explain the pathophysiology and management of Type 1 Diabetes Mellitus in children.
4. Discuss growth hormone deficiency in children: causes, clinical features, diagnosis, and treatment.
5. Describe the approach to a child with short stature, including key investigations.

### *Answers to Critical Thinking Questions*

1. (b); 2. (b); 3. (b); 4. (c); 5. (c)

## REFERENCES


1. Yeşilkaya, E., Bereket, A., Darendeliler, F., Baş, F., Poyrazoğlu, Ş., Küçükemre Aydın, B., Darcan, Ş., Dündar, B., Büyükinan, M., Kara, C., Sarı, E., Adal, E., Akıncı, A., Atabek, M. E., Demirel, F., Çelik, N., Özkan, B., Özhan, B., Orbak, Z., Ersoy, B., ... Bondy, C. (2015). Turner syndrome and associated problems in Turkish children: a multicenter study. *Journal of clinical research in pediatric endocrinology*, *7*(1), 27–36. https://doi.org/10.4274/jcrpe.1771 (accessed on 16th June 2025).
2. Acerini, C. L., Lehwalder, D., Wac, K., & Bang, P. (2017). Optimizing patient management and adherence for children receiving growth hormone. https://core.ac.uk/download/146491367.pdf (accessed on 16th June 2025).
3. Aguilar Briseño, A., Moser, J., & Rodenhuis-Zybert, I. (2020). Understanding immunopathology of severe dengue: Lessons learnt from sepsis. https://core.ac.uk/download/345434492.pdf (accessed on 16th June 2025).
4. Cox, K., Bryce, J., Jiang, J., Rodie, M., Sinnott, R., Alkhawari, M., Arlt, W., Audi, L., Balsamo, A., Bertelloni, S., Cools, M., Darendeliler, F., Drop, S., Ellaithi, M., Guran, T., Hiort, O., Holterhus, P. M., Hughes, I., Krone, N., Lisa, L., ... Ahmed, S. F. (2014). Novel associations in disorders of sex development: findings from the I-DSD Registry. *The Journal of clinical endocrinology and metabolism*, *99*(2), E348–E355. https://doi.org/10.1210/jc.2013-2918 (accessed on 16th June 2025).
5. Ahmid, M., Perry, C. G., Ahmed, S. F., & Shaikh, M. G. (2016). Growth hormone deficiency during young adulthood and the benefits of growth hormone replacement. *Endocrine connections*, *5*(3), R1–R11. https://doi.org/10.1530/EC-16-0024(accessed on 16th June 2025).
6. AlAsmi, R. (2025). *Hormonal Dysfunction and Male Infertility: A Comprehensive Review of Current Treatment Options*. https://core.ac.uk/download/640070691.pdf (accessed on 16th June 2025).
7. Gkourogianni, A., Sinaii, N., Jackson, S. H., Karageorgiadis, A. S., Lyssikatos, C., Belyavskaya, E., Keil, M. F., Zilbermint, M., Chittiboina, P., Stratakis, C. A., & Lodish, M. B. (2017). Pediatric Cushing disease: disparities in disease severity and outcomes in the Hispanic and African-American populations. *Pediatric research*, *82*(2), 272–277. https://doi.org/10.1038/pr.2017.58(accessed on 16th June 2025).
8. Ameer, B., & Weintraub, H. (2018). Pediatric obesity: Influence on drug dosing and therapeutics. https://core.ac.uk/download/155271623.pdf (accessed on 16th June 2025).
9. Panvino, F., Paparella, R., Gambuti, L., Cerrito, A., Menghi, M., Micangeli, G., Petrella, C., Fiore, M., Tarani, L., & Ardizzone, I. (2024). Klinefelter Syndrome: A Genetic Disorder Leading to Neuroendocrine Modifications and Psychopathological Vulnerabilities in Children-A Literature Review and Case Report. *Children (Basel, Switzerland)*, *11*(5), 509. https://doi.org/10.3390/children11050509(accessed on 16th June 2025).
10. Assié, G., Balsalobre, A., Bertherat, J., Chittiboina, P., et al. (2017). Loss-of-function mutations in the *CABLES1* gene are a novel cause of Cushing's disease. https://core.ac.uk/download/323066133.pdf (accessed on 16th June 2025).
11. Bagnall, A., Day, R., & Kime, N. H. (2013). *Systematic Review of Transition Models for Young People with Long-Term Conditions: A Report for NHS Diabetes*. https://core.ac.uk/download/29018738.pdf (accessed on 16th June 2025).

12. Behdani, F., Ghaemi, N., Mohareri, F., Noroozi Asl, S., et al. (2018). Evaluating of psychiatric behavior in obese children and adolescents. https://core.ac.uk/download/483633583.pdf (accessed on 16th June 2025).

13. Bonfig, W., Schmidt, H., & Schwarz, H. P. (2011). Growth patterns in the first three years of life in children with classical congenital adrenal hyperplasia diagnosed by newborn screening and treated with low doses of hydrocortisone. *Hormone research in paediatrics*, *75*(1), 32–37. https://doi.org/10.1159/000316973 (accessed on 16th June 2025).

14. Cano González, D. A., Flores Martínez, Á., & Venegas Moreno, E. (2019). AIP and MEN1 mutations and AIP immunohistochemistry in pituitary adenomas in a tertiary referral center. https://core.ac.uk/download/299806478.pdf (accessed on 16th June 2025).

15. Hanna, E. S., Cheetham, T., Fearon, K., Herbrand, C., Hudson, N., McEleny, K., Quinton, R., Stevenson, E., & Wilkes, S. (2019). The Lived Experience of Klinefelter Syndrome: A Narrative Review of the Literature. *Frontiers in endocrinology*, *10*, 825. https://doi.org/10.3389/fendo.2019.00825(accessed on 16th June 2025).

16. Ernst, M., Green-Golan, L., Leschek, E., Merke, D. P., et al. (2010). Psychiatric characterization of children with genetic causes of hyperandrogenism. https://core.ac.uk/download/55802070.pdf (accessed on 16th June 2025).

17. Madsen, T. & Hitchcock, E. (2011). *Growing Up Toxic: Chemical Exposures and Increases in Developmental Disease*. US PIRG Education Fund. https://core.ac.uk/download/71358334.pdf (accessed on 16th June 2025).

# PEDIATRIC NEUROLOGY

# 11

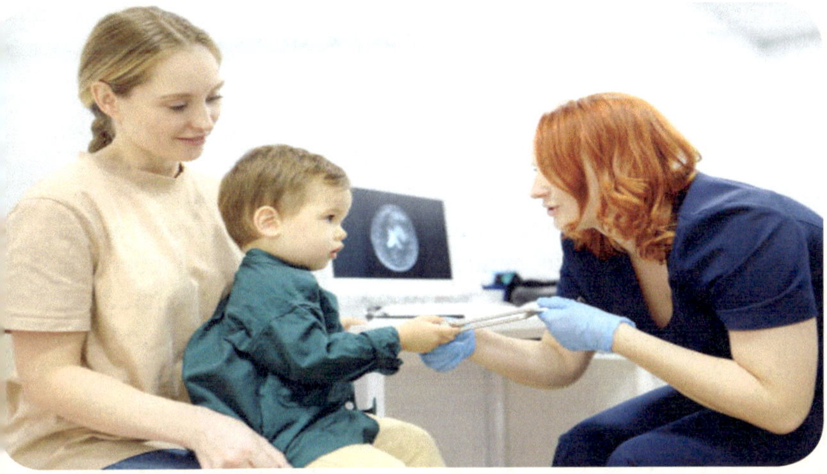

## Introduction

Pediatric neurology is a key sub-specialty of the overall branch of neurology, encompassing the diagnosis and treatment of neurological ailments of children. Because the nervous system develops vastly in children between infancy and adolescence, there is a very important need to grasp the basics of pediatric neurology. Pediatric neurology encompasses an enormous variety of diseases, including congenital malformations, neurogenetic syndromes, epilepsy, and acquired brain damage. The individualized needs of these conditions call for a particular response that not only addresses the physiological but also psychological and social determinants in young patients and their families. Complete training in pediatric neurology gives medical professionals the know-how to fight these varied problems while acquiring expertise in the complex developmental milestones of their patients. The utility of embracing the International Classification of Functioning, Disabilityand Health (ICF) cannot be overstressed in pediatric

### LEARNING OBJECTIVES

**After studying this chapter, you will be able to:**

1. Discuss the developmental milestones and neurological assessment;
2. Explain the common pediatric neurological disorders;
3. Focus on diagnostic tools and techniques;
4. Learn about treatment approaches in pediatric neurology;
5. Know challenges in pediatric neurology;
6. Understand recent advances in pediatric neurology.

neurology. The ICF framework provides a systematic method of analyzing and classifying children's neurological conditions regarding the impact of these diseases on functioning and quality of life (Bruyere et al., 2005). As pediatric neurologists contend with the various levels of disability their patients go through, the ICFs utility comes in how it can facilitate an effective communication between multidisciplinary health teams. This is not only in a clinical setting but also in research when standard outcomes can make studies more efficient. As new therapeutic interventions and technology come into being, the use of the ICF model in practice will certainly be an impetus to enhancing the quality of care in children with neurological conditions. Educational models and professional standards that guide practice are also forces guiding the future of pediatric neurology. Institutions like Virginia Commonwealth University highlight the importance of comprehensive training programs that equip prospective neurologists with the necessary skills and information required to practice in this specialist field (Virginia Commonwealth University, 2018).

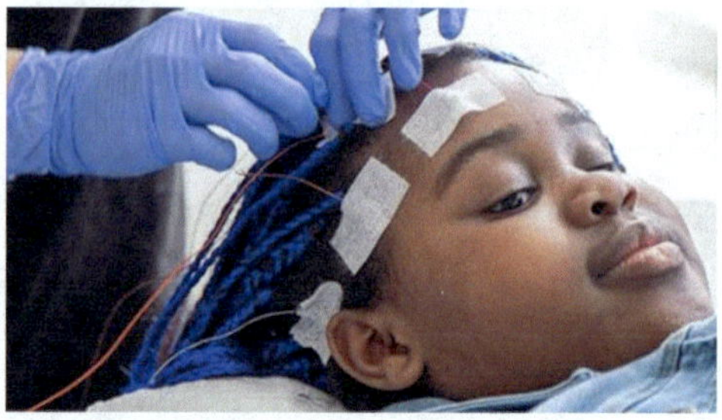

**Figure 11.1.** Pediatric neurology serves as a critical subfield within the broader discipline of neurology.

*Source:* https://www.saanvihealthcare.com/wp-content/uploads/2024/06/CHLA-Pediatric-Neurology-Program-2a.jpg.

These types of education programs cover not only the medical topics of pediatric neurology but also the vital aspects of family-centered care, advocacy, and interprofessional collaboration. The more profound the understanding of pediatric neurological disorders, the more profound the necessity for specialists to continue education and research, staying abreast of new trends and methods of treatment. The cooperative method of enhancing educational practice in pediatric neurology will ultimately lead to better outcomes for patients as well as a healthier environment for children with neurological impairment (Figure 11.1).

## Definition and Scope of Pediatric Neurology

Pediatric neurology is a medical subspecialty that is concerned with the diagnosis, treatment, and management of neurological illnesses in infants and children from birth to adolescence. Pediatric neurology is highly critical because it is concerned with many disorders, including epilepsy, cerebral palsy, and neurological congenital defects. Pediatric neurologists are capable of understanding the particular patterns of development and neurological problems that often come with their child patients, and which differentiate their practice from adult neurologists. Using sophisticated techniques of diagnosis and a wide understanding of children's development, these specialists aim to give individualized treatment strategies that are customized to meet the distinctive needs of children. Recent literature has also emphasized the multidimensionality of pediatric neurological conditions, such that effective treatment is dependent on a common, multidisciplinary endeavor with input from a variety of health professionals (Bowers et al., 2009). Pediatric neurology practice extends beyond mere diagnosis to include a more holistic understanding of the socio-emotional impact of neurological conditions on children and families. For instance, the management of a condition , such as epilepsy goes beyond the simple issue of managing medication but extends to overcoming education-related obstacles, psychosocial issues, and potential stigma to families. Pediatric neurologists are now becoming more aware that a child's health cannot simply be measured by the neurological presentation of the child, but must incorporate the overall well-being and quality of life of the child. Besides, the field is evolving to include newer treatments and technologies , such as genetic therapy and neurostimulation. As researchers continue to study the long-term effects on the child with complex chronic conditions, the importance of integrated care that addresses both physical and mental health grows more evident (Zimmermann, 2016). New areas of inquiry are progressively broadening the knowledge base regarding childhood neurological conditions, justifying the need for specialty care in this age group. The evolving definition and scope of pediatric neurology impose considerations on medical education, policymaking, and resource distribution in healthcare systems. For example, with the rising incidence of neurodevelopmental disorders and child mortality from neurological complications, there is a continuously increasing demand for training courses and funding in pediatric neurology. There is more emphasis on heightened awareness among medical practitioners and society about the special problems affecting this population that can feed into more effective intervention methods. Additionally, ongoing advancements in telemedicine and digital health are poised to significantly expand the penetration of pediatric neurology services, extending to offer access to children in underserved communities and thereby addressing gaps in treatment and care (Bowers et al., 2009).

## Importance of Studying Neurological Disorders in Children

In order to appreciate the profound implications of research on children's neurological disorders, one must accept that early recognition and treatment are key to optimizing developmental achievement. Neurological disorders, , such as epilepsy, autism spectrum disorders, and attention-deficit/hyperactivity disorder, can significantly influence a child's cognitive, affective, and social development. Because children are forging their identity and skills, disruption caused by such disorders can be detrimental over the long term. Pediatric neurology studies give us a better opportunity for early detection of these disorders, thus facilitating timely therapeutic and medical intervention. Timely intervention is a critical component in the avoidance of the negative effect of these disorders and fostering better educational and social functioning and enhancing the quality of life of affected children. Moreover, studies on neurological conditions in pediatric populations advance the larger discipline of neuroscience and mental health. Multisite collaborative studies, like those undertaken by the ENIGMA Consortium, recognize the importance of aggregating data across a variety of cohorts to understand the underlying neurobiological mechanisms of these diseases. By selecting to focus on specific diseases that present in childhood, researchers are able to study genes, environment, and psychosocial factors that may be responsible for the simultaneous emergence of symptoms. This integrative framework accommodates a sophisticated understanding of the disorders that finally culminates into tailored therapeutic interventions to address the biological and psychosocial factors of children's health. Specifically, this integrative framework is crucial in developing effective prevention and intervention programs that can be adapted across diverse demographic contexts (Adhikari et al., 2020). Besides advocating for treatment approaches, studies on childhood neurological disorders raise awareness on the dangers and lasting effects of childhood injuries, particularly in environments like sporting activity. Questions on diseases like Chronic Traumatic Encephalopathy (CTE) have fueled more interest in the neurological health of child athletes. Examining the long-term cognitive consequences of concussions, particularly in contact sports, uncovers fundamental shortcomings in our knowledge of non-catastrophic brain trauma among children. Most existing research focuses on professional athletes, ignoring the large number of children participating in contact sports. By bridging the knowledge gap, researchers will be in a position to inform communities about the potential injuries of sports among young people and improve prevention interventions and strategies for child athletes, which will ultimately lead to better health outcomes for children who engage in physical exercise (Sage, 2018) (Figure 11.2).

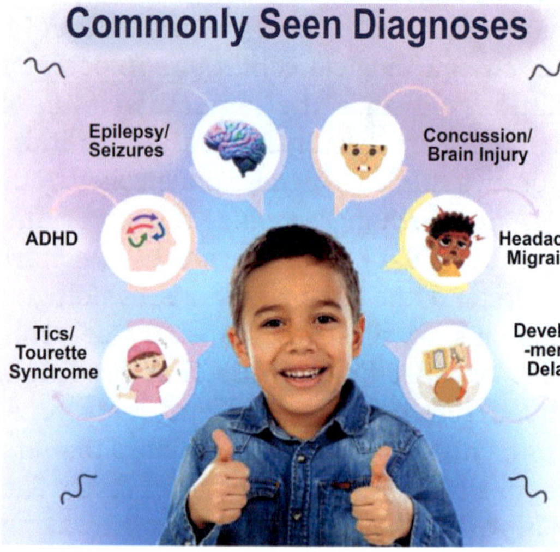


**Figure 11.2.** Importance of studying neurological disorders in children.

*Source:* https://neurologydallas.com/wp-content/uploads/elementor/thumbs/Daniel-Gossett-Welcome-2-qovunsu52vq208p5h8lz7k9j8pyl8euqc3mzvcsmfc.png.

## Overview of Common Conditions Treated in Pediatric Neurology

Pediatric neurology addresses a wide range of neurological illnesses that have the potential to profoundly affect the growth and general well-being of children. Ataxia, or a loss of coordination and balance due to the impairment of more than one nerve pathway, is a common disorder encountered in the specialty. Ataxia is secondary to numerous varied underlying diseases, including genetic syndromes and neurodevelopmental disorders. The diagnosis is made on the basis of sound history-taking, physical examination, and specific clinical maneuvers to identify the etiology. While some etiologies of ataxia may have a benign course, others are disabling and progressive and need urgent treatment in pediatric neurological clinics. Because ataxia results from multifactorial etiology, interdisciplinary collaboration among pediatric neurologists, physical therapists, and rehabilitation professionals is crucial to optimize outcome in involved children and emphasize the need for early recognition and clinical examination for successful treatment intervention (Falsaperla et al., 2017). Another extremely prevalent issue confronted by pediatric neurology is identification and management of developmental delays, which are not only prevalent but most often underdetected early in childhood. These delays can also be found in various areas, including motor skills, language, and social-emotional development. The criticality of detection at an early point cannot be overestimated because early intervention significantly improves long-term result. Pediatric neurologists are important providers of diagnosis and care of such conditions, often collaborating with primary care clinicians to improve developmental monitoring and screening processes. Studies have indicated that enhancing early intervention measures and increasing communication among healthcare workers can significantly reduce the prevalence of undiagnosed developmental disorders, therefore enabling children to reach their full potential in development and growth (Sices, 2007). Seizure disorders are another region of keen interest in pediatric neurology, with diseases like epilepsy affecting a significant percentage of children across the globe. Epilepsy management must be properly diagnosed, which could include prolonged electroencephalogram (EEG) monitoring and neuroimaging to determine the seizure type and etiology. Treatment can include antiepileptic medication, diet therapy, or surgery if epilepsy is refractory. It is challenging in pediatric epilepsy management to find a balance between drug efficacy and side effects, as well as with psychosocial impacts on the child and family. In addition, ongoing research on the environmental and genetic factors behind epilepsy works to improve modalities of treatment and improve the quality of life for survivors. Lastly, pediatric neurologists are a vital part of multimodal care, which emphasizes patient-specific treatment programs that modify to each child's unique situation and needs.

## 11.1. Developmental Milestones and Neurological Assessment

**Learning Outcome**

1. Key developmental milestones in childhood;
2. Techniques for neurological assessment in children;
3. Importance of early detection and intervention.

Familiarity with developmental milestones is necessary in pediatric neurology since these milestones provide insight into the neurological development and health of a child. Developmental milestones are age-related behavioral and physical milestones that children should typically achieve within expected time frames. For instance, at the age of two, most kids are able to say several words and possess basic motor skills , such as running and jumping. These milestones serve not only as markers of healthy development but also as significant markers for potential developmental delays or neurological impairment. A baseline on these milestones allows healthcare providers to monitor progress effectively and identify children who should be further evaluated or treated. Detection and intervention early on have a significantly positive effect on outcomes for children who may have developmental challenges. Neurological testing is imperative in determining compliance with developmental milestones in children. With a complete test, underlying neurological conditions that can affect a child's motor, intellectual, and social development are highlighted. Trace devices , such as accelerometry have emerged to quantify motor behavior accurately, yielding real-life information that is particularly valuable for identifying abnormal patterns of movement. The study noted that bilateral upper limb movements traced with accelerometry can differentiate between children who are developing normally and those at risk for motor impairment (Dosenbach et al., 2019). This new method shifts the focus away from subjective commenting towards quantifiable, measurable data, making tests more reliable.

These advancements enable clinicians to make informed decisions regarding early intervention strategies based on evidence. Also, specific conditions , such as Stereotypic Movement Disorder (SMD) point out the complexities of neurological assessments in children. From research, children with primary SMD show a significant impairment of gross and fine motor function, as indicated in scores in tests , such as the Movement Assessment Battery for Children-Second Edition (Baglioni et al., 2019). These findings suggest that interventions must be specially tailored for children with specific disorders and not just derived from generalized developmental milestones. It is possible for clinicians to develop individualized treatment plans by understanding the precision of these psychomotor profiles and thereby gaining a clearer understanding of each child's developmental pathway and that assistance is individually tailored to their needs (Figure 11.3).

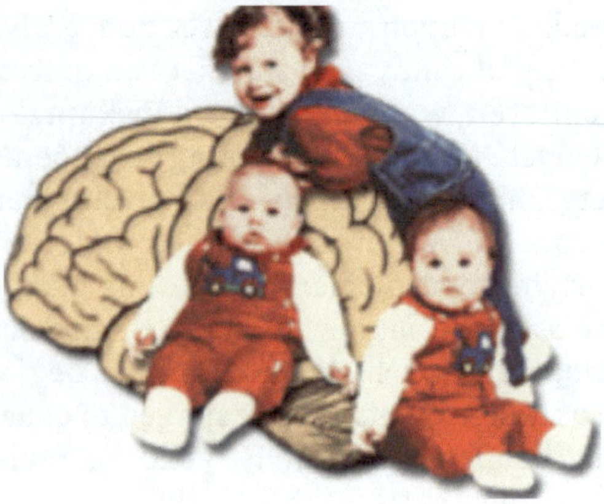

**Figure 11.3.** The focus on pediatric neurological development and assessment.

*Source:* https://neurologicexam.med.utah.edu/pediatric/images/neurologicchildren.gif.

### 11.1.1. Key Developmental Milestones in Childhood

The pathway of childhood development involves a sequence of critical milestones that are measurements of neurological well-being and general wellness. These milestones are usually grouped into areas like motor skills, language development, social-emotional development, and cognitive function. In infancy, babies start to display rudimentary motor skills, including rolling over, sitting up, and later on, crawling. These physical achievements are milestones; they do not only reflect the maturation of the nervous system but also encourage mental engagement as children figure out their worlds. As toddlers approach, anticipated development in language skills, like first words, displays the intricate interplay of neurodevelopment and communication. Early detection of delays in these milestones is able to assist with on-time interventions, and thus there is a need to monitor development within pediatric health care settings (Sices, 2007). At this time, as children transition into preschool age, social/emotional milestones become increasingly important. It is the time in which key skills , such as sharing, turn-taking, and recognizing one's own feelings and those of others are developed. By interactive play, not only are children becoming more social in competence, but they are also constructing language and thinking.

To cope with social interaction at this age is to lay the foundation upon which interpersonal relationship abilities will be based later on in life, and how physical, mental, and emotional development all coalesce. Far more significant, however, are severe delays in the achievement of these milestones as signs of underlying neurologic issues, which should be explored by medical specialists. Research shows that intervention at an early age will improve outcomes for children at risk of developmental challenges, and therefore parents and providers need to be vigilant in monitoring these crucial social-emotional markers (Brickler et al., 2017). In school age, milestones shift to more advanced cognitive and academic skills. These involve the development of literacy and numeracy skills, which underpin academic success and effective learning throughout life. At this point, the child begins to arrive at problems with a sense of independence and imagination, both as a result of developing cognitive growth as well as heightened sensitivity to the world around them. These abilities are directly related to neurological development; as the brain develops through profound changes, it also allows for greater learning and memory capabilities. Failure to reach educational benchmarks can also indicate neurological disorders that must be researched further and treated. Therefore, pediatric health professionals have a significant role to play in recognizing and addressing these developmental factors for the optimization of children's educational success and neurological health, offering a whole-person model of pediatric care (Sices, 2007) (Figure 11.4).

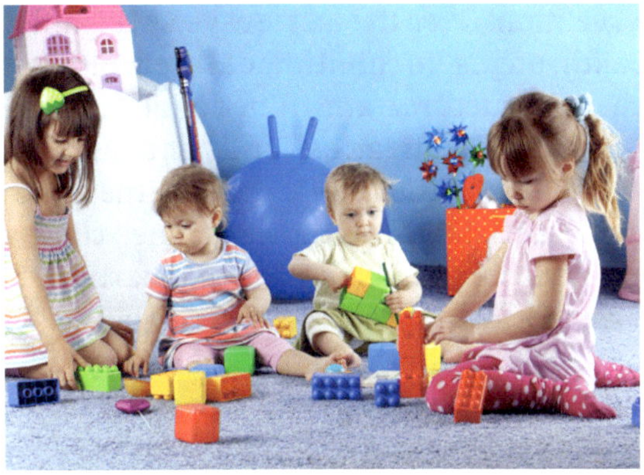

**Figure 11.4.** Key developmental milestones in childhood.

*Source:* https://elmpediatrics.com/wp-content/uploads/2023/08/Depositphotos_3098360_XL-1024x740.jpg.

### 11.1.2. Techniques for Neurological Assessment in Children

Assessment of neurological function in children has specific challenges, needing a variety of specific techniques to accurately determine their cognitive, motor, and sensory functions. One such anchoring method is to utilize developmental screening tools to track milestones and identify delays in these areas' indicative of neurological issues. These tools, , such as the Ages and Stages Questionnaire, provide a structured process for clinicians to evaluate development across various domains, from language function to gross motor. Since pediatric patients may not possess the ability or verbal facility for describing their experiences, these measures can guide further investigation into causative factors, facilitating early intervention and management strategies. By integrating parental report and observational data, professionals are better able to form a higher comprehension of a child's neurological status and provide appropriate and timely intervention (Brickler et al., 2017). Aside from developmental screening, direct neurological assessment continues to be a part of assessing children's neurological status. Through a combination of observational and physical examination techniques, reflexes, muscle tone, coordination, and sensation are examined. Tests , such as the pediatric neurological exam allow professionals to identify unusual reflexes or motor patterns that may be symptoms of cerebral palsy or neurogenetic disorders.

Particularly, the test focuses on age-comparable responses to stimulation and reflex reactions fundamental to assessing the integrity of the nervous system. Technological advances , such as computer systems that track movements are increasingly being utilized in these tests, which offer higher sensitivity to detect subtle abnormalities that may be lost with conventional methods (Brickler et al., 2017). Testing behavior is another key aspect of neurologic examination in children, especially when cognitive or emotional disorders are being evaluated. Tests like standardized psychological tests can be employed to assess attention, capacity for learning, and behavior regulation and guide regarding conditions , such as attention deficit hyperactivity disorder (ADHD) or autism spectrum disorder.

These tests would usually consist of a combination of direct observation, interviewing the parents and teachers with the aid of structured interviews, and rating scales reflecting the child's behavior across different settings. Incorporation of such measures into the neurological assessment process can help to develop an entire profile of a child's functioning, integrating behavioral observations with neurological health and leading to customized interventions. As a multi-faceted process, it ensures that professionals are able to approach the complexity of pediatric neurology in an entirety, thus improving outcomes for child patients (Brickler et al., 2017) (Figure 11.5).

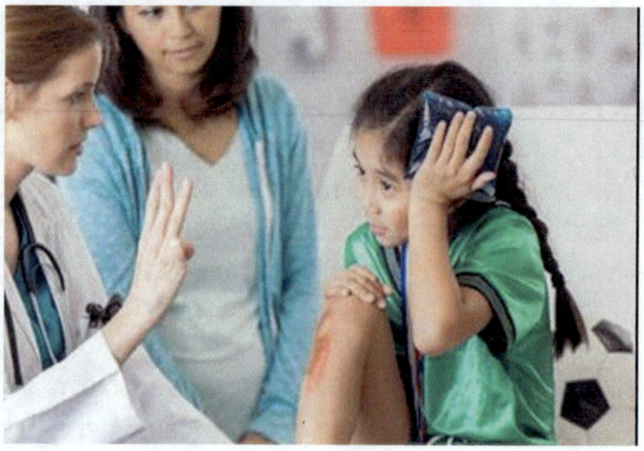

**Figure 11.5.** Techniques for neurological assessment in children.

*Source:* https://images.squarespace-cdn.com/content/v1/5be0663b620b8515f3a9f2b6/1611155154518-6LTU20ZLSUN9VOIBATC6/girlcuncuss.JPG.

## 11.1.3. Importance of Early Detection and Intervention

The necessity of early diagnosis and treatment in pediatric neurology cannot be emphasized enough. Early detection of neurological issues in early childhood is critical to achieving maximum developmental capability. Various studies delineate that developmental delays are underdetected by the primary care providers and that this leads to opportunities for successful intervention being missed. Delays are minimized dramatically through the intervention of early with taking fullest benefit of the developing brain's remarkable neuroplasticity potential in childhood. Where developmental screening and monitoring are absolutely implemented, it allows the provision of supportive services that can be able to facilitate the formation of cognitive, motor, and social skills, complementing the position that early detection is imperative not only as a treatment, but also in order to improve quality of life in general for these children (Sices, 2007). In addition to developmental delays, children with a traumatic brain injury (TBI) diagnosis place a high premium on early identification and intervention. Over the last few years, significant breakthroughs in multimodal neuroimaging, such as structural and functional MRI, have enhanced visualization and understanding of TBI complexities. By applying these novel imaging modalities in a timely manner, clinicians can establish predictors and biomarkers that inform treatment protocols and prognosis. With knowledge of the structural integrity of the brains and the results of network changes, there are opportunities for strategic intervention in therapy that can significantly decrease long-term disability. Hence, the inclusioSn of advanced imaging in initial assessment is an important consideration in optimizing treatment efficacy and results for pediatric TBI patients (Aylward et al., 2012).

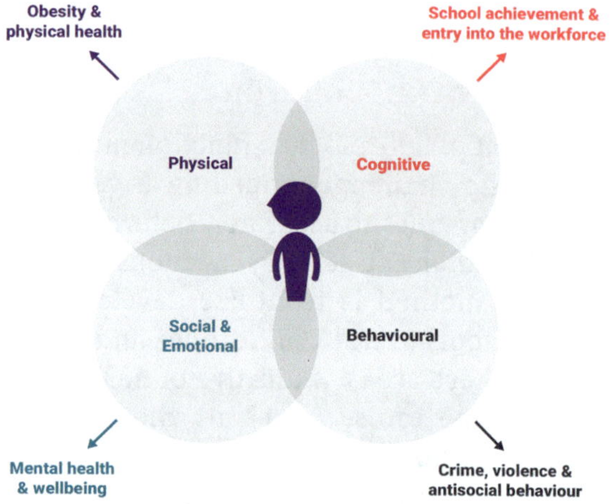


**Figure 11.6.** The significance of early detection and intervention in pediatric neurology cannot be overstated.

*Source:* https://www.eif.org.uk/files/image/about/mtc-four-domains.png.

Secondly, the inclusion of early detection has serious and wide-reaching consequences. Delays in diagnosis of neurologic disorders can result in a chain reaction of developmental, academic, and social complications. The longer the child remains undiagnosed, the greater the risk of secondary complications, including worsened behavioral difficulties and diminished school performance. Furthermore, the financial burden on families and the health care system grows as the need for intensive intervention and remediation accumulates over time. By aiming at early diagnosis and tailored therapies, we not only address the here-and-now needs but also pave the way for healthier, more productive futures for youngsters. Prioritizing future-oriented approaches in pediatric neurology is part of an effort toward more integrated care that appreciates the importance of early intervention based on both clinical expertise and technological expertise (Figure 11.6).

## Test Your Knowledge

1. What are key developmental milestones in early childhood, and why are they important in neurological assessment?
2. What techniques are commonly used for neurological assessment in children?

## 11.2. Common Pediatric Neurological Disorders

**Learning Outcome**

1. Epilepsy and seizure disorders;
2. Cerebral palsy and its implications;
3. Neurogenetic disorders and their impact.

In pediatric neurology, many disorders are characterized by being particularly prevalent, significantly impacting the lives of the affected children and families. Of these conditions, epilepsy is among the most prevalent, occurring approximately 27.6% of the patients with whom specialist clinics deal. Epilepsy is a neurological disorder characterized by recurring seizures with variable presentation and severity and possibly needing early and effective intervention. Diagnosis is often a blending of clinical evaluation, imaging, and electroencephalographic tests that aid in the determination of the exact type of epilepsy and inform treatment options. The severity of this disorder is attributable to its ability to bring normal children's development and everyday activities to a standstill and therefore warrants timely and informed intervention by medical specialists in the field of pediatric neurology. Along with epilepsy, global developmental delay occurs as a most prominent concern in about 17.03% of children's neurological cases. Global developmental delay is a condition that encompasses a range of defects of cognitive, social, and physical development that manifest in various regions. Global developmental delay's etiology is the toughest, as it may occur from genetic, environmental, or psychological reasons. Intervention at this point is essential since timely intervention can significantly affect long-term outcomes. Health practitioners often utilize a multidisciplinary framework, incorporating educational, treatment, and family resources in addition to maximizing the developmental trajectory of affected children. By effective counteract to global developmental delay's multi-dimensional dynamics, pediatric neurologists can maximize quality of life and subsequent achievement potential in young patients (Wirrell et al., 2005). Besides these prevalent disorders, pediatric neurology also deals with various other disorders including metabolic disorders and cerebral palsy. Metabolic disorders are responsible for about

10.7% of the cases and may at times have diagnostic challenges because, in most cases, there is the need for special laboratory tests and ongoing management. The children with such disorders may come with various neurological signs according to the biochemical disturbance of the underlying condition.

The other significant condition is cerebral palsy, affecting around 7.24% of the children with pediatric neurology and referring to a variety of disorders involving movement and posture due to brain damage during early life. The heterogeneity of the issues such disorders create emphasizes the importance of ongoing research and communication among practitioners. Moreover, other techniques , such as complementary and alternative medicine (CAM) have come into the scene, as studies indicate that a high percentage of families utilizing them report perceived benefits, thereby necessitating a broad discussion around choice in treatment in pediatric diseases (Wirrell et al., 2005) (Figure 11.7).

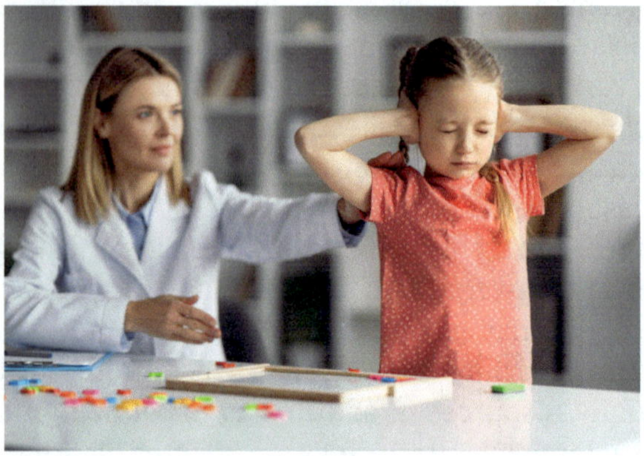

**Figure 11.7.** Demonstrating the assessment of pediatric neurological or developmental conditions.

*Source:* https://lonestarneurology.net/wp-content/uploads/2024/08/1-Pediatric-Neurology-Disorders-Common-Among-Children.jpg.

### 11.2.1. Epilepsy and Seizure Disorders

Epilepsy and seizure disorders are a major component of pediatric neurology, occurring in a significant number of children globally. Seizures can occur at any age and have multiple etiology and presentation. Of all such conditions, Lennox-Gastaut syndrome (LGS) is unique due to the severity of the condition and the complexity of its underlying pathophysiology. LGS usually occurs between 1 and 8 years of age, most often due to multiple neurological insults, , such as hypoxic-ischemic injury and cortical malformations. The multidimensional presentation of LGS reflects the complexity of issues in pediatric neurology, with clinicians required to follow complicated treatment regimens to target both the seizures as well as the resultant cognitive dysfunction (Mastrangelo et al., 2017). Despite advances in therapeutic strategies, including pharmacologic and dietary interventions, long-term outcome for patients with LGS remains poor and invites more research and innovation in this field. Another profound disorder among childhood epilepsy is tuberous sclerosis complex (TSC), which has a propensity to appear early in childhood as infantile spasms. Infantile spasms may inhibit neurodevelopment and thus drive the utility of early detection and intervention. Better management modalities have been enhanced over time, with vigabatrin and adrenocorticotropic hormone being regard as cornerstone pharmacologic therapy. Recent advances in the understanding of the molecular mechanisms of TSC have targeted specifically the mammalian target of rapamycin (mTOR) inhibitors as therapeutic adjuncts in seizure control and management of the tumors associated with TSC, , such as subependymal giant cell astrocytomas (Wang & Fallah, 2014). This evolving therapeutic scenario emphasizes the importance of early identification and customized treatment modalities, stressing the need for integrated care in pediatric neurology. The extreme prevalence of epilepsy and seizure disorders in the pediatric population necessitates a multi-disciplinary approach to management involving medical, surgical, as well as dietary methods. Surgical therapies, , such as resective surgery, corpus callosotomy, or vagus nerve stimulation, might be unavoidable in certain medically intractable seizure patients. Of special mention, resective surgery, when indicated, provides a potential cure for the majority of patients, demonstrating the importance of finding the zone of seizure generation early (Wang & Fallah, 2014). Additionally, the ketogenic diet continues to gain wider acceptance as an invaluable therapeutic agent, particularly in those not responsive to standard antiepileptic drug therapy. Future research to continue to improve the understanding of the pathophysiology of these diseases is essential. Such studies have the ability to move treatment forward and eventually to improved quality of life for pediatric patients burdened with the effects of epilepsy and seizure disorders (Figure 11.8).

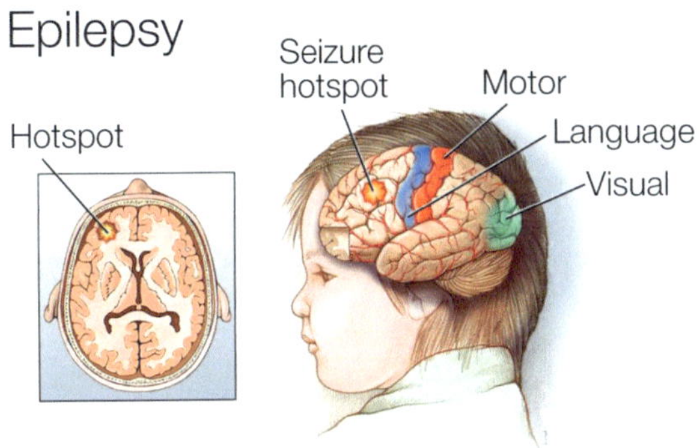


**Figure 11.8.** Epilepsy and seizure disorders represent a significant aspect of pediatric neurology.

*Source:* https://nurseslabs.com/wp-content/uploads/2018/08/Seizures.jpg.

## 11.2.2. Cerebral Palsy and Its Implications

Cerebral palsy (CP) is a complex neurological disorder that primarily impacts movement and muscle coordination because of the abnormal development of the brain or damage to the developing brain, generally before or during birth. The effects of CP are more than mere impairment of the motor system; they comprise a number of cognitive, emotional, and communicative challenges. Most children with CP have impairment of mobility and disabled daily function, along with secondary conditions , such as muscle spasticity and joint deformity. Furthermore, the spectrum of severity in CP, ranging from mild impairment of motor function to extreme disability, adds to the complexity of the condition, requiring case-specific care strategies and interventions in accordance with the specific needs of each child. With the development of knowledge in medicine, advancing the multidisciplinary policy remains crucial in the management of the diverse implications of CP in pediatric neurology. There is multidimensional treatment for children suffering from CP that is typically presented by utilizing physical therapy, occupational therapy, and orthotics in a bid to improve mobility and general quality of living. Current best practice guidelines note the importance of individualized treatments, specifically the use of ankle-foot orthoses (AFOs) for enhancing gait economy in children with Gross Motor Function Classification System (GMFCS) I-III. AFO use demonstrates that successful orthotic intervention can lead to impressive ambulatory gains, allowing children with CP to engage in functional daily activity (Morris et al., 2011). However, existing evidence recognizes gaps, foremost among them being the long-term effectiveness of various interventions and a lack of high-level evidence for the application of orthoses to other body segments , such as the hip and spine. Thus, best practice demands continuous monitoring and re-evaluation of therapeutic interventions based on evolving clinical evidence and patient response. The need for continuous research and innovation in the management of CP cannot be overstressed. Despite the advancement in therapeutic techniques and technology, there remain major challenges as far as evidence-based interventions and clinical implementation of interventions are concerned. Systematic literature review between the earlier consensus conference report of 1994 and 2008 revealed the necessity to enhance the quality of studies concerning orthopedic interventions in CP (Bowers et al., 2009). Patient population heterogeneity and heterogeneity of intervention design often complicate it to create normalized treatment protocols. Thus, with the development of the specialty of pediatric neurology, it will become a requirement that healthcare providers engage in collaborative research efforts to develop more efficient, evidence-based interventions. Through these efforts, ultimately, children with CP are given the most appropriate and most comprehensive care specific to their needs (Figure 11.9).

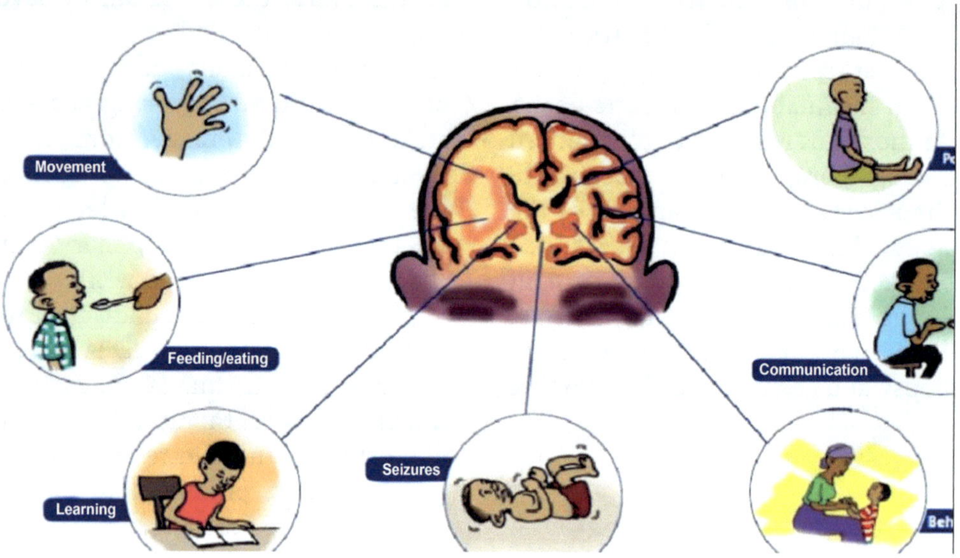


**Figure 11.9.** Cerebral palsy and its implications.

*Source:* https://www.physio-pedia.com/images/thumb/d/dd/Problems_in_CP_children.jpg/800px-Problems_in_CP_children.jpg.

## 11.2.3. Neurogenetic Disorders and Their Impact

The similarity between neurogenetic disorders, especially among children, indicates the strain on global healthcare systems. The disorders are caused by mutations in genetic structures that can influence neurological development and function to manifest with varied clinical manifestations. In the North of England, for example, evidence indicates that monogenic neurological disorders are present in a minimum of 90.9 per 100,000 people, which equates to approximately 1 in 1,100 of the population (Bargiela et al., 2015). What this figure indicates is not only how prevalent these disorders are but also the imperative upon health professionals to be aware and to include genetics within their differential diagnoses. While pediatric neurologists grapple with the complexities of diagnosis and management of such diseases, the need for wide-ranging genetic screening becomes increasingly apparent to ensure timely and accurate interventions in the affected children. Additionally, where there are limited healthcare resources, as in Tanzania, economic challenges compound the misery of pediatric patients with neurogenetic disorders. Patients usually experience systemic barriers including overall mistrust of healthcare providers, stigmatization, and limited access to specialty health care services (Alimohamed et al., 2024). These barriers disproportionately hit children who may require ongoing specialty care that is not readily available in their neighborhoods. The struggle to achieve respect for neurogenetic disorders in low and middle-income countries illustrates the urgent need for programs that aim to integrate genetic testing and diagnosis into clinical practice overall. The technical as well as the social elements of healthcare provision need to be tackled by policymakers to improve the outcomes of children with these diseases. The necessity to combat the impact of neurogenetic disorders calls for a comprehensive approach including the advancement of genetic testing technology and creating public awareness. The actions should include the establishment of properly characterized patient cohorts, enhancing diagnostic facilities, and advocating healthcare reforms that accord priority to genetic testing in routine practice (Alimohamed et al., 2024). In addition, collaboration between governments, healthcare providers, and research organizations can lead to more breakthroughs in discovering the genetic origins of neurological diseases. By investing in the training of healthcare workers in molecular diagnostics and bioinformatics, countries can build capacity for effective diagnosis and treatment. Lastly, an integrated strategy on the basis of medical research, public health policy, and community outreach can effectively minimize the impact of neurogenetic disorders in children to improve diagnosis and treatment.

## Test Your Knowledge

1. What are the key features of epilepsy, cerebral palsy, and their impact on a child's development?
2. How do neurogenetic disorders affect children, and what challenges do they present in management?

## 11.3. Diagnostic Tools and Techniques

**Learning Outcome**

1. Imaging techniques: MRI and CT scans;
2. Electroencephalography (EEG) in diagnosis;
3. Genetic testing and its role in pediatric neurology.

In pediatric neurology, diagnostic accuracy is of the greatest importance, and a spectrum of diagnostic methods and techniques are critical in achieving this. The most commonly used methods include neuroimaging modalities, like magnetic resonance imaging (MRI) and computed tomography (CT) scans. These technologies provide clinicians with detailed visualizations of brain structure, allowing for the identification of abnormalities , such as tumors, structural malformations, or signs of traumatic injuries. The non-invasive nature and high-resolution images of MRI have proven particularly advantageous in children, minimizing the need for more invasive procedures. With every technological advancement, the role of advanced imaging modalities in the early diagnosis is augmented, making the role of accurate assessments crucial for effective treatment modalities in pediatric neurology. Electroencephalography (EEG) not only remains a crucial diagnostic modality in pediatric neurology but also an essential assessment tool for the diagnosis of seizure disorders. EEG captures the brain's electrical activity, enabling clinicians to characterize seizure types, monitor brain function, and assess neurological disorders , such as epilepsy. Although the value of EEG in children also lies in the fact that it is able to provide real-time information, its comparatively quick application is also useful for the timely diagnosis of acute neurological disorders. Because children may show symptoms differently from adults, EEG offers specific information that aids in creating therapeutic approaches and anticipating potential developmental problems. This emphasis on early diagnosis underscores the use of reliable diagnostic techniques to avoid long-term effects on mental and physical growth. In addition, state-of-the-art genetic testing is now a critical diagnostic tool in pediatric neurological diseases.

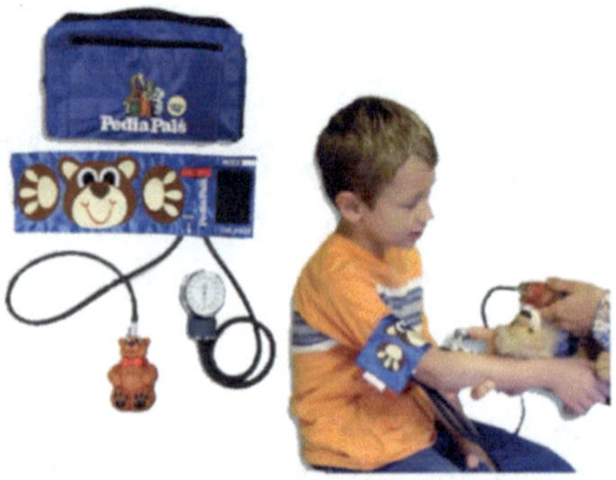


**Figure 11.10.** Diagnostic tools and techniques.

*Source:* https://cdn.shopify.com/s/files/1/0728/6754/5379/files/PED600002-Pediatric-Clinic-Kit_480x480.jpg?v=1734678568.

Advancements in the genetic sequencing technologies enable the identification of specific genetic mutations associated with conditions , such as muscular dystrophy, neurogenetic disorders, and genetic epilepsy. With this new diagnostic technology, clinicians are able to provide a more precise diagnosis, opening the way for intervention with directed therapy and bespoke treatment strategies. Understanding the genetic basis of these diseases not only facilitates effective treatment regimens but also informs the family about the nature of the disease, probable outcomes, and risks for future offspring. As technology in genetic testing continues to improve, the establishment of routine diagnostic procedures incorporating it will, in all likelihood, revolutionalize pediatric neurology, allowing for improved overall care and management of affected children and families (Figure 11.10).

### 11.3.1. Imaging Techniques: MRI and CT Scans

Magnetic Resonance Imaging (MRI) and Computed Tomography (CT) scans are basic diagnostic tools used in pediatric neurology, both with their own respective advantages in assessing neurological disorders. MRI uses very strong magnetic fields and radio waves for the production of high-resolution images of the brain and spinal cord, providing better contrast between different tissue types. This non-surgical technique is particularly useful for the evaluation of soft tissues, determination of lesions, and diagnosis of diseases , such as tumors, congenital malformations, and demyelinating diseases. Given the high prevalence of neurological disorders among the pediatric population, MRI has become a vital tool for clinicians who want total information regarding brain structure and function. Conversely, CT scans also have a second role of utilizing X-ray technology to create cross-sectional images of the brain more quickly than MRI. This quick imaging makes rapid imaging technology a favorite in the acute environment because it is effective at generating diagnoses in acute situations, like bleeding or fracture. Although CT scans allow for quick decision-making, they expose patients to ionizing radiation, and thus repeated imaging is applied with care. The mutual contrasting qualities of MRI and CT scans optimize diagnostic precision to enable healthcare providers to modify their plans according to the individualized needs of patients and specific clinical environments, further enhancing pediatric neurologys potential. The combination of advanced imaging tests like MRI and CT scans continues to develop with advancing technology so that pediatric neurological disorders can be diagnosed even more accurately. The recent developments, , such as functional MRI (fMRI) and diffusion tensor imaging (DTI), have extended the scope of traditional imaging by providing data regarding brain activity and connectivity. For instance, fMRI can be highly useful to interpret neural response in children with epilepsy or neurodevelopmental disorder, while DTI can explain white matter integrity in various pathologies. As pediatricians increasingly rely on these imaging modalities, ongoing research and clinical practice guidelines, , such as those articulated in recent publications, will become essential to optimizing pediatric patient management and monitoring plans for disorders like tuberous sclerosis complex (Northrup et al., 2021) and congenital heart disease (Rychik et al., 2019).

### 11.3.2. Electroencephalography (EEG) in Diagnosis

Electroencephalography (EEG) is a key investigative modality in childhood neurology, notably in diagnosing and managing epilepsy in children. Visualization of brain electrical activity is indispensable for seizure pattern and other neurological conditions. EEG has particular utility in the differentiation of epileptic seizures from other events because the clinical presentation of pediatric seizures is typically nonspecific. The specificity of this test allows for early intervention, which is critical in reducing risk of potential cognitive impairment and improving quality of life in inflected children. Additionally, advancements in EEG machines have allowed extended monitoring, thereby augmenting detection rates of unusual types of seizures and allowing comprehensive assessment of the child's neurological status. In drug-refractory epilepsy, the value of EEG in a presurgical evaluation process that involves multiple disciplines cannot be overstressed. Methodical evaluation by EEG, especially if supplemented by neuroimaging techniques, is extremely valuable in determining surgical candidacy for children with resistant seizures. Extensive EEG assessments can define the epileptogenic areas in the brain, keeping neurosurgeons in the loop regarding the specific areas that need to be removed in order to obtain maximum outcomes. EEG's capacity for improving surgical performance is already present in neurosurgery selection, as it eliminates myths about the adequacy of surgical intervention for drug-refractory focal epilepsies.

Continued advancement in EEG techniques will likely expand this role, advance the field's understanding of epilepsy and improve treatment options for children. Recent studies highlight the importance of using specific diagnostic tools like video-EEG in accurately classifying uncharacteristic neurological occurrences in children. The difficulty of concurrence that an uncharacteristic event is a seizure highlights the necessity for solid strategies in differentiating seizures from non-seizure occurrences in children. Studies have indicated that event frequency prior to video-EEG testing is positively related to the likelihood of successful seizure activity diagnosis, reinforcing the value of thorough clinical evaluation. While long recording times on EEG have not been associated with a high success rate of diagnoses, situation and recorded event frequency remain crucial. With the advancement of pediatric neurology, the integration of sophisticated EEG methods will enable clinicians to have reliable data, leading to enhanced diagnostic precision and treatment outcomes in managing epilepsy (James et al., 2017; Vakharia et al., 2018) (Figure 11.11).

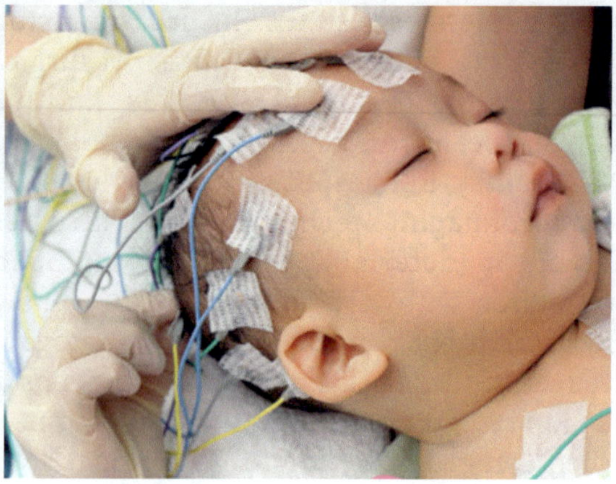

**Figure 11.11.** Electroencephalography (EEG) in diagnosis.

*Source:* https://paediatricneuro.com/wp-content/uploads/2024/04/eeg-scan.jpg.

## 11.3.3. Genetic Testing and Its Role in Pediatric Neurology

Genetic testing has emerged as an invaluable tool in pediatric neurology in the recent years, providing novel information that significantly enhances diagnostic accuracy and therapeutic choices in infants and children with neurological disorders. The use of genetic testing is not limited to diagnosis because it can guide clinicians regarding prognosis and potential response to intervention. Such disorders as epilepsy, cerebral palsy, and genetic syndromes frequently encountered in pediatric patients tend to have multi-factorial genetic etiologies. Clarification of these genetic factors allows the healthcare provider to make more precise therapeutic decision-making about approaches with the potential to modify the disease course or symptom relief. Additionally, genetic testing contributes to common knowledge of neurological disorders and makes it possible to more precisely detect rare genetic diseases that may manifest in early childhood, as shown in the intricacies of diagnosing and managing complicated diseases. Progress of genetic testing technologies, , such as whole exome sequencing and gene panels, has revolutionized pediatric neurology. These technologies provide an unprecedented ability to detect even rare genetic mutations which otherwise would have gone unnoticed in traditional diagnostic approaches. Detection of patient-specific genetic alterations allows the design of personalized treatment regimens for targeting the root biological pathways. This specific therapy approach is particularly beneficial with genetic disorders like Niemann-Pick diseases, in which lipids are stored, leading to crippling neurological symptoms (Abubakar et al., 2012). Practitioners utilize the understanding of these genetic pathways to enhance the quality of life of the children and assist the families in making informed healthcare decisions. In addition, translation of genetic findings into the clinical setting has encouraged multidisciplinary treatment, uniting genetics, neurology, and other subspecialties to offer optimal patient care. While the advantages of genetic testing are self-evident, ethical dilemmas and challenges continue to be at the forefront in pediatric neurology. Concerns , such as impact of genetic findings on family dynamics, risk for discrimination, and psychological effect of genetic diagnosis must be skillfully negotiated. Further, there were also significant differences in the availability of genetic testing across and within different socioeconomic and geographic regions and these highlighted concerns of unequal provision of healthcare. These concerns require frank discussion and policy making to create frameworks that address the ethical concerns surrounding genetic testing in children. As pediatric neurology advances, it will be essential to strike a balance between technological advancements and ethical obligations to ensure that every child has access to such pioneering developments in genetic medicine (Abubakar et al., 2012).

## Test Your Knowledge

1. What roles do MRI, CT scans, and EEG play in diagnosing pediatric neurological disorders?
2. How does genetic testing contribute to the diagnosis and management of pediatric neurological conditions?

# 11.4. Treatment Approaches in Pediatric Neurology

**Learning Outcome**

1. Pharmacological treatments and their effectiveness;
2. Surgical interventions for neurological conditions;
3. Role of rehabilitation therapies in recovery.

In pediatric neurology, the treatment of neurological conditions in children must be holistic and individualized because of the unique developmental phases and variations in disease presentation. Of primary concern is the treatment of intracranial vascular anomalies, which have a significant impact on neurological development. The anomalies range from incidental and benign lesions to severe lesions with possibilities for serious neurological impairment and even heart failure. The treatment risks and benefits must be weighed by the clinicians because therapy can potentially impact normal brain development. It is therefore imperative to understand the natural history of conditions , such as brain arteriovenous malformations and dural arteriovenous fistulas when developing optimal treatment strategies while being cognizant of long-term developmental outcomes (Morshed et al., 2020). Among the most important aspects of treatment regimens in pediatric neurology is seizure disorder control, , such as febrile seizures, which are critical concerns for parents and carers. A study indicates that early risk factor detection , such as fever and age below two years can prevent additional seizures. By studying causative reasons for febrile seizures, medical practitioners can implement preventive strategies that alleviate anxiety among families and minimize the risk of long-term complications. The importance attached to education, family support, and implementing management plans is an inclusive process that deals with physical and psychological factors of the condition in children (Fuadi et al., 2010). Furthermore, multidisciplinary care is required in the successful management of pediatric neurological illness.

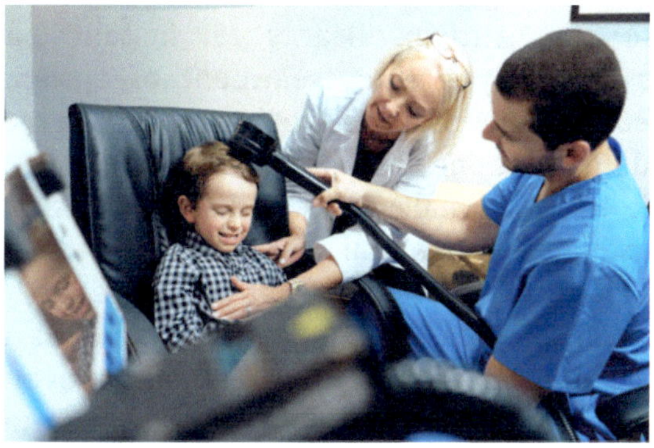

**Figure 11.12.** Treatment approaches in pediatric neurology.

*Source:* https://dramitvatkar.com/assets/images/services/best-child-neurologist-in-mumbai.jpg.

Through the integration of input from neurologists, psychologists, social workers, and teachers, a more comprehensive care plan can be constructed that addresses the diverse needs of the child. For instance, children suffering from chronic neurological illness not only require medical interventions but also some educational support to enhance their academic performance and social functioning. This integrated approach ensures that the overall well-being of the child is prioritized, preventing secondary complications arising from their neurological condition. Lastly, encouraging good communication between caregivers and health workers is essential in treating children for optimal outcomes in pediatric neurology (Figure 11.12).

### 11.4.1. Pharmacological Treatments and Their Effectiveness

The investigation of pharmacological therapies in pediatric neurology underscores the intricacies of treating neurological diseases in the pediatric population, especially in how to maximize therapeutic benefit at a minimal cost of side effects. Pharmacological drugs are used in treating a broad range of conditions, including epilepsy, migraines, and neurodevelopmental disorders. Anticonvulsants, for instance, are the mainstay in the treatment of epilepsy, effectively decreasing seizure frequency in most pediatric patients. Yet the difficulty lies in being able to individualize the medication selection to a child's individual metabolic profiles and possible comorbidities. The effectiveness of pharmacological treatment thus depends on a thorough appreciation of the child's overall medical situation, requiring close observation and possibly regular modifications to dosages in order to optimize results without inducing side effects. Despite pharmacotherapy advancements, the role of psychological and behavioral management is an important component of the integral management of pediatric neurological illnesses. Studies indicate that the application of pharmacological agents can be effective in achieving clinical outcomes, but they are not effective in addressing the complex experiences of pain and suffering in children with neurological diseases. This is particularly observed in chronic pain disorders when medications occasionally fall short in providing relief. The inclusion of psychological interventions, , such as Cognitive-Behavioral Therapy (CBT), has shown to be effective in improving the rate of treatment success and quality of life of teenagers. With coping and psychosocial issues addressed, such interventions can lead to better therapeutic outcomes (Brickler et al., 2017). Furthermore, pharmacotherapy assessment should consider the long-term implications on child development, specifically negative effects. Behavioral treatments have been found to work in conjunction with pharmacotherapy effectively, most importantly for the treatment of such conditions as headaches among children and adolescents who can play a significant role in daily function. Research determines how these treatments can reduce symptoms, reduce medication dependence, and promote compliance with treatment (Arruda et al., 2016). The dual model not only reduces side effects related to drugs but also increases the general therapeutic context, which supports a multifaceted strategy in the treatment of pediatric patients. The analysis of pharmacological therapy must thus be tightly integrated with behavioral approaches to guarantee all-round care and accommodate children with varied needs of neurological development.

### 11.4.2. Surgical Interventions for Neurological Conditions

Neurosurgical interventions for neurological disease in the pediatric age group are critical in the management of many conditions affecting brain function and the quality of life. They range from minimal procedure techniques to full open surgical procedures, depending on the condition of the neurological disorder. Conditions like epilepsy, brain tumors, and traumatic brain injuries may need surgical interventions after pharmacological and rehabilitation management have been unsuccessful. The goal of surgical procedures in these situations is to eliminate blockage or enhance neurological function, hence alleviating the symptom burden. Particularly in children, whose developmental trajectories are susceptible to disruption, early and effective surgical intervention can significantly improve long-term results and facilitate healthier development and growth patterns. Additionally, combining surgical methods with multidisciplinary teams of healthcare experts maximizes the effectiveness of neurological therapy. Surgical teams often work together with neurologists, rehabilitation therapists, psychologists, and other experts to formulate personalized treatment plans that address the multifaceted aspects of pediatric neurological disorders. One study highlighted the importance of psychological therapy combined with surgery in treating pain in neurological rehabilitation, illustrating how teamwork leads to more comprehensive care for children. Cognitive-Behavioral Therapy and mindfulness techniques are increasingly recognized as crucial in enhancing post-surgery recovery (Brickler et al., 2017). Although it serves to optimize surgical results, such interdisciplinarity also promotes the overall well-being of pediatric patients and ensures they receive the full spectrum of care necessary for effective rehabilitation. In addition, disparities in the presence of surgical intervention for neurological diseases in high-income versus low- to middle-income countries (LMIC) are of significant concern. Greater awareness is present that numerous children in LMIC suffer from diseases , such as epilepsy that could be benefited from functional neurosurgical procedures, yet the treatment is not used effectively. Scarcity of resources and the cost factor hinder the delivery of quality surgical care in these centers, and conditions that are treatable are exceedingly common (Fezeu et al., 2018). Together with increasing awareness on these disparities, concerted efforts towards establishing partnerships between high-income and low-income health centers are becoming increasingly important. These collaborations attempt to bolster understanding of the distinct disease burdens in LMIC as they devise context-specific guidelines to more easily enable access to life-changing surgical care for disadvantaged pediatric patients (Figure 11.13).

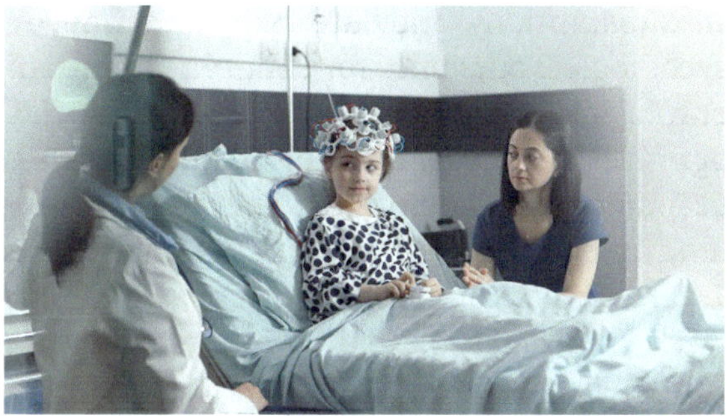

**Figure 11.13.** Surgical interventions for neurological conditions in the pediatric population.

*Source:* https://drdhanrajginnavaram.com/assets/img/services/pediatric-neurosurgery.webp.

## 11.4.3. Role of Rehabilitation Therapies in Recovery

The role of rehabilitation therapies in pediatric neurology is complex, dealing with most aspects of recovery in children with neurological impairments. Rehabilitation encompasses a continuum of interventions including physical therapy, occupational therapy, and psychological support aimed at enhancing functional independence and quality of life. In children with disability due to traumatic brain injury (TBI), these therapies are essential as they support retraining of the motor functions, improve cognitive function, and facilitate emotional adaptation. The blending of various therapeutic modalities creates a multidisciplinary practice that is required for dealing with the complex needs of children. Effective rehabilitation not just mitigates the short-term consequences of neurological illnesses but helps long-term growth in such a way that affected children can be reintegrated into their environments—a core aspect of their general well-being. Psychological therapies being such an important part of rehabilitation processes cannot be emphasized enough. Research indicates psychological interventions can substantially alleviate pain and improve psychological outcomes for children undergoing neurological rehabilitation. Techniques , such as Cognitive-Behavioral Therapy, mindfulness, and Acceptance and Commitment Therapy have been found to be effective in alleviating pain caused by various neurological disorders (Brickler et al., 2017). Besides, these therapies provide some coping techniques to the children to handle the emotional problems arising out of their diseases. Integrating psychological rehabilitation in rehabilitation programs can increase the efficacy of physical and occupational therapies as a whole, eventually facilitating a better integrated process of recovery. Therefore, the inclusion of psychological therapies is a step forward in pediatric neurology that highlights the importance of treating physical and emotional well-being during rehabilitation. Rehabilitation therapy also plays an important part in solving the particular problems encountered by children with specific neurological diseases. For example, survivors of TBI typically exhibit a range of functional impairments and therefore must be offered specialized rehabilitation methods that are suited to their specific needs and concerns (Brickler et al., 2017). Such coordination between doctors, parents, and the patients themselves is extremely critical in developing effective rehabilitation strategies. Family participation in rehabilitation promotes the development of an enabling setting where children become motivated to take part in their recovery process. In addition, continuous monitoring and treatment mode changes ensure interventions remain relevant and effective as the child grows. In general, rehabilitation therapies are crucial to optimizing recovery outcomes in pediatric neurology, pointing to their significance to an integrated model of healthcare.

## Test Your Knowledge

1. What are common pharmacological treatments used in pediatric neurology, and how effective are they?
2. When are surgical interventions considered in pediatric neurological conditions, and what are some examples?

## 11.5. Challenges in Pediatric Neurology

**Learning Outcome**

1. Ethical considerations in treatment decisions;
2. Access to care and disparities in treatment;
3. Psychological impact on patients and families.

The field of child neurology is plagued by a myriad of challenges that have a direct impact on diagnosis, treatment, and management of neurological conditions in children. The first problem is the unavailability of specialized caregivers. The global shortage of trained pediatric neurologists hinders access to timely treatment, which presents a potential delay in diagnosis and intervention of serious disease. Even countries with robust medical infrastructures suffer from this shortage, highlighting a systemic deficit that is worrying in light of the rising incidence of neurological disease in children. This burden is therefore left in the hands of general practitioners or non-specialists, who are not necessarily equipped with the specialist training needed to properly identify advanced neurological conditions. Such a state not only renders the process of diagnosis complicated but can lead to a higher risk for misdiagnosis, with long-term effects on the child's development and quality of life. Another area of special challenge in pediatric neurology is the difficulty of diagnosing and treating disorders with overlapping presenting symptoms. Disorders , such as epilepsy, cerebral palsy, and neuromuscular disorders have overlapping presentations, making differential diagnosis particularly challenging. This complexity is further exacerbated by symptom variation in children due to the phase of development and individual health profiles. New diagnostic decision support software (DDSS) has emerged as a good approach for addressing this complexity, as demonstrated in the recently established evidence from studies demonstrating its effectiveness for improving diagnostic accuracy in generalists. With Bayesian pattern matching and appropriate clinical data, such a technology can augment the diagnostic capabilities of non-specialists to the extent that misdiagnosis is reduced from 28% to 15% in certain situations. This technology has the potential to significantly improve patient outcomes through educating healthcare specialists with better instruments for challenging cases, something that is required in the field of pediatric neurology. Second, the implementation of research and advances in technology into day-to-day clinical practice poses another problem in pediatric neurology. Even though technological advancements , such as imaging studies and genetic studies have the potential to revolutionize the diagnosis and treatment of neurological conditions, there is a deficit in applying this research for clinical use. Pediatric neurologists may also face funding issues, resource limitations, and rigid regulatory frameworks that may impede the use of new approaches. Additionally, the discrepancies in availability of new modes of treatment based on geographic or socioeconomic location widen already prevailing disparities in care. Emphasizing the need for institutional reforms, , such as increased training for the general practitioners and increased integration of DDSS tools into clinical practice, can facilitate further growth of the pediatric neurology field and eventually enhance care for the affected children, guaranteeing that advancements are properly translated to clinical gains (Brickler et al., 2017) (Figure 11.14).

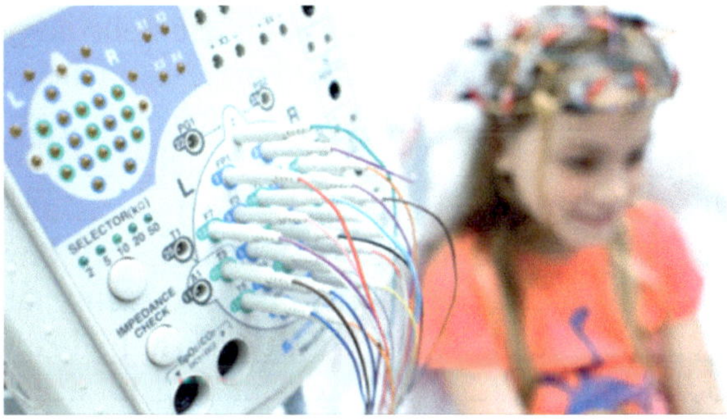

**Figure 11.14.** The field of pediatric neurology faces numerous challenges that significantly impact diagnosis.

*Source:* https://www.thelancet.com/cms/asset/520df83e-251c-4c1e-b6fa-d2afe8deaba2/fx1.jpg.

## 11.5.1. Ethical Considerations in Treatment Decisions

In pediatric neurology, therapeutic options are guided primarily by ethical issues, most notably with the resolution of complex cases , such as medically intractable epilepsy in children. Employing new advanced surgical techniques, , such as the use of high frequency oscillations (HFOs) for surgical resections, is a graphic example of one significant ethical issue. While HFOs might better manage seizures and enhance the health of younger patients, the physician has to walk a fine balance between therapeutic efficacy and the novelty of new risks. The ethical decision-making process very often entails weighing what limited evidence there is against what standards of current practice exist, and thus clinicians must take into account not only patient safety but also what the implications are likely to be for future research and clinical practice in pediatric neurology (Ibrahim et al., 2012). Moreover, when deciding on treatment, the doctrine of informed consent arises. Such children and their caregivers must be adequately informed of the uncertainties, risks, and benefits of intended treatments and the hoped-for outcomes. Such an obligation is particularly challenging in pediatric neurology, where patients may lack adequate capacity to understand complex medical details. The ethical obligation to inform caregivers includes fully discussing the impact of medical decisions, including potential unexpected complications. There is a call for clinicians to develop an environment of support that will help bring about collaborative decision-making in which families have opportunities to actively discuss the treatment options. This collaborative approach is central to helping build trust and help ensure the psychological and emotional concerns of both the patient and the family are respected (Drove et al., 2019). In addition to informed consent, access to healthcare equity has emerged as a significant ethical concern in pediatric neurology. Neurological disorders are often exposed to inequities in the quantity and quality of care based on socioeconomic status, geographical location, and system health inequities. Ethical decision-making for therapy demands reversing the inequities so that novel treatments and procedures are equitably accessible. Novel technologies, , such as those linked to HFOs, must be seriously weighed to prevent exacerbating healthcare inequities. Clinicians must call for fair resource distribution and availability of complex interventions to every child patient, so that ethical considerations are realized to transcend particular patient cases to the larger image of health care equity and justice in pediatric neurology (Ibrahim et al., 2012).

### 11.5.2. Access to Care and Disparities in Treatment

Availability of pediatric neurology care has emerged as an influential determinant of treatment effectiveness among children afflicted with neurological disorders. This inequality is generally described across spectrums of race, ethnicity, and socioeconomic status, wherein minority populations frequently experience more debilitating representations of these disorders. For instance, in a study of children with Cushing disease, Hispanic and African American children had significantly higher severity scores compared to their non-Hispanic White counterparts, demonstrating that care accessibility and quality of treatment may vary widely based on racial groups (Gkourogianni et al., 2017). Higher levels of cortisol and larger tumor sizes were established as risk factors for this disparity, indicating the need for targeted interventions to act upon these disparities. This data continues to solidify the broad consensus that equal access to healthcare resources will be needed to improve clinical outcomes in diverse pediatric populations. Furthermore, the impact of limited access to pediatric neurology goes beyond early treatment disparities in the disease process; it also touches on long-term health and quality of life. In the majority of the low- and middle-income countries (LMIC), the relative scarcity of functional neurosurgical procedures adds to the issue since these nations carry a higher burden of treatable illnesses , such as epilepsy and cerebral palsy. The excessively prohibitive fees of advanced neurosurgical interventions typically render it impossible for such families to afford them (Fezeu et al., 2018). Combined with the lack of proper data regarding the prevalence of these ailments in LMIC, health providers cannot adopt relevant and evidence-based treatment strategies. Unless financial and infrastructural barriers to care are overcome, the treatment course of children with neurological disorders will remain unequal to further exacerbating disparities across levels of socio-economic status. Reducing such disparities will require attempts to enhance the accessibility and quality of child neurological care. This requires innovative solutions, , such as the development of alliances between high-income countries (HIC) and their LMIC counterparts, development of a transfer of knowledge, and context-specific intervention design that is responsive to the unique needs of different populations. Joint action is also required to develop global guidelines that are geared towards ensuring equitable access to treatment possibilities, and high-level neurosurgical procedures do not concentrate in affluent regions (Fezeu et al., 2018). Overcoming the different barriers to care will allow healthcare systems to develop a context for all children, irrespective of socio-economic status or race, to access the neurological care they should have. Furthermore, enhancing community education and sensitization regarding neurological disorders is likely to empower families to seek timely treatment and exercise their right to health, in the end leading to improved outcomes for children with neurological disorders (Figure 11.15).

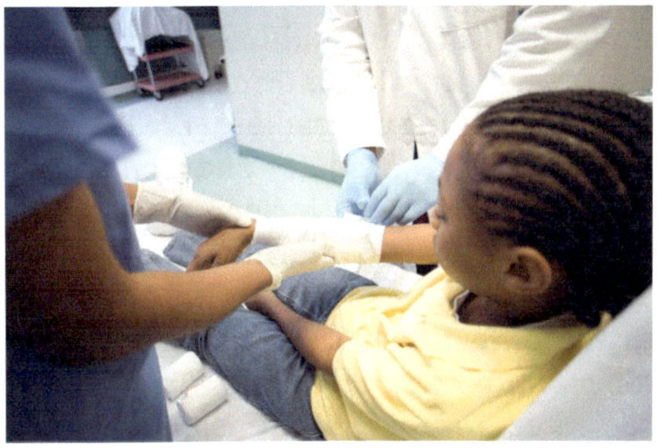

**Figure 11.15.** Pediatric emergency care and injury management.

*Source:* https://media.npr.org/assets/img/2024/01/17/gettyimages-124205732_custom-3bf73461fe935efe643f244466aee800ba7529e9.jpg.

## 11.5.3. Psychological Impact on Patients and Families

The psychological impact of pediatric neurological conditions extends well beyond the patient and into the areas of family life and emotional functioning. Families will frequently manage diagnostic stress, treatment stress, and uncertainty of long-term outcome. Parents will feel helpless as they struggle to navigate medical systems and try to advocate for their child. This can lead to increased stress and anxiety, which in turn can affect family relationships. Notably, children's neurological disorders are often socially limiting, both isolating the patients and their families. More than simple medical management is required; addressing the emotional and psychological needs is a complex issue that requires an integrated treatment approach as an integral part of the pediatric neurology service. Headaches, which are the most prevalent neurological symptom in children, are a prime example of how psychological complaints influence not just the individual patient but also the family of the patient. Research has established that psychosocial processes, , such as family stressors and social environment, are strongly associated with headache frequency and intensity. Because headaches significantly impair quality of life, it is necessary to adopt a multidisciplinary approach involving the application of behavioral interventions as well as pharmacological interventions. Such a strategy aims not only to decrease pain but also to manage the psychological components of headache disorders and therefore enhance the overall well-being of patients. Through the augmentation of coping skills and the relief of anxiety with effective behavioral treatments, families can observe stress reduction, allowing them to have healthful family interactions and improve quality of life for all members involved (Arruda et al., 2016). Furthermore, awareness of the nuances of how chronic illness affects quality of life is integral to the determination of its psychological influence on children and families. With Duchenne muscular dystrophy, patients have rated poorer physical activity and social relationship quality of life. This may be partly due to the emotional burden of having a progressive disease. Interestingly, parental ratings are more likely to indicate a poorer quality of life in their child than the children themselves do. This gap highlights the importance of facilitating open communication and parent education in order to foster a more supportive environment. By raising parental awareness of their child's condition and outlooks, families can build a more supportive and optimistic atmosphere, which ultimately contributes to the mental welfare of all concerned (Ashrafi et al., 2016).

## Test Your Knowledge

1. What are some ethical considerations in making treatment decisions for children with neurological disorders?
2. How do access to care and healthcare disparities affect treatment outcomes in pediatric neurology?

## 11.6. Recent Advances in Pediatric Neurology

**Learning Outcome**

1. Innovations in treatment methodologies;
2. Research trends in pediatric neurological disorders;
3. The role of technology in enhancing patient care.

Advances in pediatric neurology in recent times have significantly advanced knowledge and management of many neurological disorders among children. Among the key advances is an enhancement in diagnosis methods, e.g., for viral encephalitis in children. The detection of new viruses like Chandipura virus (CHPV) has served to underscore the importance of rapid and accurate diagnosis. By using the diagnostic tests , such as reverse transcription–polymerase chain reaction (RT-PCR) and enzyme-linked immunosorbent assay (ELISA), physicians can diagnose CHPV more easily, allowing them to take action immediately in individuals who are developing acute encephalitis syndrome (AES) with high mortality. With the growing number of cases of CHPV, especially in regions , such as India, the development of diagnostic capability is a must to improve clinical outcomes and utilize targeted public health interventions (Akingbola et al., 2025). In addition to developments in diagnosis, pediatric neurology therapeutic paradigms are shifting to include state-of-the-art therapies tailored specifically to the individual needs of younger patients. As an example, the therapeutic world of multiple sclerosis (MS) has grown with the introduction of novel disease-modifying therapies (DMTs). While MS is primarily an adult condition, there is growing awareness of incidence in children. Recent evidence has clarified the necessity for age-specific treatment protocols in mind with the differential presentation of diseases among children and youths. The practice-based integration of recommendations based on practice acknowledges the necessity of maximizing treatment algorithms for various forms of MS in a manner that children receive the optimal possible care (Capela et al., 2025). It stresses the necessary pediatric-focused research to address the gaps that exist presently in treatment efficacy and selection. In addition, recent studies emphasize the need for integrated care models of child neurology to manage all forms of neurological conditions. This means not only taking into consideration medication treatment but encompassing psychological treatment and educational interventions according to the needs of the child. For instance, interdisciplinary approaches whereby neurologists, psychologists, and educators work together are established to create the overall health of children who suffer from chronic neurological diseases. By fostering collaboration among specialists, pediatric neurology is ideally positioned to supply children with multi-dimensional care that maximizes both neurological and cognitive health. As increasingly sophisticated studies continue to reveal the complexities of pediatric neurological illness, these collaborative models will be pivotal in shaping the future of pediatric neurology and improving long-term outcomes in affected children (Figure 11.16).

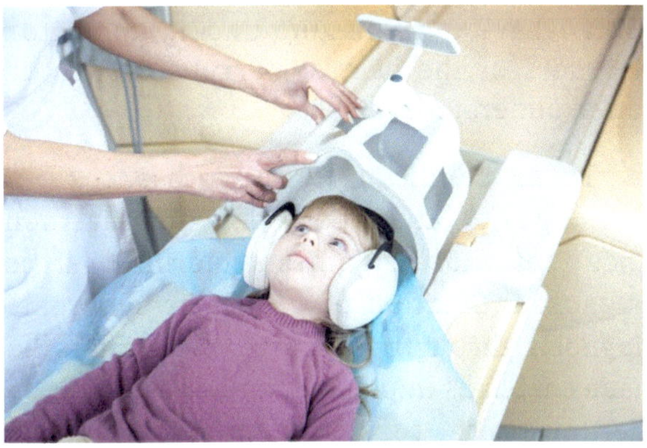

**Figure 11.16.** Recent advances in pediatric neurology have significantly improved the understanding and management of various neurological disorders affecting children.

*Source:* https://drvivekmundada.com/wp-content/uploads/2024/12/radiologist-prepares-little-girl-mri-brain-examination_179755-10374.jpg.

### 11.6.1. Innovations in Treatment Methodologies

Paragraph 26 explores the revolutionary function of technology in improving treatment strategies in pediatric neurology. Technologies like telemedicine have transformed care access for children with neurological disorders. It allows medical professionals to diagnose and treat conditions at a distance, thereby bridging gaps between geographies of specialists and patients. For example, the improvement in mobile health technologies makes it possible to monitor neurological signs in young patients in real time, enabling timely interventions. Furthermore, data-sharing platforms between different healthcare providers ensure a comprehensive knowledge of the status of each child and therefore maximize more personalized treatment regimens. Since pediatric neurology is increasingly fluent in the utilization of data, the technologies not only maximize patient engagement but also make available a vast amount of data that can be utilized to fuel precision research and developments in new therapeutic interventions (Baron et al., 2016). Among treatment developments, collaborative frameworks have been key forces behind the evolution of pediatric neurology. These are generally collaborative work that brings research into practice to implement practical interventions in children with neurological disorders. An example is the collaboration between therapists in Trinidad and America to enhance training in pediatric constraint-induced movement therapy (CIMT). This partnership employed a translational strategy, providing both educational training and hands-on instruction, ultimately leading to the design of a locally applicable type of pediatric CIMT. The effectiveness of the project demonstrates the benefit of partnership and resources in addressing the complex needs of pediatric patients. Through the cultivation of practice in teamwork, medical practitioners are able to adopt innovations in treatment methods and make it possible for children to receive effective and context-related care (Coker-Bolt et al., 2023). Finally, biologic treatments are another field for enhancement in pediatric neurology, which has significant implications for managing complex conditions , such as epilepsy and neurodegenerative disorders. The emerging technology of gene therapy holds the promise of attacking the genetic roots of these diseases, with the potential for more permanent cures. In experiments, therapies using engineered viruses to deliver therapeutic genes have proven to be capable of suppressing, and even reversing, disease in animal models, providing encouraging data for potential human therapies. In addition, as more research is conducted, regulatory frameworks are being adapted to accommodate these new therapies, making a path for clinical application. Advances in biologic therapy not only enhance the armory available to pediatric neurologists but also hold promise for improved outcome and quality of life in affected children (Baron et al., 2016) (Figure 11.17).

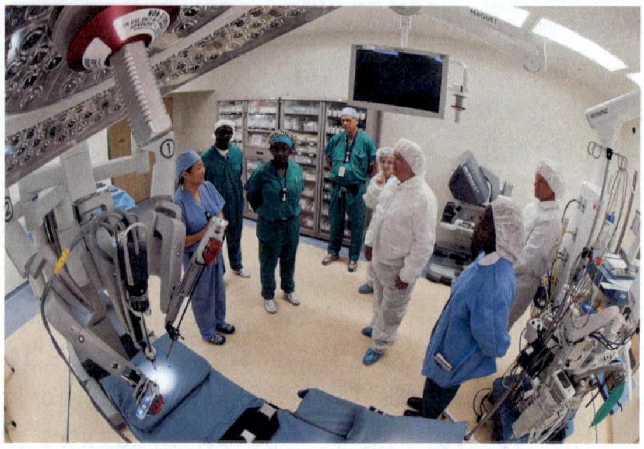

**Figure 11.17.** Innovations in treatment methodologies.

*Source:* By Staff Sgt. Bernardo Fuller - https://www.dvidshub.net/image/593562/fort-belvoir-community-hospital-astounds-with-groundbreaking-technology-and-devotion-patient-care, Public Domain, https://commons.wikimedia.org/w/index.php?curid=51702977

## 11.6.2. Research Trends in Pediatric Neurological Disorders

Current research highlights an increasing interest in elucidating the complex relationship between psychosocial factors and pediatric neurological disorders, especially headache disorders. Among the most prevalent neurological complaints in children, migraine has been found to manifest in about 60% of children and adolescents globally and significantly interferes with their daytime functioning, like schooling and social performance. This has prompted researchers to study cognitive functions, i.e., metacognitive abilities, which comprise self-monitoring and cognitive process control. These metacognitive functions show a strong relation with co-occurring conditions , such as anxiety and depression, which have a tendency to co-exist in migraine children. Through investigation of these interplays, recent studies aim to maximize treatment modalities by not just treating the physical symptom but also investigating the cognitive and emotional triggers of headache attacks (Faedda et al., 2017). Moreover, the field of pediatric neurology has matured to a point where autoimmune and inflammatory disorders of the central nervous system are better understood.

These conditions often present a real challenge to diagnosis and management since they cause significant morbidity if not diagnosed. Creation of particular syndromes diagnosis through diagnostic biomarkers has made clinicians implement immunosuppressive therapy, with resulting improved patient outcomes. The decision to treat continues to be problematic and requires careful consideration of the advantages and disadvantages of therapy. Awareness of the natural history of the diseases, the probability of causing disability, and the risk of relapse is crucial in tailoring care to individual patients. The current research aims at distinguishing between disorders with more favorable prognoses, , such as Sydenham chorea, and those with tragic consequences, like neuromyelitis optica, highlighting the call for sophisticated models of treatment (Dale et al., 2016). Finally, the present focus on multidisciplinary strategies also reflects shifting research trends in pediatric neurology. When addressing the broad spectrum of pediatric neurology disorders, researchers opt for an interdisciplinary approach that integrates multiple disciplinary orientations like neuropsychology, pediatrics, and neurology. This is particularly significant for addressing comorbid disorders related to primary neurological disorders, e.g., anxiety and depression as comorbid disorders with primary epilepsy disorders. By promoting efforts directed towards the psychosocial component of such disorders, such as, , such as building resilience and coping techniques, treatment gains can be optimized by clinicians. Even studies on research studies involving integrative management plans have been shown to improve both quality of life in children with the condition and their caregivers, a paradigm shift in treatment for pediatric neurology (Faedda et al., 2017) (Figure 11.18).

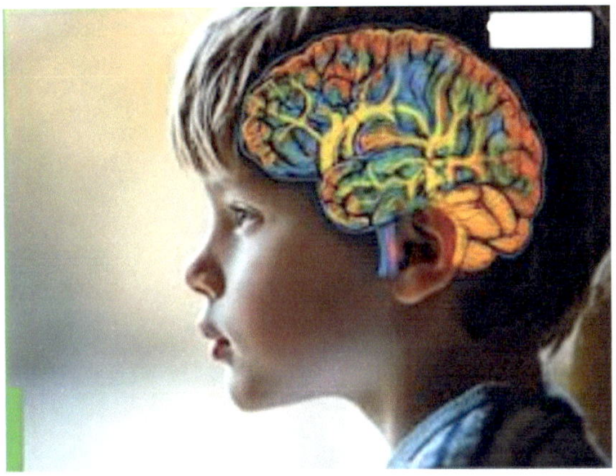

**Figure 11.18.** Pediatric neurological development and the complexity of brain function in early childhood.

*Source:* https://encrypted-tbn0.gstatic.com/images?q=tbn:ANd9GcSko7fP7KpeoF9pR6YcpYMIoU8aGU89EnXamg&s.

### 11.6.3. The Role of Technology in Enhancing Patient Care

Technology is at the heart of pediatric neurology in its role to enhance care for patients, particularly in treatment and diagnosis. The evolution of advanced imaging technologies , such as magnetic resonance imaging (MRI) and computed tomography (CT) allows physicians to obtain precise images of the underlying neurological structures of kids. This is especially significant because children that appear as pediatric patients have a tendency to pose special challenges in accurately diagnosing neurological diseases in accordance with their growth stages.

These imaging tools do not only enable the early diagnosis of ailments like brain tumors or congenital malformations, but they also provide valuable information about the progress of neurological diseases. Using these technologies, neurologists are able to design specific treatment protocols that significantly improve the quality of care for the young patients. Besides, the integration of telehealth services into pediatric neurology is a shift in paradigm in care delivery. Telemedicine makes it possible for specialists to reach patients in under-served or remote areas, thus filling the gap that often exists between the availability of specialized neurological care and those communities with reduced access. Not only has the virtual method of consultation facilitated easier follow-up care for families but has also minimized travel-related stress and economic burden on families. I

n addition, telehealth technology supports real-time monitoring of a patient's symptoms and treatment response so that early intervention can be made to their treatment plans. It supports continuous communication between specialists and families, with an open environment conducive to collaboration, support for caregivers, and facilitation of patients' active participation in managing their neurologic diseases. EHR has also revolutionized data management in pediatric neurology with seamless access to patient histories and treatment modalities across different healthcare platforms. The electronic system enhances the ability of healthcare providers to track longitudinal outcomes, enabling in-depth analyses of the efficacy of treatments. Neurologists can identify patterns that may inform treatment decisions as well as improve patient outcomes through data analytics. In addition, electronic health records (EHR) systems enable communication among healthcare teams, a feature highly critical in pediatric cases with numerous specialists. Enhanced coordination of care not only means effective management of complex diseases but also aids the integration of a holistic approach suited to the unique needs of pediatric patients. With all such technology advancements, patient care in pediatric neurology also continues to evolve, reflecting on a commitment towards improving the well-being of children suffering from neurological conditions.

## Test Your Knowledge

1. What are some current research trends in pediatric neurological disorders?
2. How is technology improving patient care in pediatric neurology?

## SUMMARY

The pediatric neurology is a critical division that addresses complex neurological diseases that significantly influence children's lives. Development in the field of genetics information and technology has passed through the ages to advance our understanding of diseases , such as developmental and epileptic encephalopathies (DEEs) and cerebral palsy (CP). Studies fueled by such research as those that have focused on DEEs have highlighted the imperative need for individualized psychosocial intervention to families undergoing diagnoses that are oftentimes complicated by emotional distress and uncertainty. The intersection of medical reports and psychosocial interventions is important since it is able to help caregivers handle the conditions of their children and address their particular needs, which makes an integrative practice of pediatric neurology very important. Furthermore, their implications are not only confined to the practice of medical therapy but also reach out to affect therapeutic practice and family support mechanisms. Caregivers also play an influential role in shaping the arena of pediatric neurology as examined in studies of the psychosocial existence of caregivers and children with DEEs. The emphasis is placed on requiring individualized care coordination to adapt resources for families' particular needs. Of particular significance, the absence of available psychosocial support mentioned throughout literature warrants immediate response and action from medical professionals. This need underlines the demand for novel methods that recognize the multidimensional aspect of treatment and care within pediatric neurology, especially as it pertains to improving quality of life in children and their families. Ultimately, continued research and collaboration among disciplines are necessary to further the field of pediatric neurology. As our knowledge of neurological impairments expands, so too must our measures for evaluating and treating these impairments. The thorough analysis of motor function in children with CP is one such area where complexity exists around both assessment measures and therapeutic interventions, as revealed through studies within the past decade. There is a clear trend for blending technological innovation and early intervention practice with the promise of improved outcomes for participating children. The practice of pediatric neurology is based on proactive and integrative approaches that put children and families center stage, and that innovative therapies, and necessary supports, are introduced into the available mainstream for all who need them.

Pediatric neurology deals with a wide spectrum of medical conditions of the nervous system in children and mandates extensive understanding of various factors in diagnosis and treatment. The most significant lesson from recent controversies is to emphasize the multidimensional nature of pediatric neurological illnesses. Understanding these disorders requires not only a good knowledge of their etiology but also an appreciation of the social, cultural, and psychological determinants that may influence treatment success. For instance, assessment of a child's neuromaturation can be highly influenced by the environment and the family situation and thus must involve a comprehensive approach to patient care. Such an integrative strategy enables practitioners to modify interventions that appeal most strongly to the specific situations involved in a patient, thus enhancing the quality of care in pediatric neurology. Another central topic of discussion has been the growing importance of successful communication strategies between providers and families. As pediatric neurologists treat mostly chronic illnesses, it is important to maintain open and continuous channels of communication. This demand is heightened by the requirements of reducing after-visit question-related workload, hence preventing clinician burnout and influencing patient satisfaction. Studies indicate that the application of quality improvement (QI) techniques can efficiently reduce the number of after-visit messages. By employing interventions to improve workflows and educational outreach, clinics saw a dramatic decrease in parent phone calls, thus making time available for neurologists to respond to patient needs. This shows the integral role played by structured models of communication towards optimizing pediatric neurological practice (Thara, 2024). Also, the ongoing need for updated and improved clinical practice guidelines cannot be overstated. The debates also brought forth a suggestion by the International Network for Orofacial Pain and Related Disorders to build a formal set of key points on which practitioners can reference in treating Temporomandibular Disorders (TMDs) and pediatric neurological conditions. These recommendations underscore the importance of staying congruent with current standards of care and specialty treatment programs, thereby preventing misappropriation of resources and ineffective treatment protocols. This kind of collaborative and evidence-based policy can serve as a model for pediatric neurology, guiding practitioners to best practices that can be translated to a variety of healthcare systems and cultures (Manfredini et al., 2024).

## KEY TERMS FROM THIS CHAPTER

- Adoption
- Ataxia
- Attention deficit hyperactivity disorder (ADHD)
- Chronic traumatic encephalopathy (CTE)
- Complementary and alternative medicine (CAM)
- Disability
- Electroencephalogram
- Emotional development
- Epilepsy
- Genetic
- Neurological disorders
- Neurological function
- Socio-emotional impacts
- Stereotypic movement disorder (SMD)
- Traumatic brain injury (TBI)

## CRITICAL THINKING QUESTIONS

1. **The most common type of seizure in children is:**
   a. Absence seizure
   b. Tonic-clonic seizure
   c. Febrile seizure
   d. Myoclonic seizure
2. **Cerebral palsy is caused by:**
   a. A progressive neurodegenerative disorder
   b. A non-progressive brain injury or malformation
   c. Autoimmune disease
   d. Brain tumor
3. **The most common causative organism of bacterial meningitis in children under 5 years is:**
   a. *Streptococcus pneumoniae*
   b. *Escherichia coli*
   c. *Hemophilus influenzae type B*
   d. *Neisseria meningitidis*
4. **A bulging anterior fontanelle in an infant may indicate:**
   a. Dehydration
   b. Increased intracranial pressure
   c. Malnutrition
   d. Anemia
5. **In hydrocephalus, cerebrospinal fluid (CSF) accumulates in the:**
   a. Blood vessels
   b. Ventricular system of the brain
   c. Spinal cord
   d. Skull bones

### Short Answer Questions

1. Describe the classification, causes, and management of seizures in children.
2. What is a febrile seizure? How is it different from epilepsy?
3. Discuss hydrocephalus in children – causes, clinical signs, investigations, and treatment options.
4. Explain the diagnosis and management of meningitis in infants and young children.
5. Describe the approach to a child with developmental delay. Include history, examination, and investigations.

### Answers to Critical Thinking Questions

1. (c); 2. (b); 3. (a); 4. (b); 5. (b)

# REFERENCES


1. Morshed, R. A., Winkler, E. A., Kim, H., Braunstein, S., Cooke, D. L., Hetts, S. W., Abla, A. A., Fullerton, H. J., & Gupta, N. (2020). High-Flow Vascular Malformations in Children. *Seminars in neurology*, *40*(3), 303–314. https://doi.org/10.1055/s-0040-1708869 (accessed on 16th June 2025).
2. Abubakar, I., Atun, R., Chakaya, J., Cox, H., et al. (2012). Drug-resistant tuberculosis—Current dilemmas, unanswered questions, challenges and priority needs. https://core.ac.uk/download/9839026.pdf (accessed on 16th June 2025).
3. Adhikari, B. M., Agartz, I., Aghajani, M., Aleman, A., et al. (2020). ENIGMA and global neuroscience: A decade of large-scale studies of the brain in health and disease across more than 40 countries. https://core.ac.uk/download/323076217.pdf (accessed on 16th June 2025).
4. Gkourogianni, A., Sinaii, N., Jackson, S. H., Karageorgiadis, A. S., Lyssikatos, C., Belyavskaya, E., Keil, M. F., Zilbermint, M., Chittiboina, P., Stratakis, C. A., & Lodish, M. B. (2017). Pediatric Cushing disease: disparities in disease severity and outcomes in the Hispanic and African-American populations. *Pediatric research*, *82*(2), 272–277. https://doi.org/10.1038/pr.2017.58(accessed on 16th June 2025).
5. Alimohamed, M. Z., Manji, M., & Siima, A. A. (2024). Advancing genetic testing for neurological disorders in Tanzania: Importance, challenges, and strategies for implementation. https://core.ac.uk/download/620145621.pdf (accessed on 16th June 2025).
6. Baglioni, V., Caravale, B., Cardona, F., Chiarotti, F., et al. (2019). Developmental motor profile in preschool children with primary stereotypic movement disorder. https://core.ac.uk/download/195777959.pdf (accessed on 16th June 2025).
7. Bargiela, D., Chinnery, P. F., Horvath, R., Keogh, M., et al. (2015). Prevalence of neurogenetic disorders in the North of England. https://core.ac.uk/download/162912848.pdf (accessed on 16th June 2025).
8. Ibrahim, G. M., Fallah, A., Snead, O. C., 3rd, Drake, J. M., Rutka, J. T., & Bernstein, M. (2012). The use of high frequency oscillations to guide neocortical resections in children with medically-intractable epilepsy: how do we ethically apply surgical innovations to patient care?. *Seizure*, *21*(10), 743–747. https://doi.org/10.1016/j.seizure.2012.07.013(accessed on 16th June 2025).
9. Bowers, R., Ross, K., & ISPO (Funder) (2009). A review of the effectiveness of lower limb orthoses used in cerebral palsy. In Recent Developments in Healthcare for Cerebral Palsy: Implications and Opportunities for Orthotics (pp. 235-297)(accessed on 16th June 2025).
10. Morris, C., Bowers, R., Ross, K., Stevens, P., & Phillips, D. (2011). Orthotic management of cerebral palsy: recommendations from a consensus conference. *NeuroRehabilitation*, *28*(1), 37–46. https://doi.org/10.3233/NRE-2011-0630(accessed on 16th June 2025).
11. Brickler, T., Morton, P., Hazy, A., & Theus, M. H. (2018). Age-Dependent Responses Following Traumatic Brain Injury. InTech. doi: 10.5772/intechopen.71344(accessed on 16th June 2025).
12. Bruyere, S. M., Peterson, D., & VanLooy, S. (2005). The International Classification of Functioning, Disability and Health: Contemporary literature overview. https://core.ac.uk/download/5124461.pdf (accessed on 16th June 2025).

13. Faedda N, Natalucci G, Calderoni D, Cerutti R, Verdecchia P and Guidetti V (2017) Metacognition and Headache: Which Is the Role in Childhood and Adolescence? Front. Neurol. 8:650. doi: 10.3389/fneur.2017.00650(accessed on 16th June 2025).

14. James, F. M. K., Cortez, M. A., Monteith, G., Jokinen, T. S., Sanders, S., Wielaender, F., Fischer, A., & Lohi, H. (2017). Diagnostic Utility of Wireless Video-Electroencephalography in Unsedated Dogs. *Journal of veterinary internal medicine*, *31*(5), 1469–1476. https://doi.org/10.1111/jvim.14789(accessed on 16th June 2025).

15. Dale, R. C., Nosadini, M., & Lim, M. (2016). Therapeutic decision making in autoimmune and inflammatory disorders of the central nervous system in children. https://core.ac.uk/download/154325209.pdf (accessed on 16th June 2025).

16. Dosenbach, N. U. F., Everett, E. A., Hoyt, C. R., Koller, J. M., et al. (2019). Detection of pediatric upper extremity motor activity and deficits with accelerometry. https://core.ac.uk/download/287888133.pdf (accessed on 16th June 2025).

17. Drove, B., Gifford, K. L., Gonzalez-Meijome, J. M., Gray, L., et al. (2019). IMI–Industry guidelines and ethical considerations for myopia control report. https://core.ac.uk/download/293867276.pdf (accessed on 16th June 2025).

18. Vakharia, V. N., Duncan, J. S., Witt, J. A., Elger, C. E., Staba, R., & Engel, J., Jr (2018). Getting the best outcomes from epilepsy surgery. *Annals of neurology*, *83*(4), 676–690. https://doi.org/10.1002/ana.25205(accessed on 16th June 2025).

19. Wang, S., & Fallah, A. (2014). Optimal management of seizures associated with tuberous sclerosis complex: current and emerging options. *Neuropsychiatric disease and treatment*, *10*, 2021–2030. https://doi.org/10.2147/NDT.S51789 (accessed on 16th June 2025).

20. Falsaperla, R., Lubrano, R., Pavone, P., Pavone, L., et al. (2017). Ataxia in children: Early recognition and clinical evaluation. https://core.ac.uk/download/80315257.pdf (accessed on 16th June 2025).

21. Fezeu, F., Ramesh, A., Melmer, P. D., Moosa, S., Larson, P. S., & Henderson, F., Jr (2018). Challenges and Solutions for Functional Neurosurgery in Developing Countries. *Cureus*, *10*(9), e3314. https://doi.org/10.7759/cureus.3314(accessed on 16th June 2025).

22. Mashaal, A. H. (2024). *A Comprehensive Study on The Assessment of Motor Functions Development in Children with Cerebral Palsy*. https://core.ac.uk/download/640069952.pdf (accessed on 16th June 2025).

23. Mastrangelo, M. (2017). Lennox-Gastaut syndrome: A state-of-the-art review. https://core.ac.uk/download/98337284.pdf (accessed on 16th June 2025).

24. Naffadi, H. M. (2024). *Neimann-Pick Diseases: Beyond Lipid Accumulation–Genetic, Diagnostics, and Therapeutic Strategies*. https://core.ac.uk/download/622109115.pdf (accessed on 16th June 2025).

25. Sage, M. (2018). *Neurocognitive Findings in Adults Who Played Youth Football*. https://open.bu.edu/bitstream/2144/33032/5/Sage_bu_0017N_14075.pdf (accessed on 16th June 2025).

26. Sices, L. (2007). *Developmental Screening in Primary Care: The Effectiveness of Current Practice and Recommendations for Improvement*. https://core.ac.uk/download/71350769.pdf (accessed on 16th June 2025).

27. Virginia Commonwealth University. (2018). *Virginia Commonwealth University Professional Bulletin.* https://bulletin.vcu.edu/professional-studies/. https://core.ac.uk/download/215485746.pdf (accessed on 16th June 2025).

28. Zimmermann, K. (2016). *Pediatric End-of-Life Care Needs in Switzerland (PELICAN): Current End-of-Life Care Practices and the Perspectives of Bereaved Parents.* https://core.ac.uk/download/84007654.pdf (accessed on 16th June 2025).

# PEDIATRIC CARDIOVASCULAR DISORDERS

# 12

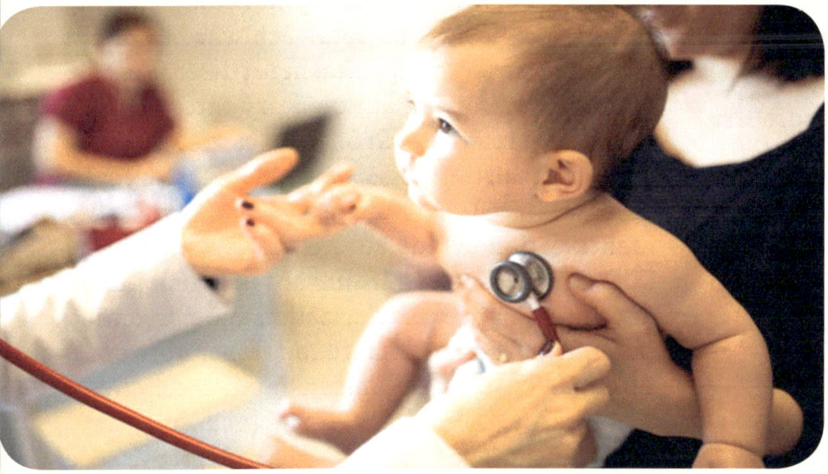

## LEARNING OBJECTIVES

**After studying this chapter, you will be able to:**

1. Discuss the common pediatric cardiovascular disorders;
2. Explain the clinical presentation and diagnosis;
3. Focus on management and treatment strategies;
4. Know prevention and education.

## Introduction

Pediatric cardiovascular disorders are a critical field of concern in pediatric medicine, which needs to be addressed at once since they can threaten lives at any given time. Pediatric cardiovascular disorders comprise a wide range of disorders, including congenital heart defects, arrhythmias, and myocarditis, which may present in any form, hence timely diagnosis and treatment. The unique anatomical and physiological composition of children renders them particularly vulnerable to cardiovascular crises, where the intervention modalities must be highly individualized and quite dissimilar from those used in adults. In addition, prompt detection of signs and symptoms is of paramount value since earliest possible medical intervention can significantly enhance outcomes and reduce morbidity. This opening provides the context for an in-depth analysis of pediatric cardiovascular disorders with special focus on the criticality of early diagnosis, interventional measures, and the necessity for healthcare providers to be well-trained to tackle these serious health issues efficiently (Figure 12.1).

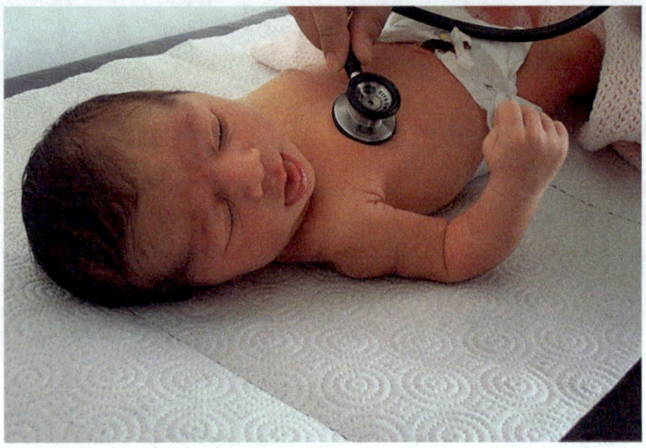

**Figure 12.1.** Pediatric cardiovascular disorders.

*Source:* By Nevit Dilmen - Own work, CC BY-SA 3.0, https://commons.wikimedia.org/w/index.php?curid=1428959

## Definition of Pediatric Cardiovascular Disorders

It is necessary to understand pediatric cardiovascular disorders because they are a group of acute health crises that severely compromise the cardiovascular system in children. These disorders, and others, are acute heart failure, cardiac arrest, and life-threatening arrhythmias and may be due to congenital heart defects, myocarditis, or severe hypertension, the latter more and more of an acknowledged significant health problem among the pediatric population. Its growing prevalence among children has elicited a good deal of study, with emphasis on early detection and management of elevated blood pressure to prevent its contribution to chronic cardiovascular disease (Lurbe et al., 2016). Patients' psychological issues, like dental anxiety, are also pertinent to the management of disorders in the framework of general health care; understanding patient behavior is imperative to the delivery of effective treatment (Abrahamsson et al., 2017). Hence, definition of pediatric cardiovascular disorders should be holistic, incorporating physiological and also psychosocial elements.

## Importance of Timely Recognition and Intervention

The importance of early diagnosis and intervention in pediatric cardiovascular disorders cannot be overestimated, given the enormous expense of taking care of diseases, such as congenital heart diseases. Early detection of these disorders is very effective in improving clinical outcome, as a high proportion of involved neonates develop severe illness shortly after birth. Through the use of sophisticated imaging techniques, , such as fetal echocardiography, prenatally severe congenital heart disease can be diagnosed, allowing anticipatory interventions to enhance readiness in offering care to the baby soon after birth (Moisa et al., 2024). Moreover, illnesses like Wellens syndrome show how early identification avoids severe consequences; the ECG signs of this syndrome are instrumental in initiating early revascularization and preventing potential myocardial infarction (Liberatore et al., 2024). Overall, an organized, multi-disciplinary team-based approach with a focus on rapid intervention can do much to improve the prognosis for pediatric patients with cardiac disorders, ultimately leading to better health outcomes.

## Overview of Common Pediatric Cardiovascular Conditions

The pediatric cardiovascular environment is heterogeneous and comprises a wide spectrum of acquired and congenital disorders with the potential to have a deep impact on a child's health. Two of the most frequent congenital cardiac abnormalities and necessitate careful monitoring, in a high proportion of cases, surgical intervention, are ventricular septal defects and tetralogy of Fallot. Moreover, the incidence of hypertension in children is also an issue of concern, with evidence indicating a rising prevalence of elevated blood pressure among children and adolescents (Lurbe et al., 2016). This is of concern because hypertension is documented to cause lifelong cardiovascular morbidities when left untreated, further making it a reason for identification and management at an early stage. Arrhythmias and cardiomyopathies are also some other common conditions that may arise acutely through cardiovascular disorders. Knowledge of these common ailments constitutes the context for successful response measures in emergency care that address the intrinsic difficulty in treating children with cardiovascular disorders (Figure 12.2).

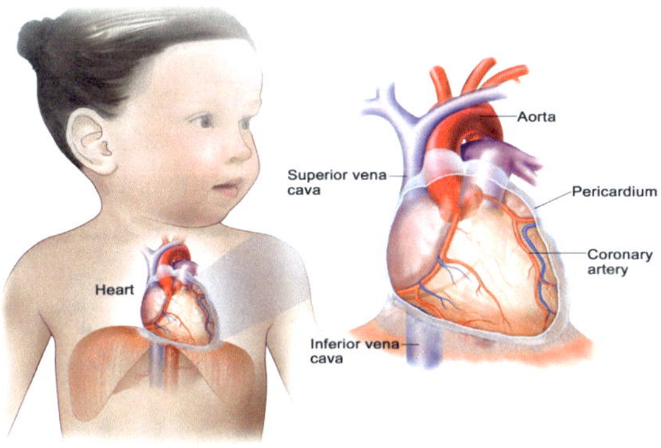


**Figure 12.2.** The common pediatric cardiovascular conditions.

*Source:* https://nci-media.cancer.gov/pdq/media/images/804602.jpg.

## Statistics on Incidence and Outcomes

The incidence of child cardiovascular disorders, that of sudden cardiac arrest (SCA), indicates a critical need within the healthcare community. Statistics indicate early intervention as a key determining factor in outcome; with the immediate application of cardiopulmonary resuscitation (CPR) an integral contributing factor in survival. Literature shows that effective administration of SCA in school contexts is often hindered by insufficient resources, even though 44% of school nurses said they felt prepared to handle such disorders (Dahlen et al., 2014). In sporting contexts, where coaches are often first responders, their competence in providing high-standard CPR is paramount. Studies have shown enhanced CPR performance post-intensive training, with a strong positive relationship between self-efficacy and the quality of CPR administered (Martinez et al., 2022). The inclusion of intensive training programs and the allocation of resources is thus pivotal in enhancing readiness and outcome improvement in pediatric cardiovascular disorders.

## Role of Healthcare Professionals in Management

In pediatric cardiovascular disorders, the contribution of healthcare providers towards management is critical to the achievement of optimal results. Some of these healthcare providers are pediatricians, emergency nurses, and cardiologists, who work together to evaluate and stabilize the condition of the child in a timely manner. Their diverse tasks include not only the provision of immediate clinical interventions but also continuous education and training, which is critical to care delivery. For instance, continuous education programs, as highlighted in newsletters created by the Iowa Board of Nursing, play an important role in keeping the nursing personnel updated with the current best practices and trends in pediatric practice (Lurbe et al., 2016). Additionally, management of such disorders demands effective communication and coordination among members of the healthcare team to ensure that they are all informed of his or her role during emergency incidents. With their experience and governance, healthcare practitioners play a key role in the creation of a responsive healthcare climate that encourages pediatric patient safety (Lurbe et al., 2016).

## Significance of Research and Advancements in Treatment

In pediatric cardiovascular disorders, ongoing research and development in treatment modalities are essential to enhance clinical outcome and safety in patients. The introduction of technologies , such as Point-of-Care Ultrasonography (POCUS) has significantly enhanced the diagnostic potential, allowing for increased speed and accuracy in assessment of cardiovascular disease in children. POCUS not only results in increased diagnostic accuracy but also affects significant patient management decisions, hence optimizing care interventions in emergency situations (Tamimi et al., 2023). Moreover, innovative developments in sensor technology, as highlighted by new strain sensors for real-time infant respiration monitoring, constitute a groundbreaking approach towards addressing challenges of daily living in pediatric care (Bastawrous et al., 2023). These advances underscore the necessity of a persistent commitment to research, which ultimately enhances therapeutic intervention and equips healthcare practitioners with better tools to cope with pediatric cardiovascular disorders (Figure 12.3).

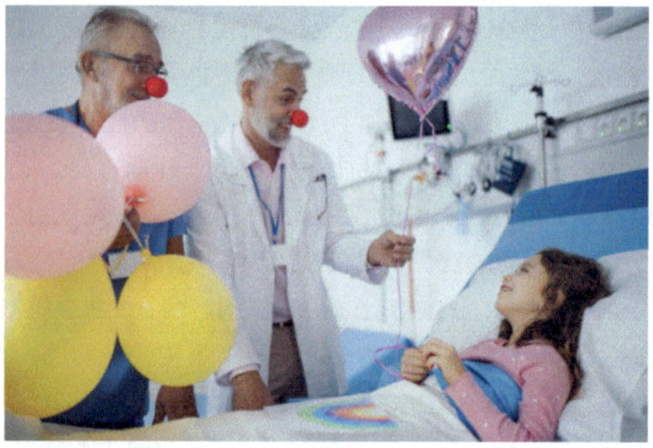

**Figure 12.3.** Significance of research and advancements in treatment.

*Source:* https://centellahealthtech.com/wp-content/uploads/2024/09/Screenshot-2024-09-30-152625.png.

### *Call to Action for Increased Awareness and Education*

Pediatric cardiovascular disorders need a strong call to action for increased awareness and education among healthcare providers, families, and society at large. The challenges that come with diagnosing and treating these disorders can lead to extreme morbidity and mortality if not addressed effectively. To minimize this risk, educational programs need to emphasize detection of early signs and symptoms of cardiovascular distress in children and the significance of effective interventions in a timely way. Besides, ongoing education (CE) and training among healthcare workers are necessary in maintaining proficiency in this dynamically evolving field. Resources , such as the Nursing Newsletter, which is issued quarterly by the Iowa Board of Nursing, can aid in the propagation of essential details regarding CE courses and updates required in pediatric care (Lurbe et al., 2016). Collegial efforts to include education in pediatric cardiovascular disorders in nursing curricula are also imperative as they ensure that future practitioners are properly prepared to perform well (Lurbe et al., 2016).

## 12.1. Common Pediatric Cardiovascular Disorders

**Learning Outcome**

1. Congenital heart defects;
2. Myocarditis and pericarditis;
3. Arrhythmias in children;
4. Cardiogenic shock;
5. Pulmonary embolism;
6. Aortic dissection;
7 Hypertrophic cardiomyopathy;
8. Heart failure in pediatric patients;
9. Cardiac arrest in children.

The rising incidence of cardiovascular disorders in children highlights the need for proper identification and management. Acute rheumatic fever, myocarditis, and Kawasaki disease are among the most frequent disorders that occur in the pediatric population. These conditions often have nonspecific presentations, rendering early detection and treatment difficult, which is required to prevent sequelae. Notably, childhood hypertension is more and more recognized as a priority public health issue to a great degree responsible for the exploding cardiovascular disease epidemic. Synthesis of guidelines from recent scientific evidence emphasizes the central role of early detection and intervention in the management of high blood pressure and cardiovascular complications prevention in adult life (Lurbe et al., 2016). Whereas pediatricians and healthcare workers are faced with such challenges, an integrated approach that includes ongoing research and public health interventions is needed to mitigate the impact of such disorders (Lurbe et al., 2016).

## 12.1.1. Congenital Heart Defects

Congenital heart defects (CHDs) present formidable challenges to pediatric cardiovascular disorders, which mandate prompt and special care. They are structural defects that disrupt normal heart action and can lead to severe complications , such as heart failure, cyanosis, and arrhythmias. Retrospective data identified that a large percentage of unsuspected CHD children present to emergency departments with serious conditions, primarily due to symptoms like cyanosis and heart failure, which indicate the need for proper diagnosis and management (Akhtar et al., 2020). Besides, adult emergency admissions due to congenital cardiac defects also replicate this trend, with cardiovascular complications leading as the most frequent reasons for urgent care, and it underscores the ongoing threats by these defects throughout life (Bauer et al., 2003). Clinicians must thus maintain a high index of suspicion of CHDs to facilitate prompt diagnosis and optimal management within the emergency department to facilitate better outcomes among such patients (Figure 12.4).

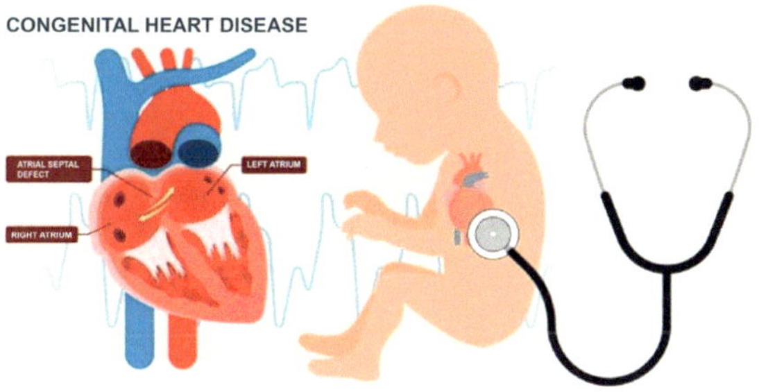


**Figure 12.4.** Congenital heart defects in children.

*Source:* https://punecardiologist.com/images/Congential-Heart-Disease.webp.

## 12.1.2. Myocarditis and Pericarditis

In pediatric cardiovascular disorders, myocarditis and pericarditis have emerged as significant concerns due to their potential to significantly impair cardiovascular function in children. Myocarditis, an inflammation of the heart muscle, can be caused by viral infection, autoimmune disorder, or even some drugs and can manifest from mild malaise to severe heart failure. Likewise, pericarditis entails inflammation of the pericardial sac, usually accompanied by pain and distress in the chest.

Importantly, both conditions can precipitate cardiovascular complications, including arrhythmias and, in serious situations, cardiac tamponade (Carvalho et al., 2005). Though their prevalence is relatively lower in the pediatric population than in adults, their impact cannot be underestimated, particularly when associated with underlying conditions , such as congenital heart disease or infections like Kawasaki disease complicating the clinical situation (Balik et al., 2018). The early diagnosis and timely intervention hold the secret to a favorable prognosis for affected children (Figure 12.5).

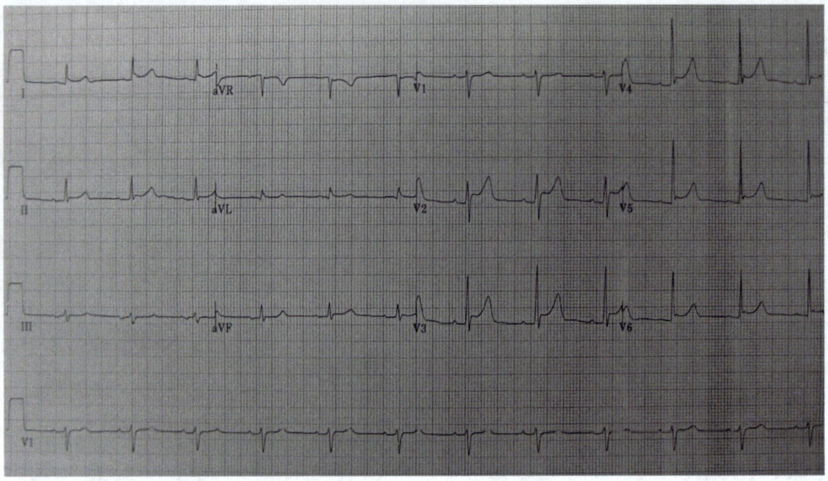


**Figure 12.5.** Pediatric pericarditis.

*Source:* By James Heilman, MD - Own work, CC BY-SA 3.0, https://commons.wikimedia.org/w/index.php?curid=8334574

## 12.1.3. Arrhythmias in Children

Children's arrhythmias are a significant problem in the scenario of pediatric cardiovascular disorders that are prone to having catastrophic clinical implications unless properly diagnosed and treated timely. These aberrations in rhythm may be as innocuous as benign or fatal conditions like ventricular fibrillation or tachycardia, leading to cardiac arrest. Of special mention is the increased complexity of arrhythmia diagnosis in this population owing to the fluctuation of normal heart rate with age and the often subtle nature of presenting signs.

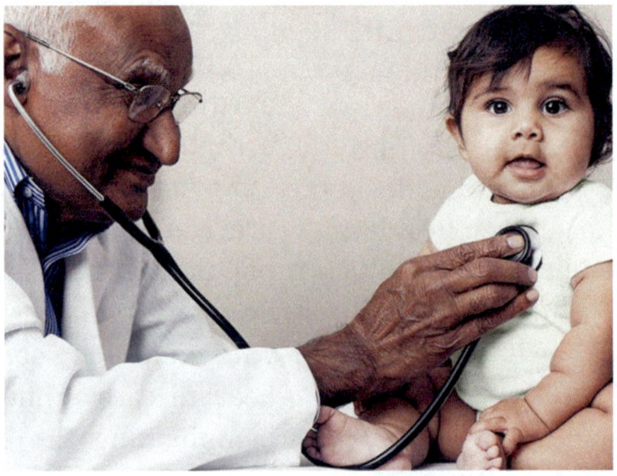

**Figure 12.6.** Arrhythmias in children.

*Source:* https://external-content.duckduckgo.com/iu/?u=https%3A%2F%2Fpost.medicalnewstoday.com%2Fwp-content%2Fuploads%2Fsites%2F3%2F2022%2F01%2FArrhythmia_children_GettyImages467653839_Thumb.jpg&f=1&nofb=1&ipt=935947c516f0464f9a42d1979c5fd9510ba944afd3038a97231c31704c292828&ipo=images.

Timely recognition is necessary, as it is postulated that early treatment can have a profound impact on prognosis in the context of sudden cardiac arrest. According to ILCOR Pediatric Task Force guidelines, the latest studies lay much emphasis on the identification of precipitating pathologies leading to predisposition towards arrhythmias in children, including genetic predispositions and structural heart disease (Kleinman et al., 2010). Moreover, continuous training in the identification and management of latent arrhythmias is essential for healthcare providers (Kleinman et al., 2010) (Figure 12.6).

## 12.1.4. Cardiogenic Shock

Pediatric cardiogenic shock (CS) is a complex issue, and it requires a detailed understanding of its etiology as well as its management. The acute condition of the heart's failure to maintain adequate blood circulation can have several causes behind it, including myocarditis, congenital heart disease, or cardiomyopathies. Early diagnosis of CS is crucial as delayed treatment can rise morbidity and mortality. Most crucially, underlying heart failure may be a significant complicating factor in the clinical presentation, as attested by heterogeneity among patients with CS presenting; for example, those with chronic deteriorating heart failure have a higher mortality than those with new-onset heart failure (Schurtz et al., 2023). Advanced treatments, including cardiac resynchronization therapy, have also emerged as life-saving measures in advanced stages of CS, and this highlights the importance of individualized interventions based on patient profiles (Mbisike et al., 2024). All these details are necessary to comprehend while making a sincere attempt to improve outcomes for pediatric cardiovascular disorders.

## 12.1.5. Pulmonary Embolism

Among pediatric cardiovascular disease, pulmonary embolism (PE) is a severe though often underappreciated disease that may have a detrimental impact on the well-being of children. Although presentation is relatively rare among children, consequences can be dire as PE continues to remain one of the leading causes of cardiovascular morbidity and mortality. Research has shown that acute pulmonary embolism is the third most common cause of cardiovascular death, after stroke and myocardial infarction (Costa et al., 2024). Chronic complications , such as post-pulmonary embolism syndrome (PPES) are notable, as the majority of the survivors may not reach baseline function, with long-term impacts on quality of life (Gonz et al., 2024). Optimal care involves an individualized strategy with risk stratification and concomitant use of both anticoagulation modalities and adjunctive treatments, including catheter-directed therapies, to limit the unique challenges of PE in children (Figure 12.7).

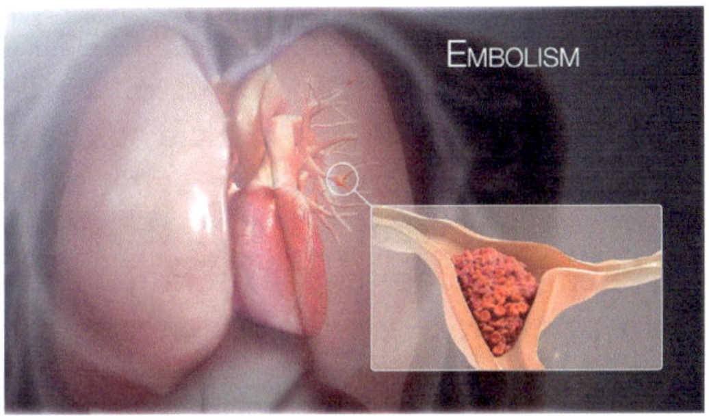


**Figure 12.7.** Pulmonary embolism.

*Source:* By https://www.scientificanimations.com - https://www.scientificanimations.com/wiki-images/, CC BY-SA 4.0, https://commons.wikimedia.org/w/index.php?curid=96876070

## 12.1.6. Aortic Dissection

Aortic dissection in pediatric cardiovascular disorders is a rare but life-threatening condition that, if not diagnosed and treated promptly, can lead to severe morbidity and mortality. It typically occurs with intimal tear of the aorta leading to separation of the vessel wall layers, which may be precipitated by underlying disorders of connective tissue or injury. Adult presentation of aortic dissection is well-characterized, while that in the pediatric patient has distinct challenges owing to their heterogeneous hemodynamic profile and anatomy. Notably, an early diagnosis is important because signs of acute chest pain, hypertension, and syncope may be imitated by other benign conditions of presentation in children and thus are delayed specific therapy (Bauer et al., 2003). Reforms in education curricula, , such as the flipped classroom model, have emphasized improving emergency medicine professionals' ability to diagnose and treat such life-threatening cardiovascular disorders effectively (Aziz et al., 2018).

## 12.1.7. Hypertrophic Cardiomyopathy

Hypertrophic cardiomyopathy (HCM) is a severe risk factor in the case of pediatric cardiovascular disorders, particularly due to its genetic basis and the potential for sudden cardiac death. Defined as abnormal heart muscle thickening, this can become an obstruction of blood flow and arrhythmias, showing symptoms , such as dyspnea, syncope, and palpitations, often with no prior warning. Genetic susceptibility is particularly relevant, as illustrated by the identification of pathogenic variants in genes related to cardiac function like myosin binding protein C3 and myosin heavy chain 7 (McBenedict et al., 2024).

HCM normally is diagnosed by echocardiography or cardiac magnetic resonance imaging, which reflect the pathognomonic myocardial hypertrophy, reported in clinical cases of patients with apparently no cardiovascular risk factors (Marraki et al., 2022). Early diagnosis and treatment of HCM thus significantly can improve patient outcomes, and it thus is a significant target in children's emergency departments (Figure 12.8).

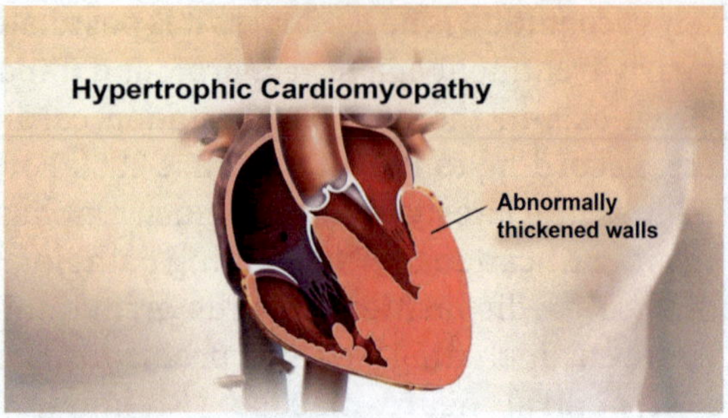


**Figure 12.8.** Hypertrophic cardiomyopathy.

*Source:* https://external-content.duckduckgo.com/iu/?u=https%3A%2F%2Fi.ytimg.com%2Fvi%2FvqWp86YVWjU%2Fmaxresdefault.jpg&f=1&nofb=1&ipt=378fe382d1e3daaaf5bc6773b1d97603934ae6bb2484b027162ec770e82ff9b7&ipo=images.

## 12.1.8. Heart Failure in Pediatric Patients

Pediatric heart failure is a cause of great concern in pediatric cardiovascular disorders that needs to be diagnosed and treated immediately. Unlike in the adult patient population, where heart failure is most often due to atherosclerotic disease, pediatric heart failure is most often due to congenital heart malformations, cardiomyopathies, or arrhythmias, which present certain diagnostic and therapeutic difficulties. Current research identifies the prognostic value of biomarkers like soluble suppression of tumorigenicity 2 (sST2), which has demonstrated clinical heart failure prognosis in children, with its predictive value for advanced cardiovascular events still limited (Sulu et al., 2024). Furthermore, the role of key fatty acids, i.e., eicosapentaenoic acid (EPA) and docosahexaenoic acid (DHA), suggests a therapeutic intervention potential through their ability to modulate oxidative stress pathways involved in cardiac dysfunction (Seth et al., 2024). Thus, an integrated approach, whereby both clinical care and new biological markers are followed, is crucial for improved results in pediatric heart failure (Figure 12.9).

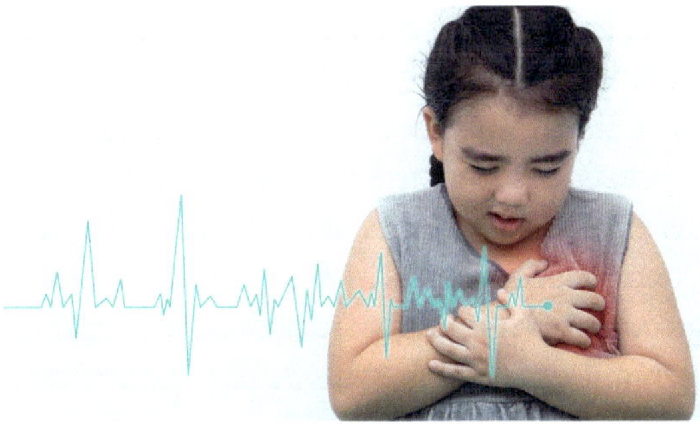

**Figure 12.9.** Heart failure in pediatric patients.

*Source:* https://www.pediatricexperts.com/wp-content/uploads/2023/05/congestive_heart_failure-1024x585-1.jpg.

### 12.1.9. Cardiac Arrest in Children

The incidence of cardiac arrest among children, although relatively rare in relation to adults, remains a critical aspect of pediatric healthcare management, with far-reaching consequences on both short- and long-term outcomes. One of the disturbing factors behind pediatric mortality is the racial disparity that has been shown in pediatric emergency departments. Research indicates that Black children are disproportionately affected, with higher adjusted risks of death from conditions , such as sudden cardiac arrest, when controlling for severity of illness and sociodemographic factors, than Whites (Colleen et al., 2023). The disparity highlights serious systemic issues in the healthcare system. Against such challenges, the International Liaison Committee on Resuscitation has emphasized the necessity of including child-oriented approaches in resuscitation guidelines to optimize outcomes in all children with cardiac disorders (Wyckoff et al., 2022). Addressing such imbalances is essential in realizing the efficacy of treatment protocols as well as in maintaining uniform care in homogeneous populations.

## Test Your Knowledge

1. What are common types of congenital heart defects in children, and how do they typically present?
2. What are the signs and causes of cardiogenic shock in pediatric patients?

## 12.2. Clinical Presentation and Diagnosis

**Learning Outcome**

1. Signs and symptoms of cardiovascular disorders;
2. Importance of history-taking in pediatric patients;
3. Physical examination techniques;
4. Diagnostic imaging modalities;
5. Laboratory tests and biomarkers;
6. Differential diagnosis considerations;
7. Role of telemedicine in diagnosis;
8. Challenges in diagnosing pediatric patients;
9. Importance of early diagnosis for outcomes.

Early diagnosis and clinical presentation are vital in pediatric cardiovascular disorders to ensure successful treatment. Unique signs , such as cyanosis, tachypnea, and poor feeding may be manifestations of serious congenital heart defects that need prompt evaluation. For instance, unlike other cardiovascular disorders, congenital heart diseases (CHDs) have the potential to rapidly worsen in a brief period following birth, underlining the need for early detection and treatment (Moisa et al., 2024). Central to this process is the multidisciplinary consultation of medical practitioners, enhancing diagnostic accuracy and expediting treatment decisions. Furthermore, point-of-care ultrasound (POCUS) has been greatly beneficial in these settings, being very sensitive and specific for common cardiovascular disorders (Putri et al., 2024). Thus, a general comprehension of clinical presentations, along with advanced imaging modalities, takes center stage in navigating the complex arena of pediatric cardiovascular disorders towards improved patient outcomes.

### 12.2.1. Signs and Symptoms of Cardiovascular Disorders

Identification of the signs and symptoms of pediatric patients with cardiovascular disorders is important for early management and intervention. Tachycardia, hypotension, and fever are common indicators, which might also be related to severe diseases , such as multisystem inflammatory syndrome in children (MIS-C) after COVID-19.

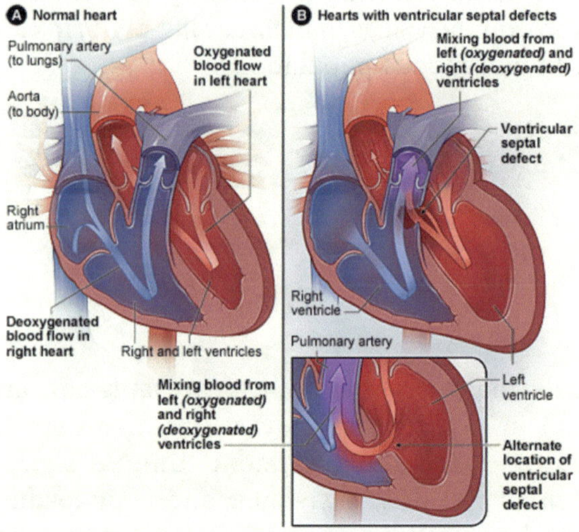


**Figure 12.10.** Signs and symptoms of cardiovascular disorders.

*Source:* By National Heart Lung and Blood Institute - http://www.nhlbi.nih.gov/health/dci/Diseases/chd/chd_types.html, Public Domain, https://commons.wikimedia.org/w/index.php?curid=11069905

In Kawasaki disease, Kawasaki disease-like presentation was observed in patients with accompanying gastrointestinal issues, where 100% of the cases presented with cardiovascular abnormalities like myocardial dysfunction and shock (El-Samman et al., 2024). Infants are also presented in emergency departments to follow up on complaints, and cyanosis, seizures, and cough are presenting symptoms in those diagnosed with significant cardiovascular abnormalities (Öztürk et al., 2023). Identification of such diverse presentations is important as early identification can have a significant impact on the management and outcomes of pediatric patients with cardiovascular disorders. Clinicians should, therefore, be observant in their assessments to effectively manage these life-threatening disorders (Figure 12.10).

### 12.2.2. Importance of History-Taking in Pediatric Patients

In pediatric patients, the clinical art of good history-taking is paramount to good diagnosis and treatment, particularly in cardiovascular disorders. Good medical history may reveal such critical information about underlying conditions , such as hypertension, increasingly identified as a public health problem in children and adolescents.

The rising prevalence of hypertension underscores the significance of consideration by clinicians of not only presenting symptoms, but also historical risk factors like family medical history and lifestyle to effectively guide treatment interventions (Lurbe et al., 2016). Moreover, an understanding of a child's health history allows for targeted intervention, especially in acute presentations like sudden cardiac arrest, where every minute matters (Dahlen et al., 2014). An accurate and detailed history gives healthcare practitioners the background they need to implement effective and timely medical care, ultimately improving patient outcomes in pediatric cardiovascular treatment.

### 12.2.3. Physical Examination Techniques

There is a proper physical examination in the diagnosis of pediatric cardiovascular disorders, particularly with the rise of hypertension in children. An effective examination procedure should include precise measurement of blood pressure, which has also evolved with new guidelines giving greater significance to out-of-office measurement for correct figures. For instance, the ability to diagnose primary arterial hypertension (PAH) in teenagers is of importance, where the widespread lifestyle adjustment manifesting as obesity and reduced activity levels exacerbates the condition (Lurbe et al., 2016). Secondly, familiarity with hypertensive emergencies, characterized by sudden increases in blood pressure, necessitates understanding of its classification into disorders and urgencies, and this can significantly impact morbidity (Akingbola et al., 2012). Therefore, expertise in physical examination skills not only aids early detection of these conditions but also directs appropriate management strategies, ultimately contributing to positive results in the treatment of pediatric cardiovascular patients.

### 12.2.4. Diagnostic Imaging Modalities

The selection and use of diagnostic imaging modalities gain profound significance in delivering timely and correct intervention. Methods , such as echocardiography, MRI, and CT scans provide essential information about cardiac structure and function in order to detect conditions like congenital heart defects or myocardial infarctions. For instance, in evaluating acute ischemic stroke in children, neuroimaging can potentially yield significant data regarding potential underlying vascular abnormalities. As has been noted by Au et al. (2020), imaging findings should be accurately interpreted, since subtle findings can be linked with severe clinical presentations. Also, as relentless advances in imaging technology continue to enhance diagnostic capability, pediatric patients can receive comprehensive investigation at little risk. Hence, having a good understanding of these modalities and their consequences is of vital importance to healthcare practitioners working with pediatric cardiovascular disorders, ultimately impacting patient safety and treatment results (Figure 12.11).

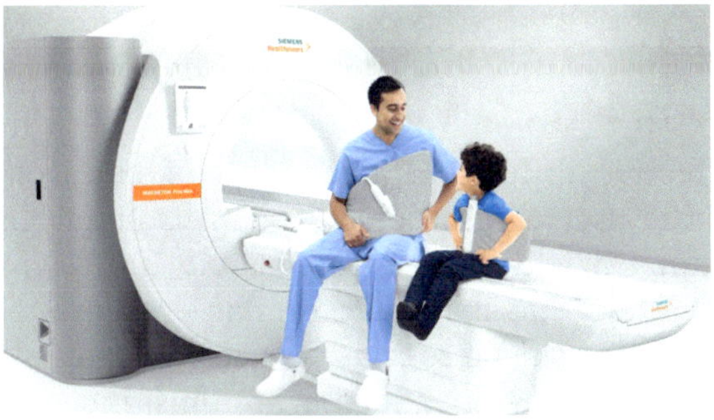

**Figure 12.11.** The use of pediatric-friendly imaging technology for a comfortable diagnostic experience.

*Source:* https://marketing.webassets.siemens-healthineers.com/71880bc8564c624b/1e80d2068543/v/0b0f11132cfe/siemens-healthineers_mri_pediatric_patient-friendliness-light-weight-coils.jpg.

### 12.2.5. Laboratory Tests and Biomarkers

In pediatric cardiac disorders, biomarkers and laboratory tests have a critical function in timely diagnosis and management. The tests allow clinicians to quantify various physiological and biochemical parameters that are likely related to cardiac conditions. For instance, elevated troponins are indicative of myocardial damage and can be utilized for early identification of disorders , such as myocarditis or ischemia in children. In addition, recognition of hypertension (HTN) as the forerunner of cardiovascular disease underscores the importance of periodic laboratory tests, particularly in screening among young patients who may not present evident symptoms (Lurbe et al., 2016). Biomarkers , such as B-type natriuretic peptide (BNP) are equally important in measuring heart failure, and use should be made necessary if required. The application of these laboratory tests in the clinical setting not only enhances diagnosis but also informs critical treatment decisions, in the end, improving outcomes for pediatric patients with cardiovascular disorders (Prylińska et al., 2019).

### 12.2.6. Differential Diagnosis Considerations

Effective differential diagnosis of children's cardiovascular disorders is vital in distinguishing among a wide range of possible underlying disorders that may have similar presentation. Physicians should consider varied etiologies that can present with sudden symptoms, including congenital cardiac abnormalities, arrhythmias, and vasculitis, among many others. The pediatric presentation polymorphism needs a strong foundation in physiological and pathophysiologic differences between children and adults, as defined in present education curricula to enhance emergency medicine training (Aziz et al., 2018). In addition, an especial emphasis should be laid on concomitant conditions, especially in neonates and infants, who are prone to present with multiple anomalies and complicating their diagnostic workup (Caliskan et al., 2016). By using a methodical system for differential diagnosis, medical practitioners are able to provide timely interventions, ultimately leading to better outcomes in pediatric patients with cardiovascular crises. Therefore, careful consideration of all potential diagnoses continues to be a foundation of effective emergency care in this susceptible population.

### 12.2.7. Role of Telemedicine in Diagnosis

Telemedicine usage in the diagnosis of pediatric cardiovascular disorders has been a game-changer, with on-demand access to specialist services that are so very needed in emergency cases. Teleconsultation tools, , such as those developed in the HINT project, enable real-time communication between specialists and general practitioners so that they can make timely assessments and referrals. This convergence supports the general sharing of digital clinical information, , such as important diagnostic images, required for accurate assessment and treatment of pediatric cardiac diseases. The use of innovative technologies, , such as the Hub and Spoke model, enhances remote communication efficiency and enables telemonitoring efficiently, thereby preventing delay in emergency diagnoses and treatments (Caforio et al., 2022). Furthermore, the adoption of international healthcare standards makes handling data easier, enabling health practitioners to remain current and be ready to handle intricate clinical scenarios in a timely fashion (Prylińska et al., 2019). Telemedicine is hence a relevant part of modern pediatric cardiovascular care, particularly in disorders (Figure 12.12).

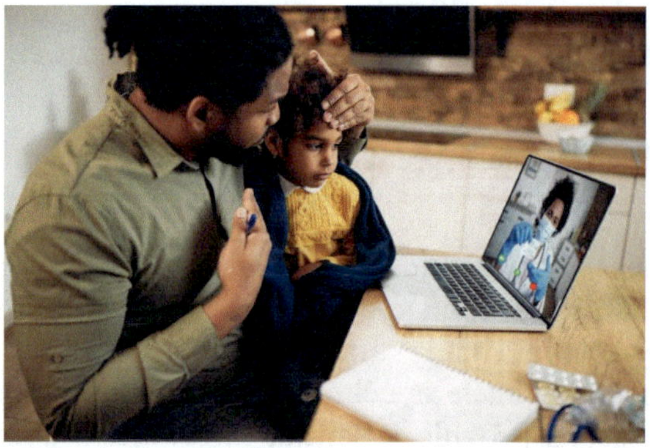

**Figure 12.12.** The role of telemedicine in the diagnosis of pediatric cardiovascular disorders has been transformative.

*Source:* https://sa1s3optim.patientpop.com/assets/images/provider/photos/2499739.jpg.

### 12.2.8. Challenges in Diagnosing Pediatric Patients

The complexity involved in pediatric patient diagnosis is significant, particularly for pediatric cardiovascular disorders. The pediatric patients are more likely to present abnormal clinical presentations compared to adults, thus complicating the diagnosis of such dire conditions as acute chest pain or dyspnea. In addition, the application of diagnostic tools like Point-of-Care Ultrasonography (POCUS) has proven to provide higher accuracy; however, because of variations in the levels of training among emergency experts (Tamimi et al., 2023), integration into routine pediatric assessment is not uniform. Further, studies on prehospital seizure care point out the potential delay and mismanagement due to poor clinical assessment, which is surprisingly evidenced in failure to appropriately record children's vital signs (Bester et al., 2020). The issue, therefore, is not only symptom identification but also that all the information relevant to it is utilized appropriately to direct timely and appropriate clinical interventions.

### 12.2.9. Importance of Early Diagnosis for Outcomes

The value of early pediatric cardiovascular disorders diagnosis cannot be overstated, as early detection can contribute greatly to improved patient outcomes. It has been shown that disorders like hypertension, which are increasingly occurring in children and adolescents, can have the potential to lead to severe cardiovascular complications if left untreated (Lurbe et al., 2016). Early screening and intervention strategies are thus crucial in reducing the burden of long-term cardiovascular disease in this category of patients. Moreover, proper response planning with well-trained health workers can optimize the management of acute incidents, , such as unexpected cardiac arrest, in schools (Dahlen et al., 2014). Through well-coordinated communication networks and adequate allocation of resources, health practitioners can ensure that children receive the immediate attention they need. On the whole, emphasis on early diagnosis and treatment not only enhances survivorship but also brings a better quality of life to pediatric patients with cardiovascular issues.

## Test Your Knowledge

1. What are common signs and symptoms indicating cardiovascular disorders in children?
2. Which diagnostic imaging modalities are commonly used in pediatric cardiovascular disorders, and what challenges exist in diagnosis?

## 12.3. Management and Treatment Strategies

**Learning Outcome**

1. Understand the insanity defense
2. Explain the role of mental illness in sentencing
3. Know the impact of forensic evaluations on legal outcomes
4. Discuss confidentiality and privilege in forensic settings
5. Focus on the intersection of mental health and criminal law
6. Learn case law influencing forensic psychiatry
7. Describe ethical dilemmas in legal contexts
8. Know the role of forensic psychiatry in civil cases
9. Explain legislative changes affecting forensic practices

Effective treatment and management of childhood cardiovascular disorders mandate a multidimensional approach, highlighting early diagnosis and intervention. Enhanced determination of hypertension in children and teenagers plays a central role in this aspect, owing to the increased prevalence of elevated blood pressure as an important aspect of public health (Lurbe et al., 2016). These interventions are not only the acute clinical interventions, i.e., hypertensive emergencies pharmacotherapy, but also the long-term lifestyle modifications to avert future cardiovascular risk. The merging of rigorous clinical guidelines assists healthcare providers in making the most optimal decisions based on deep scientific evidence and clinical expertise. These programs aim at the necessity for intensified blood pressure screening as well as out-of-office measurement, thus enabling early detection of cardiovascular abnormality (Prylińska et al., 2019). By developing an intersectoral collaborative framework for families, healthcare providers, and policymakers, care for pediatric cardiovascular disorders can contain the rising trend of related disease burdens (Figure 12.13).

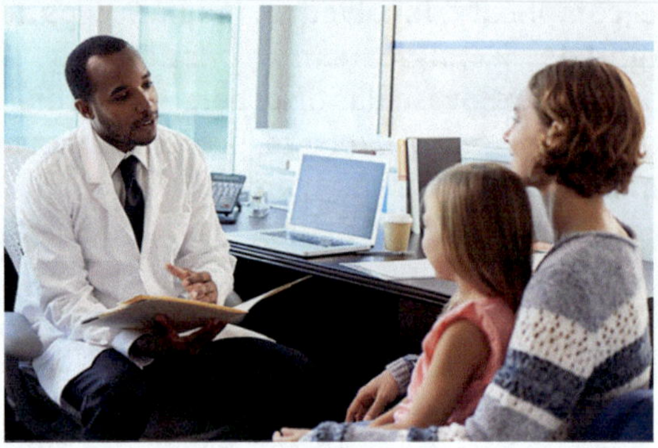

**Figure 12.13.** Management and treatment strategies.

*Source:* https://clf1.medpagetoday.com/assets/images/resource-center/cs-ADHD-myths-600x400.jpg.

### 12.3.1. Initial Assessment and Stabilization

In pediatric cardiovascular disorders, early evaluation and stabilization of the patient are crucial so that further deterioration has not taken place. This is then followed by an immediate assessment of the child's airway, breathing, and circulation or the ABCs of emergency. Early recognition of clinical deterioration is also crucial, as delay can lead to worse outcomes. Research indicates that healthcare professionals , such as nurses, indicate that they require specialized training during emergencies with an emphasis on the significance of being prepared in such high-risk environments (Clancy-Burgess et al., 2024). Further, incorporating specialized training in pediatric-focused emergency care can enhance the competence of medical professionals to perform effective initial assessments (Altschuld et al., 2017). In the end, well-designed educational programs can lead to timely interventions, thus enhancing survival and long-term health benefits in children suffering from cardiovascular disorders.

### 12.3.2. Pharmacological Interventions

Pharmacologic treatment is an important component in pediatric cardiovascular disorders, treating hypertension, arrhythmias, and heart failure effectively and safely. The increasing prevalence of hypertension in children requires a highly coordinated therapeutic response since it is a significant contributor to lifetime cardiovascular risks (Lurbe et al., 2016). Angiotensin-converting enzyme inhibitors and beta-blockers are used most commonly to manage blood pressure and cardiac function. In addition, emergent response in cases of emergency often involves medication to manage acute arrhythmias of the heart, with benzodiazepines like Diazepam often used because they act rapidly and are potent (Bester et al., 2020). Prescription and dosing of these medications are particularly important, given the unique physiological differences in pediatric patients, which underscores the necessity for ongoing education and protocol establishment among healthcare providers treating pediatric cardiovascular disorders.

### 12.3.3. Role of Advanced Cardiac Life Support (ACLS)

The role of Advanced Cardiac Life Support (ACLS) in pediatric cardiovascular disorders is indispensable since it provides an organized framework for medical professionals to act fast in response to emergent conditions. ACLS is a system of protocols and interventions specifically designed to be used on cardiac arrest or acute cardiovascular events in children, emphasizing the early recognition and rapid intervention. At the center of success is the incorporation of high-quality cardiopulmonary resuscitation (CPR), which significantly improves prognosis if instituted promptly. Also integrated into the use of ACLS algorithms is advanced airway management together with the administration of life-saving medications, and these are critical factors for stabilizing a child patient. The continuous education and inter-professional communication among medical providers, as emphasized by publications , such as the Iowa Board of Nursing newsletters, ensure that practitioners are current with such life-saving skills and, in turn, improve outcomes for children in emergency care (Prylińska et al., 2019) (Figure 12.14).

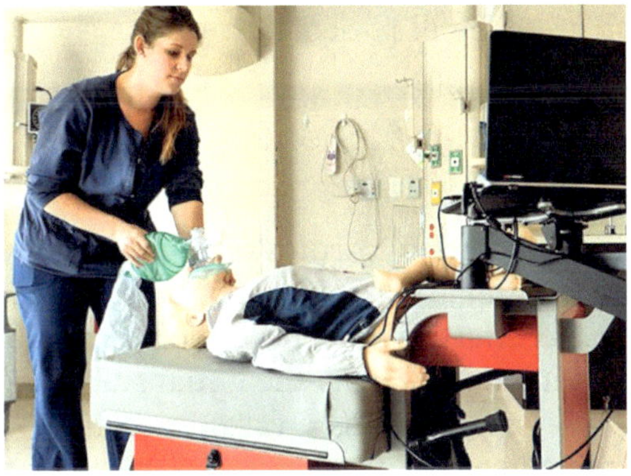

**Figure 12.14.** The role of advanced cardiac life support (ACLS) in pediatric cardiovascular disorders.

*Source:* https://rqipartners.com/wp-content/uploads/blog-featured-image-your-guide-to-bls-vs.-acls-and-pals-600x440.jpg.

### 12.3.4. Surgical Interventions and Procedures

In pediatric cardiovascular diseases, surgical interventions and procedures are often crucial in controlling life-threatening congenital cardiac malformations and acute cardiac conditions. Multidisciplinary practice is needed to cater to the complexity of the procedures that involve working in tandem by neonatologists, pediatric surgeons, and specialist cardiologists. Specifically, the necessity for intervention highlights the importance of prenatal checks because they might assist in the identification of congenital malformations at an earlier stage and better prepare for immediate postnatal treatment (Moisa et al., 2024). Moreover, complications like hospital-acquired infection are significant threats to patients who undergo surgical procedures. For instance, increased frequency of *Stenotrophomonas maltophilia* bloodstream infections in pediatric cardiovascular surgery ICUs is indicative of the complexity of postoperative care (Karaagac et al., 2024). Therefore, it is imperative to frame proper infection control procedures alongside surgical interventions to enhance outcomes in these critically ill patients.

### 12.3.5. Post-Emergency Care and Monitoring

Within pediatric cardiovascular disorders, monitoring and follow-up after an emergency are also crucial components of successful patient management. Following the initial stabilization of a child experiencing a cardiovascular event, there is a need to finish an intensive evaluation and individualized monitoring program to avoid complications and achieve optimal recovery. It is marked by the observation of vital signs, cardiac function, and any developing symptoms that may indicate worsening, as timely intervention is paramount to avoiding relapses. In addition, effective communication with caregivers on signs of distress and the need for further treatment can go a long way in enhancing the prognosis of the child. Also, adherence to mandated protocols for surveillance can reduce variability in care and improve adherence to best practices, as with comparable structures in other areas of medical practice that emphasize systematic approaches to management and surveillance (Canning, 2020; Howard et al., 2023). Overall, solid post-emergency protocols directly influence the long-term health of pediatric patients who have recovered from cardiovascular emergencies.

### 12.3.6. Family Involvement in Treatment Decisions

In the case of pediatric cardiovascular disorders, a family member involved in treatment planning is what ensures comprehensive care and productive outcomes. Family involvement creates an open environment in which health care practitioners can share vital information about the health status of a child and therapeutic interventions. This kind of communication helps alleviate the fear usually involved in such medical crises and enables relatives to make informed choices that best appeal to their values and tastes. Additionally, new recommendations for the management of conditions like hypertension also underscore the necessity for involving families since they call for a trend towards patient-focused care in pediatricians (Lurbe et al., 2016). Such an interaction not only enhances compliance with treatments but also unites several perspectives, thus enriching the process of decision-making and overall patient care (Johnson, 2018). Lastly, recognizing and identifying the family's role in all such crucial decisions is pivotal in developing effective treatment regimens in pediatric cardiovascular disorders (Figure 12.15).

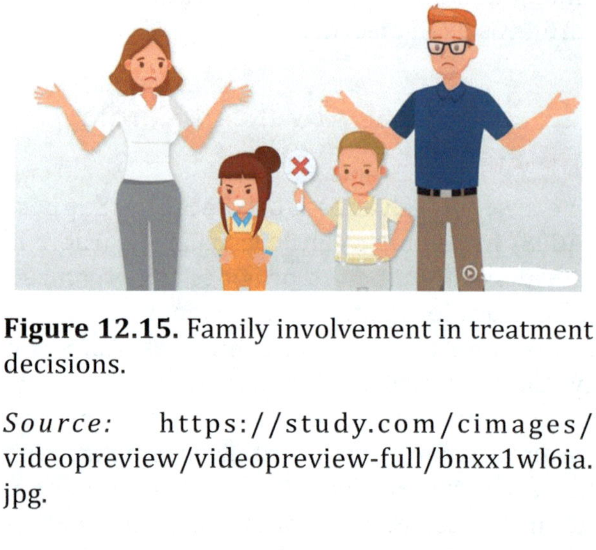

**Figure 12.15.** Family involvement in treatment decisions.

*Source:* https://study.com/cimages/videopreview/videopreview-full/bnxx1wl6ia.jpg.

### 12.3.7. Multidisciplinary Approach to Care

The rarity of pediatric cardiovascular disorders demands a multidisciplinary delivery model that merges the services of various healthcare providers. As has been highlighted in recent literature, the success mostly relies on early intervention and proper diagnosis, most notably in the situation of congenital heart diseases (CHDs), where speedy identification is critical. Multidisciplinary care, including neonatologists, cardiologists, pediatricians, and surgeons, permits comprehensive evaluation and management, so that all aspects of the child's illness are thoroughly addressed (Moisa et al., 2024). In addition, illnesses , such as Marfan syndrome show the benefits of multidisciplinary care, as these usually affect more than a single organ system; therefore, clinical management in children becomes more complex (Baban et al., 2024). By facilitating interaction and coordination among specialists, medical teams can build personalized management plans that not just solve acute crises but look toward long-term goals, ultimately enhancing children's cardiovascular disorders care quality.

## 12.3.8. Long-Term Management and Follow-Up

Effective long-term follow-up and management are critical components in the treatment of pediatric cardiovascular disorders. Because earlier intervention in health greatly reduces morbidity and mortality, continuous surveillance becomes unavoidable to assess clinical improvement and solve emerging complications. This measure is particularly important in light of the rising prevalence of hypertension in youth that has been linked to increased risk for cardiovascular disease in the long run (Lurbe et al., 2016). Additionally, data about adults with congenital heart disease typically experiencing serious complications necessitate strict follow-up treatment to prevent long-term risks associated with their conditions (Bauer et al., 2003). A well-planned follow-up strategy should involve individualized treatment plans, ongoing evaluation of cardiovascular function, and active lifestyle modifications to ensure maximal results. Lastly, establishing congruent collaboration between healthcare providers, patients, and families is the key sto achieving successful long-term control in this high-risk population.

## 12.3.9. Ethical Considerations in Treatment

In pediatric cardiovascular disorders, ethical issues are at the forefront since medical practitioners are exposed to complex decision-making scenarios that encroach on the vulnerable group. The situation is extremely dire when one considers the scarce availability of resources in rural hospitals, under which emergency nurses may be forced to administer critical care without the intensive backup typically offered in cities.

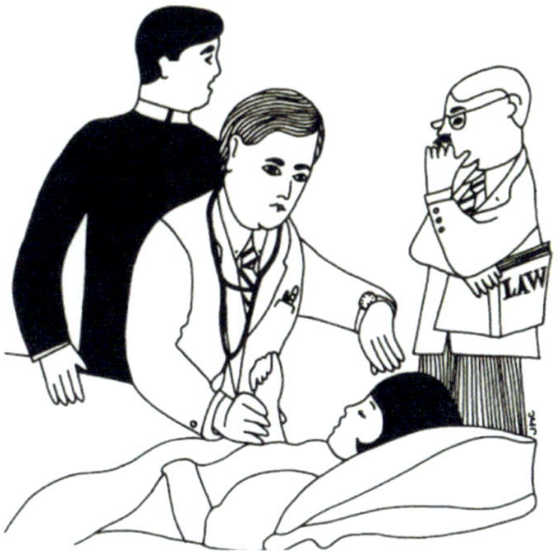


**Figure 12.16.** An illustration portrays a physician examining a child while a clergyman and a lawyer observe, symbolizing the ethical, spiritual, and legal dimensions involved in pediatric medical decision-making.

*Source:* https://journals.healio.com/cms/asset/963bcccd-6b7d-448a-a1fb-71afe2cf1e2e/10.3928_00904481-19731001-07-fig1.jpg.

This conflict highlights nurses' imperative to possess quality clinical judgment and competence since patient outcomes rest in their hands. Ethical practice also necessitates that healthcare practitioners maintain effective communication with families, ensuring informed consent and promoting the child's best interests. As understood in newer quality improvement projects aimed at rural nursing, there is a need to enhance critical thinking and clinical decision-making skills, particularly where the need for speed of care and limited resources complicate ethical decisions (Plano, 2022). Ultimately, these ethical concerns in these disorders work towards highlighting continued training and intervention for healthcare professionals to uphold care standards (Lurbe et al., 2016) (Figure 12.16).

## Test Your Knowledge

1. What are the key steps in the initial assessment and stabilization of a child presenting with a cardiovascular emergency?
2. What is the role of Advanced Cardiac Life Support (ACLS) and when are surgical interventions indicated in pediatric cardiovascular care?

## 12.4. Prevention and Education

**Learning Outcome**

1. Importance of preventive care in pediatrics;
2. Screening for congenital heart disease;
3. Parental education on warning signs;
4. Community awareness programs;
5. Role of schools in health education;
6. Guidelines for physical activity in children;
7. Vaccination and its impact on cardiovascular health;
8. Research on prevention strategies;
9. Future directions in pediatric cardiovascular health.

A multidisciplinary approach to the prevention and education of pediatric cardiovascular disorders is essential in order to minimize risk and enhance outcomes. Behind this effort is a need to be aware of the increasing prevalence of hypertension in children and adolescents as a major public health problem. Education programs directed towards healthcare providers and parents can foster the awareness of risk factors, symptoms, and early diagnosis. Specifically, the development of guidelines for the management of hypertension offers an emergent framework that is bringing into focus the necessity of routine screening and monitoring protocols to identify isolated systolic hypertension in early childhood (Lurbe et al., 2016). Besides, use of learning programs, including programs distributed by channels like the Nursing Newsletter, can keep nursing professionals current with practice developments in care and public health policy to assist their role in preventative health care (Lurbe et al., 2016). Targeted prevention and education efforts ultimately foster a proactive environment for managing pediatric cardiovascular health.

### 12.4.1. Importance of Preventive Care in Pediatrics

Pediatric preventative care is crucial to address emerging health problems, particularly in the instance of cardiovascular conditions. Since hypertension increases among youths, there is a need to diagnose and intervene early to manage long-term health risks, particularly because these conditions are amongst the causative agents of increasing cardiovascular disorders among children (Lurbe et al., 2016). Regular screenings and tests are needed not only to monitor blood pressure but also to assess lifestyle factors that predispose children to heart-related complications. Furthermore, the addition of dental care to preventive services indicates its broader importance in the care of children; oral health has been linked to many systemic diseases, including cardiovascular disease (Thursby et al., 2016). Thus, by prioritizing preventive care, healthcare professionals can efficiently control risk factors as well as encourage healthier lifestyles that bring better health outcomes and fewer incidents of emergency cases relating to pediatric cardiovascular complications.

## 12.4.2. Screening for Congenital Heart Disease

Congenital heart disease (CHD) screening in children is crucial for early detection and intervention, resulting in improved outcomes for the affected individuals. The occurrence of non-sustained ventricular tachycardia (NSVT) among pediatric patients has been increasing, with evidence showing that up to 6% of such patients show the arrhythmia, particularly in those with underlying cardiac conditions, i.e., CHD (Assaad et al., 2024).

This draws attention to the importance of proper management and monitoring plans in pediatric cardiovascular disorders. Furthermore, with heightened medical and surgical intervention, the number of cases of adults with CHD has superseded cases occurring in pediatric patients, highlighting the need for ongoing screening and evaluation as patients progress through different stages of their lifespan (Robb et al., 2024). Thus, establishing sound screening guidelines not only enables the diagnosis of congenital heart disease in a timely manner but also enables preparation for potential complications during a person's lifetime and eventually enhances overall cardiovascular care (Figure 12.17).

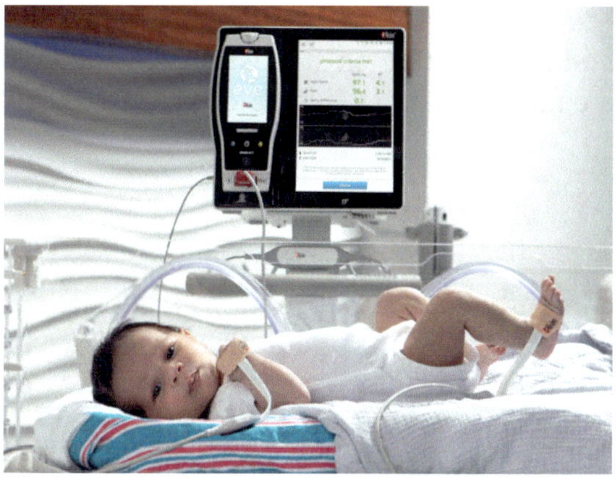

**Figure 12.17.** Screening for congenital heart disease.

*Source:* https://www.masimo.co.uk/siteassets/uk/images/clinical-solution/newborn/neonatal_dual_oximetry1918_123121.png.

## 12.4.3. Parental Education on Warning Signs

The role of parents' education to assess warning signs related to pediatric cardiovascular disorders is vital. Recognition of symptoms , such as unexplained fatigue, cyanosis, or shortness of breath will significantly influence early intervention. Well-educated parents about their child's specific cardiac disorder show enhanced confidence regarding their abilities to care for their child, leading to effective monitoring of their child's health status upon discharge, especially following cardiac surgery. Research has established that educational interventions, in the form of developing extensive informational materials, can minimize parental anxiety and maximize an appreciation for potential complications, thus maximizing the treatment outcomes of children with congenital cardiac malformations (Barsella et al., 2020). Additionally, educative briefing of parents regarding symptoms of a downturn can assist in ensuring timely access to medical consultations in an effort to avoid tragic consequences. Therefore, educationally structured programs aimed at critical warning signs should be prioritized in healthcare systems, resulting in a positive outcome for the child and family (Lurbe et al., 2016).

### 12.4.4. Community Awareness Programs

Community education programs play a key role in the battle against pediatric cardiovascular disorders through parental, teacher, and healthcare worker education on symptoms and signs of disorders like sudden cardiac arrest (SCA) in children. Programs foster an environment where rapid intervention can be prompted, therefore enhancing survival. For instance, a review of literature on pediatric SCA is concerned with the need to provide school nurses with proper resources and education to handle such disorders efficiently within educational institutions (Dahlen et al., 2014). CPR and automated external defibrillator (AED) instructional programs are required to make an educated community. With growing awareness comes a higher likelihood of early response, ultimately reversing the impact of cardiovascular disorders in children (Lurbe et al., 2016). By ongoing community participation and educational initiatives, awareness campaigns empower individuals to act instantaneously in times of crisis.

### 12.4.5. Role of Schools in Health Education

Schools are well placed to assist in health education, in particular, in pediatric cardiovascular health issues. Schools can educate young people in the essential information regarding risk factors of hypertension and cardiovascular disease that have become increasingly common in children and youth. As highlighted by recent research on the determinants of youth hypertension, schools represent strategic locations for early identification and education about cardiovascular risk (Lurbe et al., 2016). Through the promotion of healthy lifestyles through initiatives , such as nutrition and regular exercise, schools can directly influence the long-term health potential of students. In addition, through tight coordination with medical practitioners, schools can deliver vital information and material resources to families, hence empowering them to access preventive care. Ultimately, school life plays an important role in constructing awareness as well as active participation in health actions, which is vital to combat the escalating public health issue of pediatric cardiovascular disorders (Lurbe et al., 2016) (Figure 12.18).

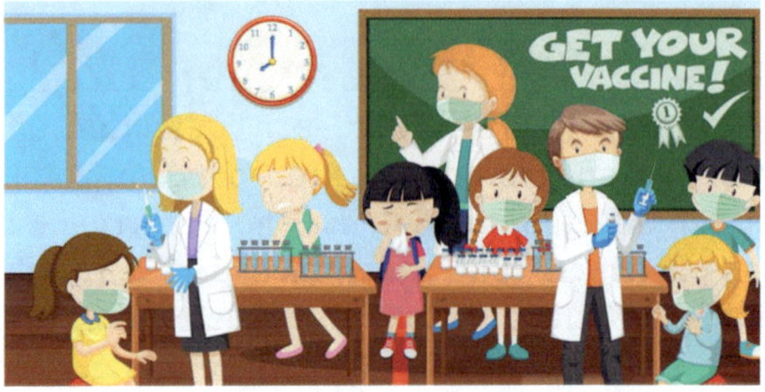


**Figure 12.18.** Role of schools in health education.

*Source:* https://www.billabonghighschool.com/blogs/wp-content/uploads/2024/06/How-Schools-Promote-Better-Health-for-the-Students.jpg.

### 12.4.6. Guidelines for Physical Activity in Children

Effective management of pediatric cardiovascular disorders requires the implementation of universal standards of physical activity among children. Regular physical activity is a must to maintain cardiovascular health, develop a strong heart and vascular system among children, and reduce the risk of diseases , such as hypertension, which has seen a shocking rise among the pediatric population. As has been recommended by the American College of Cardiology and the American Heart Association, physical activity guidelines stress that children should engage in a minimum of 60 minutes of moderate to vigorous physical activity sdaily, which not only facilitates fitness but also prevents hypertension and other cardiovascular risk factors (Lurbe et al., 2016). Furthermore, the management of increased hypertension in children demands better sensitization of these guidelines, leading parents and educators to put weight behind physical exercise as a component of child health promotion (Lurbe et al., 2016). By promoting an active lifestyle, we are able to prevent cardiovascular disorders in this vulnerable group.

### 12.4.7. Vaccination and Its Impact on Cardiovascular Health

Vaccination and cardiovascular health, particularly in children, have been a matter of growing concern in recent years, notably in the time of the COVID-19 pandemic. Vaccination plays a central role in the prevention of severe adverse effects of viral infections on cardiovascular function. For instance, older adults are viewed as a high-risk group for severe complications of COVID-19, and hence vaccination has been prioritized in efforts to reduce mortality. This is particularly pertinent to children presenting with system infection-exacerbated illness. While life-threatening reactions to vaccinations , such as anaphylaxis, are very rare, familiarity with their management is very important in the pediatric population. Furthermore, data obtained from recent studies affirm the shifting clinical approach to vaccination based on accessibility and prevention for the health of children (Lurbe et al., 2016). Overall, vaccination is a critical aspect of ensuring protection against infectious disease and its cardiovascular aftermath.

### 12.4.8. Research on Prevention Strategies

Over the past several years, the burgeoning rate of hypertension among children and adolescents has emphasized the utmost importance of the prevention strategies that would minimize pediatric cardiovascular disorders. Studies show that improving our current understanding of the definition of hypertension and its clinical implications in children is paramount for early recognition and treatment. For instance, detection of isolated systolic hypertension as a risk factor demands advanced measurement methods, including out-of-office blood pressure determination and determination of vascular phenotypes (Lurbe et al., 2016). Further, emphasis on the central clustering of cardiovascular risk factors allows for comprehensive prevention strategies, enabling healthcare workers and families to preemptively address underlying health issues. There is also a need for public health programming and policy development to address enhancing diagnosis and treatment of hypertension in this high-risk group through the dissemination of evidence-based recommendations and educational resources readily accessible to meet the rising danger of pediatric cardiovascular health (Lurbe et al., 2016) (Figure 12.19).

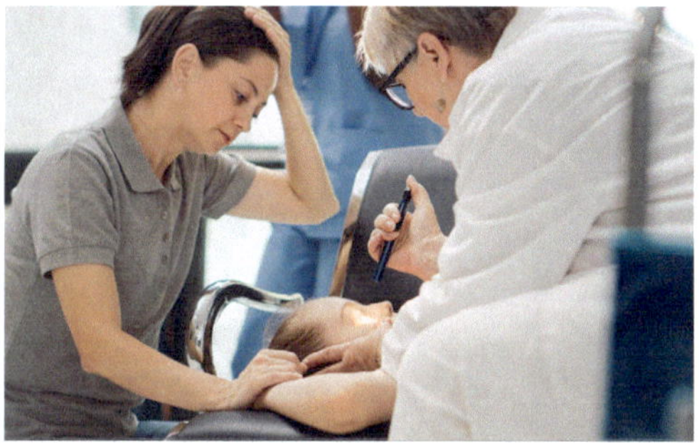

**Figure 12.19.** Emergency care for pediatric heat-related illness.

*Source:* https://nortonhealthcareprovider.com/wp-content/uploads/pediatric-heat-illness.png.

### 12.4.9. Future Directions in Pediatric Cardiovascular Health

With continuing advances in pediatric cardiovascular wellness, efforts in the future need to be directed toward the incorporation of new technologies and individualized care to enhance patient outcomes in disorders. Advances in telemedicine promise much, as they will allow for rapid assessment and intervention in acute cardiovascular diseases, which can potentially reduce morbidity from late intervention. Additionally, genetic testing is at the forefront of preventive care, where individuals can determine vulnerable children even prior to the onset of symptoms, enabling forward-looking planning that can avert crises. Putting in place stringent training programs for healthcare personnel is also crucial, so that staff are properly trained to detect and treat pediatric cardiovascular disorders efficiently. Finally, establishing an interdisciplinary climate of cooperation amongst cardiologists, emergency medicine physicians, and primary care doctors will render delivery of care efficient at last, and thus improve the prognosis for children. Such innovative steps represent a crucial shift towards a more proactive and integrative system in pediatric cardiovascular health, as evidenced Lurbe et al., 2016.

## Test Your Knowledge

1. Why is preventive care important in pediatric cardiovascular health, and what role does parental education play?
2. How does vaccination impact cardiovascular health in children?

## SUMMARY

It is of crucial importance to differentiate the urgency and complexity of such cases. Effective control relies on rapid decision-making and applying expert knowledge to minimize risks associated with congenital cardiac disease, posing catastrophic threats to pediatric patients. As noted, adults with congenital heart disease pose a serious challenge, with emergency presentation having a high mid-term and in-hospital mortality rate, and thus the importance of specialist management in this population (Bauer et al., 2003). Also, in children's resuscitations, where vascular access is sometimes challenging due to anatomical constraints, intraosseous (IO) access seems an essential device. The ease of use of equipment like the EZ-IO® allows for fast drug and fluid administration, improving results in disorders (Kikodze et al., 2019). Thus, a well-coordinated approach that incorporates advanced techniques and expertise is needed for proper management of pediatric cardiovascular disorders.

Prevention and management in pediatric cardiovascular disorders involve a multifaceted strategy, with emphasis laid upon mounting concerns , such as high blood pressure among children and adolescents. The increasing incidence of hypertension (HTN) has sparked extensive research that has explained its clinical significance, including isolated systolic hypertension and the necessity for advanced measurement tools for enhanced diagnosis and control strategies (Lurbe et al., 2016). Besides, the discussion is advanced to cognitive aids applied in resuscitation and has proven to be variously effective in various provider settings. According to research, while healthcare providers are assisted by cognitive aids to maintain CPR quality, their use among lay providers has been found to pose a potential to generate adverse effects because of the absence of adequate training (Abelairas-Gomez et al., 2024). Together, they underscore the need for specialized protocols to improve disorders identification, care, and outcomes.

## KEY TERMS FROM THIS CHAPTER

- Arrhythmias
- Cardiogenic shock (CS)
- Cardiovascular
- Congenital heart defects (CHDs)
- Echocardiography
- Hypertrophic cardiomyopathy (HCM)
- Kawasaki disease
- Point-of-care ultrasonography (POCUS)
- Cardiac magnetic
- Cardiopulmonary resuscitation
- Cardiovascular diseases
- Docosahexaenoic acid (DHA)
- Eicosapentaenoic acid (EPA)
- Infant respiration
- Morbidity
- Pulmonary embolism (PE)

## CRITICAL THINKING QUESTIONS

1. **The most common congenital heart disease is:**
   a. Patent ductus arteriosus
   b. Ventricular septal defect
   c. Atrial septal defect
   d. Tetralogy of Fallot
2. **Cyanotic heart disease in children includes:**
   a. Atrial septal defect
   b. Ventricular septal defect
   c. Patent ductus arteriosus
   d. Tetralogy of Fallot
3. **A machinery-like continuous murmur is characteristic of:**
   a. Aortic stenosis
   b. Pulmonary stenosis
   c. Patent ductus arteriosus
   d. Mitral valves prolapse
4. **Which of the following is a sign of congestive heart failure in infants?**
   a. Fever
   b. Poor feeding and sweating during feeds
   c. Constipation
   d. Skin rash
5. **"Boot-shaped heart" on chest X-ray is associated with:**
   a. Atrial septal defect
   b. Coarctation of aorta
   c. Tetralogy of Fallot
   d. Patent foramen ovale

### Short Answer Questions

1. Describe the pathophysiology, clinical features, diagnosis, and management of Tetralogy of Fallot.
2. Explain congestive heart failure in infants and children – causes, signs, and treatment.
3. Discuss the clinical presentation and management of patent ductus arteriosus.
4. Describe coarctation of the aorta – pathogenesis, clinical findings, and surgical treatment.
5. Explain the nursing care plan for a child with congenital heart disease.

### *Answers to Critical Thinking Questions*

1. (b); 2. (d); 3. (c); 4. (b); 5. (c)

## REFERENCES

1. Abdul Aziz Abdullah Al Tamimi, A. M. S. Alruwaili, E. M. Alruwaili, F. M. Alenazi, N. A. Almoammar, N. S. Alwayli, & T. A. Alfayer. (2023). The utility of point-of-care ultrasound (POCUS) in the emergency department: A systematic review. https://core.ac.uk/download/603897418.pdf (accessed on 16th June 2025).
2. Abdul Latiff, A. H., Agache, I., Akdis, C. A., Al-Ahmad, M., et al. (2021). Management of anaphylaxis due to COVID-19 vaccines in the elderly. https://core.ac.uk/download/512009419.pdf (accessed on 16th June 2025).
3. Abelairas-Gomez, C., Gilfoyle, E., Greif, R., Koota, J., et al. (2024). Cognitive aids used in simulated resuscitation: A systematic review. https://core.ac.uk/download/618390409.pdf (accessed on 16th June 2025).
4. Abrahamsson, A., Abramiuk, A., Aitken, P., Ajram, L., Akers, J., Aldhouse-Green, S., Andrews-Hanna, J., et al. (2017). The odyssey of dental anxiety: From prehistory to the present. A narrative review. https://core.ac.uk/download/84923580.pdf (accessed on 16th June 2025).
5. Lurbe, E., Agabiti-Rosei, E., Cruickshank, J. K., Dominiczak, A., Erdine, S., Hirth, A., Invitti, C., Litwin, M., Mancia, G., Pall, D., Rascher, W., Redon, J., Schaefer, F., Seeman, T., Sinha, M., Stabouli, S., Webb, N. J., Wühl, E., & Zanchetti, A. (2016). 2016 European Society of Hypertension guidelines for the management of high blood pressure in children and adolescents. *Journal of hypertension, 34*(10), 1887–1920. https://doi.org/10.1097/HJH.0000000000001039 (accessed on 16th June 2025).
6. Akhtar, S., Bano, S., & Khan, U. R. (2020). Pediatric congenital heart diseases: Patterns of presentation to the emergency department of a tertiary care hospital. https://core.ac.uk/download/322820432.pdf (accessed on 16th June 2025).
7. Akingbola, O., El-Dahr, S., Singh, D., Yosypiv, I., et al. (2012). Emergency management of hypertension in children. https://core.ac.uk/download/pdf/8723168.pdf (accessed on 16th June 2025).
8. Artenstein, A. (2016). *Baystate Medical Practices Annual Report–2016*. https://core.ac.uk/download/234573495.pdf (accessed on 16th June 2025).
9. Aziz, F., Bachmann, D., Barrie, M., Bubolz, B., et al. (2018). Novel emergency medicine curriculum utilizing self-directed learning and the flipped classroom method: Cardiovascular disorders small group module. https://core.ac.uk/download/484274721.pdf (accessed on 16th June 2025).
10. Baban, G., Parlapiano, M., Cicenia, M., Armando, M., Franceschini, A., Pacifico, C., Panfili, A., et al. (2024). Unique features of cardiovascular involvement and progression in children with Marfan syndrome justify dedicated multidisciplinary care. *Journal of Cardiovascular Development and Disease, 11*. https://www.semanticscholar.org/paper/99c27d2714b7363407a3632228a32f08da900c13 (accessed on 16th June 2025).
11. Balik, H., Bilici, M., & Ture, M. (2018). Myocardial infarction in children. https://core.ac.uk/download/322435882.pdf (accessed on 16th June 2025).
12. Biban, P., Santuz, P., & Soffiati, M. (2009). Neonatal resuscitation in the ward: The role of nurses. https://core.ac.uk/download/326651736.pdf (accessed on 16th June 2025).
13. Bozzola, E., Caffarelli, C., Corsello, G., & Santamaria, F. (2022). The year 2021 in COVID-19

pandemic in children. https://core.ac.uk/download/546074563.pdf (accessed on 16th June 2025).

14. Prylińska, M., Piątkowska, P., Porada, M., Skierkowska, N., Kubiak, K., Szewczak, D., Bryfczyńska, M., Osiak, J., Trawka, P., Kliszewska, P., Nieciecka, A., & Kędziora-Kornatowska, K. (2019). Laboratory tests in geriatric patients - an overview of the latest reports. https://doi.org/10.5281/zenodo.3382422(accessed on 16th June 2025).
15. Caliskan, E. (2016). Anesthetic management of neonatal emergency abdominal surgery. https://core.ac.uk/download/322427131.pdf (accessed on 16th June 2025).
16. Carvalho, A. C., Diógenes, M. S. B., Machado, D. M., Moisés, R. S., et al. (2005). Cardiac longitudinal study of children perinatally exposed to human immunodeficiency virus type 1. https://core.ac.uk/download/37706053.pdf (accessed on 16th June 2025).
17. Clancy-Burgess, S. C. (2024). *Implementing Change: Training For Adult Emergency Assessment, Recognition, And Stabilization for Novice and Non-Critical Care Nurses*. https://core.ac.uk/download/619611553.pdf (accessed on 16th June 2025).
18. Diane M. Horm, H. E. Brophy-Herb, & C. A. Peterson. (2024). Optimizing health services for young children in poverty: Enhanced collaboration between Early Head Start and pediatric health care. *Frontiers in Public Health, 12*. https://www.semanticscholar.org/paper/be131e6e2838d72ae93be75a0e51c2f3a5ef0f16 (accessed on 16th June 2025).
19. Istiqomah Putri, & R. D. Astuti. (2024). The role of ultrasound in the diagnosis and management of pediatric abdominal disorders in Jakarta, Indonesia. *Sriwijaya Journal of Radiology and Imaging Research*. https://www.semanticscholar.org/paper/f7b3017c875211a5b5390975e1661bdad8576760 (accessed on 16th June 2025).
20. Johnson, T. (2018). Development and evaluation of an emergency department-based nurse practitioner care delivery model. https://core.ac.uk/download/220128500.pdf (accessed on 16th June 2025).
21. Kikodze, N., Tvildiani, D., & Nemsadze, K. (2019). Pediatric Emergency Cases Managed with Intraosseous Access: Indications, Complication and Outcomes. *International Journal of Sciences: Basic and Applied Research (IJSBAR)*, *47*(2), 22-30. https://gssrr.org/JournalOfBasicAndApplied/article/view/10124(accessed on 16th June 2025).
22. Plano, Denise, "Identifying and Enhancing Key Competencies for Emergency Nursing in Rural Alaska: A Quality Improvement Project" (2022). DNP Scholarly Projects. 62. https://scholars.unh.edu/scholarly_projects/62(accessed on 16th June 2025).
23. Sulu, G. U., Kosger, P., & Ucar, B. (2024). Does the ST2 level in pediatric heart failure patients correlate with cardiovascular events and mortality? *Children, 11*. https://www.semanticscholar.org/paper/2b403dd63793a16af47d8ecc972239f8495a6951 (accessed on 16th June 2025).

# INDEX


## A

Abnormal endocrine function 312
Accurate diagnosis 169, 183
Acute health 352
Acute lymphoblastic leukemia (ALL) 280, 281
Adolescence 53
Adoption 346
Adverse childhood experiences (ACEs) 23
Advocacy 318
Antimicrobial stewardship programs (ASPs) 183
Aortic dissection 354, 357
Arrhythmia diagnosis 356
Arrhythmias 351, 352, 353, 354, 355, 356, 357, 358, 362, 365, 373
Asthma 187, 188, 189, 190, 191, 192, 193, 195, 196, 197, 200, 201, 202, 203, 204, 207, 208, 209, 211, 214, 215, 216, 217
Ataxia 320, 346, 349
Attention deficit hyperactivity disorder (ADHD) 323, 346

## B

Bacteria 183, 184
Behavioral health 1
Biological development 31
Body mass index (BMI) 53
Breastfeeding 88
Bronchitis 187, 188, 189, 193, 195, 215

## C

Cardiac anomalies 312
Cardiac magnetic 373
Cardiac tamponade 355
Cardiogenic shock 354, 373
Cardiogenic shock (CS) 373
cardiopulmonary resuscitation (CPR) 353, 365
Cardiovascular 351, 352, 354, 360, 371, 373, 375
Cardiovascular disease 352, 354, 355, 357, 361, 363, 367, 369, 370
Cardiovascular diseases 373
Cardiovascular disorders 351, 352, 353, 354, 355, 356, 357, 358, 359, 360, 361, 362, 363, 364, 365, 366, 367, 368, 369, 370, 371, 372, 373
Celiac disease (CeD) 229, 248
Central nervous system (CNS) 183
Central nervous system disorders 312
Chemotherapy 269, 280, 283
Chickenpox 164, 165, 183
Childhood 10, 13, 23, 25
Chronic conditions 53
Chronic health 53
Chronic myeloid leukemia (CML) 259, 280, 281
Chronic traumatic encephalopathy (CTE) 346
Cognitive advancements 53
Cognitive development 5, 6, 23
Cognitive function 88
Cognitive skills 53

Collaboration 248
Collective health 93
Communication skills 221
Complementary and alternative medicine (CAM) 346
Complex health landscapes 312
Complex landscape 183
Computed tomography (CT) 183
Congenital adrenal hyperplasia (CAH) 312
Congenital anomalies 187, 190
Congenital heart defects (CHDs) 355, 373
Congenital heart disease (CHD) 53

**D**

Deoxygenation 215
Diabetes 285, 286, 287, 288, 293, 294, 296, 301, 302, 306, 308, 309, 312, 313, 314
Diabetes Mellitus 221
Diagnose 1, 23
Diagnostic accuracy 183
Digital health 319
Diphtheria 120, 121, 154
Disability 346, 348
Disabilityand Health 317
Diseases 352, 359, 360, 362, 365, 367, 369, 370, 372, 375
Disorders of gut-brain interaction (DGBIs) 248
Disorders of sex development (DSD) 287, 289, 312
Disruption 319, 334
Docosahexaenoic acid (DHA) 373
Dysphagia 88

**E**

Echocardiography 373
Effective administration 353
Effective treatment 352, 366
Eicosapentaenoic acid (EPA) 373
Electroencephalogram 320, 346
Emotional development 346
Emotional growth 53
Emotional skills 53
Endocrine disorders 285, 287, 293, 296, 297, 298, 299, 300, 301, 302, 303, 304, 305, 306, 307, 308, 309, 310, 311
Endocrinology 285, 286, 300, 307, 308, 312
Energy demands 60, 61
Epilepsy 320, 325, 326, 327, 346
Epilepsy management 321
Essential component 2
Etiology 183

**F**

Family-centered care 318
Family interaction macro-coding system (FIMS) 312
Feeding and swallowing difficulties (FSD) 215
Fetal echocardiography 352
Follicle-stimulating hormone (FSH) 312
forensic psychiatry 364
Fostering optimal development 53
Functional gastrointestinal disorders (FGIDs) 222, 246, 248
Fungi 183

**G**

Gastric acid production 248
Gastroenterology 219, 220, 225, 230, 231, 235, 237, 243, 248, 251
Gastroesophageal reflux disease (GERD) 248
Genetic 329, 332, 346, 349
Genetic factors 215
Genetic influences 53
Genetic syndromes 320, 332
Global health security 120, 154
Growth hormone deficiency (GHD) 288, 294, 295, 312

**H**

Healthcare 3, 14, 17, 23, 28
Healthcare professionals 162, 181
Health education 23
Health equity 23
Health interventions 23
Health measures 23
Health monitoring 120, 154
health problems 2

Health professionals 23, 88
Healthy development 3, 7, 20
Hematology 253, 254, 268, 275, 280
Hemophilia 280
Herpes simplex virus (HSV) 168, 183
Human existence 31
Human papillomavirus (HPV) 120, 154
Hyper-reactive immune system 187
Hypertension 221
Hypertrophic cardiomyopathy (HCM) 358, 373
Hypothalamus-pituitary-gonadal (HPG) 312

## I

Immunization 93, 94, 95, 96, 97, 98, 99, 100, 101, 102, 103, 104, 105, 106, 107, 108, 109, 110, 111, 112, 113, 114, 115, 116, 117, 118, 119, 120, 121, 154
Impetus 318
Infancy 36, 53
Infections 133, 136, 168, 183, 186
Infectious diseases 120, 154
Inflammatory bowel disease (IBD) 229, 248
Integrative medicine modalities (IMMs) 280
Intrauterine growth restriction (IUGR) 23

## K

Kawasaki disease 354, 355, 360, 373

## L

Leukemia 280
Lower respiratory tract infections (LRTI) 215
Luteinizing hormone (LH) 312
Lymphomas 280

## M

Machine learning 120, 154
Macro-coding system 286, 312
Macronutrients 88
Magnetic resonance imaging (MRI) 183, 233, 248
Malignancy 280
Malnutrition 68, 88
Measles, mumps, and rubella (MMR) 120, 154
Medicine 2, 4, 6, 14, 17, 19, 22, 23, 24, 25, 26, 27, 28
Mental health 9, 23, 27, 248
Metabolism 312
Microbial populations 248
Micronutrients 88
Milestones 5, 6, 23
Minerals 53
Morbidity 373
Multiple sclerosis (MS) 53
Myocardial infarction 352, 357
Myocarditis 351, 352, 354, 355, 357, 361

## N

Necrotizing enterocolitis (NEC) 88
Neonatal intensive care unit (NICU) 145, 149
Neurodevelopmental 319, 320, 331, 334
Neurological 317, 318, 319, 320, 321, 322, 323, 324, 325, 326, 327, 328, 329, 330, 331, 332, 333, 334, 335, 336, 337, 338, 339, 340, 341, 342, 343, 344, 345, 346, 348
Neurological assessment 317, 321, 323, 324
Neurological disorders 319, 338, 346
Neurological function 346
Neurology 23, 317, 318, 319, 320, 321, 323, 324, 325, 326, 327, 328, 329, 330, 331, 332, 333, 334, 335, 336, 337, 338, 339, 340, 341, 342, 343, 344, 345, 346, 348, 349
Neuroplasticity potential 324
Nutritional intake 53
Nutrition literacy 60
Nutrition management 88

## O

Oncology 23, 25, 253, 254, 266, 272, 275, 280, 283

## P

Pathogens 183
Patient management 188, 199, 354, 366
Patients 261, 271, 275, 280, 283
Pediatric cardiovascular disorders 351, 352, 354
Pediatric care 3
Pediatric feeding disorders (PFDs) 88
Pediatric growth 32, 37, 53
Pediatric health 322

Pediatric hematology-oncology (PHO) 280
Pediatricians 2, 3
Pediatric infectious 161, 162, 169
Pediatric mental health 1
Pediatric neurologists 318, 320, 321, 325, 328, 336, 342, 345
Pediatric neurology 317, 318, 319, 320, 345
Pediatric nutrition 60, 81, 88
Pediatric populations 319, 338
Pediatric respiratory illness 187
Pediatrics 1, 2, 4, 5, 8, 9, 10, 11, 12, 16, 17, 18, 24, 25, 26, 27, 28, 29
Physiological 2, 3, 4, 12, 22
Physiology 187, 191, 192, 194, 215
Pneumonia 187, 188, 189, 190, 192, 195, 198, 200, 201, 203, 204, 207, 215, 216
Point-of-Care Ultrasonography (POCUS) 354, 363
Point-of-care ultrasound (POCUS) 170, 183
Population immunity 105, 120, 154
Potential injuries 320
Potential misdiagnosis 183
Promote optimal growth 88
Psychological health 312
Psychological patterns 31
Psychomotor 321
Public health 98, 106, 116, 120, 154
Public health strategies 88
Pulmonary embolism 354, 357, 373

## R

Reduce morbidity 351, 372
Reproduction 312
Respiratory disorders 215
Respiratory distress syndrome (RDS) 128, 133, 134
Respiratory illnesses 215
Respiratory syncytial virus (RSV) 120, 154, 215
Respiratory tract 215
Robust health 120, 154

## S

Sensitization 188
Sickle cell disease (SCD) 255, 280
Social-emotional development 320, 322
Socio-emotional impacts 346
Stereotypic Movement Disorder (SMD) 321
Sudden cardiac arrest (SCA) 353, 370

## T

Thrombocytopenia 280
Toxicity 280
traumatic brain injury (TBI) 324, 335
Treatment 19, 22, 24
Tyrosine kinase inhibitor (TKI) 280

## U

Undernutrition 88
Understand the oncological disorders in children\; 253

## V

Vaccination programs 94, 96, 103, 104, 105, 106, 107, 113, 114, 117, 119
Vaccine hesitancy 106, 107, 120, 154
Vaccine-preventable diseases 120, 154
Vulnerable population 215